SURGICAL COMPLICATIONS AND WOUND HEALING IN THE SMALL ANIMAL PRACTICE

SURGICAL COMPLICATIONS AND WOUND HEALING IN THE SMALL ANIMAL PRACTICE

JOSEPH HARARI, MS, DVM, Diplomate ACVS

Assistant Professor
Department of Veterinary Clinical Medicine and Surgery
College of Veterinary Medicine
Washington State University
Pullman, Washington

W.B. SAUNDERS COMPANY
Harcourt Brace Jovanovich, Inc.
Philadelphia   London   Toronto   Montreal   Sydney   Tokyo

W. B. SAUNDERS COMPANY
Harcourt Brace Jovanovich, Inc.

The Curtis Center
Independence Square West
Philadelphia, Pennsylvania 19106

Library of Congress Cataloging-in-Publication Data

Surgical complications and wound healing in the small animal practice / [edited by] Joseph Harari.

    p.   cm.

ISBN 0–7216–3984–4

    1. Dogs—Surgery—Complications.   2. Dogs—Wounds and injuries—Treatment.   3. Cats—Surgery—Complications.   4. Cats—Wounds and injuries—Treatment.   5. Veterinary surgery—Complications.   6. Veterinary traumatology.   7. Wound healing.   I. Harari, Joseph.

SF991.S89   1993

636.7′089701—dc20   92-20695
                                             CIP

SURGICAL COMPLICATIONS AND WOUND HEALING
IN THE SMALL ANIMAL PRACTICE   ISBN 0–7216–3984–4

Printed in Mexico.

Last digit is the print number: 9   8   7   6   5   4   3   2   1

For my parents,
Ruth and Paul Harari,
who brought our family to this country
in search of the American Dream.

CONTRIBUTORS

WILLIAM S. DERNELL, DVM
Surgical Resident, Washington State University College of Veterinary Medicine, Pullman, Washington
Surgical Devices and Wound Healing

DAVID FOWLER, DVM, MVSc, DIPLOMATE, ACVS
Professor, Small Animal Surgery, Western College of Veterinary Medicine, University of Saskatchewan, Saskatoon, Saskatchewan
Principles of Wound Healing

STEPHEN A. GREENE, DVM, MS, DIPLOMATE, ACVA
Assistant Professor and Chief of Anesthesiology, Department of Veterinary Clinical Medicine and Surgery, Washington State University College of Veterinary Medicine, Pullman, Washington
Perioperative Complications of Anesthesia

SCOTT GUSTAFSON, DVM, MS
Former Clinical Instructor, Washington State University; Senior Veterinary Surgeon, Davis and Geck Division, American Cyanamid Co., Pearl River, New York
Traumatic, Septic, and Immune-Mediated Joint Diseases

NANCY L. HAMPEL, DVM, MS, DIPLOMATE ACVS
Staff Surgeon, Broadway Animal Hospital, El Cajon, California
Surgical Drains

JOSEPH HARARI, MS, DVM
Assistant Professor, Department of Veterinary Clinical Medicine and Surgery, Washington State University College of Veterinary Medicine, Pullman, Washington
Perioperative Antibiotic Therapy; Surgical Devices and Wound Healing

CARLOS C. HODGES, DVM, MS
Clinical Assistant Professor, Department of Small Animal Medicine and Surgery, Texas A & M University College of Veterinary Medicine, College Station, Texas
Postoperative Physical Therapy

CHERYL R. KILLINGSWORTH, DVM, PhD
Research Associate, Harvard University School of Public Health, Boston, Massachusetts
Repair of Injured Peripheral Nerves, Tendons, and Muscles

KARL H. KRAUS, DVM, MS
Assistant Professor, Tufts University School of Veterinary Medicine; Attending Orthopedic Surgeon, Foster Hospital for Small Animals, North Grafton, Massachusetts
Healing of Bone Fractures

ELIZABETH J. LAING, DVM, DVSc, Diplomate, ACVS
Surgical Referral Service, Stoughton, Wisconsin
The Effects of Chemotherapy and Radiation on Wound Healing

CANDACE E. LAYTON, DVM, MS, Diplomate, ACVS
Associate Professor, Department of Clinical Sciences, College of Veterinary Medicine, Kansas State University, Manhattan, Kansas
Nutritional Support of the Surgical Patient

SCOTT M. LOZIER, DVM, MS
Clinical Instructor, Department of Veterinary Clinical Medicine and Surgery, Washington State University College of Veterinary Medicine, Pullman, Washington
Topical Wound Therapy

L. KAY MASON, DVM, Diplomate, ACVS
Director of Surgery, Delaware Veterinary Speciality Group, Newark Animal Hospital, Newark, Delaware
Treatment of Contaminated Wounds, Including Wounds of the Abdomen and Thorax

ROSS H. PALMER, DVM, MS, Diplomate, ACVS
Staff Surgeon, Santa Cruz Veterinary Hospital, Santa Cruz, California
Postoperative Physical Therapy

JOHN T. PAYNE, DVM, MS, Diplomate, ACVS
Assistant Professor, Department of Veterinary Medicine and Surgery, College of Veterinary Medicine, University of Missouri—Columbia, Columbia, Missouri
Pathophysiology and Treatment of Thermal Burns

ERIC R. POPE, DVM, MS, Diplomate, ACVS
Associate Professor, Department of Veterinary Medicine and Surgery, College of Veterinary Medicine, University of Missouri—Columbia, Columbia, Missouri
Pathophysiology and Treatment of Thermal Burns

ROBERT M. RADASCH, DVM, MS, Diplomate, ACVS
Staff Surgeon, Dallas Veterinary Surgical Center, Dallas, Texas
Osteomyelitis

JAMES K. ROUSH, DVM, MS, Diplomate, ACVS
Assistant Professor, Department of Clinical Sciences, College of Veterinary Medicine, Kansas State University, Manhattan, Kansas
Nosocomial Infections

DON R. WALDRON, DVM
Associate Professor, Department of Small Animal Sciences, Virginia—Maryland Regional College of Veterinary Medicine, Virginia Polytechnic Institute, Blacksburg, Virginia
Detection of Sepsis in the Postoperative Patient

PREFACE

Proper management of surgical wounds, treatment of infections, and avoidance of complications are serious concerns for practicing veterinarians. In the field of surgery, the goals are to obtain a successful recovery from disease and to reduce patient morbidity and mortality. The objective of this book, therefore, is to provide veterinary clinicians, students, and technicians with sound practical knowledge for management of wounds, infections, and surgical complications in injured animals.

The chapters in this book include important topics about problems in surgical patients. The chapters are organized into body systems (skin, bone, joints, muscles, body cavities) and perioperative protocols (antibiotic, wound and burn therapies, surgical drains and devices, anesthesia, and physical therapy). Other clinical areas of interest affecting the surgical patient such as nutrition, chemotherapy, nosocomial infections, and detection of postoperative sepsis are also presented. The contributors for the chapters are specialists from academic and private practices who were asked to provide current and relevant information for the reader.

I am indebted to the authors who contributed their time and expertise for this textbook. Linda Mills and the staff at W.B. Saunders Company are commended for assisting me with the genesis, development, and completion of this project. Finally, my colleagues and the staff and students at Washington State University should be recognized for creating a stimulating professional environment.

JOSEPH HARARI, MS, DVM
Pullman, Washington

CONTENTS

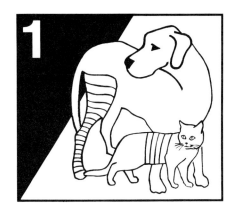

PRINCIPLES OF WOUND HEALING

DAVID FOWLER

HISTORICAL PERSPECTIVES ON WOUND REPAIR

Wounds and their management have long been of concern, with evidence of traumatic wounds dating back to fossil records of prehistoric humans.[1] From the time of earliest recorded history into the first part of the nineteenth century, principles of wound management revolved around gross observations of healing. The classic features of inflammation following wounding were described in ancient times,[1] leading to the realization that patients who developed a watery brown discharge following wounding characteristically progressed to gangrene and death. Conversely, patients who developed a thick, whitish discharge generally healed and survived. An early and intense inflammatory response was considered essential to the successful healing of traumatic wounds, and treatments that favored generation of "laudable pus" were subsequently developed.[1, 2]

In the 19th and early 20th centuries, causative agents in infectious processes were identified through the work of Semmelweiss, Pasteur, Lister, Koch, and others. It is upon this work that modern theories of antisepsis and asepsis are founded. Elucidation of the etiologies of wound infection rapidly led to the realization that wound infection and wound healing were separate entities and that wounds were, in fact, capable of healing with very little outward evidence of the healing process.

The modern era of understanding the mechanisms of wound healing began with the description by Metchnikoff in the early 1900s of the initial cellular response to injury.[3, 4] Investigations into the specific roles of various cells in the healing process began in the 1950s and continue to the present.[5] There has been an explosive increase in our knowledge of the cellular and molecular biology of wound healing over the past 20 years, and investigations into the molecular events in normal and abnormal wound healing continue to add to our current understanding of wound healing. The modern surgeon must be aware of the basic tenets of wound healing in order to provide an environment suitable for optimal healing.

PHASES OF WOUND HEALING

The process and results of wound repair depend somewhat on the tissues that are injured and the species in which the injury occurs. Two processes are involved to varying extents: repair and regeneration.

Regeneration involves the replacement of lost cells or tissues with normal, functioning cells of the same type. Only tissues that maintain a cell population capable of undergoing mitotic division are able to regenerate. Bone and liver characteristically heal by regeneration, with the final result of healing being the restoration of a tissue nearly identical to that lost or disrupted in the initial injury. Epithelial and endothelial tissues also regenerate following injury. The ultimate in regeneration occurs in amphibians with the restoration of extremities following amputation. Cutaneous injuries in the fetus regenerate without the formation of a scar, whereas identical injuries post-natally result in scar formation. The mechanisms that control repair versus regeneration of tissues are not completely understood.

Despite the potential for many tissues to regenerate, mammalian wounds characteristically heal through the formation of a relatively avascular scar that serves to bind surrounding tissues together. The phases of wound *repair* have been arbitrarily divided on a time scale into inflammation (substrate), fibroplasia (proliferation), and remodeling (Fig. 1–1).

Inflammation

An acute inflammatory reaction follows every injury. The severity of the inflammatory response is directly correlated with the severity of the trauma and is initially directed at controlling hemorrhage at the site of injury. Subsequent to coagulation, cellular elements of inflammation are attracted to and migrate into injured tissues. Thus, the inflammatory reaction can be subdivided into an early vascular phase and a late cellular (inflammatory) phase.

The immediate response of blood vessels to injury is vasoconstriction, which serves to limit blood loss at the site of injury. Vasoconstriction, however, is short-lived (lasting only 5 to 10 minutes) and is followed by active vasodilation. Blood vessel disruption at the time of injury results in the extravasation of blood elements into the surrounding tissues. Platelets adhere and aggregate following exposure to subendothelial collagen and form a

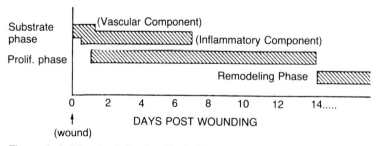

Figure 1–1. The classically described phases of wound healing are divided into inflammation (substrate), fibroplasia (proliferation), and remodeling. The substrate phase can be further subdivided into early vascular and subsequent inflammatory components. These phases of wound healing are not distinct entities but overlap on a time scale. (Reprinted with permission from Kanzler MH, Gorsulowsky DC, Swanson NA: Basic mechanisms in the healing cutaneous wound. J Dermatol Surg Oncol 12 (11):1156–1164, 1986.)

hemostatic plug. Injured cells also release thromboplastin, which activates the extrinsic coagulation system. The end result of the coagulation cascade is the formation of thrombin, which cleaves fibrinogen into fibrin monomers that polymerize to form a reinforcing fibrin network.

Following initial vasoconstriction, postcapillary venules undergo changes resulting in "leaking" of plasma constituents. Histamine, 5-hydroxytryptamine (serotonin), kinins, leukotrienes, substance P, and fibrin-derived peptides contribute to alterations of these vessels in response to injury.[6] Upon exposure to these substances, endothelial cells within postcapillary venules contract and form intercellular gaps.[7, 8] Plasma and its macromolecular constituents are then able to cross the endothelial boundary, forming the wheal typical of acute inflammatory reactions.

The cellular phase of inflammation is characterized by the appearance of neutrophils, macrophages, and lymphocytes (Fig. 1–2). Neutrophils, the first inflammatory cells to appear within the wound, are typically present approximately 6 hours following injury and increase to maximum numbers over 2 to 3 days.[9] The primary roles of the neutrophil are prevention of infection and debridement. Lymphocytes are somewhat slower to appear in the wound, reaching maximum numbers in approximately 6 days. Although lymphocytes are probably not vital to wound healing, certain subpopulations of T cells have been shown to have a positive effect on the rate and quality of tissue repair. Macrophages are the key cell in mediating the transition from the inflammatory to the fibroplastic phase of wound healing. The appearance of macrophages in the wound lags behind the appearance of neutrophils by 24 to 48 hours. Macrophages are important in wound debridement and induction of fibroplastic activity. During the first 3 to 4 days after injury, the collagenolytic activity of macrophages predominates. Subsequently, macrophages synthesize and secrete numerous growth factors that induce the migration of fibroblasts into the wound and the synthesis of matrix by wound fibroblasts.

Fibroplasia

The fibroplastic (proliferative) phase of wound healing is characterized by fibroblast migration and matrix synthesis, neovascularization, and reestablishment of the epidermis.

Epithelial migration begins approximately 12 hours after injury. The rate

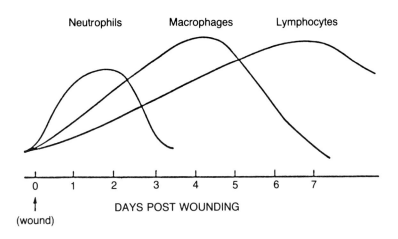

Figure 1–2. The major cellular components of the inflammatory phase of wound healing. Neutrophils are the first inflammatory cell to appear in the wound, followed by macrophages and lymphocytes. (Reprinted with permission from Kanzler MH, Gorsulowsky DC, Swanson NA: Basic mechanisms in the healing cutaneous wound. J Dermatol Surg Oncol 12(11): 1156–1164, 1986.)

Neutrophils   Macrophages   Lymphocytes

0   1   2   3   4   5   6   7

↑
(wound)

DAYS POST WOUNDING

of epithelialization and the time to achieve complete coverage of the wound are variable. The local wound environment is of considerable importance, since epithelial cells require adequate oxygen tensions and a suitable substrate for migration. The time required for epithelialization also varies with the size of the wound. Primarily sutured wounds such as surgical incisions are typically bridged by migrating epithelial cells within 48 hours of injury. Epithelialization of open wounds progresses more slowly.

Fibroblasts appear in concert with new vascular elements, migrating into the wound just ahead of the newly advancing blood vessels as the inflammatory phase subsides in 2 to 3 days. Fibroblasts begin synthesizing matrix components (collagen, elastin, proteoglycans) shortly after their appearance in the wound. A slightly acidic environment and oxygen tension of approximately 20 mmHg are required for optimal collagen synthesis. Matrix synthesis then proceeds at a rapid rate with associated increases in wound tensile strength. The total amount of collagen reaches a maximum 2 to 3 weeks after wounding. Despite this fact, wounds achieve only a small percentage of their original tensile strength by the end of the fibroplastic period. Remodeling of the wound matrix is responsible for continued increases in tensile strength.

Remodeling

The remodeling phase is characterized by a balance of collagenolysis and new collagen production, as well as a regression of vascular elements. Remodeling continues for up to 1 year or more. There is a gradual decrease in collagen type III and a corresponding increase in collagen type I. Collagen fibers form stable cross-links through covalent bond formation and reorient along lines of stress.[10] Cutaneous wounds achieve approximately 80% of their original strength by the completion of this phase.

Wound Contraction

The process of wound contraction deserves special mention. Contraction is particularly important in most animals because large wounds on the trunk are capable of undergoing relatively rapid functional and cosmetic repair through this process (Fig. 1–3). The ability of wounds to contract in animals is related to the panniculus carnosus muscle under the skin and the lack of restrictive cutaneous attachments to inelastic underlying tissues.

Wound contraction should be differentiated from wound contracture. Contracture implies a loss of function or mobility resulting from wound contraction or tissue fibrosis. The fine details of wound contraction continue to be controversial. However, it is apparent that contraction is mediated by an interaction of wound myofibroblasts and matrix components. Wound contraction begins approximately 1 week after injury and progresses at a fairly constant rate of 0.6 to 0.7 mm/day.[9]

FACTORS AFFECTING WOUND HEALING

Wound healing is often taken for granted in this era of modern surgical technique. It is, however, important to recognize factors that may adversely affect wound healing. These may be classified as local factors (factors within

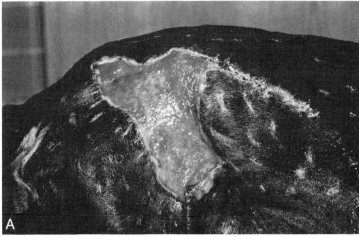
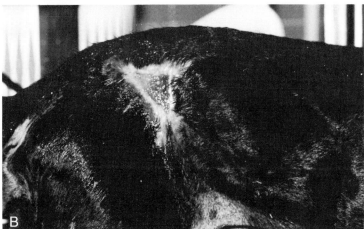

Figure 1-3. Open wound, subsequent to tumor excision, of the gluteal region in a Doberman pinscher. *A,* Appearance following 2 weeks of open wound management. The granulation bed is well established. *B,* Appearance 6 weeks after surgery. Wound contraction has greatly reduced the surface area of the wound.

the wound environment), systemic factors (those affecting the whole animal), and organ and species variability in response to injury. Many of these factors will be discussed at length in subsequent chapters.

Local Factors

Foreign Material. Only a small percentage of wounds have the advantage of being created in a sterile, controlled environment. Animals frequently are presented with wounds resulting from trauma. Because of the environment in which these wounds occur, contamination with foreign particles is expected. Foreign particles exacerbate the inflammatory response to injury and increase the resulting migration of neutrophils and macrophages into the wound. The release of degradative enzymes into the wound results in destruction of the wound matrix, prolongation of the inflammatory phase, and delay in the fibroplastic phase of tissue repair. Judicious surgical debridement of contaminated wounds is required to avoid these undesirable sequelae (Fig. 1-4).

Soils rich in organic matter and clay also contain highly charged particles termed *infection-potentiating fractions (IPFs)*. Wounds contaminated with IPFs require thorough evaluation and meticulous debridement because these

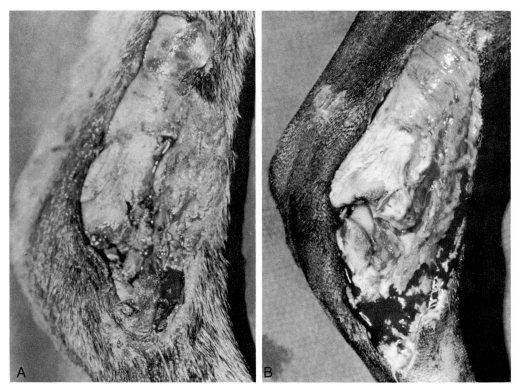

Figure 1–4. Shearing injury, due to motor vehicle–related trauma, of the medial aspect of the tibia and tarsus. *A*, The wound is heavily contaminated with foreign material and debris. Continued presence of debris in the wound exacerbates the inflammatory response and increases the risk of infection. *B*, Meticulous surgical debridement and lavage have been performed. Repeated assessment and debridement are required to provide an environment optimal for tissue repair.

particles will inhibit the activity of antibiotics, leukocytes, and antibodies and are therefore associated with an increased risk of wound infection.[11, 12]

Sutures. Suture material is used to reduce dead space and approximate tissues within wounds. In an optimal environment, this decreases the wound area that must undergo repair and hastens healing. Sutures, however, should be considered as foreign material introduced into the wound. It has been demonstrated experimentally and clinically that the presence of more than 10^5 bacteria per gram of tissue produces infection in the majority of primarily closed wounds. The presence of buried suture within a wound greatly decreases the critical number of bacteria required to cause infection. The deleterious effects of sutures result from direct irritation, harboring of bacteria, and generation of ischemic islands of tissue within the wound (Fig. 1–5).

Oxygenation. It has long been recognized that wounds in poorly vascularized tissue heal slowly or not at all. Reparative cells are metabolically active and require adequate oxygen and nutrient levels for their synthetic functions. Macrophages are resistant to hypoxia, but epithelialization and protein synthesis by fibroblasts are oxygen-dependent. Collagen synthesis requires a critical level of 20 mmHg PO_2.

Artificial increases in oxygen within a wound are associated with more rapid gains in wound strength. Collagen synthesis, collagen cross-linkage, and reparative cell differentiation are augmented in this situation, with a

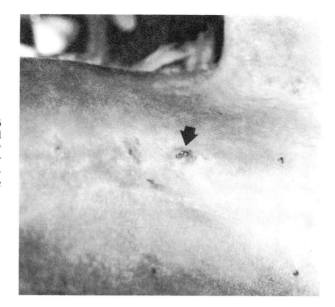

Figure 1–5. Draining suture tract (*arrow*) 6 weeks following laparotomy. Suture material may interfere with optimal wound healing by acting as a direct irritant, harboring bacteria, or causing ischemic foci within the wound. Exploration and removal of the offending suture material were curative in this case.

maximum effect being seen in animals breathing pure oxygen under hyperbaric conditions.[13, 14] Hyperbaric oxygen therapy also has been utilized to facilitate the healing of chronic wounds such as decubital ulcers.

Factors that interfere with the delivery of nutrients or oxygen to a wound result in a dampened reparative process (Fig. 1–6). Severe hypovolemia results in a temporary cessation of progressive healing. Continued hypovolemia or dehydration results in a decreased rate of gain of wound tensile strength.[15, 16]

Devitalized Tissue. Devitalized tissue within a wound must be removed prior to the onset of fibroplasia. Removal of devitalized tissue is most appropriately completed by prompt and thorough surgical debridement. In the absence of surgical debridement, phagocytic cells must clear the wound of devitalized tissue. This results in a prolongation of the inflammatory phase of healing.

Dead Space. Excessive dead space within a wound leads to the accumulation of fluid, or seroma formation (Fig. 1–7). Seroma formation is particularly problematic in tissues that are subject to excessive movement. Reparative cells, as previously discussed, require a provisional matrix for migration. The hypoxic fluid environment of the seroma, therefore, inhibits migration of reparative cells into the wound and delays healing.

In situations where dead space exists, and where seroma formation is likely to occur, active obliteration of dead space is beneficial. Techniques for the management of dead space include deep sutures, passive and active drainage systems, and open wound management. These techniques are discussed in subsequent chapters.

Infection. Infection has a deleterious effect on wound repair. Infection within the wound exacerbates the inflammatory process. In addition, many bacteria produce destructive enzymes that further degrade wound matrix and result in ongoing tissue necrosis.

Systemic Factors

Systemic factors, including age, obesity, associated disease, malnutrition, uremia, hypoproteinemia, and severe trauma, have a negative impact on

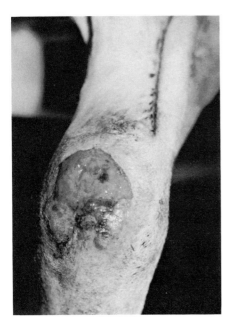

Figure 1–6. Chronic decubital ulcer of the caudal aspect of the elbow in an Irish wolfhound. This ulcer resulted from repeated trauma and ischemic injury to the affected area. Continued restriction of nutrient and oxygen delivery to the wound prohibits healing. Prevention of continued injury through the use of protective splints and bandages and reconstruction using a vascularized tissue flap are required in this case.

tissue repair. It is well established that wound repair is an anabolic process. Serious traumatic injury substantially increases total-body protein–calorie requirements and may overwhelm the reparative process. Hypoproteinemia, protein–calorie malnutrition, and specific nutritional deficiencies (e.g., of vitamin A or zinc) also have adverse effects on the rate and quality of wound repair.

Medications that directly or indirectly affect the activity of cells involved in the repair process may adversely affect wound healing. Corticosteroids and antineoplastic drugs are common examples of medications administered during periods of tissue repair. Corticosteroids, if given in anti-inflammatory doses prior to the migration of macrophages into the wound, will cause a delay in wound healing. Administration of corticosteroids following the appearance of macrophages in a wound is of far less consequence. Many antineoplastic agents have a negative effect on activity and protein synthesis by reparative cells, thereby resulting in decreased matrix production.

Organ-Specific Variations

The basic principles of wound healing outlined in this chapter apply to all tissues. However, certain tissues, such as bone, characteristically heal through a complex process resulting in regeneration of tissue similar or identical to that initially injured. Injuries in most tissues and organ systems heal by formation of a relatively avascular scar that binds the injured tissue together. Injuries in tissues and organs that normally have a high cellular activity and vascularity heal rapidly. Wounds involving oral mucous membranes or the upper gastrointestinal tract are examples. Wounds that are isolated from a rich vascular supply, such as those in sheathed tendons, are typically slow to heal unless allowed access to a new vascular supply.

The unique environment of organs such as the lower urinary tract or large bowel also may affect wound healing. The large bowel, owing to its high numbers of resident bacteria, characteristically has increased collagenase activity following injury, with a subsequent delay in the development of

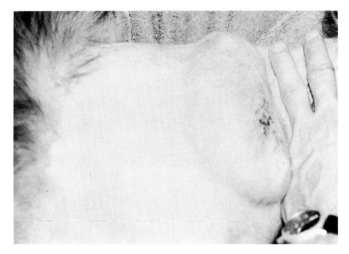

Figure 1–7. Seroma formation following extensive surgery of the lateral neck region. Dead space in the wound was difficult to close, and the area was subject to excessive movement. The hypoxic environment of the seroma inhibits migration of reparative cells into the wound and results in delayed healing.

wound tensile strength. Urine produces a marked inflammatory response in interstitial tissues, and this may lead to an increased incidence of complications.

Species-Specific Variations

The basic mechanisms and principles of healing apply to all mammalian species. However, species-specific differences in the quality of repair and complications of wound healing are seen. Distal extremity wounds in horses are often characterized by production of excessive or exuberant granulation tissue (Fig. 1–8). The reasons for this phenomenon are poorly understood but may relate to the wound environment or the inelasticity and paucity of tissues surrounding the wound. It is also intriguing to consider that differences in the elaboration of growth factors, matrix, or the cellular responses to these factors may be present in the horse.

Open wounds involving the trunk in dogs and cats close rapidly through wound contraction. The rapidity of open wound closure in these species is likely not due to differences (compared with horses) in matrix or myofibroblast function but rather is due to elasticity of the surrounding skin and soft tissues.

Vitamin C is required for collagen maturation in all species. The vast majority of domestic animals are capable of endogenous vitamin C synthesis; however, guinea pigs (and humans) require a dietary source of this vitamin. A deficiency in dietary vitamin C in guinea pigs is associated with abnormal wound healing.

CELLULAR RESPONSES IN WOUND HEALING

The classically described phases of wound healing involve inflammation, fibroplasia, and remodeling. It should be recognized that these phases are arbitrary and that they overlap in time. A predictable cascade of complex cellular and biochemical events is initiated at the time of injury and progresses to completion of repair. The cellular responses to wounding were first described by Metchnikoff early in this century.[2, 3] The specific roles of cells in the healing process continue to be elucidated, particularly with respect to

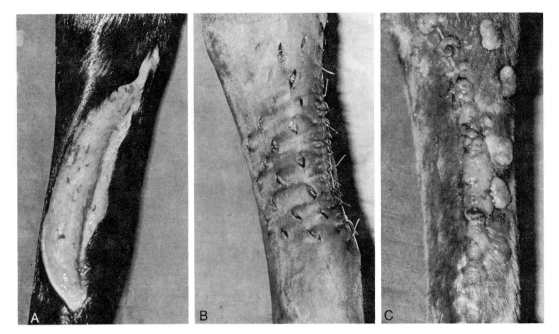

Figure 1–8. Traumatic skin wound of the distal aspect of a limb in a horse. *A*, Appearance of the wound following ten days of open wound management. *B*, The wound has been closed, following final debridement, using a mesh expansion technique. *C*, Appearance of the wound after two weeks in a cast. Exuberant granulation tissue has formed at the mesh expansion sites. The causes of excessive granulation tissue production in the horse are not well understood.

mechanisms that initiate, modulate, and terminate cellular functions such as migration and protein synthesis.

Platelets

Platelets appear in the wound immediately following injury. The primary role of the platelet is coagulation. However, it is becoming increasingly evident that platelets also play a vital role in other inflammatory and wound-healing processes through the release of numerous peptide mediators (Table 1–1).

Platelets are anucleate, discoid fragments derived from budding megakaryocytes within bone marrow.[17] They have a life span of 7 to 10 days and are specialized for adhesion, aggregation, and subsequent secretion. Following vascular injury, platelets adhere to exposed subendothelial collagen in damaged vessels.[9, 18] Arachidonic acid, released from platelet membrane phospholipids, is metabolized into thromboxane A_2, which stimulates further platelet aggregation.[19] Stimulated platelets subsequently undergo a secretion reaction and release mediators that promote continued platelet aggregation, vasoconstriction, and changes in vascular permeability. Several mitogenic or growth factors important in wound healing are also released from platelets.[20–22]

The majority of mediators released by platelets are concentrated in storage organelles. In addition, platelets are capable of synthesizing metabolites of arachidonic acid.[23] Platelet alpha-granules contain four adhesive glycoproteins—fibrinogen, fibronectin, von Willebrand factor, and thrombospondin—that contribute to coagulation and provisional matrix formation through

TABLE 1–1. Platelet-Derived Mediators of Inflammation

CLASS	MEDIATOR	ACTIONS
I. Cyclooxygenase dependent	Thromboxane A_2	Vasoconstrictor, proaggregant, increased neutrophil adherence
	Thromboxane B_2	More stable thromboxane A_2 derivative
	Prostaglandins D_2, E_2, F_2	Vasoactive, modulates hemostasis and leukocyte function
	HHT	Chemotactic
II. Lipoxygenase dependent	12-HPETE	Vasoconstrictor
	LTB_4 synthesis	Inhibitor, stimulates leukocyte
	12-HETE	Chemotactic
III. Dense-body contents	Serotonin	Vasoconstrictor, increases vascular permeability, fibrogenic
IV. Alpha-granule contents	Thrombospondin	Endogenous platelet lectin, inhibits fibrinolysis, binds to matrix constituents
	Growth factors: e.g., platelet-derived growth factor (PDGF)	Connective-tissue mitogen, cell-transforming factor, chemotactic
	Platelet factor 4 (PF4)	Proaggregant, chemotactic, inhibits neutral proteases, induces basophil histamine release
V. Granule contents	Cationic permeability factor release	Stimulates mast cell histamine
	Serum-activating enzymes	Generate C5a in serum
	Cathepsins A,C,D,E	Acid proteinases
	Elastase	Neutral proteinase
	Collagenase	Neutral proteinase
	α_1-Antitrypsin, α_2-macroglobulin	Proteinase inhibitors
	α_2-Antiplasmin	Primary plasmin inhibitor

Source: Reprinted with permission from Terkeltaub RA, Ginsberg MH. Platelets and response to injury. In Clark RAF, Henson PM (eds): The Molecular and Cellular Biology of Wound Repair. New York, Plenum Press, 1988.

their ability to form contact interactions with platelet membrane proteins, vessel wall proteins, and each other. Fibronectin is of particular importance in wound healing. In addition, platelet alpha-granules release four factors essential for wound repair: platelet-derived growth factor, transforming growth factor β, the transforming growth factor α family (including epidermal growth factor), and platelet factor 4.[24] Platelets also release platelet-derived angiogenesis factor, a nonmitogenic chemoattractant for endothelial cells that produces dose-dependent, noninflammatory angiogenesis in the rabbit corneal assay.[25]

The release of growth factors by stimulated platelets is thought to be the initiator of the reparative process in all healing wounds. Platelet-origin growth factors signal local mesenchymal cells and epidermal cells to move, divide, and increase their synthesis of collagen and glycosaminoglycans. These growth factors are capable of inducing all the biologic activity required for the production of granulation tissue.

Neutrophils

Neutrophils appear in the wound within several hours. Neutrophil numbers usually peak between 24 and 48 hours and then rapidly decline in noninfected wounds.[9, 26] Neutrophils are attracted to sites of inflammation by a number of chemoattractants, including kallikrein, fibrinopeptides, C5a from complement activation, leukotriene B_4 from other activated neutrophils, bacterial formyl–methionyl peptides, and platelet-release products.[27] Once at the site of the injury, neutrophils must adhere to the vessel wall, migrate between vascular endothelial cells, penetrate the basement membrane, and migrate through the interstitium. Neutrophil–endothelial cell adhesion is apparently mediated by cell surface glycoprotein adhesion molecules that are upregulated in response to soluble inflammatory mediators at the wound site. Migration of neutrophils occurs in a directed fashion in response to chemotactic gradients within the wound.[27]

Noncontaminated wounds in animals with experimentally induced neutropenia undergo normal cellular repair sequences and heal at a normal rate.[28, 29] However, in the presence of infection, wounds in severely neutropenic animals develop infection with subsequent septicemia and death. These observations suggest that the neutrophil plays little direct role in orchestrating the biochemical and cellular events in the healing wound. The primary role of the neutrophil appears to be one of creating a favorable wound environment in the event of bacterial contamination. The neutrophil is not essential to the wound-healing process per se.

Macrophages

Tissue macrophages appear in the wound shortly after neutrophils. Macrophage numbers generally peak 24 to 48 hours following neutrophils and then gradually decrease.[26, 30, 31] The macrophage's role as a "housekeeper" in wounds has long been recognized. The macrophage is adapted for the ingestion and subsequent destruction of foreign debris within the cellular phagosomes. The tissue macrophage works, therefore, in conjunction with neutrophils to provide an optimal wound environment for the ensuing proliferative phase of wound healing.

Macrophages are derived from circulating blood monocytes, which, in turn, are formed from precursor cells within the bone marrow. Following vascular disruption, monocytes are attracted to the site of injury by a number of chemoattractants, including collagen fragments, fibronectin fragments, lymphokines, bacterial endotoxins, and complement components.[32] One of the most sensitive of the monocyte chemoattractants is transforming growth factor β, a product of stimulated platelets.[33]

In addition to their role in wound debridement, tissue macrophages are critical in affecting cellular events throughout the proliferative phase of wound healing. Macrophages are thus integrally involved in the degradative and reparative phases of wound healing. Experiments on wounds depleted of macrophages have demonstrated a marked delay in the onset and extent of granulation tissue formation.[34] Corticosteroids, when given at the time of wounding, interfere with macrophage migration into the wound and result in a delay in wound healing. The negative effects of corticosteroids on the rate of wound healing are largely prevented if their administration is delayed until after macrophages appear in the wound.

Macrophages have recently been shown to produce a number of polypeptide growth factors important in the recruitment and regulation of cellular elements in the reparative process.[33, 35, 36] The growth factors produced by wound macrophages are collectively known as *macrophage-derived growth factor (MDGF)*.[37] The exact nature of MDGF remains to be fully elucidated, but it undoubtedly represents multiple growth factors. Included among the identified regulatory proteins produced by macrophages are platelet-derived growth factor, fibroblast growth factor, transforming growth factor β, interleukin 1, and arachidonic acid metabolites.[36] The secretion of growth factors by macrophages differs from that of platelets because macrophages are induced to synthesize and directly secrete growth factors into the wound environment, whereas platelet-derived growth factors are storage products released during the secretion reaction.

Stimulation of macrophages is apparently required prior to their production and release of growth factors. Nonstimulated macrophages are incapable of inducing fibroblastic and angiogenic activity. Inactive macrophages harvested from the peritoneal cavity and injected into the cornea of animals induce no fibroblastic activity. However, stimulated macrophages injected into the cornea induce fibroplasia, collagen synthesis, and neovascularization.[35, 38] It also has been demonstrated that addition of supernatant from medium in which macrophage phagocytic activity has been induced is capable of inducing proliferation of quiescent fibroblasts in tissue culture.[39] Addition of macrophage-depleted medium to tissue-repair fibroblasts obtained from postoperative peritoneal fluid in rabbits suggests a differential, time-dependent effect characterized by initial stimulation of fibroblasts and subsequent modulation of fibroblast differentiation.[36] This suggests that postoperative macrophages may alter the composition of their secretory products over time.

Macrophages have a stimulatory effect on neovascularization following wounding. The addition of macrophages to wounds prior to the time of their normal appearance results in an ingrowth of vessels at a correspondingly earlier time interval.[40] Reduced oxygen tension in the wound is thought to stimulate the secretion of angiogenesis factor(s) by wound macrophages.[37] Elimination of the oxygen gradient present within wounds inhibits neovascularization.[37, 41] In addition to their ability to recruit mesenchymal cells and induce neovascularization, wound macrophages also produce factors that modulate the production of connective-tissue matrix proteins by other cells such as the wound fibroblast.

The wound macrophage is the central figure in the control of cellular and biochemical events resulting in tissue repair. How the macrophage is regulated to fulfill its multiple functions in wound healing is largely unknown. There is little doubt, however, of the role of the macrophage in initial wound debridement, recruitment of mesenchymal cells, stimulation of angiogenesis, and modulation of matrix production within a wound.

Lymphocytes

The role of lymphocytes in tissue repair has only recently been critically examined. Lymphocyte numbers within a wound peak 6 days following injury.[42] Activated lymphocytes secrete soluble factors, or lymphokines, that are capable of stimulating fibroblast migration, replication, and collagen synthesis *in vitro*.[43] Conversely, T-lymphocytes also secrete soluble factors that are capable of inhibiting the migration, replication, and protein synthesizing abilities of fibroblasts *in vitro*.[43] Interferons also inhibit fibroblast collagen synthesis.[44] The specific subsets of lymphocytes that contribute to wound healing have not been identified with certainty. It has been demonstrated that depletion of all T-lymphocytes by specific monoclonal antibodies leads to delayed wound healing, as measured by wound breaking strength and collagen synthesis.[45, 46] Selective depletion of the T-helper/effector lymphocyte population has no effect on wound healing. Depletion of the T-suppressor/cytotoxic subset, however, results in enhanced wound healing, thus implying a negative effect on wound healing expressed by this population of cells.[45, 47]

Results of these experiments suggest the presence of a T-lymphocyte population distinct from the T-helper/effector and T-suppressor/cytotoxic subsets. Depletion of these cells results in a marked perturbation of wound healing. The exact identity of this cell population has not been determined.

In summary, it is now apparent that lymphocytes play an integral role in regulating wound-healing processes, probably through the elaboration of soluble mediators that are capable of either stimulating or inhibiting migration and protein synthesis by other cells. T-suppressor cells have an apparent inhibitory effect on wound healing. On the whole, however, lymphocytes have a positive effect on wound healing and their absence results in a decrease in collagen synthesis and wound tensile strength. A subset of T-lymphocytes distinct from T-suppressor and T-helper cells is responsible for the positive regulation of wound healing.

Mast Cells and Eosinophils

The specific roles of mast cells and eosinophils in the process of wound healing are not well understood. Recent research, however, has suggested that both cell types have a contributory effect.

Mast cells are high-affinity IgE receptor–bearing cells present in increased numbers in many chronic inflammatory and allergic conditions, often accompanied by fibrosis.[48, 49] Upon activation, mast cells release mediators such as histamine, proteoglycans, proteolytic enzymes, and chemotactic factors that are stored within cytoplasmic granules. They also synthesize and release plasma membrane phospholipid products such as prostaglandins, leukotrienes, and platelet-activating factor. The presence of mast cells in fibrosing inflammatory processes has led to recent investigations into their role in normal wound healing. It has been shown that rat peritoneal mast cells enhance migration and proliferation of "wounded" fibroblasts in tissue culture.[47] Immunologic activation of mast cells further enhances this effect. Despite the apparent positive effect of mast cells on fibroblasts in tissue culture, *in vivo* research techniques have not yet defined the role for mast cells in wound healing.[50, 51]

Eosinophils are present in healing wounds, reaching peak numbers 7 days following injury and maintaining their presence thereafter. The exact role of eosinophils in wound healing has been questioned, although they have been implicated in the modulation of collagen metabolism.[52, 53] It has been shown recently that eosinophils in an open cutaneous wound-healing model in rabbits contain transforming growth factor α mRNA and protein.[54] Furthermore, the eosinophil appeared to be the primary source of transforming growth factor α in these wounds after day 7. This suggests that the eosinophil may play a role in the induction of epithelial-cell migration, angiogenesis, and organization of the wound-healing materials.

Fibroblasts

Fibroblasts are specialized cells derived from embryonic mesenchyme. In the embryo and adult, fibroblasts have multiple functions, with apparent functional heterogeneity demonstrated by specific subpopulations.[55] These cells are critical in embryonic morphogenesis, dictating skeletal structure, muscle-cell location, cutaneous organization, and nerve development.[56, 57]

In adult animals, fibroblasts are responsible for the production and reorganization of connective-tissue matrix components, such as collagen, fibronectin, and proteoglycans. Fibroblasts produce and secrete degradative collagenases, proteoglycanases, glycosaminidases, and other proteases that contribute to their role in continuously turning over and remodeling the connective-tissue matrix. In the case of connective-tissue injury, fibroblasts migrate into the wound site, proliferate, synthesize, and remodel the newly formed connective-tissue matrix.[58, 59]

Wound fibroblasts are derived from local undifferentiated mesenchymal cells.[31, 60] The factors responsible for their recruitment are not completely understood, but it is apparent that fibroblast migration and activity depend on cellular elements (e.g., macrophages, T-lymphocytes), noncellular elements (e.g., fibronectin), and environmental factors (e.g., oxygen tension) within the wound. At the end of the inflammatory phase, fibroblasts begin migrating into the wound and undergo phenotypic alterations to produce elevated levels of collagen types I and III.[56] There is approximately a 2-day delay between the appearance of fibroblasts within a wound and production of significant amounts of collagen, the so-called lag phase.[61]

Fibroblasts migrate into the wound by means of cytoplasmic extensions termed *lamellipodia*, or *ruffled membranes*.[56] The lamellipodium forms along the leading edge of the fibroblast and adheres to underlying fibronectin-coated fibrin and collagen.[62, 63] Activation of contractile proteins within the fibroblast is responsible for drawing the cell to new adhesion sites.

Three mechanisms may be involved in the induction and coordination of fibroblast migration into wounds: chemotaxis, haptotaxis, and contact guidance.[64] *Chemotaxis* is defined as the migration of cells in response to a concentration of soluble factors. A number of chemoattractants responsible for fibroblast migration have been identified, including a T-lymphocyte–derived protein, a complement-derived cleavage product from C5a, leukotriene B_4, and platelet-derived growth factor.[56] Sources of these chemoattractants are diverse and include platelets, macrophages, and T-lymphocytes.

Haptotaxis is the directional migration of cells along an adhesion gradient that comes from the substratum rather than fluid surrounding the cell.[64] Fibroblasts migrating by haptotaxis initially extend randomly oriented lamellipodia, which tend to stabilize along the leading edge of the cell as adhesion gradients increase along the substratum. Many matrix constituents are apparently capable of inducing haptotactic migration via interaction with cell receptors, including collagen types I, II, and III, hydroxyproline-containing peptides, heparan sulfate proteoglycan, hyaluronate, laminin, and fibronectin.[56, 64] Fibronectin-coated fibrin and collagen are of particular importance in the directional guidance of migrating fibroblasts.

Fibroblasts also may be guided in their migration by a process of *contact guidance.* Contact guidance is closely related to haptotaxis but refers to the tendency of cells to align along discontinuities within the underlying substratum. Fibroblasts first migrate into a wound along randomly oriented fibrils from the initial clot, and new collagen is also deposited in a random pattern. As healing progresses, patterns of orientation develop parallel to lines of stress in the wound.[65] *In vitro* experiments with motile fibroblasts cultured on fibronectin-covered coverslips indicate that cells adhere to the fibronectin substratum, remove it from the surface, and subsequently develop it into relatively parallel substratum-associated fibrils.[64] Fibroblast migration then continues along these patterns of orientation via contact guidance.

Oxygen tension and oxygen gradients are important in inducing stimuli necessary for fibroblast migration. The sequence of cellular migration into wounds is well established, with macrophages leading the order, followed by fibroblasts and then new vascular buds (Fig. 1–9). Fibroblasts require a critical oxygen tension of 20 mmHg for collagen production.[14] Cells in the low oxygen tension zone at the leading edge of advancement primarily produce and secrete degradative enzymes, whereas those in areas of higher oxygen tension produce collagen and matrix proteins.[66]

Myofibroblasts

During healing of tissue defects, the edges of the wound are progressively brought into closer apposition by a process of wound contraction dependent on transitional granulation tissue in the wound.[67] Although wound contraction is of considerable importance in the healing of open wounds, it also can result in undesirable sequelae, such as disfigurement, excessive scarring, and impaired function.[68] Historically, it was believed that collagen provided the contractile force within the granulation tissue, but subsequent research indicated that contraction occurred in vitamin C–deficient guinea pigs despite defective collagen synthesis.[69] Ultrastructural and biochemical evaluation of fibroblasts within granulating wounds has revealed that they possess characteristics intermediate between fibroblasts and smooth muscle cells. These

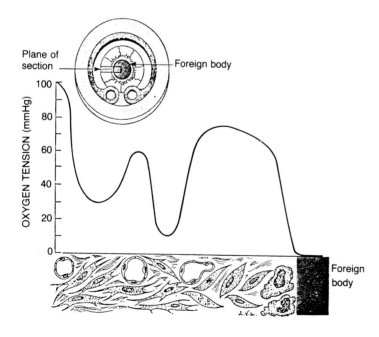

Figure 1–9. Diagrammatic representation of cellular migration and corresponding oxygen tensions in a healing rabbit ear chamber into which a well-tolerated foreign body has been placed. Macrophages lead the cellular migration into the wound, followed by fibroblasts and vascular endothelium. Elevation in tissue oxygen corresponds to the area of advancing capillary bud formation. (Reprinted with permission from Hunt TK: Wound healing: Disorders of repair. In Dunphy JE (ed): Fundamentals of Wound Management in Surgery. South Plainfield, NJ, Chirurgecon, Inc, 1976.)

cells were termed *myofibroblasts* and were suggested as the contractile force in granulation tissue.[70]

Myofibroblasts are characterized by the presence of multiple bundles of microfilaments, termed *stress fibers*, that measure up to 2 μm in length and branch or radiate from focal points.[71] Indirect immunofluorescence studies indicate that stress fibers contain actin-associated proteins such as myosin and tropomyosin. Actin concentration is significantly higher in cultured human myofibroblasts from granulating wounds than in normal dermal fibroblasts.[72–74] Granulation tissue myofibroblasts contract or relax in response to pharmacologic agents such as serotonin, angiotensin, and papaverine in a manner similar to smooth muscle cells.[75]

Gap junctions between myofibroblasts have been described, and the interconnection between myofibroblasts and extracellular matrix, termed the *fibronexus*, has been identified.[76] It is speculated that myofibroblasts modify and reorient the extracellular matrix via the fibronexus, thereby mediating the process of wound contraction. It appears as if the myofibroblast has both synthetic and contractile properties that may generate the forces responsible for wound contraction. The fibronexus serves to link stress fibers in wound myofibroblasts with collagen via fibronectin. In addition, intercellular gap junctions likely synchronize or coordinate myofibroblast activity.

Myofibroblasts reach maximum numbers during wound contraction and decrease as the need for wound contraction subsides. It is likely that transition from fibroblast to myofibroblast is reversible, accounting for the differential numbers of myofibroblasts compared with fibroblasts in wounds at varying stages of repair. The factors that induce this transition and reversal of the fibroblast phenotype are not known.

Endothelium and Angiogenesis

Healing of wounds requires the formation of new capillary buds and their invasion into the site of injury. Once wound healing is complete, regression of newly formed capillary buds results in the formation of a relatively avascular scar. The factors responsible for control of angiogenesis are poorly understood, but mast cells, macrophages, neutrophils, matrix components, and endothelial cells all play a role.[77, 78] In order for angiogenesis to occur, endothelial cells must undergo stimulation, migration and proliferation, tube formation and stabilization, and finally, regression.

Serotonin and histamine, derived from local mast cells, are among the first factors to induce endothelial cell stimulation. These compounds selectively bind to membrane surface receptors on postcapillary venule endothelial cells, causing separation of cell-to-cell junctions and retraction of the endothelial cells.[79] The resulting increase in flow of fluids from the vessel lumen into the interstitial tissues is a well-recognized component of inflammatory reactions. Endothelial cells, once stimulated, also upregulate surface receptors for leukocytes, resulting in enhanced margination of leukocytes at the site of injury and subsequent migration of these cells into the wound.[80, 81] Stimulated endothelial cells synthesize and release enzymes, such as plasminogen activator, plasmin, and collagenases, that are capable of disrupting their surrounding basement membrane. It is possible that degradative enzymes from migrated leukocytes also play a role in disruption of endothelial cell basement membranes.[82, 83]

Migration and proliferation of endothelial cells are required following stimulation. Endothelial cells in the presence of an intact basement membrane are metabolically active, mitotically quiescent, and nonmigratory. In the absence of a basement membrane or in the presence of interstitial connective-tissue components, endothelial cells express elevated rates of mitosis and cell migration.[78] Chemotactic factors produced by leukocytes and matrix components are probably responsible for inducing endothelial cell migration. Endothelial cells also form stress lines that interact with matrix fibrils much in the same manner as previously described for migrating fibroblasts. Thus endothelial cells not only are responsive to their environment but are capable of modifying that environment as well, a phenomenon termed *dynamic reciprocity*.[84]

Endothelial cells at the leading edge of migration are not actively proliferating since cell migration precedes cell proliferation by 24 hours.[85] Proliferating cells are located just behind the leading edge of endothelial cell migration.[86] Proliferative stimuli are probably similar to the migratory stimuli suggested above, including mitogenic factors produced by leukocytes and matrix components. Thrombin also triggers endothelial cell proliferation.[87]

Following migration and proliferation, endothelial cells begin to form complex three-dimensional structures with lumina. The local matrix environment appears important in this process. Endothelial cells cultured *in vitro* on interstitial collagen types I and II form confluent monolayers, whereas cells cultured on collagen types IV and V, typical of basement membranes, form tubelike structures.[88] As mentioned previously, migrating endothelial cells modify their matrix environment through synthesis of specific components. Biosynthesis of collagen types IV and V is favored by migrating endothelial cells. It is therefore likely that the migrating endothelial cell itself modifies the local microenvironment to favor formation of tubelike structures.

Once wound healing is complete, newly formed capillaries begin to regress. The stimuli that trigger endothelial cell death and capillary regression are not well understood. It is possible that the absence of a continued positive stimulus for migration and proliferation leads to some degree of capillary regression, but it also has been suggested that transforming growth factor β produced by epithelial and mesenchymal cells serves to downregulate endothelial cells.

Epithelium

Reepithelialization is of critical importance to the wound-healing process. Rapid establishment of an intact epidermis is required to prevent continued loss of body fluids to the environment and entry of environmental elements, such as microorganisms, into the body. Reepithelialization begins shortly after clot formation, with phenotypic alterations of the epithelial cells at the wound margin becoming apparent in 12 hours and epithelial cell migration present 24 hours following injury.[9, 89]

Epithelial cell motility and mitosis are not interdependent. Migrating epithelial cells arise from the wound periphery, and cell motility is noted even in the presence of agents that block cell division.[90] Epithelial cells appear to migrate in sheets across the wound while maintaining desmosomal attachments to neighboring cells. This may be of functional importance in maintaining an environmental barrier during wound reepithelialization. Cells at the leading edge of the migrating sheet are responsible for "pulling" the sheet across the defect. When the defect is large, cells must be added to the migrating sheet. Mitotic activity noted in cells somewhat distant from the wound margin serves this purpose.

Within 12 hours of wounding, epithelial cells in the stratum spinosum or basale undergo phenotypic changes in preparation for migration. These marginal cells flatten out parallel to the defect and develop pseudopod-like or lamellipodial projections, similar to those described in migrating fibroblasts.[91] The number of desmosomal contacts decreases, and the underlying basement membrane loses definition. Peripherally positioned microfilament bundles appear, and the cytoplasm of the migrating cells stains with antiactin and antimyosin. Accompanying the loss of desmosomal attachments is a relative increase in the number of gap junctions between cells, thus supporting the concept of a coordinated migration of epithelial sheets.[92]

Two mechanisms have been proposed for epithelial cell migration, and both may be operational within mammalian species. The first mechanism, the *sliding model*, is well documented in amphibians and involves a pulling force exerted by the leading epithelial cells.[93] It has been shown in tissue culture that release of the leading cells in a migrating epithelial sheet results in retraction of the entire sheet. Similarly, in amphibians, the formation of an epithelial defect with an intact underlying basement membrane results in the rapid formation of lamellipodial projections from neighboring cells. These lamellipodia anchor along the substrate, and contraction of actin microfilaments within the cytoplasm then draws the cell into the defect. Movement of this cell results in the formation of intercellular gaps. Neighboring cells produce lamellipodia and advance in a similar fashion. Mammalian skin offers a more complex picture, since epithelial sheet migration is multilayered. In the *leapfrog model*, epithelial cells appear to migrate by rolling over one another, with suprabasal cells rolling over attached basal cells, making contact with the basal lamina, and attaching to the basal lamina via formation of hemidesmosomes.[94] Successive submarginal suprabasal cells then roll over the newly anchored basal cells. In deep wounds, where there is a loss of the basal lamina, a thickened provisional matrix containing fibrin and fibronectin is formed that promotes migration of epithelial cells in much the same manner as described for migrating fibroblasts and endothelium. Approximately 7 to 9 days after wounding, the basement membrane zone loses its thickened appearance, and type IV collagen and laminin, typical of normal basement membrane, reappear.

Epithelial cells require a favorable environment for migration to occur. Epithelialization progresses most rapidly in a moist and well-oxygenated environment and will progress only over viable tissue.[9] Epithelial cells are capable of phagocytic activity, an activity that may be enhanced by fibronectin and which assists the ability of epithelial cells to burrow beneath the coagulum on the wound surface.[95]

Once migrating epithelial cells reach cells moving from the opposite side of the wound, they form desmosomal attachments and migration ceases. The rate of epithelial cell mitosis decreases, but it continues at an elevated rate as compared with resting cells (3 to 4 times normal). This poorly understood phenomenon has been termed *contact inhibition*.

MOLECULAR EVENTS IN WOUND HEALING

Growth Factors

Normal wound healing is characterized by the sequential appearance of many cell types within the wound. As previously described, all these cells have specific functions within the wound, varying from debridement to synthesis of repair tissue. Current concepts suggest that the recruitment, proliferation, and function of these cells are largely under the control of growth factors.[96] Growth factors are derived primarily from cells involved in the repair process. Platelets are known to release several chemoattractant and mitogenic factors following stimulation. It is plausible that each population of cells that enters the wound is responsible for secreting growth factors that attract and modulate the function of subsequent cell populations.

Growth factors are proteins that can be classified according to their mode of action. Growth factors may act in an endocrine, paracrine, or autocrine fashion. Insulin-like growth factors 1 and 2 are delivered into the bloodstream and act on target cells in an endocrine fashion. More common in wound healing is paracrine delivery of growth factors. Platelet-derived growth factor and the transforming growth factors, for example, are produced by one cell and used by other cells in the immediate wound environment. In other situations, reparative cells are known to regulate their own function via autocrine delivery of growth factors. Cellular stimulation by growth factors depends on their binding to specific high-affinity receptor sites on the membranes of target cells.

Growth factors also may serve as either competence or progression factors. *Competence factors* act early in the cell cycle and serve to move cells out of the resting phase. Platelet-derived growth factor and fibroblast growth factor are examples of competence factors. *Progression factors*, such as insulin-like growth factors 1 and 2, act later in the cell cycle and stimulate cellular activity. Competence and progression factors may act synergistically in inducing cell proliferation. Progression factors alone are incapable of promoting cell division, unlike competence factors, which are capable of this activity.[96, 97]

Synthesis and release of growth factors have been ascribed to virtually all cells involved in wound healing. The specific effects of growth factors depend on the target cell and the wound environment. The terminology of growth factors is somewhat misleading because, for the most part, they are named after the cell of original isolation. Thus platelet-derived growth factor was originally isolated from platelets but is also produced by macrophages, endothelial cells, and smooth muscle cells. Transforming growth factors were originally isolated from purified tumor cells but are now recognized to be produced by many normal cells regulating a variety of normal cellular processes.[96, 98] Terminology is also confusing because some growth factors characterized from diverse sources and named accordingly are now found to be closely related or identical. For example, acidic fibroblast growth factor and endothelial cell growth factor are identical.

A detailed description of growth factors is beyond the scope of this chapter. Some of the better-characterized and important growth factors in wound healing (platelet-derived growth factor, epidermal growth factor, fibroblast growth factor, and type β transforming growth factor) are discussed.

PLATELET-DERIVED GROWTH FACTOR

It is recognized that serum is required for the successful culture of fibroblasts grown *in vitro*. The specific component of serum required for fibroblast culture was not known, however, until recently. The source of this factor has been isolated to the alpha granules of platelets and termed *platelet-derived growth factor (PDGF)*.[99] PDGF consists of two polypeptide chains, an A chain and a B chain, both of which must be present for biologic activity.[100, 101] Cultured endothelial cells and activated monocytes also produce PDGF-like molecules that bind to PDGF receptors, although it is not clear whether their biologic activity is identical to PDGF of platelet origin.

PDGF acts as both a chemoattractant and a mitogen.[102, 103] It is the most potent mitogen known for mesenchymal cells, including fibroblasts, glial cells, and smooth muscle cells. Its mitogenic activity is mediated through receptors on the cell surfaces of target cells. PDGF acts as a chemoattractant for neutrophils and monocytes, as well as fibroblasts and smooth cells, although it does not express mitogenic activity for inflammatory cells. The concentration of PDGF required for maximal chemotactic activity varies with cell type. Peak neutrophil chemotaxis occurs at concentrations of 1 to 5 ng/ml, whereas monocyte chemotaxis peaks at a concentration of approximately 20 ng/ml.[102] Different receptors are likely responsible for PDGF's chemotactic versus mitogenic effects. In addition to acting as a chemoattractant, PDGF also activates neutrophils and monocytes at a concentration of 20 to 40 ng/ml.

Target cells are exquisitely sensitive to the effects of PDGF. Excess PDGF released from platelets at the site of injury and gaining access to the circulation system could have undesirable systemic effects. However, free PDGF rapidly forms complexes with plasma α_2-macroglobulin and is subsequently cleared from the circulation (estimated half-life of 2 minutes).[104]

In wound healing, PDGF has several effects. PDGF released from platelets first acts as a chemoattractant for neutrophils and macrophages. Once at the site of injury, PDGF and other local factors stimulate neutrophils to release lysosomal enzymes and neutral proteases that aid in the degradative processes prior to wound repair. Macrophages are similarly activated. PDGF-like factors are subsequently produced by activated macrophages, smooth muscle cells, and endothelial cells and, along with platelet-origin PDGF, serve to recruit fibroblasts into the wound. Fibroblasts, in turn, are stimulated by PDGF to produce and secrete collagenases, which are important in matrix degradation and remodeling.

FIBROBLAST GROWTH FACTOR

Fibroblast growth factors were first isolated from bovine brain and pituitary gland and named because of their mitogenic activity for fibroblasts and endothelial cells.[105] Two classes of fibroblast growth factor with identical biologic activity but different isoelectric points were subsequently identified and termed *acidic* and *basic fibroblast growth factor (aFGF and bFGF)*. Growth factors isolated from multiple tissues, including cartilage-derived growth factor, astroglial growth factor, β-heparin–binding growth factor, retina-derived growth factor, and endothelial cell growth factor, have since been identified as either acidic or basic FGF.[106] Basic FGF and acidic FGF share a common cell receptor and the ability to bind strongly to heparin. Basic FGF is 20 times more potent than acidic FGF in mitogenic activity.

There is evidence that FGF is important in the processes of angiogenesis, mesodermal cell recruitment, and substrate synthesis. FGF injected into the cornea with a carrier induces a noninflammatory angiogenic response in animal models.[107] The angiogenic activity of FGF is enhanced by binding to heparin, and it is speculated that binding to heparan sulfate, the major glycosaminoglycan of endothelial surfaces, is important in the angiogenic activity of FGF.[108] FGF has been demonstrated *in vitro* to have mitogenic activity for many mesodermal cell types, including fibroblasts, endothelial cells, and vascular smooth muscle cells. Finally, there is evidence that FGF modulates the synthesis of fibronectin and collagen by vascular endothelial cells.[106]

FGF has been used in wound-healing models to assess the effect of exogenous FGF on the reparative process. Exogenously applied FGF increases migration of mesenchymal cells into the wound, increases protein and collagen synthesis, and promotes angiogenesis.[108–112]

EPIDERMAL GROWTH FACTOR

Epidermal growth factor (EGF) was first isolated from mouse submaxillary salivary glands.[113] Other identified sources of epidermal growth factor include human urine, milk, and Brunner's glands of the small intestine. Transforming growth factor α is a naturally occurring growth factor related to EGF, binds to EGF receptors, and has activity similar to EGF.[114] EGF receptors have been identified on nearly all mammalian cell types but are particularly abundant on epithelial cells, fibroblasts, endothelial cells, and smooth muscle cells.[115–117]

The primary effect of EGF is stimulation of cell growth; proliferation of essentially all mammalian cell types is effected by EGF. However, EGF acts as a progression factor requiring the presence of other competence factors prior to exerting its effect on cell growth.[114] Following binding to receptors, EGF induces a dedifferentiation of phenotype and an increase in mitotic activity. *In vitro* and *in vivo* experiments using EGF indicate that it has a positive effect in the healing of skin wounds, corneal wounds, deep tissue injury, and bone injury.[114]

TYPE β TRANSFORMING GROWTH FACTOR

Transforming growth factors were initially identified in tissue cultures from transformed cells. It was noted that transformed cells produced a factor not detectable in normal tissue cultures and capable of inducing phenotypic changes when added to normal cell cultures.[118] Subsequent analysis revealed that this transforming factor was actually composed of two distinct factors, termed *transforming growth factor* α and *transforming growth factor* β (*TGF-α, TGF-β*). TGF-α, as previously discussed, is closely related to EGF. TGF-β, however, binds to a distinct receptor site on target cells.[119]

TGF-β is stored in platelet alpha-granules and is released following platelet stimulation with thrombin. Activated lymphocytes also synthesize and secrete TGF-β following wounding.[120] Administration of exogenous TGF-β in *in vivo* wound-healing models leads to enhancement of granulation tissue formation.[121] With *in vitro* models, TGF-β has been shown to stimulate the production of collagen and fibronectin by fibroblasts.[122] The primary effect of TGF-β, therefore, is its ability to modulate matrix production. The effects of TGF-β are augmented in the presence of EGF and PDGF.[121]

Fibronectin

Fibronectins are glycoproteins critical to the process of wound healing because of their ability to stimulate cell attachment and migration.[123–126] Fibronectins may be found in soluble form in plasma or insoluble forms in connective-tissue matrix. Fibronectin first appears in sites of injury as a result of deposition of plasma fibronectin during hemostasis. It is believed that fibronectin in the coagulum assists in the initial migration of cellular elements, such as macrophages and epithelium, into the wound. Many cells involved in the wound-healing process have the ability to synthesize and secrete fibronectin. Secretion of fibronectin by macrophages, endothelium, fibroblasts, and epithelium is probably important in the interaction of these cells with their underlying matrix.[127]

Fibronectin is a large molecule with multiple binding sites capable of binding bacterial cell wall components, collagens, actin, thrombospondin, heparan sulfate, hyaluronic acid, fibrin, cell surface receptors, and other fibronectin molecules.[128] These binding sites appear to be specific and independent of one another. Thus fibronectin may play an important role in the provision of an early wound-healing matrix and in interlinking cellular and matrix components during wound healing. The cell surface receptors that bind fibronectin are intimately associated with cytoskeletal components within the cell, implying a role for fibronectin in cell migration through the wound matrix.[129, 130] Exogenously administered fibronectin has been demonstrated to increase healing of chronic corneal ulcers *in vivo*.[131]

In addition to fibronectin's ability to provide an early wound matrix and facilitate cell migration, it also stimulates and modulates collagen production and deposition. *In vitro* studies indicate that inhibition of fibronectin matrix formation subsequently inhibits deposition of collagen types I and III by cultured lung fibroblasts.[132] The fibronectin matrix also serves as a scaffold for the subsequent formation of collagen matrices via fibronectin's collagen-binding domains.

As wound healing nears completion, the amount of fibronectin in the matrix decreases. The mechanisms responsible for this decrease are not understood.

Proteoglycans and Glycosaminoglycans

Proteoglycans are complex polyanionic molecules consisting of a protein core to which linear polysaccharides, called *glycosaminoglycans*, are covalently linked (Fig. 1–10). Several classes of proteoglycans have been characterized. Proteoglycans are present in varying degrees within the matrix ground substance of virtually all connective tissues and serve important functions during wound healing. In addition, proteoglycans have been described as cell surface–associated molecules.

Proteoglycans vary enormously in size, composition, and probably in function. Proteoglycans have traditionally been classified according to their attached glycosaminoglycans. The two major groups of glycosaminoglycans are chondroitin and heparan sulfates. Other glycosaminoglycans include keratan sulfates and hyaluronic acid. Hyaluronic acid is not found biologically linked to a protein core and therefore functions as a free glycosaminoglycan rather than part of a larger proteoglycan molecule. The overall proteoglycan structure is determined by the type, number, and length of the polysaccharide side chains as well as the composition of the protein core. It should be noted that although proteoglycans are traditionally classified according to their glycosaminoglycan side chains, single proteoglycan molecules may contain more than one type of glycosaminoglycan.

Cell surface–associated proteoglycans are important in cell adhesion to matrix proteins. Heparan sulfates are associated with the cell surfaces of many cell types and, in this location, are capable of binding fibronectin.[133]

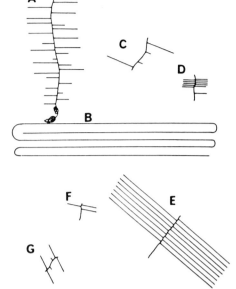

Figure 1–10. Diagrammatic representation, drawn to approximate scale, of several proteoglycan and glycosaminoglycan molecules. Proteoglycans are structurally diverse molecules but share the feature of glycosaminoglycan side chains attached to a central protein core. *A,* Large keratan sulfate–bearing cartilage proteoglycan. *B,* Hyaluronic acid. *C,* Dermatan sulfate proteoglycan of type isolated from loose connective tissue. *D,* Dermatan sulfate synthesized by PYS-2 cells in culture. *E,* Heparin proteoglycan. *F,* Liver cell surface heparan sulfate proteoglycan. *G,* Small heparan sulfate proteoglycan isolated from the EHS tumor. (Reprinted with permission from Couchman JR, Hook M: Proteoglycans and wound repair. In Clark RAF, Henson PM (eds): The Molecular and Cellular Biology of Wound Repair. New York, Plenum Press, 1988.)

These molecules also have an intracellular domain that interacts directly with the cellular cytoskeleton.[134] Heparan sulfates may be intimately associated with formation of stable adhesions between cellular elements and matrix proteins during wound healing and are critical in the process of wound contraction mediated by myofibroblasts.

While heparan sulfate–fibronectin interactions tend to stabilize cell–matrix adhesions, there is evidence that chondroitin sulfate proteoglycans destabilize such adhesions.[135–137] This phenomenon may be important in promoting cell migration. Migrating cells may produce chondroitin sulfates that bind to the fibronectin matrix but not to the cellular cytoskeleton, thus preventing formation of stable adhesions between fibronectin and heparan sulfates and allowing cell migration.[138]

Hyaluronic acid is present in elevated quantities in areas of active cell migration and is produced by proliferating cells.[139–141] As the wound matures and granulation tissue begins to form, levels of hyaluronic acid decrease. Hyaluronic acid is important in maintaining a hydrated milieu due to its hydrophilic properties. This property may provide a matrix with decreased resistance to cell migration. Hyaluronate also maintains cells in a relatively dedifferentiated phenotype consistent with cell migration. However, the exact mechanisms through which hyaluronate facilitates migration are unknown.

In summary, proteoglycans are important in all phases of wound healing. The matrix during cell migration contains elevated concentrations of non-sulfated glycosaminoglycans such as hyaluronate. As maturation of the wound progresses, relatively more sulfated species of glycosaminoglycans appear, such as chondroitin sulfate and heparan sulfate. Heparan sulfate, in particular, is characteristic of mature granulation tissue.

Collagen

Collagens are large glycoproteins that serve a structural function in a vast array of tissues. They are a diverse group of molecules consisting of at least

11 distinct types.[142] Type I collagen is the major structural component of skin, tendon, and bone. Type III collagen is also present in dermis, but less is known of its specific function relative to type I collagen. Type II collagen is the major collagen of cartilage, whereas type IV collagen is an important component of basement membranes. The important players in the process of wound healing appear to be collagen types I, III, and IV.

All collagens have some common features.[143] All consist of three linear peptide chains (alpha chains) of equal length arranged parallel to each other and assembled into a left-handed superhelix. Glycine is present in every third position along each peptide chain. Collagen molecules contain the amino acids hydroxylysine and hydroxyproline. Differences in the composition of the alpha chains account for the variability in collagen types.

The details of collagen synthesis are complex. Intracellular ribosomal synthesis results in the production of pro-alpha chains. These chains subsequently undergo hydroxylation and glycosylation, a process dependent on the presence of Fe^{2+}, α-ketoglutarate, oxygen, and ascorbic acid as enzyme cofactors. Disulfide links form between pro-alpha chains within the endoplasmic reticulum. This cross-linking results in formation of the triple-helical procollagen that is subsequently secreted from the cell. Within the extracellular environment, terminal peptides are cleaved from the procollagen molecules, resulting in the formation of tropocollagen. Tropocollagen spontaneously polymerizes and forms intermolecular cross-links in a quarter-stagger array, resulting in the quaternary structure of the collagen filament. Collagen filaments are further grouped into fibrils, fibrils are grouped into a primitive fiber, and primitive fibers are grouped into the mature collagen fiber or bundle as remodeling progresses (Fig. 1–11).

Collagen interacts in the wound-healing process at all levels: inflammation, neomatrix formation, contraction, and reepithelialization.[142] In the event of vascular injury, exposure to interstitial collagen first stimulates platelets to adhere and undergo the release reaction. Collagen is synthesized and secreted into the wound matrix shortly after the appearance of the first migrating fibroblasts, usually 3 to 5 days after wounding. Collagen synthesis continues at a rapid rate for 10 to 12 days in most wounds, at which time the rate begins to subside. The synthesis of collagen during this time period is directly correlated with increases in tensile wound strength.[144] Collagenolysis and collagen synthesis subsequently equalize in the wound and continued remodeling progresses for up to 2 years. During remodeling, collagen bundles are formed that align along lines of stress, thus providing a gradual increase in wound strength. Preexisting and newly synthesized collagen in the wound matrix serve an important function in providing anchoring points for myofibroblasts during wound contraction. Finally, it appears as if migration of epithelial cells depends on the loss of the basement membrane, including type IV collagen. Once epithelial migration is complete, type IV collagen is produced, the basement membrane is reconstructed, and epithelium resumes a more differentiated phenotype.[145]

SUMMARY

Knowledge of the cellular and molecular interactions that regulate wound healing is expanding at a rapid rate. It is important for the surgeon to understand the basics of these interactions to provide an optimal wound

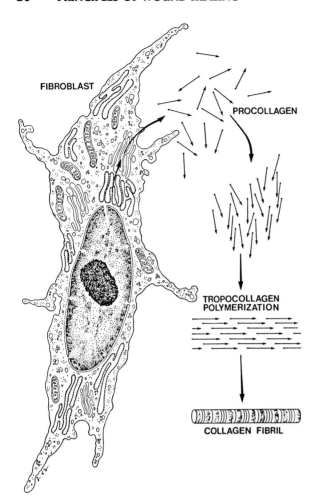

FIBROBLAST

PROCOLLAGEN

TROPOCOLLAGEN
POLYMERIZATION

COLLAGEN FIBRIL

Figure 1–11. Diagrammatic representation of collagen synthesis. Triple-helical procollagen is synthesized intracellularly within the endoplasmic reticulum. Following secretion from the cell, terminal peptides are cleaved from the procollagen, resulting in the formation of tropocollagen. Tropocollagen spontaneously polymerizes in a quarter-stagger array to form the characteristic collagen fibril. (Reprinted with permission from Hunt TK: Wound healing: Disorders of repair. In Dunphy JE (ed): Fundamentals of Wound Management in Surgery. South Plainfield, NJ, Chirurgecon, Inc, 1976.)

environment for repair. Even more critical is the ability to intervene with appropriate therapy in instances of abnormal wound repair. The concept that optimal wound healing occurs in the absence of complicating factors is now being challenged. Numerous growth factors are now produced through recombinant technology, and studies investigating the effects of exogenously applied growth factors in clinical wounds are under way.[20, 110, 146] The obvious economic incentive for drug companies to pursue the use of growth factors for wound treatment will undoubtedly lead to their eventual application in routine clinical settings. The future of pharmacologic intervention in wound treatment should prove exciting. It should be stressed, however, that advances in the field of wound pharmacology are unlikely to offset the importance of surgical judgment in providing an optimal environment for tissue repair.

REFERENCES

1. Majno G: The Healing Hand, Man and Wound in the Ancient World. Cambridge, Mass., Harvard University Press, 1975, pp 1–29
2. Hunt TK, Halliday B: Inflammation in wounds; from "laudable pus" to primary repair and beyond. In Hunt TK (ed): Wound Healing and Wound Infection: Theory and Surgical Practice. New York, Appleton-Century-Crofts, 1980, pp 281–295

3. Metchnikoff E: Immunity in Infective Diseases, Binnie FG (trans). London, Cambridge University Press, 1905
4. Metchnikoff E: Lectures on the Comparative Pathology of Inflammation, Starling FA, Starling IH (trans). New York, Dover, 1891
5. Edwards LC, Dunphy JE: Wound healing: I. Injury and wound repair. N Engl J Med 1958; 259:224–233
6. Williams TJ: Factors that affect vessel reactivity and leukocyte emigration. In Clark RAF, Henson PM (eds): The Molecular and Cellular Biology of Wound Repair. New York, Plenum Press, 1988, pp 115–147
7. Majno G, Shea SM, Leventhal M: Endothelial contraction induced by histamine-type mediators: An electron microscopic study. J Cell Biol 1969; 42:647–672
8. Joris I, Majno G, Ryan GB: Endothelial contraction in vivo: A study of the rat mesentery. Virchows Arch 1972; 12:73–83
9. Kanzler MH, Gorsulowsky DC, Swanson NA: Basic mechanisms in the healing cutaneous wound. J Dermatol Surg Oncol 1986; 12(11):1156–1164
10. Bailey AJ, Bazin S, Delawney A: Changes in the nature of the collagen during development and resorption of granulation tissue. Biochem Biophys Acta 1973; 328:383–390
11. Rodeheaver GT, Pettry D, Turnbull V, et al: Identification of the wound infection–potentiating factors in soil. Am J Surg 1974; 128:8–14
12. Haury BB, Rodeheaver GT, Pettry D, et al: Inhibition of nonspecific defenses by soil infection-potentiating factors. Surg Gynecol Obstet 1977; 144:19–24
13. Niinkoski J: Effect of oxygen supply on wound healing and formation of experimental granulation tissue. Acta Physiol Scand 1969; 334:1–72
14. Niinkoski J: The effect of blood and oxygen supply on the biochemistry of repair. In Hunt TK (ed): Wound Healing and Wound Infection: Theory and Surgical Practice. New York, Appleton-Century-Crofts, 1980, pp 56–70
15. Hunt TK, Zederfeld B, Goldstick TK: Tissue oxygen tensions during controlled hemorrhage. Surg Forum 1967; 18:3–4
16. Sandberg N, Zederfeld B: Influence of acute hemorrhage on wound healing in the rabbit. Acta Chir Scand 1960; 118:367–371
17. Penington DG: Formation of platelets. In Gordon JL (ed): Platelets in Biology and Pathology, vol 2. Amsterdam, Elsevier/North-Holland, 1981, pp 19–42
18. Barnhart MI, Walsh RT, Robinson JA: A three-dimensional view of platelet responses to chemical stimuli. Ann NY Acad Sci 1972; 210:360–390
19. Dodds WJ: Physiology of hemostasis. In Slatter DH (ed): Textbook of Small Animal Surgery, vol 1. Philadelphia, WB Saunders, 1985, pp 71–74
20. Knighton DR, Doucette M, Fiegel VD, et al: The use of platelet-derived wound healing formula in human clinical trials. In Barbul A, Pines E, Caldwell M, Hunt TK (eds): Growth Factors and Other Aspects of Wound Healing: Biological and Clinical Implications. New York, Liss, 1988, pp 319–329
21. Ksander GA, Sawamura BS, Ogawa Y, et al: The effect of platelet releasate on wound healing in animal models. J Am Acad Dermatol 1990; 22(5):781–791
22. Pierce GF, Mustoe TA, Altrock BW, et al: Role of platelet-derived growth factor in wound healing. J Cell Biochem 1991; 45:319–326
23. Weksler BB, Goldstein IM: Prostaglandins: Interactions with platelets and polymorphonuclear leukocytes in hemostasis and inflammation. Am J Med 1980; 68:419–428
24. Terkeltaub RA, Ginsberg MH: Platelets and response to injury. In Clark RAF, Henson PM (eds): The Molecular and Cellular Biology of Wound Repair. New York, Plenum Press, 1988, pp 35–55
25. Hunt TK, Knighton DR, Thakral KK, et al: Studies on inflammation and wound healing: angiogenesis and collagen synthesis stimulated in vivo by resident and activated wound macrophages. Surgery 1984; 96:48–54
26. Ross R. Inflammation, cell proliferation, and connective tissue formation in wound repair. In Hunt TK (ed): Wound Healing and Wound Infection: Theory and Surgical Practice. New York, Appleton-Century-Crofts, 1980, pp 1–8
27. Tonnesen MG, Worthen GS, Johnston RB: Neutrophil emigration, activation, and tissue damage. In Clark RAF, Henson PM (eds): The Molecular and Cellular Biology of Wound Repair. New York, Plenum Press, 1988, pp 149–183
28. Simpson D, Ross R: The neutrophilic leukocyte in wound repair: A study with antineutrophil serum. J Clin Invest 1972; 51:2009–2023
29. Dale DC, Wolff SM: Skin window studies of the acute inflammatory responses of neutropenic patients. Blood 1971; 38:138–142
30. Irvin TT: Wound Healing: Principles and Practice. London, Chapman and Hall, 1981, pp 1–34
31. Peacock EE: Wound Repair. Philadelphia, WB Saunders, 1984, pp 1–102
32. Postlethwaite A, Kang A: Collagen and collagen peptide induced chemotaxis of human blood monocytes. J Exp Med 1976; 143:1299–1307
33. Leibovich SJ, Wiseman DM: Macrophages, wound repair and angiogenesis. In Barbul A,

Pines E, Caldwell M, Hunt TK (eds): Growth Factors and Other Aspects of Wound Healing: Biological and Clinical Implications. New York, Liss, 1988, pp 131–145

34. Leibovich SJ, Ross R: The role of the macrophage in wound repair. Am J Pathol 1975; 84:71–100

35. Polverini PJ, Cotran RS, Gimbrone MA, Unanue ER: Activated macrophages induce vascular proliferation. Nature 1977; 269:804–806

36. Fukasawa M, Campeau JD, Yanagihara DL, et al: Regulation of proliferation of peritoneal tissue repair cells by peritoneal macrophages. J Surg Res 1990; 49:81–87

37. Riches DWH: The multiple roles of macrophages in wound healing. In Clark RAF, Henson PM (eds): The Molecular and Cellular Biology of Wound Repair. New York, Plenum Press, 1988, pp 213–239

38. Clark RA, Stone RD, Leung DYK: Role of macrophages in wound healing. Surg Forum 1976; 27:16–18

39. Leibovich SJ, Ross R: A macrophage dependent factor that stimulates the proliferation of fibroblasts in vitro. Am J Pathol 1976; 84:501–514

40. Thakral KK, Goodson WH III, Hunt TK: Stimulation of wound blood vessel growth by wound macrophages. J Surg Res 1979; 26:430–436

41. Knighton DR, Hunt TK, Scheuenstuhl H, et al: Oxygen tension regulates the expression of angiogenesis factor by macrophages. Science 1983; 221:1283–1285

42. Ross R, Benditt EP: Wound healing and collagen formation: I. Sequential changes in components of guinea pig skin wounds observed in the electron microscope. J Biophys Biochem Cytol 1961; 11:677–700

43. Barbul A: Role of T cell–dependent immune system in wound healing. In Barbul A, Pines E, Caldwell M, Hunt TK (eds): Growth Factors and Other Aspects of Wound Healing: Biological and Clinical Implications. New York, Liss, 1988, pp 161–171

44. Jimenez SA, Freundlich B, Rosenblood J: Selective inhibition of human diploid fibroblast collagen synthesis by interferons. J Clin Invest 1984; 74:1112–1116

45. Efron JE, Frankel HL, Lazarou SA, et al: Wound healing and T-lymphocytes. J Surg Res 1990; 48:460–463

46. Petersen JM, Barbul A, Breslin RJ, et al: Significance of T-lymphocytes in wound healing. Surgery 1987; 102:300–305

47. Barbul A, Breslin RJ, Woodyard JP, et al: The effect of in vivo T-helper and T-suppressor lymphocyte depletion on wound healing. Ann Surg 1989; 209:479–483

48. Levi-Schaffer F, Kupietzky A: Mast cells enhance migration and proliferation of fibroblasts into an in vitro wound. Exp Cell Res 1990; 188:42–49

49. Galli SJ, Lichtenstein LM: Biology of mast cells and basophils. In Middleton E, Reed CF, Ellis EF, et al (eds): Allergy, Principles and Practice, 3d ed. St. Louis, Mosby, 1988, pp 106–134

50. Persinger MA, Lepage P, Simard JP, Parker GH: Mast cell numbers in incisional wounds in rat skin as a function of distance, time and treatment. Br J Dermatol 1983; 108:179–187

51. Schittek A, Demetrioy AA, Padawar J, et al: Compound 48/80 and the healing of wounds in rats: The effect of timing of drug injections. Agents Actions 1984; 15:172–176

52. Basset EG, Baker JR, De Souza P: A light microscopical study of healing incised dermal wounds in rats, with special reference to eosinophil leucocytes and to the collagenous fibers of the periwound areas. Br J Exp Pathol 1977; 58:581–605

53. Hibbs MS, Mainardi CL, Kang AH: Type-specific collagen degradation by eosinophils. Biochem J 1982; 207:621–624

54. Todd R, Donoff BR, Chiang T, et al: The eosinophil as a cellular source of transforming growth factor alpha in healing cutaneous wounds. Am J Pathol 1991; 138(6):1307–1313

55. Sloan P: Current concepts of the role of fibroblasts and extracellular matrix in wound healing and their relevance to oral implantology. J Dent 1991; 19:107–109

56. Postlethwaite AE, Kang AH: Fibroblast chemoattractants. Methods Enzymol 1988; 163:694–707

57. Lewis J, Chevalier A, Kienny M, Wolpert I: Muscle nerve branches do not develop in chick wings devoid of muscle. J Embryol Exp Morphol 1981; 64:211–232

58. Baum JL: Source of the fibroblast in central corneal wound healing. Arch Ophthalmol 1971; 85:473–477

59. Cohen K, Moore CD, Diegelmann RF: Onset and localization of collagen synthesis during wound healing in open rat skin sounds. Proc Soc Exp Biol Med 1979; 160:458–462

60. Ross R: The fibroblast and wound repair. Biol Rev 1968; 43:51–96

61. Stewart R, Duley JA, Allardyce RA: The migration of fibroblasts into an in vitro wound. Br J Exp Pathol 1979; 60:582–588

62. Abercrombie M, Heaysman JEM, Pegrum SM: The locomotion of fibroblasts in culture: IV. Electron microscopy of the leading lamella. Exp Cell Res 1971; 67:359–367

63. Abercrombie M, Heaysman JEM, Pegrum SM: Locomotion of fibroblasts in culture: V. Surface marking with concanavalin A. Exp Cell Res 1972; 73:536–539

64. McCarthy JB, Sas DF, Furcht LT: Mechanisms of parenchymal cell migration into wounds.

In Clark RAF, Henson PM (eds): The Molecular and Cellular Biology of Wound Repair. New York, Plenum Press, 1988, pp 281–319

65. Repesh LA, Fitzgerald TJ, Furcht LT: Fibronectin involvement in granulation tissue and wound healing in rabbits. J Histochem Cytochem 1982; 30:351–358

66. McGrath MH, Hundhal SA: The spatial and temporal quantification of myofibroblasts. Plast Reconstr Surg 1982; 69:975–976

67. Skalli O, Gabbiani G: The biology of the myofibroblast relationship to wound contraction and fibrocontractive diseases. In Clark RAF, Henson PM (eds): The Molecular and Cellular Biology of Wound Repair. New York, Plenum Press, 1988, pp 373–404

68. Montandan D, Gabbiani G, Ryan GB, Majno G: The contractile fibroblast: Its relevance in plastic surgery. Plast Reconstr Surg 1973; 52:286–290

69. Abercrombie M, Flint MH, Janes DW: Wound contraction in relation to collagen formation in scorbutic guinea pigs. J Embryol Exp Morphol 1956; 4:167–175

70. Gabbiani G, Ryan GB, Majno G: Presence of modified fibroblasts in granulation tissue and their possible role in wound contraction. Experientia 1971; 27:549–550

71. Skalli O, Gabbiani G: The biology of the myofibroblast relationship to wound contraction and fibrocontractive diseases. In Clark RAF, Henson PM (eds): The Molecular and Cellular Biology of Wound Repair. New York, Plenum Press, 1988, pp 373–402

72. Vande Berg JS, Rudolph R, Poolman WL, Disharoon DR: Comparative growth dynamics and actin concentration between cultured human myofibroblasts from granulating wounds and dermal fibroblasts from normal skin. Lab Invest 1989; 61(5):532–538

73. Fujiwara K, Pollard TD: Fluorescent antibody localization of myosin in the cytoplasm, cleavage furrow, and mitotic spindle of human cells. J Cell Biol 1976; 71:848–875

74. Lazarides E: Tropomyosin antibody: The specific localization of tropomyosin in nonmuscle cells. J Cell Biol 1975; 65:549–561

75. Ryan GB, Cliff WJ, Gabbiani G, et al: Myofibroblasts in human granulation tissue. Hum Pathol 1974; 5:55–67

76. Singer II, Kawka DW, Kazazis DM, Clark RAF: In vivo codistribution of fibronectin and actin fibers in granulation tissue: Immunofluorescence and electron microscopic studies of the fibronexus at the myofibroblast surface. J Cell Biol 1984; 98:2091–2106

77. Madri JA, Pratt BM: Angiogenesis. In Clark RAF, Henson PM (eds): The Molecular and Cellular Biology of Wound Repair. New York, Plenum Press, 1988, pp 337–358

78. Madri JA, Pratt BM: Endothelial cell–matrix interactions: In vitro models of angiogenesis. J Histochem Cytochem 1986; 34:85–91

79. Simionescu N, Heltianu C, Antohe F, Simionescu M: Endothelial receptors for histamine. In Fishman AP (ed): Endothelium, vol 401. New York, New York Academy of Science, 1982, pp 132–148

80. Pober JS, Gimbrone MA: Expression of Ia-like antigens by human vascular endothelial cells is inducible in vitro: Demonstration by monoclonal antibody binding and immunoprecipitation. Proc Natl Acad Sci USA 1982; 79:6641–6645

81. Pober JS, Gimbrone MA, Cotran RS, et al: Ia expression by vascular endothelial cells is inducible by activated T cells and by human gamma interferon. J Exp Med 1983; 157:1339–1353

82. Gross JL, Moscatelly D, Rifkin DB: Increased capillary endothelial cell protease activity in response to angiogenic stimuli in vitro. Proc Natl Acad Sci USA 1983; 880:2623–2627

83. Kalebic T, Garbisa S, Glaser B, Liotta L: Basement membrane collagen: Degradation by migrating endothelial cells. J Cell Biol 1983; 221:281–283

84. Bornstein P, McPherson J, Sage H: Synthesis and secretion of thrombospondin and fibronectin by cultured human endothelial cells. In Nossel H, Vogel H (eds): Pathobiology of the Endothelial Cell (P and S Biomedical Sciences Symposia Series), vol 6. New York, Academic Press, 1982, pp 215–228

85. Sholley MM, Ferguson GP, Seibel HR, et al: Mechanisms of neovascularization: Vascular sprouting can occur without proliferation of endothelial cells. Lab Invest 1984; 51:624–634

86. Burger PC, Klintworth GK: Autoradiographic study of corneal neovascularization induced by chemical cautery. Lab Invest 1981; 45:328–335

87. Nicosia RF, Madri JA: The microvascular extracellular matrix: Developmental changes during angiogenesis in the aortic ring–plasma clot model. Am J Pathol 1987; 128:78–90

88. Madri JA, Williams SK: Capillary endothelial cell cultures: Phenotypic modulation by matrix components. J Cell Biol 1983; 97:153–165

89. Dillman T, Penn J: Studies on repair of cutaneous wounds: II. The healing of wounds involving loss of superficial portions of the skin. Med Proc 1956; 2:150–158

90. Gipson IK, Wescott MJ, Brooksby NG: Effects of cytochalasins B and D and colchicine on migration of the corneal epithelium. Invest Ophthalmol Vis Sci 1982; 22:633–642

91. Stenn KS, Depalma L: Reepithelialization. In Clark RAF, Henson PM (eds): The Molecular and Cellular Biology of Wound Repair. New York, Plenum Press, 1988, pp 321–336

92. Gabbiani G, Chaponnier C, Huttner I: Cytoplasmic filament and gap functions in epithelial cells and myofibroblasts during wound healing. J Cell Biol 1978; 76:561–568

93. Radice G: The spreading of epithelial cells during wound closure in Xenopus larvae. Dev Biol 1980; 76:26–46

94. Winter GD: Movement of epidermal cells over the wound surface. Adv Biol Skin 1964; 5:113–127

95. Takashima A, Grinnell F: Human keratinocyte adhesion and phagocytosis promoted by fibronectin. J Invest Dermatol 1984; 83:352–358

96. Nemeth GG, Bolander ME, Martin GR: Growth factors and their role in wound and fracture healing. In Barbul A, Pines E, Caldwell M, Hunt TK (eds): Growth Factors and Other Aspects of Wound Healing: Biological and Clinical Implications. New York, Liss, 1988, pp 1–17

97. Clemmons DR, Underwood LE, VanWyk JJ: Hormonal control of immunoreactive somatomedin produced by cultured human fibroblasts. J Clin Invest 1981; 67:10–19

98. Salo T, Lyons JG, Rahamtulla F, et al: Transforming growth factor-β1 up-regulates type IV collagen expression in cultured human keratinocytes. J Biol Chem 1991; 266(18):11436–11441

99. Ross R, Glomset JA, Kartya B, Harker L: A platelet-dependent serum factor that stimulates the proliferation of arterial smooth muscle cells in vitro. Proc Natl Acad Sci USA 1974; 71:1207–1210

100. Betsholtz C, Johnsson A, Heldin CH, et al: cDNA sequence and chromosomal localization of human platelet-derived growth factor A-chain and its expression in tumour cell lines. Nature 1986; 320:695–699

101. Deuel TF, Huang JS, Proffitt RT, et al: Human platelet-derived growth factor: Purification and resolution into two active protein fractions. J Biol Chem 1981; 256:8896–8899

102. Deuel TF, Senior RM, Huang JS, Griffin GL: Chemotaxis of monocytes and neutrophils to platelet-derived growth factor. J Clin Invest 1982; 69:1046–1049

103. Tzeng DY, Deuel TF, Huang JS, et al: Platelet-derived growth factor promotes polymorphonuclear leukocyte activation. Blood 1984; 64:1123–1128

104. Bowen-Pope DF, Malpass TW, Fowter DM, Ross R: Platelet-derived growth factor in vivo: Levels, activity, and rate of clearance. Blood 1984; 64:458–469

105. Gosposdarowicz D: Localization of a fibroblast growth factor and its effect alone and with hydrocortisone on 3T3 cell growth. Nature 1974; 249:123–127

106. Fox GM: The role of growth factors in tissue repair: III. Fibroblast growth factor. In Clark RAF, Henson PM (eds): The Molecular and Cellular Biology of Wound Repair. New York, Plenum Press, 1988, pp 265–271

107. Gospodarowicz D, Bialecki H, Thakral TK: The angiogenic activity of the fibroblast and epidermal growth factor. Exp Eye Res 1979; 28:501–514

108. Shing Y, Folkmann J, Sullivan R, et al: Heparin affinity: Purification of a tumor-derived capillary endothelial cell growth factor. Science 1984; 223:1296–1299

109. Davidson J, Buckley A, Woodward S, et al: Mechanisms of accelerated wound repair using epidermal growth factor and basic fibroblast growth factor. In Barbul A, Pines E, Caldwell M, Hunt TK (eds): Growth Factors and Other Aspects of Wound Healing: Biological and Clinical Implications. New York, Liss, 1988, pp 63–75

110. Davidson J, Klagsbrun M, Hills K, et al: Accelerated wound repair, cell proliferation, and collagen accumulation are produced by a cartilage-derived growth factor. J Cell Biol 1985; 100:1219–1227

111. Buntrock P, Jentzsch KD, Heder G: Stimulation of wound healing, using brain extract with fibroblast growth factor (FGF) activity: I. Quantitative and biochemical studies into formation of granulation tissue. Exp Pathol 1982; 21:46–53

112. Buntrock P, Jentzsch KD, Heder G: Stimulation of wound healing, using brain extract with fibroblast growth factor (FGF) activity: II. Histological and morphometric examination of cells and capillaries. Exp Pathol 1982; 21:62–67

113. Cohen S: Isolation of a mouse submaxillary gland protein accelerating incisor eruption and eyelid opening in the new-born animal. J Biol Chem 1962; 237:1555–1562

114. Banks AR: The role of growth factors in tissue repair: II. Epidermal growth factor. In Clark RAF, Henson PM (eds): The Molecular and Cellular Biology of Wound Repair. New York, Plenum Press, 1988, pp 253–263

115. Toyoda S, Lee PC, Lebenthal E: Interaction of epidermal growth factor with specific binding sites of enterocytes isolated from rat small intestine during development. Biochem Biophys Res Commun 1986; 886:295–301

116. Chabot JG, Walker P, Pelletier G: Distribution of epidermal growth factor binding sites in the adult rat liver. Am J Physiol 1986; 250:G760

117. Lim RW, Hauschka SD: A rapid decrease in epidermal growth factor–binding capacity accompanies the terminal differentiation of mouse myoblasts in vitro. J Cell Biol 1984; 98:739–747

118. DeLarco JE, Todaro GJ: Growth factors from murine sarcoma virus–transformed cells. Proc Natl Acad Sci USA 1978; 75:4001–4005

119. Assoian RK: The role of growth factors in tissue repair: IV. Type β transforming growth factor and stimulation of fibrosis. In Clark RAF, Henson PM (eds): The Molecular and Cellular Biology of Wound Repair. New York, Plenum Press, 1988, pp 273–280

120. Kehrl JH, Wakefield LM, Roberts AB, et al: Production of transforming growth factor-beta by human T-lymphocytes and its potential role in the regulation of T cell growth. J Exp Med 1986; 163:1037–1050
121. Lawrence WT, Sporn MB, Gorxchboth C, et al: The reversal of an Adriamycin-induced healing impairment with chemoattractants and growth factors. Ann Surg 1986; 203:142–147
122. Ignotz RA, Massague J: Transforming growth factor-beta stimulates the expression of fibronectin and collagen and their incorporation into the extracellular matrix. J Biol Chem 1986; 261:4337–4345
123. Yamada KM, Akiyama SK, Hasegawa T, et al: Recent advances in research on fibronectin and other cell attachment proteins. J Cell Biochem 1985; 28:79–97
124. Brotchie H, Wakefield D: Fibronectin: Structure, function and significance in wound healing. Australas J Dermatol 1990; 31:47–56
125. Clark RAF: Fibronectin matrix deposition and fibronectin receptor expression in healing and normal skin. Soc Invest Dermatol 1990; 94(6):128S–134S
126. Luomanen M, Virtanen I: Fibronectins in healing incision, excision, and laser wounds. J Oral Pathol Med 1991; 20:133–138
127. Oh E, Pierschbacher M, Ryoslahti E: Deposition of plasma fibronectin in tissues. Proc Natl Acad Sci USA 1981; 78:3218–3221
128. McDonald JA: Fibronectin: A primitive matrix. In Clark RAF, Henson PM (eds): The Molecular and Cellular Biology of Wound Repair. New York, Plenum Press, 1988, pp 405–435
129. Chen WT, Hasegawa E, Hasegawa T, et al: Development of cell surface linkage complexes in cultured fibroblasts. J Cell Biol 1985; 100:1103–1114
130. Chen WT, Wang J, Hasegawa T, et al: Regulation of fibronectin receptor distribution by transformation, exogenous fibronectin, and synthetic peptides. J Cell Biol 1986; 100:1649–1661
131. Nishida T, Nakagawa S, Awate T, et al: Fibronectin promotes epithelial migration of cultured rabbit cornea in situ. J Cell Biol 1983; 97:1653–1657
132. McDonald JA, Kelley DG, Broekelmann TJ: Role of fibronectin in collagen deposition: Fab' to the gelatin-binding domain of fibronectin inhibits both fibronectin and collagen organization in fibroblast extracellular matrix. J Cell Biol 1982; 92:485–492
133. Yamada KM: Cell surface interaction with extracellular matrix materials. Annu Rev Biochem 1983; 52:761–799
134. Rapraeger A, Bernfield M: An integral membrane proteoglycan is capable of binding components of the cytoskeleton and the extracellular matrix. In Hawkes SP, Wang JL (eds): Extracellular Matrix. New York, Academic Press, 1982, pp 265–269
135. Laterra MW, Ansbacher R, Culp LA: Glycosaminoglycans that bind cold-insoluble globulin in cell-substratum adhesion sites of murine fibroblasts. Proc Natl Acad Sci USA 1980; 77:6662–6666
136. Brennan MJ, Oldberg A, Hayman EG, Ruoslahti E: Effect of a proteoglycan produced by rat tumor cells on their adhesion to fibronectin-collagen substrata. Cancer Res 1983; 43:4302–4307
137. Yeo TK, Brown L, Dvorak HF: Alterations in proteoglycan synthesis common to healing wounds and tumors. Am J Pathol 1991; 138(6):1437–1450
138. Funderburg FM, Markwald RR: Conditioning of native substrates by chondroitin sulfate proteoglycan during cardiac mesenchymal cell migration. J Cell Biol 1986; 103:2475–2487
139. Alexander SA, Donoff RB: The glycosaminoglycans of open wounds. J Surg Res 1980; 29:422–429
140. Grimes NL: The role of hyaluronate and hyaluronidase in cell migration during the rabbit ear regenerative healing response (abst). Anat Rec 1981; 199:100
141. Docherty R, Forrester JV, Lackie JM, Gregory DW: Glycosaminoglycans facilitate the movement of fibroblasts through three-dimensional collagen matrices. J Cell Sci 1989; 92:263–270
142. McPherson JM, Piez KA: Collagen in dermal wound repair. In Clark RAF, Henson PM (eds): The Molecular and Cellular Biology of Wound Repair. New York, Plenum Press, 1988, pp 471–496
143. Peacock EE: Wound Repair, 3d ed. Philadelphia, WB Saunders, 1984, pp 56–101
144. Heughan C, Hunt T: Some aspects of wound healing research: A review. Can J Surg 1975; 18:118–126
145. Woodley DT, O'Keefe EJ, Prunieras M: Cutaneous wound healing: a model for cell–matrix interactions. J Am Acad Dermatol 1985; 12:420–433
146. Carter DM, Balin AK, Gottlieb AB, et al: Clinical experience with crude preparations of growth factors in healing of chronic wounds in human subjects. In Barbul A, Pines E, Caldwell M, Hunt TK (eds): Growth Factors and Other Aspects of Wound Healing: Biological and Clinical Implications. New York, Liss, 1988, pp 303–317

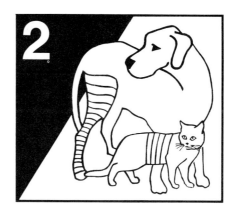

TREATMENT OF CONTAMINATED WOUNDS, INCLUDING WOUNDS OF THE ABDOMEN AND THORAX

L. KAY MASON

CLASSIFICATION OF WOUNDS

Veterinarians are frequently faced with the challenge of managing many types of contaminated wounds. These range from a traumatic wound in which dirt and hair are embedded to rupture of a hollow abdominal viscus. The goals in managing a contaminated wound are to prevent its development into an infected wound and to provide the environment necessary for healing. The application of sound principles, including thorough evaluation of the patient and the wound, appropriate cleansing and debridement of the wound, proper use of drains, and adequate patient nutrition and wound care during the healing period, is necessary to prevent contamination from developing into infection. An understanding of the factors affecting infection and wound healing is also required. Wound healing may be affected by factors specific to the patient, such as age, nutritional status, behavior, medications, and concurrent diseases (e.g., hyperadrenocorticism and diabetes), that negatively affect wound healing and increase susceptibility to infection. Healing is also affected by factors specific to the wound, such as blood supply, species and number of bacteria, hydration, location, and the manner in which the wound was inflicted. By thoroughly evaluating the patient and the nature of the wound, a treatment plan can be applied that will prevent the development of infection and allow healing to proceed in a rapid and uncomplicated manner.

Wounds may be classified by degree of contamination (Table 2–1), location

TABLE 2–1. Classification of Wounds by Degree of Bacterial Contamination

CATEGORY	DEFINITION OR EXAMPLE
Clean	Elective procedure not involving respiratory, urogenital, or gastrointestinal system with primary closure No break in asepsis
Clean-contaminated	Surgery involving respiratory, urogenital, or gastrointestinal tract without significant contamination Minor break in asepsis
Contaminated	Fresh traumatic wound, less than 4 to 6 hours old Surgery of respiratory, urogenital, or gastrointestinal tract with significant contamination Surgery in the presence of inflammation
Dirty	Old traumatic wound, more than 4 to 6 hours old Traumatic wound with foreign material and significant devitalized tissue Perforated hollow viscus Surgery in the presence of abscessation

on the body (Table 2–2), or the manner in which they were inflicted. These classification schemes allow us to identify factors that will affect the choice of treatment and the expected course of healing for a given wound. They also highlight the most common causes of complications of wound healing for individual types of wounds. For example, a fresh wound made by a clipper blade over the flank area can be treated by immediate cleansing and closure and will heal quickly. In contrast, the surgeon presented with an open bite wound to the carpus that is 3 days old must consider the presence of infection and tissue damage, lack of tissue for closure, and the possibility of joint or bone involvement. In planning a treatment regimen, the surgeon must therefore consider problems associated with the wound's location, cause, and degree of contamination.

Contaminated wounds are often traumatic injuries, such as dog bites, lacerations, and abrasion injuries caused by automobile accidents. However, many of the routine surgical procedures performed daily in a general veterinary practice also involve contaminated wounds. Procedures involving the respiratory, alimentary, or urogenital tract and those performed on inflamed or infected tissue (e.g., lateral ear canal resection in the presence of otitis) are examples of treatment of contaminated tissues. A general classification system of the degree of expected contamination in specific surgical wounds was established in 1964 by the Committee on Trauma of the National Academy of Sciences–National Research Council[1] (see Table 2–1). Because wound infection rates are directly affected by the degree of contamination present, this system allows prediction of infection of a surgical procedure. For example, in a recent study, the infection rate for wounds classified as clean was only 2.5%, whereas an 18.1% infection rate was observed in those classified as dirty.[2] All traumatic wounds fall into the category of contaminated or dirty; reported infection rates are 5.8% for contaminated wounds and 18.1% for dirty wounds.[2] Although bacterial contamination increases the likelihood of infection, appropriate surgical treatment can usually prevent wound infection. *Traditionally, a "golden period" of 6 hours after injury exists in which a contaminated wound may be cleaned and primarily closed without development of infection.*[3, 4] This is because fresh wounds

TABLE 2–2. Classification of Wounds by Location

LOCATION	CONCERNS IN MANAGEMENT	FACTORS CONDUCIVE TO RECOVERY
Head	CNS trauma Cosmetic result important Anesthetic risk Minimal loose skin for closure	Excellent healing of oral cavity
Neck	Tracheal or esophageal injury Damage to vagosympathetic trunk Damage to carotid arteries	Loose skin for closure
Chest	Penetrating injury possible Associated trauma to pulmonary or cardiovascular system Anesthetic risk	Loose skin for closure
Abdomen	Penetrating injury possible Rupture of hollow viscus possible	Loose skin for closure
Extremity	Associated orthopedic injury Minimal loose skin for closure Hindlimb: abdominal injury Forelimb: thoracic injury	Usually not life-threatening

(4–6 hours old) are able to be cleansed of bacteria-laden debris before bacteria proliferate and invade the wound edges. After this time, bacterial colonization within the damaged tissues has usually occurred, making infection more likely. In these cases, infection must be controlled before the wound can be closed and allowed to heal.

The quantity of contaminating bacteria in a wound is an important factor affecting the likelihood of infection. *Infection* has been defined as the presence of 1 million organisms per gram of tissue.[5] Wounds contaminated with a large number of bacteria are more likely to become infected. The number of bacteria within a wound increases with time in contaminated traumatic and surgical wounds. This explains the increased infection rate after surgery requiring more than 90 minutes to complete and in wounds managed after the golden period.[2, 6]

Foreign and necrotic material contribute to infection in a contaminated wound by serving as a source of organisms and an increased surface area for bacterial proliferation. As infection develops, wound healing is delayed or inhibited. The inflammatory and debridement phases of wound healing are significantly prolonged. Foreign material such as hair, soil, gravel, and wood are directly irritating to a wound. Enzymes are released by invading neutrophils that affect capillary permeability, decrease local blood supply, and degrade newly synthesized proteins such as fibrin and collagen.[7] Bacteria within a wound also release enzymes that break down fibrin and collagen and lead to further tissue devitalization.[4] Bacteria, foreign material, and developing purulent exudate mechanically separate the wound edges and interfere with the wound's blood supply. Bacteria continue to be harbored within foreign materials and are isolated from the body's defense mechanisms. Devitalized tissue within a wound is similar to foreign material in that it provides an environment that aids bacterial growth and protects the bacteria from phagocytosis by invading neutrophils. The presence of foreign and necrotic materials in wounds thus promotes the development of infection and increases the incidence of wound complications, sepsis, and even death.[8]

The location of a wound is another means of evaluating its severity and factors affecting its management. Wounds over the extremities are less likely to involve life-threatening injury. However, significant orthopedic injury may be present, and associated skin loss often makes primary closure impossible. Conversely, wounds over the thorax can be associated with severe life-threatening internal injury such as pulmonary contusion and pneumothorax but rarely involve skin deficits that cannot be closed. Considerations for specific wound location are summarized in Table 2–2 and will be discussed later in this chapter.

The manner in which a wound is inflicted also dictates how it should be treated. Bite wounds, lacerations, stab wounds, gunshot wounds, degloving injuries, and snake bite wounds are all examples of contaminated wounds with special concerns related to their origin. Their management is still governed by the same general principles of wound treatment, but specific considerations apply to each and will be discussed later in this chapter.

Although wounds may present in many forms, the general principles governing their treatment and healing are the same as originally defined by Halsted. *These include gentle handling of tissues, use of aseptic surgical technique, maintenance of blood supply to the tissues, hemostasis, closure of dead space, and closure without tension on the suture line.* These principles must be adhered to for proper wound management. Most postoperative complications and problems with wound healing can be traced back to violation of one or more of these principles.

GENERAL PRINCIPLES IN MANAGEMENT OF CONTAMINATED WOUNDS

Before the surgeon attempts to treat any traumatic wound, the patient must be evaluated by a thorough history, including age, breed, sex, time of injury, cause of injury, activity and treatment since injury, and any other concurrent health problems or medications that may complicate treatment. The patient should be given a complete physical examination, with special attention to cardiovascular status if severe trauma is involved. Thoracic radiographs of all patients with injuries caused by automobiles should be taken in order to rule out life-threatening chest trauma, such as a diaphragmatic hernia or pneumothorax (Fig. 2–1). In one study, thoracic injuries in

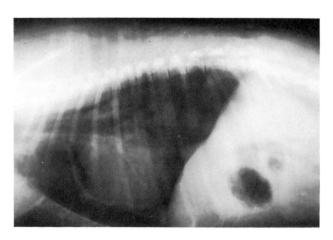

Figure 2–1. Pneumothorax in a 2-year-old Shar Pei following an automobile accident. This dog was presented for a degloving injury of the right forelimb.

dogs with hindlimb fractures following motor vehicle accidents included pulmonary contusion (52%), pneumothorax (15%), and pleural effusion (10%).[9] Although external wounds are often obvious to the owner, underlying cardiovascular, pulmonary, and internal organ injury must be assessed and treated prior to wound management. Patients also should be monitored for urine production until injury to the urinary tract, such as urinary bladder rupture, can be ruled out. Laboratory evaluation of packed cell volume (PCV), serum total solids (TS), and appropriate serum chemistries should be performed. Treatment of shock with rigorous fluid and blood replacement should be instituted if needed. If necessary, in animals requiring emergency care, wounds may be simply clipped of hair and the area gently scrubbed, flushed with sterile saline, and covered with a sterile dressing and bandage until more definitive treatment can be performed. Areas with exposed bone, such as open fractures and shear injuries, must be covered as soon as possible. These wounds should be clipped, scrubbed, flushed liberally with sterile saline, covered with skin or soft tissues in a loose closure, and placed in a sterile dressing and bandage. The goal is to cleanse the wound, rehydrate and nourish the damaged tissue, and prevent further contamination. Although definitive debridement and closure of wounds are precluded in emergency conditions and require general anesthesia, the simple act of early cleansing and protection will prevent contamination from proceeding to infection and allow primary closure beyond the golden period of 4 to 6 hours following injury.

Once the patient's condition is stable, definitive wound treatment can begin. Definitive treatment of traumatic wounds that are assumed to be contaminated consists of the following steps:

1. Thorough evaluation of the extent and nature of the wound and associated injuries
2. Preparation of the wound for treatment by clipping and scrubbing
3. Debridement of all foreign material and devitalized tissue
4. Thorough lavage and rehydration of the wound
5. Wound closure
6. Bandaging

In evaluating the extent and nature of a wound, it is helpful to know how it was inflicted. For example, a bite wound may appear to be a minor lesion, but such wounds are always contaminated with oral bacteria and may involve significant crushing injury to deeper tissues. Radiographs should be taken, if necessary, to rule out damage to underlying structures, such as fractures or internal organ damage. Penetrating wounds should be evaluated for entry and exit sites. Thoracic wounds should be evaluated by chest radiographs to determine if penetration has occurred and the extent of damage to the lungs and mediastinum. Wounds to the abdomen also should be evaluated radiographically to rule out penetration, defects of the abdominal wall, and internal organ damage. Contrast studies to determine involvement of the urinary system may be necessary. In some cases, ultrasonography may augment evaluation of body cavities for injury resulting in fluid or air accumulation. Preliminary and thorough evaluation will allow the surgeon to form an appropriate treatment plan and prevent later complications.

After evaluation of the wound, it is clipped and scrubbed in preparation for surgery. The wound should be protected during clipping by covering it with sterile petrolatum or lubricating jelly. Alternatively, the wound may be packed with sterile sponges soaked in sterile saline. Clipping should begin at the wound edges and proceed in a direction away from the wound. This will minimize further contamination of the wound with hair and debris. The clipper blades may be dipped in mineral oil or sterile jelly so that hair will adhere to the blades and refrain from falling into the wound. A generous area of skin surrounding the wound should be clipped to allow enlargement of the wound if necessary during exploration. In wounds involving skin deficits, an appropriate area of adjacent skin for mobilization or skin-flap closure also should be surgically prepared.

After clipping, a surgical scrub of the area is performed in preparation for aseptic surgery. Because contaminated wounds usually involve tremendous soilage, additional scrubbing time is required. Scrubbing should begin at the wound margins and proceed away from the wound. The wound should remain covered during this time to prevent further contamination with debris and dirt during scrubbing. The detergent and antiseptic used in the surgical scrub should not be allowed to enter the wound. The wound is then draped in preparation for surgery.

The wound can now be explored and debrided. This is the most important step in the treatment of contaminated wounds. *The most common cause of delayed wound healing and infection is inadequate debridement.*[10] Debridement of all but the most superficial wounds should be performed as a true surgical procedure with all the attendant aseptic preparations, including mask, gloves, and sterile surgical instruments, to prevent further contamination of the wound with hospital flora, which are usually more virulent than the contaminants. Debridement should be performed with sharp incision and proceed from the most superficial layer of the wound to the deepest layer.[4, 11] I prefer to use a no. 15 scalpel blade, but Metzenbaum scissors also may be used. All devitalized tissue and foreign material are removed because they provide a good bacterial substrate, which can lead to infection. Damaged tissues with a good blood supply are left in place because they resist infection and heal in the face of contamination as a result of the capillary-mediated immune response. Metal from gunshot wounds should be removed as encountered, but deep exploration into noncontaminated tissues is avoided. Metal in these areas is tolerated by the body. An exception is foreign material within joints, which should be removed. Small, avascular fragments of bone that are not important to fracture stability can be removed. Long bone fractures and joint injuries should be stabilized as soon as possible to aid healing of soft tissues and promote granulation tissue coverage of open wounds. Even severe shear injuries with extensive soft-tissue loss over the distal aspect of the extremities will heal if underlying bones and joints are stabilized.

Necrotic muscle should be debrided liberally. Muscle is removed if it is discolored, nonbleeding, friable, or embedded with foreign material. Muscle is especially susceptible to further necrosis following injury, and injured muscle is an excellent bacterial substrate. Loss of muscle mass may not deleteriously affect recovery. Conversely, tendons, ligaments, blood vessels, and nerves should be minimally debrided. Severed tendons may be sutured. These structures should be cleaned and covered with healthy tissue where possible. Infections from inadequate debridement of tendons, nerves, and blood vessels are unlikely.

Fascia and fat should be debrided liberally. Loss of these structures is well tolerated, and if damaged, they are likely to be colonized by contaminating bacteria. Skin should be debrided if it is nonbleeding, discolored, dry, or excessively thickened.

The wound should be thoroughly exposed and explored to fully determine the extent of damage and allow complete debridement of all devitalized and contaminated tissue. With bite wounds especially, underlying crushed muscle should be exposed and excised as necessary. In wounds where preservation of structure is critical and there is question as to viability of tissues, conservative debridement should be performed and the wound reevaluated in 1 to 2 days. At this time, further debridement may be performed.

During debridement, hemostasis is critical. Bleeding vessels should be ligated or cauterized. Inadequate hemostasis can lead to seroma formation, which can serve as a medium for bacteria and can mechanically interfere with wound healing.

Following thorough debridement, the final stage in contaminated wound cleansing is lavage. The purposes of lavage are to clean the wound of remaining debris and bacteria and rehydrate exposed tissues. The volume of lavage fluid and pressure of irrigation are important determinants of the efficacy of lavage. Lavage with large volumes (500–1000 ml) of fluid has been shown to decrease the incidence of infection in contaminated wounds by removal of contaminating bacteria and debris.[12, 13] High irrigation pressures also serve to mechanically increase the effectiveness of particle removal and decrease the number of contaminating bacteria in a wound.[14, 15] Effective lavage pressures as high as 8 lb/in^2 can be achieved with a simple system consisting of a 35-mm syringe attached to a 19-gauge needle.[16] Use of a pulsating-water-jet lavage can achieve even higher irrigation pressures (70 lb/in^2).[17] These have both been shown to achieve more effective bacteria and debris removal than lavage by simple irrigation alone.

The type of lavage fluid should aid in wound cleansing and rehydration without causing further damage to the tissues. This can be achieved in grossly contaminated wounds by copious lavage with tap water, followed by cleansing with sterile saline. Sterile isotonic saline is the most universally accepted lavage fluid. Because its effectiveness relies on the mechanical removal of bacteria, high volumes (500–1000 ml) at high pressures (8 lb/in^2 or above) are recommended.

Antiseptics added to the lavage fluid must be used with care. To be beneficial, they must enhance bacterial removal without causing damage to the tissues. Antiseptics combined with detergents, such as surgical scrub soaps, are not acceptable in lavage fluid because they cause chemical irritation to soft tissues, leading to decreased wound healing and impairment of defenses to bacterial infection. Detergents indiscriminately alter the surface properties of both bacteria and host cells, leading to cell injury and death.

Antiseptics alone, however, may reduce the bacterial population in contaminated wounds.[18, 19] This is useful because bacterial proliferation reduces wound healing through production of collagenases, tissue pH changes, and interference with the activity of wound fibroblasts.[4, 11] Chlorhexidine, in 0.5% and 1% solutions, has been shown to have effective antimicrobial activity with minimal tissue reaction.[19] Chlorhexidine causes bacterial cell death by altering permeability of the cell wall and has the added benefit of residual bactericidal activity in the wound bed. However, when used as an antiseptic for repeated wound cleansing over several days, it may decrease the formation of granulation tissue in the wound bed,[18] thus delaying wound healing.

Povidone-iodine is also an excellent antiseptic, but iodine may be absorbed systemically. It is toxic to fibroblasts at concentrations of 1% and 5%.[20] Povidone-iodine has minimal residual bactericidal activity and is inactivated by organic material within the wound,[19] thus making it no more beneficial than sterile isotonic saline as a lavage fluid. Irrigation of wounds with chlorhexidine diacetate at 0.005% and 0.05% was associated with less bacterial contamination than irrigation with either 0.1% and 1.0% povidone-iodine solutions or physiologic buffered saline alone and had no detrimental effects on wound tissues.[21] Chlorhexidine lavage augments mechanical cleansing with direct antibacterial action and improves wound healing by the prevention of bacterial infection.

The final step in the treatment of a contaminated wound is closure. Depending on the condition of the wound, closure may be performed immediately following debridement and lavage, or it may be delayed until infection is controlled. In some cases, the wound is left to heal without closure. The timing of closure is critical to prevent suture-line dehiscence, abscess formation, and delays in wound healing. Premature closure of contaminated and infected wounds can lead to wound breakdown, sepsis, and death.[8] Closure leading to successful healing is governed by good soft-tissue surgical principles, including gentle tissue handling, hemostasis, elimination of dead space, and closure without tension. If closure cannot be achieved within these guidelines, the wound should be left open.

Types of wound closures include primary closure, delayed primary closure, secondary closure, and healing by second intention. These are summarized in Table 2–3. The type of closure chosen for a particular wound is determined by the patient's clinical status, the amount of contamination and infection in a wound, and the amount of soft-tissue loss and adjacent skin available for closure.

Primary closure involves immediate suturing of a wound following thorough debridement and lavage. It may be performed in fresh wounds (less than 4–6 hours old) that are able to be closed without tension. If present, dead space should be eliminated by closure in layers or placement of a drain.

Delayed primary closure is closure within 5 days of injury before granulation tissue begins to form but after infection is controlled. Animals that are presented for treatment several days after injury frequently have wounds that are grossly infected and benefit from preliminary treatment to control infection for 1 to 5 days prior to closure. This permits further debridement of devitalized tissue and conversion of an infected wound to one more optimal for healing. The bacteria in a wound can be quantitated, and if less than 10^6 bacteria per gram of tissue are present, the wound can be closed.[11] When in doubt, it is best to leave a wound open.

Wound closure performed 5 days or more after injury is termed *secondary closure*. At this time, a bed of granulation tissue has formed in the wound, and the skin edges are closed over this. Adherence of the wound edges to the underlying tissue requires excision of the wound edge–granulation tissue

TABLE 2–3. Types of Wound Closure

Primary	Immediate closure
Delayed primary	1 to 5 days after injury, before granulation bed formation
Secondary	More than 5 days after injury, following granulation bed formation
Healing by second intention	No closure; healing by granulation, epithelialization, and contraction

margin with undermining and mobilization of skin over the granulation tissue. As with delayed primary closure, secondary closure allows control of wound infection and removal of devitalized tissue prior to closure, thereby improving conditions for uncomplicated wound healing.

Wounds with significant tissue loss or those requiring massive debridement are left to heal without closure. In these cases, healing occurs through granulation tissue formation, contraction, and epithelialization.[7, 22] This process is called healing by *second intention*. This may apply to any wound in which repeated debridement is necessary. The ability of open wounds in animals to heal by second intention is quite impressive (Fig. 2–2). Its disadvantages include prolonged healing time and less satisfactory cosmetic result. In areas where sufficient skin is available for healing by contraction, even large defects will close completely and leave only a small scar of fibrous tissue. A wound in which healing results in a scar that is cosmetically unacceptable can be revised and the scar excised after healing is complete (Fig. 2–3). On the distal extremities, contraction of second-intention healing is limited by the amount of available skin. Healing by epithelialization predominates, and the resulting skin is of poor quality. The scar tissue that forms is fragile, thin, and easily abraded. Open wounds over flexion surfaces allowed to heal by second intention may be complicated by contracture deformity, requiring later reconstructive surgery. Another option in managing large, open wounds is the placement of a skin flap or free graft after infection has been controlled and an adequate bed of granulation tissue has formed (Fig. 2–4).

Until the wound has healed, it must be kept clean and protected with appropriate dressings and frequent bandage changes. Wounds with exposed bone, periosteum, cartilage, and tendon should be covered with sterile

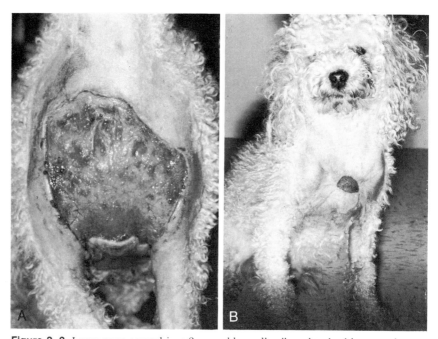

Figure 2–2. Large open wound in a 2-year-old poodle allowed to heal by second intention. *A,* Open wound following initial debridement of necrotic skin and muscle. *B,* The same wound 3 weeks later has significantly decreased in size by wound contraction.

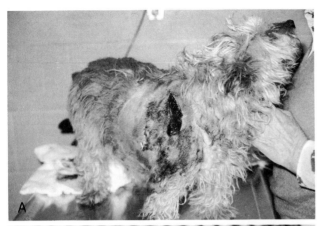

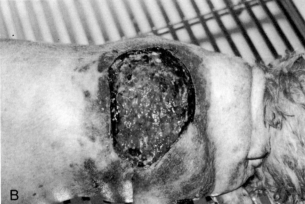

Figure 2–3. Infected wound in an 8-year-old mixed-breed dog. *A*, Wound at presentation. *B*, Wound following debridement.

dressings of petrolatum-saturated gauze. If such wounds are properly treated, granulation tissue will rapidly cover these structures, and a skin graft may then be placed. In some areas, flaps of muscle may be used to cover exposed bone, provide protection, and act as a source of early blood supply. Transposition of the cranial sartorius muscle and the cranial tibialis muscle to cover exposed areas of the tibia and tibiotarsal region, allowing improved blood supply to the area and earlier placement of skin grafts, has been described.[23, 24] Complications with muscle flaps include seroma formation, lameness, and wound infection.

When a wound is closed, the choice of suture material for closure is complicated by the presence of bacteria in contaminated wounds. Sutures are essentially foreign bodies and may serve as a scaffold for further bacterial colonization. Bacterial wound counts are actually increased in the presence of suture material.[25] However, the use of the appropriate material in a contaminated wound can minimize the potentiation of wound infection by sutures. Monofilaments of inert materials such as nylon, polypropylene, and stainless steel have the advantage of minimal tissue reaction and decreased surface area for bacterial invasion.[26] If an absorbable material is required, polyglycolic acid and polyglactin are good choices because they do not stimulate an inflammatory reaction and minimally potentiate infection.[27, 28] Catgut elicits a strong inflammatory response during absorption and is not recommended for use in contaminated wounds. Good tissue-handling tech-

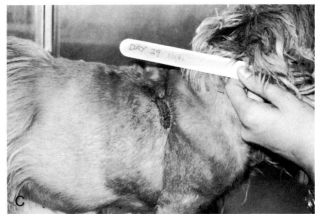

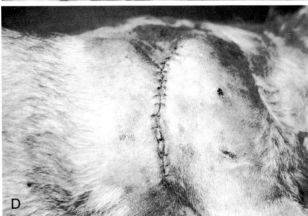

Figure 2–3 *Continued C*, Wound 4 weeks after injury showing resulting small fibrous scar and unhealed area. *D*, The scar and unhealed area have been debrided, and the wound has been closed. (Courtesy of N. L. Dykes.)

niques, use of the finest material possible, and placement of the least number of sutures also will minimize suture-associated wound infection.

Bandages should be placed on wounds that are open, require protection, contain a drain, are susceptible to seroma formation, or require immobilization. Bandages should be monitored and changed at appropriate intervals to prevent complications of wound disruption and infection. Improper management of bandages may lead to problems worse than the original wound. Ill-fitting and loose bandages may further traumatize open wounds by causing abrasion and irritation of the wound surface and delay healing by slowing epithelial migration across the granulation bed.[22] Wounds in areas of movement may benefit from immobilization to prevent stress on the wound and disruption of neovascularization and collagen synthesis. Conversely, in experimental studies, movement has been shown to be beneficial in wound healing by improving circulation, reducing infection, and increasing resulting wound strength.[4, 29] Depending on the area of the body in which a wound occurs, immobilization may aid or delay wound healing. Open wounds over flexion surfaces were shown to have improved healing by contraction when the affected area is allowed to move and decreased contraction when it is immobilized.[30] In this study, wound dressings caused increased separation of the wound edges and delayed healing. Mobility had no effect on healing in body areas that are naturally immobile. Sutured footpad lacerations should be immobilized with splints to prevent weight-bearing on the pads, which causes sutures to tear through tissue.[31] Wounds

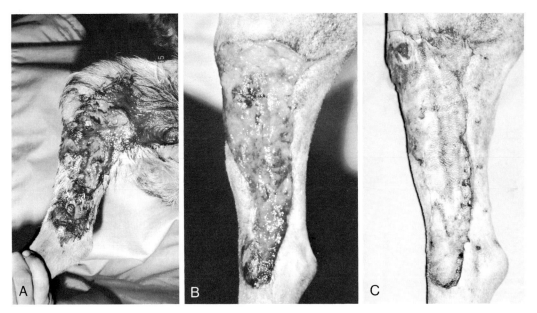

Figure 2–4. Infected wound over the medial tibia in a 5-year-old mixed-breed dog. *A,* Wound at initial presentation. *B,* Wound 3 weeks following debridement and management is now covered by a healthy bed of granulation tissue. *C,* Wound 1 week following placement of a full-thickness free skin graft over the granulation bed.

that involve tendon and ligament repairs should be immobilized for support and to reduce the tension of weight-bearing on the repaired tendon.[32]

MANAGEMENT OF CONTAMINATED WOUNDS CLASSIFIED BY LOCATION

Depending on the area of the body, there are specific considerations that affect how a contaminated wound should be managed. Frequently, there is damage to underlying structures that affects treatment (see Table 2–2). The amount of loose skin available for closure, blood and nerve supply to the area, location in a body cavity, and proximity of vital structures that may have been concurrently injured will determine the manner in which a wound should be treated.

Head

Wounds to the head are most commonly caused by bites and automobile accidents. They may involve trauma to the central nervous system, skull fractures, and damage to the sensory organs. Central nervous system trauma may be life-threatening and requires vigorous treatment. Use of systemic steroids (2 mg/kg dexamethasone sodium phosphate by slow IV infusion) or mannitol (1.5 gm/kg IV) may be indicated to reduce cerebral edema. Proptosis of the globe requires rapid replacement to salvage the eye. Patients with head injuries represent an increased anesthetic risk that may delay definitive treatment of wounds. Crushing injuries, bite wounds, and blunt trauma from automobile accidents are often associated with fractures of the skull and mandible. After patient stabilization, these must be identified by thorough examination and radiography.

In cats, contaminated wounds of the head and face are often associated with tremendous swelling of soft tissues from hematoma, edema, and inflammation. Definitive treatment of wounds should be delayed until the patient's condition is stable and swelling has subsided. A gastrostomy or pharyngostomy tube should be placed in patients with any injuries, swelling, fractures, or pain that prevent adequate food intake. Proper nutrition is critical to meet the animal's increased energy requirements for wound healing and protein synthesis. Skull fractures, especially those involving the mandible, are frequently open fractures. Because of the excellent blood supply to the oral cavity and structures of the face, however, wounds in this area usually heal well and are resistant to infection despite significant contamination.

In general, reconstruction and repair should provide the best cosmetic result. Simple skin lacerations may be closed primarily after cleansing and debridement. Fracture management and wound repair can be performed at the same time. Fractures of the hard palate should be repaired to prevent aspiration of food and water. Fractures of the maxilla and mandible are repaired to allow normal occlusion, food prehension, and mastication. Attention should be paid to the involvement of tooth roots in both the initial fracture and any method of fracture fixation used. Metal implants used in fracture repair of the mandible should not injure the tooth roots. This can lead to tooth loss and root abscessation. Interdental wiring can be used in fracture fixation and prevents tooth-root damage caused by placing large implants into the body of the mandible. When severe bone and soft-tissue injuries are present, some mandibular fractures may be managed successfully by partial mandibulectomy.[33] Mucosal lacerations usually heal rapidly and are closed only if associated with a fracture. Labial avulsions should be repaired by reattachment of the avulsed skin to the mandible with stainless steel horizontal mattress sutures and closure of the mucosa with fine absorbable suture material.[34]

Neck

Contaminated wounds of the neck are caused most commonly by dog bites and small collars that have been left on growing dogs (Fig. 2–5). Wound preparation is performed according to the general principles previously outlined. Wounds in this area must be explored thoroughly to rule out damage to the vital underlying structures. After exploration and treatment of injuries to vital structures, debridement, lavage, and closure are performed according to the general principles for treatment of contaminated wounds. The loose skin in this area aids wound closure even when large skin deficits are present.

Penetration of the esophagus causes significant wound contamination and may cause esophageal leakage. Signs of esophageal perforation include fever and subcutaneous emphysema in the cervical area and thoracic inlet. Small tears may heal spontaneously or can be debrided and closed primarily if identified at the time of wound treatment. Large lacerations should be debrided, and the mucosal and muscularis layers should be sutured carefully. Corticosteroids can be given to prevent secondary esophageal stricture formation, although controlled studies to document the efficacy of this treatment after laceration repair have not been reported. Oral prednisolone

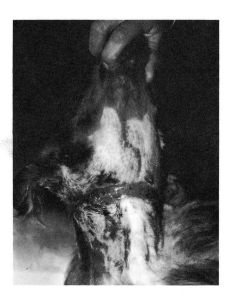

Figure 2–5. Deep, contaminated neck wound caused by a rubber band in a 9-month-old mixed-breed dog. (Courtesy of N. L. Dykes.)

at an anti-inflammatory dose (0.5 mg/kg for 7 days, tapering to alternate-day therapy) may be given for 14 to 21 days. When esophageal penetration has occurred, a cervical drain should be used and bactericidal, broad-spectrum, systemic antibiotics administered.

Tracheal injury also can cause subcutaneous emphysema. Small lacerations are usually self-limiting and do not require treatment. Laceration of the cervical trachea is not life-threatening unless obstruction or transection occurs. Animals in respiratory distress with extensive injuries must be managed swiftly. A patent airway must be maintained. The patient may be intubated through the laceration if necessary. The trachea should be debrided, and closure should be performed with fine monofilament suture material. Stenosis is least likely to occur when sutures are placed in an interrupted fashion between split rings rather than in the annular ligament between rings.[35] Administration of corticosteroids postoperatively may be helpful in reducing mucous membrane inflammation and swelling. Systemic antibiotics should be administered.

Extremities

Wounds that occur to the extremities frequently involve orthopedic injury. Fractures, dislocations, and joint instabilities must be assessed by thorough physical examination and radiography before definitive wound repair can be attempted. Extremity injuries are not life-threatening and should be addressed after the patient's condition is well stabilized and anesthesia is not a risk. Any exposed bone, however, should be cleaned immediately and covered with skin, soft tissue, or sterile dressing as part of the emergency treatment. Repair of associated orthopedic injury may be performed concurrently with wound treatment or, in cases with severe contamination, delayed until infection is controlled. Wounds with large soft-tissue deficits and underlying joint instability, such as shear injuries to the medial aspect of the tarsus and dorsal aspect of the carpus, heal most rapidly when stabilization is performed early. This allows rapid coverage with granulation tissue and subsequent epithelial cell migration over the granulation bed. Because of the paucity of redundant skin over the extremities, most of these wounds are left to heal by second intention or skin grafting.

Wounds involving the footpads require maximum tissue preservation to provide a walking surface. Normal, haired skin and the thin, fragile skin formed in wounds healing by epithelialization are inadequate to sustain the regular trauma of weight-bearing and will become mechanically abraded and worn and will bleed (Fig. 2–6). An exception is lightweight cats confined to houses with well-carpeted floors. Following injury, footpads should be minimally debrided, and if they are avulsed, they should be reattached. Toes with missing digital footpads should be amputated to prevent recurrent trauma and bleeding during weight-bearing activities. If the metacarpal or metatarsal pad is lost, one of the digital pads may be rotated into position and used to cover the major weight-bearing surface.[36] The phalangeal bones of the donor digit are removed or "filleted," leaving a skin flap containing the digital pad to fill the defect and provide an appropriate weight-bearing surface. Forelegs with loss of all digits and metacarpal pad, such as may occur with a trap injury, may be salvaged by advancement of the carpal pad over the remaining stump.[37]

Laceration of the footpads is common in dogs. In acute cases, a dramatic amount of bleeding occurs. This may be controlled by tourniquet to allow evaluation and cleansing of the wound. Superficial lacerations may be treated by a well-padded wrap without suturing. Deeper injuries with digital vessel lacerations require ligation of the vessel, thorough cleansing, lavage, and debridement. Such injuries may then be left unsutured and placed in a well-padded wrap. Footpads expand with weight-bearing, causing sutures to tear through the tissue as the pad splays out. This is the reason for the frequent wound breakdown seen in sutured footpad lacerations. If footpads are sutured, a splint should be applied within the bandage to support the pad and prevent expansion with weight-bearing.[31]

Thorax

Although indirect injury to the chest is common with trauma, an important concern is direct thoracic wounding. Common causes include motor vehicle accidents, animal fights, gunshots, stab wounds, owner abuse, and, in cats, a fall from a height.[9, 38] The chief concerns when a contaminated wound occurs over the thorax are penetration of the thoracic cavity and intrathoracic

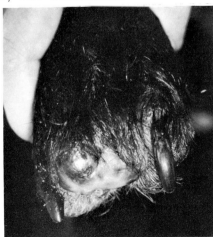

Figure 2–6. Loss of digits 3 and 4 in the rear leg allowed to heal by epithelialization resulting in coverage by a thin, fragile epithelium in a 10-year-old black Labrador retriever.

injury. Because of the loose skin in this area, trauma to deep tissues may be obscured by minimal damage to skin and superficial structures. Penetrating wounds to the thorax are severe because they disrupt intrapleural pressure, destroying the vacuum necessary for lung expansion and respiration, and they allow bacterial contamination of the thoracic cavity. Priorities are to restore intrapleural pressure and prevent infection. When an animal is presented with a wound over the thorax, a rapid assessment of respiratory status must be made. Rapid, shallow breathing, pale or blue mucous membranes, a sucking chest wound, and a flail chest-wall segment are indications that life-threatening chest injury is present. A sucking chest wound should be covered immediately with petrolatum-impregnated gauze. Immediate thoracocentesis is performed with a needle and syringe, followed by chest-tube placement for continued evacuation of air from the pleural space. The mouth and upper airway should be cleared, and oxygen should be administered by face mask, nasopharyngeal tube, endotracheal tube, or tracheostomy. In struggling critically ill patients that fight a face mask or endotracheal tube, a drop of lidocaine is instilled intranasally, followed by nasopharyngeal intubation with a small no. 4 or 5 French red rubber catheter. This is attached to the plastic adapter from an endotracheal tube, and oxygen is delivered at high flows (3–5 liters/min). The tube is sutured in placed over the bridge of the nose and top of the head. Other life-threatening conditions such as shock and loss of blood volume must also be treated.

Animals with sucking chest wounds (or any wound causing an open chest) should be intubated immediately and ventilated with positive-pressure ventilation to maintain lung expansion. Anesthesia should be administered only as necessary, and agents with minimal cardiac and respiratory depressive effects should be used. The wound is clipped and prepared for surgery, as previously described, using sterile technique. Surgery is performed in an operating room under aseptic conditions. The wound may be enlarged to allow exploration of the thoracic cavity and treatment of intrathoracic injuries. Partial or complete lung lobectomy of lacerated or severely contused lung tissue is performed as necessary. Intrathoracic hemorrhage is controlled by ligation of bleeding vessels. Rib fractures are not stabilized unless associated with a flail segment. All foreign material is removed, and the thorax is lavaged with copious amounts of sterile saline. Chest-wall muscles in the wound are debrided and closed, and a chest tube is placed through a separate incision. The subcutaneous tissues and skin are debrided, lavaged, and closed as for any other contaminated wound. Systemic antibiotics should be administered and continued for 10 to 14 days.

Any wound that involves penetration of the chest also causes intrathoracic contamination with bacteria (Fig. 2–7). If untreated, this may lead to sepsis, pyothorax, pulmonary abscess, and restrictive pleuritis. Even if the chest is not open and normal intrapleural pressures are present, thoracotomy should be performed to remove contaminating foreign material and to lavage and dilute the bacterial contamination. The lungs should be managed as for injuries even if air leakage is not present. Mild contusions will heal if left untreated, but severely damaged lung should be removed to prevent abscess formation. Systemic antibiotics should be administered. Other indications for thoracotomy in animals presented with contaminated chest wounds are listed in Table 2–4.

Animals with nonpenetrating wounds to the thorax may still have significant intrathoracic trauma. After patient stabilization, thorough physical

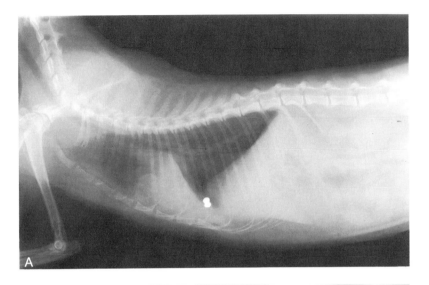

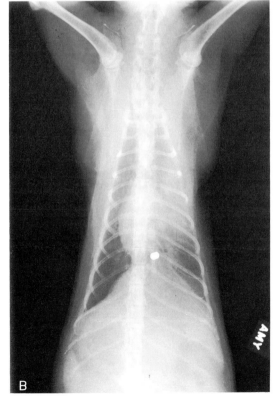

Figure 2–7. *A*, *B*, Lateral and ventrodorsal radiographs of the thorax of a 1-year-old cat with a penetrating pellet wound to the chest treated by lateral thoracotomy, partial right caudal lung lobectomy, and removal of the pellet. Staphylococci spp. were cultured from the thoracic cavity at the time of surgery.

TABLE 2–4. Indications for Thoracotomy in Animals with Contaminated Chest Wounds

Open thoracic wounds
Contamination of the pleural space with foreign bodies
Severe or persistent hemothorax
Massive hemoptysis
Recurrent cardiac tamponade
Rapid or persistent air leakage into the pleural space

examination of the wound and thorax should be performed. Chest radiographs should be taken to rule out diaphragmatic hernia, pneumothorax, hemothorax, pulmonary contusion, rib fracture, and cardiac tamponade[39-42] (Fig. 2–8). Electrocardiography and ultrasonography can be used to evaluate traumatic cardiac lesions. If significant chest-wall trauma is present, the wound should be clipped and cleaned and covered with a sterile wrap. Definitive debridement and closure are performed after treating the more severe intrathoracic problems.

Abdomen

Wounds to the abdomen occur frequently in dogs and cats. As with wounds to the thorax, priorities are to rule out internal organ injury and penetration of the abdominal wall resulting in bacterial contamination (Fig. 2–9). The most common cause is motor vehicle trauma, and up to 60% of the animals may have major organ injury.[43] Bite wounds often result in penetration and contamination of the abdominal cavity with oral bacteria. Because of the loose abdominal skin, the external wound may not indicate the extent of internal damage and contamination. Weapons such as knives and guns are also causes of contaminated abdominal wounds and usually involve penetration. A small, benign-appearing entry or exit wound may not be indicative of the amount of internal organ damage. Penetration of the gastrointestinal tract is especially dangerous and can result in rapid sepsis and death.

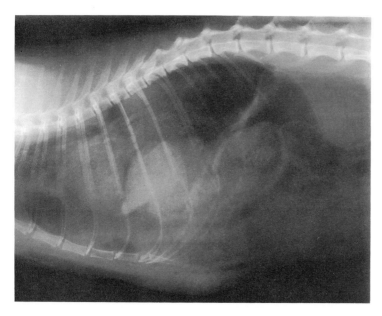

Figure 2–8. Traumatic diaphragmatic hernia in a 3-year-old Siamese cat with a nonpenetrating laceration of the thorax.

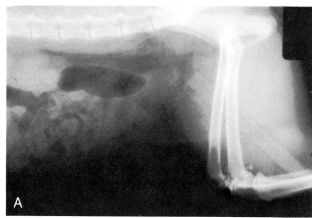

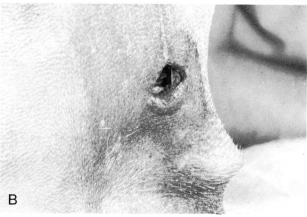

Figure 2–9. Penetrating abdominal wound in a 6-month-old cat that fell onto a tree branch. At exploratory laparotomy, a partial splenectomy and intestinal resection and anastomosis were performed. *A*, Lateral abdominal radiograph showing penetration of abdominal cavity by a large stick lodged into the epaxial muscles. *B*, Entrance wound of the penetrating foreign body.

Illustration continued on following page

Animals with abdominal wounds should be evaluated and treated initially for life-threatening problems. A thorough history aids in determining the extent of injury. Information regarding cause of injury and postinjury activity, such as urination, emesis, blood loss, and ambulation, will aid in decision making. A complete physical examination should be performed. Abdominal palpation should note areas of fluid, pain, and foreign bodies. An attempt should be made to check all abdominal organs. The abdominal wall also should be evaluated for the presence of hernias. Grossly contaminated wounds can be clipped, scrubbed, and covered with sterile antibiotic ointment or wrapped until diagnostic testing is completed. Prior to management of superficial wounds, internal organ damage and bacterial contamination of the peritoneal cavity requiring laparotomy must be ruled out. Indications for laparotomy are listed in Table 2–5. Abdominal radiographs should be evaluated for free gas, loss of contrast, ileus, peritoneal and retroperitoneal fluid, and the presence of a ruptured urinary bladder. When the integrity of the urinary tract is in question, contrast radiographic studies should be performed to rule out laceration and urine leakage. Small lacerations of the bladder and urethra will heal spontaneously with urinary diversion by catheterization for 5 to 7 days. Larger ruptures of the bladder, urethral transections, and urethral avulsions must be repaired surgically.

The differentiation between surgical and nonsurgical abdominal injury is often difficult. In these cases, peritoneal lavage is the single most accurate diagnostic tool to rule out a surgically treatable lesion and is reliable in 94.5%

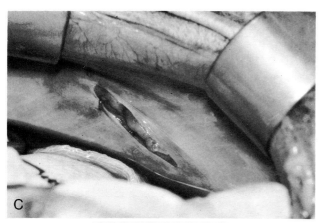

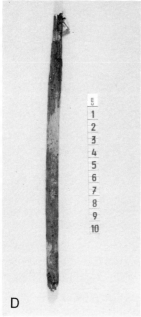

Figure 2–9 *Continued C,* Intra-abdominal view of the entrance wound at exploratory laparotomy. *D,* The penetrating stick that was removed at surgery.

of cases evaluated.[44] To perform a diagnostic peritoneal lavage, 22 ml/kg of sterile warm saline is infused into the peritoneal cavity through an over-the-needle intravenous catheter or peritoneal dialysis catheter. The infusion set is then inverted, and fluid is collected by gravity flow. Diagnostic tests, including cytology, white blood cell count, and creatinine, lipase, and bilirubin concentration determinations, are performed to rule out internal organ injury requiring laparotomy. Peritoneal lavage does not detect injuries to structures in the retroperitoneum, such as the kidneys and proximal ureter. These are better evaluated by a contrast radiographic study such as an excretory urogram. *An exploratory laparotomy may be used as a diagnostic procedure when significant internal abdominal injury is suspected or when patient deterioration occurs despite appropriate medical therapy.*

When an exploratory laparotomy is performed, all abdominal organs are examined and evaluated. Liver lacerations are generally not treated, since handling may lead to further hemorrhage and suturing the parenchyma is difficult. Major hemorrhage, however, from hepatic and portal blood vessels must be controlled. Injury to the pancreas is managed conservatively or with

TABLE 2–5. Indications for Laparotomy in Animals with Contaminated Abdominal Wounds

Any penetrating wound
Free intraperitoneal gas apparent on abdominal radiographs
Peritoneal effusion or lavage fluid containing urine, bacteria, or bile
Clinical signs of peritonitis
Persistent hemoperitoneum not responsive to fluid/blood replacement
Diagnostic procedure revealing significant injury to internal organs
Hematemesis
Proctorrhagia

debridement of necrotic areas. Splenic lacerations are difficult to suture and usually are treated by partial or complete splenectomy, if necessary, to control hemorrhage. Most injuries to the kidneys cause hematoma or parenchymal fracture and will heal without treatment. If severe injury occurs, partial or complete nephrectomy is performed. Ureteral injury, demonstrated by excretory urography, is repaired by careful suturing with very fine absorbable suture material. Rupture of the urinary bladder usually occurs at the apex. Closure is performed after debridement with sutures that do not penetrate the bladder mucosa. The abdomen is then thoroughly lavaged with sterile warm saline and closed.

Penetration of the gastrointestinal tract results in gross contamination of the abdomen with bacteria and causes rapid patient deterioration. Vigorous treatment with intravenous fluids, systemic antibiotics, and surgical exploration is indicated. Thorough debridement and closure of the injured bowel are followed by copious abdominal lavage with sterile saline. In animals with gross contamination of the abdomen with bacteria, debris, and fecal material, open peritoneal drainage may be considered. In this procedure, the linea alba is loosely closed in a continuous suture pattern that leaves a gap of 4 to 5 cm. A well-padded sterile wrap of gauze sponges, cotton, and bandage material is then placed around the body. The bandage is changed daily, with the animal under heavy sedation, and the abdomen can be lavaged. Bandage changes must be performed under absolutely aseptic conditions. When the amount of peritoneal drainage is minimal, the animal is anesthetized and the abdominal cavity is thoroughly lavaged and closed. The disadvantages of this procedure are the need for absolutely aseptic management of the patient until the abdomen is closed and hypoproteinemia from loss of plasma proteins in the draining peritoneal fluid.[45–47] The chief advantages, however, are the ability to lavage the abdomen repeatedly and the continued drainage of contaminated and infected fluid.

After management of internal abdominal injuries, superficial contaminated wounds are treated by debridement, lavage, and closure. Because of the loose, redundant skin in this area, the great majority of abdominal wounds are able to be closed primarily, even in animals with large skin deficits.

Abdominal wounds also may result in abdominal wall hernia or avulsion of the ventral abdominal wall from the pelvis. Defects or lacerations in the abdominal wall muscles are closed in layers with absorbable suture material after vigorous debridement of injured tissue. Avulsions of the caudal abdominal wall from the pubis are more difficult to manage because usually little tissue is left on the pelvis for reattachment of the avulsed musculature. Sutures can be placed through small holes drilled in the cranial ventral aspect of the pubis and passed through the fascia of the rectus muscle to bring it into normal position. Similarly, the external abdominal oblique muscles can be attached laterally. In addition, a muscle flap from the cranial sartorius muscle may be rotated into position to further close the defect and support the repair. Finally, drains are placed, and the subcutaneous tissues and skin are closed in routine fashion.

MANAGEMENT OF SPECIFIC WOUNDS CLASSIFIED BY TYPE

Bite Wounds

Animal fights are a common cause of contaminated wounds in dogs and cats. Bite wounds occur frequently around the head and neck in small dogs or cats that are picked up and shaken by a larger animal. In cat fights, wounds occur on the extremities and tail, where they may develop abscesses when bacteria become embedded below the skin surface. Important considerations in the management of bite wounds include deep bacterial contamination from the oral cavity, damage to underlying tissue despite minimal skin laceration, and possible rabies exposure.

All bite wounds are considered contaminated. The oral cavities of dogs and cats normally contain a large bacterial population, many of which colonize the tooth surfaces and contribute to bacterial plaque. When one animal bites another, these bacteria are deeply embedded into underlying soft tissues and are a potent source of infection. This is especially important in cat bites, because the long, pointed shape of the feline eyeteeth essentially causes an injection of bacteria into the wound. The oral cavity of normal dogs commonly contains *Streptococcus, Staphylococcus, Pasteurella,* and *Escherichia; Pseudomonas* and *Proteus* also have been isolated.[48] In cats, *Pasteurella* spp. are more common.[48] Appropriate debridement, copious lavage, and use of systemic antibiotics are necessary to prevent infection. Common sequelae to an untreated cat bite wound are cellulitis and abscesses. These commonly occur in outdoor cats. Because of the small size of the puncture wound to the skin, the initial injury is not detected. In time, the deep pocket of damaged tissue, combined with bacterial contamination, allows formation of a large area of inflamed and infected tissue that is warm and painful. Cellulitis alone may be present or may progress to fulminant abscess formation. The cat often becomes systemically ill at this time, showing signs of lethargy, inappetence, fever, and dehydration. Systemic antibiotics and fluids should be administered. The wound should be clipped, scrubbed, and opened to provide drainage. *Drainage is the single most important aspect in the successful management of cat bite wounds.* Although a drain may be placed within the wound to keep it open, simply opening and enlarging the wound is sufficient to allow irrigation and adequate drainage. Once the wound is opened, most cats recover quickly.

Because of the redundant and loose skin in dogs and cats, bite wounds usually result in multiple, small skin lacerations. Frequently, skin damage is minor. However, the crushing action of the jaws and teeth may cause significant damage to underlying structures. Bite wounds that occur over the chest and abdomen are potentially very serious. If penetration of the body cavity has occurred, exploration is indicated. All puncture bite wounds should be surgically enlarged to allow evaluation for damage to underlying tissues.

This is best performed by an incision in a dorsoventral direction to allow ventral drainage. Thorough debridement, especially of contused muscle, lavage, and management of specific tissue injuries are performed as previously described. Depending on the degree of underlying damage, contamination, and necessary debridement, the wound may be left open to drain or may be closed with a Penrose drain in place. The drain should be placed in the deepest part of the wound and allowed to exit through a separate ventral stab incision. The practice of placing drains with both dorsal and ventral exit sites does not improve drainage and may allow further ingress of bacteria into the wound.

When an animal with a bite wound is presented for treatment, it is important to determine the rabies vaccination status of that animal and of the attacker. Bites that occur between vaccinated animals are usually not a concern. If a vaccinated animal receives a bite wound from a wild animal or a domestic animal of unknown vaccination status, a booster rabies vaccination should be given immediately. When possible, the head of the attacking animal should be submitted for rabies evaluation. The wound also should be thoroughly lavaged as soon as possible. If the victim is unvaccinated and received a bite wound from an animal with unknown vaccination status, the local health authorities should be contacted for guidelines concerning rabies quarantine and vaccination.

Gunshot Wounds

Gunshot wounds are similar to bite wounds because they cause bacterial contamination, deep tissue destruction, and minor skin damage. In preliminary evaluation of a wound caused by a gunshot, it is helpful to know the type of weapon that caused the wound. Bullets are classified as low or high velocity. Low-velocity bullet wounds, such as those from handguns, are most common. Low-velocity bullets produce an entrance wound and missile tract with minimal damage beyond the tract. Wounds caused by low-velocity missiles, which are uncomplicated by fracture or body-cavity penetration, usually cause minimal internal tissue damage and may be treated by simply clipping the hair and cleansing of the entry and exit wounds.[49] A sterile bandage is placed and changed as needed, and systemic antibiotics are administered.

Gunshot wounds caused by high-velocity bullets are more serious. As the velocity of the bullet increases, the kinetic energy it carries rises exponentially.[49] Along with creating the entry and exit wounds and resultant missile tract, this increased kinetic energy is transmitted to adjacent soft tissues and causes extensive tissue destruction even at a distance from the bullet's path. This is referred to as *cavitation injury*. Gunshot wounds caused by high-velocity bullets should therefore be treated aggressively. The entry and exit wounds should be enlarged and thoroughly debrided. Devitalized tissue, hair, debris, and foreign bodies should be removed, taking care to preserve nerves, tendons, and blood vessels. Bullet fragments that have been scattered into tissues beyond the wound tract are not removed unless they are within joints or body cavities. If a fracture occurs, the soft tissues should be treated first and definitive orthopedic repair delayed. Exploratory laparotomy must be performed with wounds involving penetration of the thoracic and abdominal cavities. Because of the legal implications of gunshot injuries, bullets and bullet fragments that are removed should be saved.

Snake Bites

Snake bite wounds are similar to other animal bite wounds because minimal skin puncture wounds with deep crush injury are produced. They usually occur in the limbs of dogs. Snake bite wounds that occur without envenomation may be treated by clipping, cleansing, debridement of deeper crushed tissue, and application of a sterile bandage. Bites from venomous snakes are complicated by lethal toxins that are injected and become absorbed systemically by the local lymphatics. Myotoxins, neurotoxins, cardiotoxins, and hemolysins may be involved depending on the species of snake.[50] The severity of injury depends on the snake species, volume of venom injected, size of the patient, and the length of time since the bite. Whenever possible, the species of snake and potential for envenomation should be determined. The patient should be presented for treatment as soon as possible after the bite has occurred. A tourniquet may be applied above the wound to prevent further absorption of toxin if envenomation has occurred. The fang marks are evaluated for evidence of envenomation and its severity. These include pain, swelling, edema, ecchymoses, and hemorrhage. The patient also should be evaluated for systemic signs such as shock, cardiac arrhythmias, neurologic dysfunction, and respiratory distress, which may occur depending on the type of toxin injected. Systemic signs and marked swelling and ecchymoses of the puncture sites are indications that envenomation has occurred. If systemic signs are present, an intravenous catheter should be placed, and the animal should be treated for shock. Animals in respiratory distress should receive oxygen by mask or nasopharyngeal or endotracheal intubation. If the bite is less than 30 minutes old, a deep incision into subcutaneous tissues should be made, and suction and lavage should be performed to remove as much toxin as possible and to prevent absorption. If the bite is more than 30 minutes old, absorption has probably already occurred, and incision and suction are not recommended.[50] Antivenin, if available, is most effective if given early and administered intravenously. If severe pain is present, analgesics such as butorphanol, meperidine, and morphine may be given. Envenomation often leads to severe tissue necrosis, requiring further surgical debridement and management of the bite area as an open wound. Systemic antibiotics effective against gram-positive and anaerobic organisms such as ampicillin or one of the cephalosporins are recommended.

Shear Wounds

Shear wounds are caused by dragging the animal along a hard surface, usually during an automobile accident. They occur over bony prominences of the distal portion of limbs such as the lateral and medial aspects of the malleolus of the tarsus and the dorsal and medial aspects of the carpus. Wounds caused by the shearing effect of tissue dragged over pavement are often complicated by large tissue and bone deficits, severe contamination, fracture, and joint instability. After the patient has been stabilized and more serious systemic injuries addressed, the wound should be clipped, scrubbed, and evaluated. Radiographs are taken to evaluate the extent of orthopedic injury; however, the major injury is often obvious because of the severe tissue loss and the open nature of these wounds. Soft-tissue and ligamentous instability must be assessed by physical examination and stress radiography of the affected joints.

Shear wounds to the tarsus may involve loss of the lateral or medial malleolus and its collateral ligaments (Fig. 2–10). After evaluation of the injury, the wound is clipped and prepared for aseptic surgery. The joint is thoroughly lavaged and replaced into anatomic alignment. Debridement is performed to remove all debris. Often dirt is deeply embedded into the bone and tissues, making debridement difficult. Stabilization is performed at the time of wound debridement, since it is necessary for rapid granulation tissue formation and coverage of the wound. Collateral ligament repair should be performed with screws and prosthetic ligaments of wire or suture material.[51-53] A sterile bandage is placed over the wound, and the limb is placed in a support wrap. External skeletal fixators may be applied and are useful for support without interfering with wound healing. Once the wound is covered with healthy granulation tissue, skin grafting with flaps or free grafts may be performed.

Shear injuries to the carpus involve loss of skin, muscle, extensor tendon, ligament, and bone. Usually the injury occurs to the dorsal aspect of the carpus and may involve loss of the styloid processes and associated collateral ligaments.[54] Often the carpal joints are open, with large amounts of debris embedded into the tissues. As with the tarsus, the wound is managed in an open manner with early stabilization of affected joints. Under surgically aseptic conditions, debridement and lavage are performed followed by stabilization. Debridement should be extremely thorough, removing all foreign matter while preserving tendons and ligaments. If possible, ligaments and soft tissues that support the joint should be sutured. If there is isolated loss of the radial collateral ligament, a prosthetic replacement of screws and wire or suture material is made.[54] Arthrodesis of affected joints is indicated

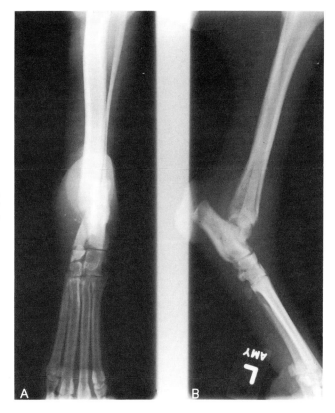

Figure 2–10. *A, B,* Shear injury to the medial aspect of the tarsus resulting in loss of the medial malleolus and medial aspect of the talus in a 2-year-old mixed-breed dog.

when the degree of soft-tissue and bone loss results in unmanageable instability (Fig. 2–11). This can be performed at the time of wound debridement. Following debridement and stabilization, the limb is placed in a sterile bandage with an external support such as a Kirschner-Ehmer device or caudal half-splint. Frequent bandage changes are usually necessary until granulation tissue formation and contraction close the skin. Skin grafting may be performed when a healthy granulation bed has formed and covers the wound, but this is rarely necessary.

Degloving Injuries

Degloving injuries are most commonly caused by automobile accidents (or animal fights) and occur when the skin is grabbed, rotated, and avulsed from its underlying attachments. This results in formation of a large flap of loose, unattached skin. In some cases, a flap may not be torn free, but a large area of skin hangs loosely with torn fascial attachments. This is termed a *physiologic degloving injury*. Often there is damage to underlying structures, especially blood vessels that normally supply the skin flap. The wound is treated according to the general principles of contaminated wound management. Skin that is devitalized is removed, and the remaining flap is closed with a drain in place. Since it may be difficult to determine the viability of tissue that has been severely traumatized, the wound should be reexamined frequently. Further debridement is performed as necessary. Intravenous administration of vital dyes such as xylenol orange or fluorescein sodium can be used to distinguish viable from nonviable flaps, but these methods have not been shown to be significantly superior to visual observation for flap viability.[55]

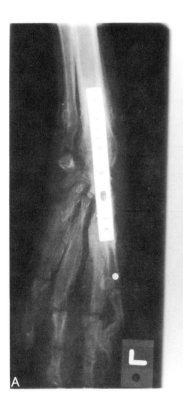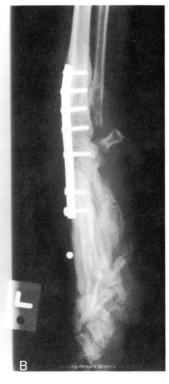

Figure 2–11. *A, B,* Severe shear injury to the antebrachial-carpal region in a 1-year-old mixed-breed dog 4 weeks following injury. A pancarpal arthrodesis was performed at the time of initial wound debridement because of severe loss of bone and soft tissues from the radius, ulna, carpal, and metacarpal bones.

COMPLICATIONS IN CONTAMINATED WOUND MANAGEMENT

Infection

Despite the presence of bacteria, debris, and devitalized tissue in contaminated wounds, with proper management, it is uncommon for infection to occur. *The most common cause of secondary infection in wounds is inadequate debridement.* Other contributing factors include improper or inadequate use of drains, improper use of dressings and bandages, poor patient health and nutrition, and poor blood supply to the wound site. Inadequate antibiotic administration is not often a cause of wound infection but can occur with misdiagnosed anaerobic bacterial conditions. When infection is present, healing will be inhibited by the bacterial production of collagenases, decreased wound pH and oxygen tension, interference with blood supply to the area, and mechanical interference by exudate. Abscessation may cause an animal to become systemically ill and, in extreme cases, can progress to septicemia.

Signs that infection is developing include copious, foul-smelling exudation and lack of progression of healing in an open wound; swelling, redness, and heat in a closed wound; and systemic signs such as fever, inappetence, and depression. When infection is suspected, dehydration and pyrexia should be treated with administration of intravenous fluids and systemic antibiotics. The wound should be reevaluated after appropriate preparation under aseptic conditions. Wounds that have been closed are reopened. Pockets of exudate and pus are drained, and further debridement of debris and damaged and necrotic tissue is performed. The wound is then thoroughly lavaged with a large volume of sterile saline. The wound may be closed with a drain in place, or it may be left open to drain and be closed at a later time when infection is under control. The wound should be examined and lavaged daily until all tissue appears healthy and healing is taking place. During this time, the wound should be protected in a sterile bandage to prevent further contamination.

Seroma

A *seroma* is the subcutaneous accumulation of a large volume of serum in a wound that has been closed. Because it is rich in proteins and isolated from the normal immune defenses of the body, it is an excellent medium for bacterial growth and thereby enhances wound infection and abscessation. Seromas are generally caused by violations of Halsted's principles, such as inadequate hemostasis, lack of obliteration of dead space through proper use of drains, and trauma to soft tissues during handling. It is best to prevent this complication by recognizing the potential for seroma formation in wounds with significant disruption of skin attachments (degloving injuries) and excessive oozing or bleeding. In these cases, wound closure should be delayed until drainage has significantly decreased or should be performed with good drain placement and use of compression bandages. Drains should be placed with an exit site separate from the incision closing the wound and at the most ventral aspect of the area requiring drainage.

Small seromas may resolve without treatment. Large ones may be treated by ventral drainage through a small stab incision. If possible, several skin sutures may be removed and drainage allowed through the incision. After drainage of the accumulated fluid, a compression bandage is placed for approximately 1 week. In recurrent cases, a Penrose drain may be placed deep into the pocket to permit continuous drainage.

Dehiscence

Wound breakdown is caused by tension on the wound closure, devitalization of the wound edges, inadequate wound debridement, and wound infection. *Most cases of wound dehiscence are due to technical error by the surgeon.* Dehiscence of a closed contaminated wound is best treated by leaving the wound open and allowing it to heal by second intention. If necessary, further debridement and lavage are performed. Any overlooked foreign material or devitalized tissue is removed. The wound may be reclosed when the cause of the dehiscence has been determined and is no longer present.

Failure to Heal

Despite thorough debridement and control of infection, some contaminated wounds may still fail to heal. A healthy granulation bed is often present that fails to progress by contraction and coverage with new epithelium. The most common instances are the cessation of contraction in wounds under tension, such as large skin defects over the distal aspect of extremities, and exhaustion of contraction due to the sheer size of the wound. Cessation of contraction is best treated by skin grafting over a healthy granulation bed with free grafts or skin flaps.

Delays in healing also may occur in granulating wounds in mobile areas that have been covered by bandages that continually abrade the wound surface. Common examples are open wounds over flexion surfaces. These may resume healing by simply being left unbandaged.

Contracture Deformity

Wound contraction is an important part of the normal process of second-intention healing. In dogs and cats, contraction will occasionally result in a large area of scar tissue that causes a deformity or loss of function. Examples include contractions that limit movement of a body part, such as formation of a fibrous band over a flexion surface, and contractions that narrow a normal body orifice, usually the anus. Both types of contracture are treated by reconstructive procedures that open or increase the size of the contracted area. These include Z-plasty, W-plasty, and the use of rotation flaps.[56]

REFERENCES

1. National Academy of Sciences–National Research Council Division of Medical Sciences Ad Hoc Committee of the Committee on Trauma: Postoperative wound infections: The influence of ultraviolet irradiation of the operating room and of various other factors. Ann Surg 1964; 160:1–192
2. Vasseur PB, Levy J, Dowd E, Eliot J: Surgical wound infection rates in dogs and cats. Vet Surg 1988; 17:60–64
3. Johnston DE: Wound healing. Arch J Am Coll Vet Surg 1974; 3:30
4. Swaim S: Management of contaminated and infected wounds. In Swaim S (ed): Surgery of Traumatized Skin: Management and Reconstruction in the Dog and Cat. Philadelphia, WB Saunders, 1980, p 119
5. Robson MC, Heggers JP: Bacterial quantification in open wounds. Mil Med 1969; 134:19

6. Cruse PJE, Foord R: The epidemiology of wound infections: A ten-year prospective study of 62,939 wounds. Surg Clin North Am 1980; 60:27–40
7. Peacock EE: Wound Repair. Philadelphia, WB Saunders, 1984, pp 1–14
8. Lees MJ, Fretz PB, Bailey JV: Factors influencing wound healing: Lessons from military wound management. Compend Contin Educ Pract Vet 1989; 7:850–856
9. Tamas PM, Paddleford RR, Krahwinkel DJ: Thoracic trauma in dogs and cats presented for limb fractures. J Am Anim Hosp Assoc 1985; 21:161–166
10. Edlich RF, Rodeheaver GT, Thacker JG: Technical factors in the prevention of wound infections. In Simmons RL, Howard KJ (eds): Surgical Infectious Diseases. New York, Appleton-Century-Crofts, 1982, pp 449–472
11. Bright RM, Probst CW: Management of superfical skin wounds. In Slatter DH (ed): Textbook of Small Animal Surgery. Philadelphia, WB Saunders, 1985, p 432
12. Singleton AO, Julian J: An experimental evaluation of methods used to prevent infection in wounds which have been contaminated with feces. Ann Surg 1960; 151:912
13. Peterson LW: Prophylaxis of wound infection: Studies with particular references to soaps with irrigation. Arch Surg 1945; 50:177
14. Madden J, Edlich RF, Schauerhamer R: Application of principles of fluid dynamics to surgical wound irrigation. Curr Top Surg Res 1971; 3:85–93
15. Rodeheaver GT, Pettry D, Thacker JG: Wound cleansing by high pressure irrigation. Surg Gynecol Obstet 1975; 141:357–362
16. Stevenson TR, Thacker JG, Rodeheaver GT: Cleansing the traumatic wound by high pressure syringe irrigation. J Am Coll Emerg Phys 1976; 5:17
17. Gross A, Cutright DE, Bhaskar S: Effectiveness of pulsating waterjet lavage in treatment of contaminated crushed wounds. Am J Surg 1972; 124:373
18. Lee AH, Swaim SF, McGuire JA, Hughes KS: Effects of chlorhexidine diacetate, povidone-iodine and polyhydroxydine on wound healing in dogs. J Am Anim Hosp Assoc 1988; 24:77–84
19. Amber EI, Henderson RA, Swaim SF, Gray BW: A comparison of antimicrobial efficacy and tissue reaction of four antiseptics on canine wounds. Vet Surg 1983; 12:63–68
20. Lineaweaver W, McMorris S, Howard R: Effects of topical disinfectants and antibiotics on human fibroblasts. Surg Forum 1982; 33:37–39
21. Sanchez IR, Swaim SF, Nusbaum KE, et al: Effects of chlorhexidine diacetate and povidone-iodine on wound healing in dogs. Vet Surg 1988; 17:291–295
22. Johnston DE: The processes in wound healing. J Am Anim Hosp Assoc 1977; 13:186–189
23. Basher AWP, Presnell KR: Muscle transposition as an aid in covering traumatic tissue defects over the canine tibia. J Am Anim Hosp Assoc 1987; 23:617–628
24. Weinstein MJ, Pavletic MM, Boudrieau RJ: Caudal sartorius muscle flap in the dog. Vet Surg 1988; 17:203–210
25. Katz S, Mordechai I, Mirelman D: Bacterial adherence to surgical sutures. Ann Surg 1981; 194:35–41
26. Smeak DD, Wendelburg K: Choosing suture materials for use in contaminated or infected wounds. Compend Contin Educ Pract Vet 1989; 11:467–475
27. Varma S, Ferguson HL, Johnson LW: Tissue reaction to suture materials in infected surgical wounds—a histopathologic evaluation. Am J Vet Res 1981; 42:563–569
28. Sharp WV, Belden TA, King PH: Suture resistance to infection. Surgery 1982; 91:61–63
29. Royen BJ, O'Driscoll SW, Wooter JA, Salt RB: A comparison of the effects of immobilization and continuous passive motion on surgical wound healing in mature rabbits. Plast Reconstr Surg 1986; 78:360–366
30. Swaim SF, Lee AH, Henderson RS: Mobility versus immobility in the healing of open wounds. J Am Anim Hosp Assoc 1989; 25:91–96
31. Swaim SF: Management and bandaging of soft tissue injuries of dog and cat feet. J Am Anim Hosp Assoc 1985; 21:329–340
32. Swaim SF, Wilhalf D: The physics, physiology and chemistry of bandaging open wounds. Compend Contin Educ Pract Vet 1985; 7:146–151
33. Lantz GC, Salisbury SK: Partial mandibulectomy for treatment of mandibular fractures in dogs: Eight cases (1981–1984). J Am Vet Med Assoc 1987; 191:243–245
34. Miller WW, Swaim SF, Pope ER: Labial avulsion repair in the dog and cat. J Am Anim Hosp Assoc 1985; 21:435–438
35. Hedlund CS: Tracheal anastomosis in the dog: Comparison of two end-to-end techniques. Vet Surg 1984; 13:135
36. Swaim SF, Garrett PD: Foot salvage techniques in dogs and cats: Options, "do's" and "don'ts." J Am Anim Hosp Assoc 1985; 21:511–519
37. Barclay CG, Fowler JD, Basher AW: Use of the carpal pad to salvage the forelimb in a dog and cat: An alternative to total limb amputation. J Am Anim Hosp Assoc 1987; 23:527–532
38. McKiernan BC, Adams WM, Huse DC: Thoracic bite wounds and associated injury in eleven dogs and one cat. J Am Vet Med Assoc 1984; 184:959–964
39. Kramek BA, Caywood DD: Pneumothorax in noncardiac surgical diseases of the thorax. Vet Clin North Am 1987; 17:285–300

40. Hunt CA: Chest trauma: Specific injuries. Compend Contin Educ Pract Vet 1979; 1:624–632
41. Kolata RJ: Management of thoracic trauma. Vet Clin North Am 1981; 11:103–120
42. Kagan KG: Thoracic trauma. Vet Clin North Am 1980; 10:641–653
43. Kolata RJ, Kraut NH, Johnston DE: Patterns of trauma in urban dogs and cats: A study of 1000 cases. J Am Vet Med Assoc 1974; 164:499–502
44. Crowe DT: Diagnostic abdominal paracentesis techniques: Clinical evaluation in 129 dogs and cats. J Am Anim Hosp Assoc 1984; 20:223–230
45. Orsher RJ, Rosin E: Open peritoneal drainage in experimental peritonitis in dogs. Vet Surg 1984; 13:222–226
46. Woolfson JM, Dulisch ML: Open abdominal drainage in the treatment of generalized peritonitis in 25 dogs and cats. Vet Surg 1986; 15:27–32
47. Greenfield CL, Walshaw R: Open peritoneal drainage for treatment of contaminated peritoneal cavity and septic peritonitis in dogs and cats: 24 cases (1980–1986). J Am Vet Med Assoc 1987; 191:100–105
48. Burrows CF, Harvey CE: Oral examination and diagnostic technique. In Harvey CE (ed): Veterinary Dentistry. Philadelphia, WB Saunders, 1985, p 29
49. Lipowitz AJ: Management of gunshot wounds of the soft tissues and extremities. J Am Anim Hosp Assoc 1976; 12:813
50. Morgan RV: Manual of Small Animal Emergencies. New York, Churchill Livingston, 1985, pp 431–448
51. Aron DN: Prosthetic ligament replacement for severe tarsocrural joint instability. J Am Anim Hosp Assoc 1987; 23:41–55
52. Aron DN, Purinton PT: Replacement of the collateral ligaments of the canine tarsocrural joint. Vet Surg 1985; 14:178–184
53. Mathiesen DT: Tarsal injuries in the dog and cat. Compend Contin Educ Pract Vet 1983; 5:548–555
54. Brinker WO, Piermattei DL, Flo GL: Handbook of Small Animal Orthopedics and Fracture Treatment, 2d ed. Philadelphia, WB Saunders, 1990, pp 524–526
55. Bellah JR, Krahwinkel DJ: Xylenol orange as a vital stain to determine the viability of skin flaps in dogs. Vet Surg 1985; 14:124–126
56. Swaim SF: Principles of plastic and reconstructive surgery. In Slatter DH (ed): Textbook of Small Animal Surgery. Philadelphia, WB Saunders, 1985, pp 443–457

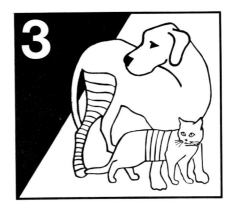

TOPICAL WOUND THERAPY

SCOTT M. LOZIER

The use of topical medications in healing wounds is a controversial subject. Objective information is often contradictory and falsely extrapolated from studies performed on nonclinically relevant species. There is an excess of topical wound medications and primary-layer dressings available to the practicing veterinarian. These compounds often have few guidelines for use. In addition, there is an uncontrollable urge by clinicians to use these products for every wound. In reality, some of these products for wound therapy may be detrimental to the healing process. With frequent assessments and basic knowledge of the healing process and available treatments, however, a rational plan can be formulated that will lead to rapid and uncomplicated healing in most wounds. The purpose of this chapter is to provide the reader with these guidelines.

WOUND ASSESSMENT

When treating a wound, numerous questions must be answered at each assessment until the wound is healed (Table 3–1). Determining the history and cause (traumatic laceration 15 minutes ago, thermal injury 2 days ago, wound puncture of unknown duration) permits determination of the wounding stage and selection of an appropriate topical agent. Most wound complications result from bacterial inoculation. Classification of the wound as clean, clean contaminated, or dirty/infected is often subjective but helps in deter-

TABLE 3–1. Wound Assessment Factors

1. Wounding history, including cause of injury or persistence
2. Wound classification based on bacterial infection
3. Wound progression (healing)
4. Stage of healing
5. Goal(s) of therapy (delayed primary closure, secondary closure, or second-intention healing)
6. Risks and benefits of therapy
7. Times of reevaluation

mining the likelihood of successful wound closure and type of topical therapy. Knowledge of the timing, location, and source of contamination will aid in selection of systemic and topical antimicrobial agents. As with antibiotics, antiseptics are often effective against specific pathogenic microbes. If the wound is healing satisfactorily, careful thought should be given to deciding if therapy is required. *Conditions that favor healing should always be preserved, and topical therapy should protect the wound and "above all, do no harm."*

WOUND STAGING

Wounds require specific treatment based on stages of repair in the wound at the time of assessment. A clinically applicable staging system for assessment and treatment of wounds is composed of wounding, inflammatory, proliferative, and maturation phases. These stages are continuous and have a certain degree of overlap. Different stages of repair also may be present in a single wound.

Injuries still in the *wounding stage* may often be presented for treatment. The skin may be intact or have only a small visible defect, yet there is underlying soft-tissue destruction. Examples of these include infiltration of tissue with toxin (extravasated caparsolate, antineoplastic agents, bacterial toxins, spider or snake bite injuries) and infected ischemic/traumatic injuries (failing skin flaps, thromboembolism, crushing injuries, constricting foreign objects). Injuries of the wounding stage require aggressive and immediate local or systemic treatment against the wounding agent. Primary topical treatment of these wounds with topical antiseptic detergents is useful prior to surgical intervention.

Inflammation occurs rapidly after wounding, so these stages may be con-current. Severe inflammation can play a major role in secondary wounding of tissue because of enzymatic and inflammatory product-mediated destruction of tissues. Dead tissues that harbor infectious agents also will elicit continued inflammation. Accumulation of inflammatory exudate perpetuates the cycle of tissue destruction. The importance of surgical debridement and drainage cannot be overemphasized in such situations. Topical therapy becomes important (and augments physical debridement) through the use of antiseptic or antibiotic lavage, debridement dressings and enzymatic agents, and dressings to maintain drainage and absorb exudate. Topical therapy may become the primary mode of therapy when surgical management is impractical, inadvisable, or not required. In these early stages of healing, selection of appropriate topical therapy is most critical to the outcome of healing. Inciting further tissue trauma and inflammation will prolong the healing process, whereas suppression of inflammation may compromise local defenses and prevent initiation of the repair process.

Cellular and chemical mediators elicited by the inflammatory stage of healing activate a proliferative response in the fibroblastic, endothelial, and epithelial cells surrounding the wound. This initiates the *repair stage* of healing. These cells are responsible for collagen production and contraction, vascularization, and resurfacing of the wound. Once granulation tissue has covered the wound, a surprisingly effective barrier to infection of deeper tissue has been reestablished, although superficial infection may still occur and inhibit the remainder of the healing process. The role of topical therapy in these wounds is to prevent infection of the healthy wound while protecting and enhancing the activity of reparative elements.

Healthy wounds contract vigorously 5 to 7 days following wounding and cease contraction when epithelial margins meet, tension equals the force of contraction, or the fibroblasts mature. Collagen production starts to decrease 2 to 4 weeks after injury. Wound *maturation* occurs as cross-linking and remodeling of collagen begins. With the onset of this stage, there is a concomitant increase in tensile strength. Infection decreases the tensile strength of healing wounds. Wounds that fail to contract and epithelialize completely can be particularly challenging to treat. Conversely, wounds that contract excessively can compromise local function. Several types of topical treatments may be utilized to manipulate wounds during this stage to decrease or increase contraction, stimulate granulation or epithelialization, and minimize bacterial contamination and infection.

GOAL OF THERAPY

The type of topical therapy is based on the ultimate treatment plan for the wound. If delayed primary or secondary closure of the defect is expected, the most important objectives are to remove dead and foreign material from the wound and reduce bacterial load to permit successful closure without abscessation. Less than 100,000 bacteria per gram of tissue should be present, although this number depends on foreign material in the wound, type and virulence of the pathogen, degree of local tissue destruction, and systemic status of the host. When planning closure, delays in epithelialization are of little concern. Debridement dressings may be used until closure. Irritating substances should be avoided because inflammation and tissue necrosis at closure will potentiate infection. When second-intention healing is desired, topical treatments should be used that protect the proliferating cell population and allow unabated contraction and epithelialization.

Topical medications should provide a specific desired effect during the appropriate stage of healing. Treatments may have untoward effects that outweigh beneficial effects. Attention must be paid to the manufacturer's instructions and pertinent veterinary literature regarding appropriate use, concentration, frequency of administration, and mode of application.

One of the most important concepts in treating wounds is to realize that they are dynamic. Treatment frequently must be modified based on the progression of the wound through the various stages of healing. During initial presentation, wounds may require aggressive treatment with enzymatic and debridement dressings that are changed several times daily. Continued use of this topical treatment as the wound progresses may inhibit later stages of healing. Conversely, continued use of an occlusive dressing changed every third day on a wound with *Pseudomonas* infection will delay the healing process and may cause patient sepsis. Frequent assessments and appropriate modifications of therapy are, therefore, required for successful wound healing.

WOUND MANAGEMENT

Contaminated wounds require initial cleansing of the wound prior to surgery or to minimize continued contamination while the wound is being treated topically. After initial inspection of the wound, exposed tissue should be protected from detergents and clipped hair. Antiseptic scrubs should not be used in open wounds because detergents cause tissue toxicity and irritation. They may inhibit host defenses, cause considerable pain, and potentiate wound infection. Sterile lubricating jelly is commonly used to protect such wounds. Saline-soaked sponges are also an effective method of protecting such wounds.

Skin Antisepsis and Wound Preparation

Once the wound is protected, an antiseptic detergent may be used to reduce contamination in the surrounding area. Chlorhexidine and povidone-iodine products are most commonly used. Both products are rapid-acting, broad-spectrum agents that reduce skin surface bacterial contamination.[1, 2] Acute contact dermatitis, however, occurs in 50% of dogs scrubbed with povidone-iodine products and in 20% of dogs scrubbed with chlorhexidine gluconate.[2, 3] No significant clinical differences in antibacterial activity has been documented between povidone-iodine and chlorhexidine gluconate skin scrubs.[1-4]

The antiseptic ability of alcohol is the standard by which the World Health Organization compares other antiseptic agents.[5] Solutions of 70% ethanol or 50% isopropyl or n-propyl alcohol are commonly used. They are broad-spectrum antiseptics with excellent activity against gram-negative and gram-positive bacteria, viruses, and many fungi.[5] They are not effective against bacterial spores, and their potency is inhibited by organic substances such as blood or mucus.[5, 6] Therefore, alcohol wipes should follow antiseptic skin scrubs used to cleanse the skin. Interestingly, a clinical trial using gauze sponges soaked with 70% isopropyl alcohol between successive chlorhexidine gluconate scrubs demonstrated reduced bacterial kill compared with sterile saline-soaked sponges used between scrubs.[1]

When diluted in water, alcohols denature protein in bacterial cells.[5] Between 95% and 99% bacterial kill occurs within 1 minute of alcohol contact, but no residual effect is present after drying.[5] Emollients may be added to alcohol to increase residual activity by slowing drying time. Alcohols are also commonly used as solvents for antiseptics. Although alcohol is a superb antiseptic, it will kill and fix exposed tissues on contact.[7] Use of products containing high concentrations of alcohol should be strictly limited to intact skin.

Numerous other agents have been used as skin disinfectants.[5] These include quaternary ammonium compounds, hexachlorophene, halogenated phenolic compounds, silver- and mercury-containing compounds, and aniline dyes. None of these possess the broad-spectrum efficacy and wide margin of safety of chlorhexidine, povidone-iodine, and alcohol products used alone or in various combinations.[5]

Topicals for Initial Wound Management

Most veterinary patients will require anesthesia for initial wound inspection and care. Trauma victims and high-anesthetic-risk patients with minor wounds may allow treatment following local anesthesia alone or in combination with sedation or neuroleptanalgesia. Lidocaine-soaked sponges may be used topically to anesthetize the wound surface. As an added advantage, lidocaine possesses significant antibacterial activity.[8] Alternatively, ring blocks or local infiltration can be used effectively.[9] A new topical anesthetic agent containing a mixture of 5% lidocaine and prilocaine (Emla Cream) has been marketed for use on intact skin.[10] Investigation of this agent revealed antibacterial activity and damage to host defenses. The anesthetic mixture potentiated wound infection in guinea pigs and was not recommended for use on wounds. Local anesthetics that contain vasoconstrictors such as epinephrine should not be used on wounds because they cause local inflammation and potentiate infection.[11]

Contaminated and infected wounds often contain foreign debris, copious exudate, and necrotic tissue. To thoroughly assess the wound and initiate therapy, the wound must be cleansed of gross contamination. Initial lavage of the wound with tap water has been recommended. In general, tap water is very low in bacterial numbers and causes less destruction of tissue than distilled water.[7] Other studies indicate that the use of sterile water on wounds does not delay wound healing compared with wounds lavaged with lactated Ringer's solution.[12] Lukewarm tap or sterile water under moderate pressure provides an excellent and cost-effective means of initially reducing the amount of gross contamination.

Scrubbing an open wound may cause harmful effects. Saline-soaked gauze sponges used to scrub wounds cause excessive inflammation and impair resistance to infection.[13] Pluronic polyols are nontoxic detergent agents with excellent wetting and surfactant properties, but they possess no antibacterial activity.[5] Gentle scrubbing of contaminated wounds with gauze coated with a pluronic polyol helps to remove gross debris and solubilize organic material.[6, 14] These agents reduce mechanical damage and inflammation caused by the sponge and experimentally have been effective in reducing infection when used alone as a wound scrub or as a solvent for iodophors.[6, 13]

WOUND IRRIGATION

Wound irrigation is an important but controversial aspect of topical management of open wounds. Principles of wound irrigation are listed in Table 3–2. Wound lavage reduces bacterial numbers mechanically by loosening and flushing away bacteria and associated necrotic debris and chemically by the addition of antimicrobial agents.

Bulb syringes are inadequate for removing contaminating bacteria and preventing wound infection.[15] High pressure, pulsatile lavage is capable of generating 70 to 80 lb/in^2 of pressure and is the most effective means of removing bacteria and foreign material. Although this method of irrigation is effective in preventing infection in experimentally contaminated wounds, spread of bacteria into loose tissue planes and significant damage to the underlying tissue can occur.[16] This method of irrigation should be confined to extremities, where systemic dissemination of bacteria may be less likely to occur.[15] Other disadvantages of this method is sterility of the pumping instrument and indirect spraying of the operator. *High-pressure syringe lavage with a 60-cc syringe and 18-gauge needle is capable of generating approximately 7*

TABLE 3–2. Principles of Wound Irrigation

1. Use of adequate pressure, volume, and frequency
2. Combination with other physical means of removing necrotic and foreign debris
3. Use of appropriate antimicrobial agents with low tissue toxicity

to 8 lb/in² of pressure and is an effective means of removing bacteria. When combined with povidone-iodine, this method of irrigation is superior to high-pressure pulsatile lavage in reducing bacteria in canine wounds.[15] The specific volume of lavage fluid required to reduce bacterial numbers has not been determined. Use of copious amounts of fluid is important in reducing bacterial numbers.[17] Frequency of lavage will depend on exudate, frequency of bandage changes, and residual activity of the antiseptic or topical agent.

ANTISEPTIC LAVAGE

Antiseptics have been shown to further reduce bacterial numbers and speed wound healing compared with saline-lavaged controls.[18] The ideal wound irrigant should (1) possess a broad spectrum of antibacterial activity; (2) be fast acting and have prolonged residual activity after a single dose; (3) be nontoxic, nonteratogenic, and noncarcinogenic to host cells; (4) be nonallergenic; (5) exhibit minimal systemic absorption; (6) be incapable of promoting bacterial resistance; and (7) be inexpensive and widely available.[6, 19]

Many antiseptics have been evaluated for use in open wounds. Commonly used agents include dilute alcohols, acetic acid, quaternary ammonium compounds, sodium hypochlorite (Dakin's solution), hydrogen peroxide, inorganic iodides, complexed iodine solutions (povidone-iodine), and different salts of chlorhexidine. Many comparative studies and reviews of these products have been published.[18–24] It must be remembered that inappropriate use of antiseptics can create severe inflammation, thereby decreasing resistance to infection, wound strength, granulation tissue formation, contractile ability, and rate of epithelialization.[25]

Iodine Compounds. Since the mid-1800s, iodine compounds have been used for their antibacterial properties.[5] They possess a broad spectrum of activity against vegetative and sporulated bacteria, fungi, viruses, protozoa, and yeast.[5, 6, 26] Free iodine (I_2) is directly responsible for the bactericidal effects of the iodinated products. The rapidity of bacterial destruction is proportional to the concentration of free iodine.[26] A variety of cell-membrane and cytoplasmic components are inactivated by iodination and subsequent oxidation. No true bacterial resistance to iodine has been reported. Earlier reports of a *Pseudomonas* resistance was due to mechanical protection of the bacteria by an organic slime coating. This emphasizes the necessity of maintaining clean storage containers.[26] Free iodine is readily bound by organic substances, which reduce its potency.[26] Drying of the iodine formulation and rapid binding by organic substances account for its short duration of activity.[5, 6, 26]

Organic iodine products are available as alcohol tinctures or aqueous solutions with molecular iodine in concentrations of 2% to 7%.[6] These substances stain tissues and have a characteristic odor. They are irritating and will potentiate infection if used at stock concentrations.[27] Dilute concentrations of 0.1% to 1% aqueous iodine are acceptable for use on exposed tissues.[6]

Iodophors are products in which iodine has been complexed with surfactants or polymers. Povidone-iodine (PI) is a water-soluble, strongly acidic (pH 3.2) iodophor produced by combining molecular iodine with polyvinylpyrrolidone. Iodophors are essentially odorless, and staining is greatly reduced. These improved characteristics of povidone-iodine compounds have made them the most popular form of iodophor used today. Most commercial products contain approximately 90% water, 8.5% polyvinylpyrrolidone, and 1% iodine.[26, 28] The iodine is complexed to polyvinylpyrrolidone by a loose ionic bond. An equilibrium exists between the providone-bound iodine and free iodine. This results in a constant release of free iodine until the iodine is depleted. This may account for povidone-iodine's residual effect of 4 to 8 hours.[5, 6, 27] The concentration of free iodine in 10% PI is approximately 1 ppm. At lower PI concentrations, iodine becomes more loosely bound, and free iodine concentration increases. The highest concentration of free iodine is 24 ppm at a PI concentration of 0.7% (0.07% iodine). Free iodine concentrations diminish at PI concentrations lower than this.[26] This concentration of PI correlates well with its greatest antibacterial efficacy.[28] Polyvinylpyrrolidone is a high-molecular-weight flexible polymer that has no inherent antibacterial activity.[26] It has an affinity for cell membranes and aids in efficient delivery of free iodine directly to the active site. This is crucial to iodine's antibacterial activity. As a result, povidone-iodine has greater antibacterial activity than some inorganic preparations (Lugol's solution) that have greater concentrations of free iodine. Although more dilute solutions of PI are more potent, the number of bacteria killed may be limited by the overall amount of available iodine in the solution.[5, 26]

Iodine affects mammalian and bacterial cells *in vitro*. The lowest concentration of PI lethal to *Staphylococcus aureus* will also kill 100% of cultured fibroblasts. Significant *Staphylococcus* survival occurs at concentrations less than 1% PI, but fibroblast survival occurs only at concentrations less than 0.3% PI.[21] Povidone-iodine, in low concentrations, also appears to cause a functional toxicity of leukocytes. Chemotaxis of human polymorphonuclear cells is inhibited by 10 μg/ml of PI and is completely arrested by 75 μg/ml.[26, 29] Lymphocyte blastogenesis and granulocyte and monocyte viability are also compromised by PI.[26] These early inflammatory cells are important mediators of wound repair, including fibroblast stimulation and migration. There are conflicting reports of the value of PI in reducing wound bacteria, preventing wound infection, and enhancing wound healing compared with saline controls. Some of the support for PI includes a study in humans in which 5% PI potentiated wound infections and inhibited leukocyte migration, whereas 1% PI decreased postoperative infections and had less effect on leukocytes.[30] In experimentally contaminated canine wounds, 0.5% PI was better in preventing overt infection than lower concentrations.[18] A slight increase (0.1% PI) and decrease (1% PI) in wound infection was demonstrated using 0.1% and 1% compared with saline controls in a canine wound-healing study.[22] *These studies, combined with* in vitro *data, have resulted in recommendations for using 1% to 0.1% PI as a wound lavage solution (1:10 to 1:100 dilutions, respectively). This has been described as a weak tea–colored solution.*

PI has been associated with some toxicity owing to its acidic pH and the systemic absorption of iodine. These effects are most pronounced when large wounds, body cavities, or mucosal surfaces are irrigated.[26] Serum iodine levels with increased use of PI normally return to baseline within 3 to 7 days.[26] Hyperthyroid or hypothyroid states may result from chronic PI use. Patients with compromised renal function are at risk for developing iodinism and metabolic acidosis because iodine is normally excreted by the kidneys. Iodine is protein-bound and may displace other protein-bound drugs. Contact hypersensitivities to PI also have been noted in humans and dogs.[1, 2, 26]

Polyhydroxydine is a new iodophor similar to povidone-iodine that is reported to have antibacterial activity and to enhance wound healing.[19] A study in dogs revealed it to be similar to PI in antibacterial activity and effects on the healing wound.[19]

Chlorhexidine. Chlorhexidine [N,N''-bis(4-chlorphenyl)-3,12-diamino-2, 4,11,13-tetraazatetradecanediimidamide] was first used in England as a preservative, topical antiseptic, and disinfectant.[31] It was later used as an antiplaque agent, surgical scrub, and eventually an antiseptic wound lavage agent.[32, 33] It is available as an acetate, gluconate, or hydrochloride salt.[33] At low concentrations, it is bacteriostatic, and at high concentrations, it is bactericidal. It is more effective at an alkaline pH, although it is still effective when diluted in mildly acidic diluents such as saline or lactated Ringer's solution.[12] Its activity is reduced in the presence of organic material, although not to the degree seen with PI and benzalkonium chloride compounds.[6] At low concentrations, chlorhexidine alters bacterial cell membranes, causing the release of K^+ and pentoses. It is also an inhibitor of adenosine triphosphatase (ATP) activity. At bactericidal concentrations, chlorhexidine induces cytoplasmic protein and nucleic acid precipitation. Chlorhexidine damages the cytoplasmic membrane of yeasts and prevents outgrowth, but not germination, of bacterial spores. Chlorhexidine possesses a broad spectrum of activity,[32] although some bacteria, including *Proteus*, *Serratia*, and *Pseudomonas* spp., may be inherently resistant or develop resistance.[31, 32]

Chlorhexidine is immediately active against bacteria.[32] A single application of chlorhexidine provides sustained activity for 2 days, and its effectiveness increases after repeated applications. It has a low potential for causing anaphylaxis, allergic contact sensitization, nonphotoallergenic contact sensitization, and phototoxicity.[1, 2, 33, 34] Systemic absorption and toxicosis appear to be minimal in humans, although it can be ototoxic when used directly in the middle ear.[27, 30]

Chlorhexidine is lethal to mammalian cells and bacteria *in vitro*. A concentration of 0.05% is 100% lethal to *Staphylococcus aureus* and canine fibroblasts.[21] Significant fibroblast survival occurred only when chlorhexidine concentrations were less than 0.006%.[21] In a study with cultured human fibroblasts and epidermal cells, chlorhexidine was toxic to all cell types, and 50% cellular survival occurred at 0.004%.[30] It also was less toxic than 0.5% sodium hypochlorite or 3% hydrogen peroxide.

Clinically, chlorhexidine is useful in reducing wound bacteria, preventing infection, and improving healing of contaminated wounds. In a canine study, 0.05% chlorhexidine lavage enhanced wound healing compared with saline or PI lavage.[22] Use of 0.05% to 0.1% chlorhexidine on experimentally infected wounds was effective in reducing bacterial numbers and decreasing wound infection.[18] In a study with guinea pigs, 0.05% chlorhexidine prevented infection better than benzalkonium chloride, PI, and saline and was the only agent effective when used before wounds were inoculated.[20]

Some reports contain conflicting data regarding chlorhexidine usefulness. In a canine wound-healing study, 0.1% chlorhexidine-soaked sponges had longer residual activity but did not reduce bacterial numbers significantly when compared with PI- or saline-soaked sponges.[19] In the same study, significant bacterial reduction was seen when 0.5% chlorhexidine-soaked gauze sponges were used; however, delayed wound contraction and granulation tissue formation occurred.

The information gained from *in vitro* and *in vivo* studies indicates that the concentration of chlorhexidine useful for wound irrigation is between 0.05%

and 0.5%. *The concentration of chlorhexidine most frequently recommended for clinical use on exposed tissue is 0.05%.*[6, 27, 35]

Experimentally, physiologic saline[22] and water[20] have been used to dilute chlorhexidine. Clinically, 0.9% sodium chloride, lactated Ringer's solution, and water are frequently used as diluents for chlorhexidine. Chlorhexidine diluted in electrolyte solutions will form a heavy precipitate in 1 to 4 hours at room temperature, although this precipitated solution can be used as a wound irrigant. Results of a recent study indicate that bacterial efficacy of 0.05% chlorhexidine acetate against *Staphylococcus intermedius* is similar when the chlorhexidine is diluted in any of these solutions, even when a precipitate forms. This study also showed no difference in wound healing when chlorhexidine, diluted in water or various electrolyte solutions, was used to treat wounds healing by second intention.[12]

Quaternary Ammonium Compounds. These are cationic detergent agents that are active against bacteria, fungi, protozoa, and viruses.[6] They act by denaturing bacterial enzyme systems and neutralizing acidic phospholipid radicals in the cell wall. Killing of bacteria occurs more slowly than with iodine compounds. Quaternary ammonium compounds are more effective against gram-positive than gram-negative organisms. They are inactivated by anionic detergents and soaps, and their activity is reduced by gauze sponges, cotton, iodine, rubber, purulence, blood, and serum. At high concentrations, these are bactericidal agents, whereas at low concentrations, they are bacteriostatic. Oral ingestion is poisonous; however, when these agents are used topically, systemic toxicities are low. Hypersensitivity and dermatitis may develop with repeated use. These agents are most effective when combined with 70% alcohol, but this form is contraindicated for use in wounds. Sterile distilled water or sterile water for injection should be used for dilution because tap water, deionized water, and saline reduce the potency.

Benzalkonium chloride is the most popular of these compounds. In a canine study, 1:2500 benzalkonium chloride was more effective than 1:5000 and 1:10,000 dilutions.[18] This concentration also was more effective than 0.1% to 0.5% povidine-iodine but less effective than 0.5% and 1% chlorhexidine in preventing infection in wounds experimentally contaminated with *Staphylococcus aureus*. None of these antiseptic solutions was shown to cause tissue irritation. In a guinea pig wound model, 0.1% benzalkonium chloride was superior to 10% povidone-iodine in preventing infection in wounds experimentally contaminated with *S. aureus* and less effective than 0.01% to 0.05% chlorhexidine gluconate.[20] *When used on wounds, an aqueous solution of 1:2500 to 1:10,000 (0.007% to 0.002%) has been recommended.*[6, 18]

Dakin's Solution. Dakin's solution (sodium hypochlorite) was used in World War I as an antiseptic agent. Its antimicrobial action is due to formation of hypochlorous acid and release of free chlorine and oxygen into the tissue. It is most effective in an acidic environment. A 0.5% solution may be prepared by a 1:10 dilution of plain laundry bleach. This concentration is capable of liquefying necrotic tissue and killing bacteria,[5, 27] although it decreases wound strength and delays epithelialization in rats.[27] In humans, half-strength (0.25%) is used most commonly, but quarter-strength (0.125%) may be used if higher concentrations cause patient discomfort.[27] In one study, 0.005% Dakin's caused 100% bacterial kill without significant toxicity to cultured human fibroblasts.[24] However, a 0.5% solution delayed epithelialization and was considered unsuitable for wound irrigation. In another study, 50% survival of cultured human fibroblasts and epidermal cells occurred only at concentrations less than 0.0004% sodium hypochlorite. No similar studies have been performed in the dog, and no studies evaluated the effects on wound healing and antibacterial activity at concentrations lower than 0.5%.

Acetic Acid. Acetic acid exerts it antibacterial effect by decreasing local wound pH. Alkalinity has been reported to slow wound healing by stabilizing oxyhemoglobin and preventing dissociation of oxygen into the wound.[36] Carbon dioxide loss in an uncovered wound and the presence of urease-producing organisms are common causes of increased wound alkalinity. Acidification of the wound with acetic acid may be of benefit, particularly in wounds containing urea-splitting organisms.[36] Acetic acid has been used primarily as an antipseudomonad agent, but it is also effective against a wide variety of gram-negative and gram-positive organisms.[36] Resistance may develop to this compound, however. In a study of rat and human skin wounds undergoing split-thickness grafting, the healing rate of wounds treated with 0.25% acetic acid was not significantly different from that of wounds treated with 10% povidone-iodine or saline.[37] Wounds treated with 0.25% acetic acid became infected less frequently than saline-treated wounds. In a study comparing the toxicities of different antiseptics, concentrations of povidone-iodine and sodium hypochlorite were bactericidal but did not cause significant toxicity to cultured human fibroblasts, although all concentrations of acetic acid were more toxic to fibroblasts than to bacteria.[24] A 0.25% concentration delayed wound epithelialization in rats and was considered unacceptable for use on open wounds.[24] *A concentration of 0.5% to 0.25% (1:10 to 1:20 dilution) has been cited for use on wounds in dogs.*[27] Stock solutions are usually 5%.

Hydrogen Peroxide. Hydrogen peroxide is an oxidizing agent found in macrophages that contributes significantly to *in vivo* bacterial killing.[38] It is an effective sporicide[27] and has shown good *in vitro* antibacterial activity at a concentration of 3%.[24] This concentration is also cytotoxic to cultured human fibroblasts and causes tissue irritation.[24] A tenfold dilution (0.3%) is neither bactericidal nor toxic to cultured fibroblasts. This antiseptic is considered unacceptable for use on wounds at the 3% concentration.[24] The effervescent action as it makes contact with tissues dislodges bacteria and debris from the wound.[27, 37] Although it did not delay wound healing in human clinical trials, bullae formation was noted under the newly formed epithelium once coverage was complete.[37] It is doubtful that effervescence is effective as a lavage technique in removing bacteria from wounds. Hydrogen peroxide is usually available in a 3% solution.

Summary of Antiseptics. Of the antiseptics currently available, povidone-iodine and chlorhexidine most closely approximate the ideal irrigant. This has lead to their wide acceptance in both human and veterinary medicine. *Chlorhexidine offers certain advantages over other antiseptics, including greater residual antibacterial activity,*[6] *better antibacterial activity in the presence of blood and other organic debris,*[6, 19, 27] *less systemic absorption and toxicity,*[6, 27] *and more rapid wound healing.*[22] Chlorhexidine is not an innocuous agent, and bacteria can become resistant to it. It has been suggested that selection of an antiseptic should be based on the organism(s) present in the wound.[39] Table 3–3 contains instructions for preparation of 1 liter of the commonly used antiseptic agents.

In vitro comparisons of antiseptics may not be reliable indicators of *in vivo*

TABLE 3–3. Formulas for Making 1 Liter of Commonly Used Antiseptics

0.05% Chlorhexidine (gluconate or diacetate)	
Chlorhexidine 2%	25 ml
Sterile water	975 ml
1% Povidone-iodine	
Povidone-iodine 10%	100 ml
Sterile water	900 ml
0.25% Dakin's solution (half-strength)	
Sodium hypochlorite 5%	50 ml
Sodium bicarbonate	30 ml
Sterile distilled water	920 ml
0.25% Acetic acid	
Acetic acid 5%	50 ml
Sterile water	950 ml

efficacy.[21, 22] A possible explanation is that host cells are compromised in cell culture and susceptible to toxic insults, whereas bacteria have developed better mechanisms for survival in an abnormal environment. The reverse situation may be occurring *in vivo*. Viable superficial host cells are protected and nourished on one surface to maintain homeostasis, while unprotected bacteria encounter humoral, cell-mediated, and antimicrobial challenges.

Within hours after wounding, bacteria become firmly engulfed in the wound coagulum and are protected from the effects of surface antiseptics. To be most effective, attempts in removing the wound coagulum and exposing (gentle scrubbing, enzymatic debridement) hidden bacteria will provide a greater reduction in bacterial numbers. These techniques are beneficial when combined with antibiotic therapy.

Antiseptics probably have little effect on bacteria that penetrated host tissues and established infection. Bacterial removal at this stage is by physical extirpation and augmentation of local defenses through gentle wound care and use of antimicrobial drugs. Antiseptics will be beneficial in these infected wounds, although their effect will be limited to superficial areas of the wound.

ANTISEPTIC CREAMS AND OINTMENTS

Several antiseptic agents (e.g., chlorhexidine, povidone-iodine) are available in cream or ointment forms. There is a paucity of information concerning indications for their use and effects on wound healing. Their therapeutic effects are based on the antiseptic constituent. They are useful at "ostomy" and drainage sites for controlling infection associated with fluid leakage.

PROPHYLACTIC ANTIBIOTIC LAVAGE

Shortly after the discovery of sulfonamides in the 1930s, their topical use in the treatment of open fractures was shown to decrease wound infection from 27% to 5%, although no controls were available.[40] Routine use of topical "sulfas" prior to wound closure was performed until the late 1940s, when it was discovered that sulfonamide powder caused tissue necrosis and increased wound infection rates.[40] The discovery of penicillin, streptomycin, and tetracycline in the 1940s also led to their wide use as topical irrigants. Controlled studies, however, failed to document a decrease in the infection rate with their use. Since these early studies, the role of topical antibiotics has remained controversial, although some progress has been made in defining the role for topical antibiotics in wound management. The potential advantages of antibiotics compared with antiseptics are selective bacterial toxicity, efficacy not reduced in the presence of organic material,[41] and combined efficacy with systemic antibiotic administration. Disadvantages include expense, reduced antimicrobial spectrum, potential for bacterial resistance, creation of superinfections, and increased nosocomial infections. Factors that must be considered prior to using topical antibiotics include antibiotic selection (spectrum, dose, pharmacokinetics, tissue and systemic toxicity), timing, route of administration, and type of preparation (lavage, ointment or cream, or powder).

Antibiotic Selection. While endogenous *Staphylococcus* and *Streptococcus* spp. are the most common pathogens found in postoperative and traumatic wounds, Gram-negative bacteria and mixed infections also may be encountered. Failure to choose a broad-spectrum antibiotic initially, when the type of infecting agent is unknown, may lead to treatment failure. Evaluation of Gram stains of smears from the wound may help predict bacterial isolates and possible antibiotic sensitivities.[13] Cephalosporins are useful for treatment of infections caused by gram-positive organisms. Aminoglycosides are useful for treatment of infections caused by gram-negative bacteria.[13] Combinations of antibiotics may be used for mixed infections. Subsequent lavage should be based on bacterial culture and antimicrobial sensitivity results.

Timing of Administration. The effective use of antibiotics in wounds depends on timing of administration. There is a decisive period after wounding when subsequent development of infection is determined.[42] During this period, open lymphatic and blood vessels allow bacterial contaminants to infiltrate deep within the wound margins. As these conduits to the deeper tissues are sealed off by hemostatic mechanisms (blood, platelet, and fibrin coagulum), subsequent bacterial infiltration is reduced.[43] If, through infiltration and replication, significant numbers of pathogenic bacteria accumulate during this period to overwhelm local host defenses, infection will result. Antibacterial agents must be present in the tissues in sufficient quantity at the time of bacterial invasion or shortly thereafter to assist host defenses in eliminating these pathogens. Systemic antibiotics given before the onset of contamination have a pronounced effect in preventing infection in wounds subsequently contaminated with bacteria. This effect occurs up to 3 hours after contamination.[42] Many clinical studies have demonstrated a prophylactic effect of topically administered antibiotics used by 1 hour after the onset of contamination.[40, 44–47] Many antibiotics have been shown to provide antibacterial activity within seconds,[48] but a minimum contact time of 1 minute is recommended for antibiotics in lavage solutions.[40] There appears to be no advantage in combining topical and systemic antibiotics for the prevention of infection in wounds with mild or moderate contamination.[41] Combined therapy is advantageous in heavily contaminated wounds compared with either route alone.[41, 49, 50]

Numerous topical antibiotics have been proven effective in *preventing* infection, including penicillin, ampicillin, carbenicillin, tetracycline, kanamycin, neomycin, bacitracin, polymyxin and cephalosporins.[40, 51] Neomycin, bacitracin, and polymyxin are used frequently in combination. However, no controlled clinical studies have been performed comparing the efficacies of different prophylactic topical antibiotic protocols.[40]

Variable concentrations of antibiotics have been used as lavage agents. No general guidelines or recommendations have been established for topical dosage or volume of lavage, and dosing often seems empirical. Table 3–4 lists antibiotic concentrations and doses used in human and veterinary studies. Well-absorbed, nontoxic antibiotics were given at a systemic total dose prior to closure and left in the wound to encourage absorption.[51] Poorly absorbed antibiotics were used several times during surgery to provide better prophylaxis than single administration.[40] If available, minimum inhibitory concentrations may help determine optimal topical concentration. Little veterinary information is available on local tissue toxicity associated with topical antibiotics,[52] and further work is needed in this area.

Locally applied cephazolin (0.2 ml/kg of 100 mg/ml solution; total dose 20 mg/kg) provides high levels of the antibiotic in wound fluid that remain above the minimum inhibitory concentration for a longer time than systemically administered cephazolin.[51] Furthermore, locally administered cephazolin was 95% bioavailable and rapidly absorbed, thus providing effective systemic levels that equaled wound fluid levels within 1 hour.[51] Powdered cephalosporins are placed in wounds to achieve higher and more prolonged tissue concentrations than solutions.[53] Other antibiotics (e.g., bacitracin, neomycin, polymyxin) are poorly absorbed from topical sites and less effective in treating established infection.[54] Even poorly absorbed antibiotics may achieve toxic systemic levels if large wound areas are treated for prolonged periods.[54] More work needs to be done to establish the tissue toxicity and pharmacokinetics of different topically applied antibiotics and antibiotic forms.

Unfortunately, many veterinary patients with contaminated wounds are treated hours or days following wounding. *Once infection has become established, there is no beneficial effect of topical or systemic antibiotics in preventing suppuration of wounds undergoing closure.*[42, 55] The presence of the wound coagulum (fibrin, necrotic tissue, foreign material, and inflammatory exudate) prevents topical antibiotics from reaching effective levels in tissues deep within the wound and prevents systemic antibiotics from reaching superficial bacteria.[43] The

TABLE 3–4. Topical Antibiotics Used in Human and Veterinary Medicine

Ampicillin (0.5–1 gm)[40]

Bacitracin (50,000 units/L)*[46]

Bacitracin (50,000 units/L), polymyxin (25 mg/ml)[40]

Bacitracin (50,000 units/L), polymyxin B sulfate (50 mg/L)[48]

Bacitracin (25,000 units/L), neomycin (5%), polymyxin B sulfate (25 mg/L)[40]

Carbenicillin indanyl sodium (0.4%)[48]

Cephalothin sodium (0.4%)[48]

Cephalothin sodium (1%)[47]

Cephazolin (20 mg/kg, 100 mg/ml)[51]

Gentamicin (1%)[48, 52]

Kanamycin (1%)[47]

Penicillin (5 million units)[40]

Neomycin sulfate (1% to 5%)[40]

Tetracycline (250 mg)[40]

*Repeated or chronic use may cause hypersensitivity.

period of effectiveness of systemic antibiotics may be extended from 3 to 24 hours with the use of gentle scrubbing of the contaminated wound with saline-moistened gauze sponges.[55] This effect also has been demonstrated with topical antibiotics. Combining topical and systemic antibiotics with gentle scrubbing may be most effective in prolonging antibiotic effectiveness in the early stages following injury.[50] Enzymatic debridement agents also will increase the effectiveness of antibiotics by dissolving the wound coagulum and increasing exposure of the bacteria to the antibacterial agent.[43] Prompt, meticulous, and repetitive (when necessary) surgical debridement and debriding bandages should never be replaced by topical antibiotic therapy but rather should be used in conjunction with these techniques. Combined use of antiseptics and antibiotics is rational. Many antiseptics (e.g., Tris-EDTA) are membrane active and may increase uptake or susceptibility of microbes to antibiotics. If used together, large volumes of antiseptic lavage should precede application of topical antibiotic.

Tris-EDTA is solution of a disodium-calcium salt of ethylenediamenetetraacetic acid (EDTA) buffered with tris(hydroxymethyl)aminomethane (Tris) (Table 3–5). This agent causes increased permeability of gram-negative bacteria to extracellular solutes and leakage of intracellular solutes.[57] As a result, treated bacteria are more susceptible to destruction by lysosymes, antiseptics, and antibiotics. *Pseudomonas aeruginosa, Escherichia coli*, and *Proteus vulgaris* are rapidly lysed by Tris-EDTA in sterile water. Used in combination with antibacterial agents, it markedly reduces minimum inhibitory concentration of antibiotics against several pathogens. Chelation of divalent cations by EDTA may account for potentiation of gentamicin against *P. vulgaris*. Trist-EDTA increases cell-wall permeability of *E. coli* to penicillins and tetracycline. Antimicrobial synergism has been noted between Tris-EDTA and penicillin, oxytetracycline, or chloramphenicol against *E. coli* and between Tris-EDTA and gentamicin, oxytetracycline, polymyxin B, nalidixic acid, or triple sulfonamide against *P. vulgaris*. Higher concentrations of penicillin and chloramphenicol have been found in *P. aeruginosa* treated with Tris-EDTA.[57] The antimicrobial efficacy of 0.01% chlorhexidine gluconate is increased 1000-fold by the addition of Tris-EDTA (1.34 mM EDTA, 0.01 M Tris).[58] Tris-EDTA does not injure tissues, although controlled studies are lacking.

THERAPEUTIC ANTIBIOTIC LAVAGE

Wounds greater than 24 hours old are frequently treated when it is impossible to completely remove infected tissue containing bacterial concentrations greater than 10^5 per gram of tissue. Methods are available to quantitate wound bacteria, but in practice, subjective judgment or the inability to close a defect will most often dictate whether a wound is closed or left open. Although closure increases a wound's ability to resist infection, open wounds rapidly become resistant to infection.[59] Experimental studies of infected open wounds have shown that by day 4 after infection, most wounds

TABLE 3–5. Tris-EDTA, 1 Liter

1.2 gm EDTA
6.05 gm Tris
1 liter sterile water for injection
Adjust pH to 8.0 with sodium hydroxide

will not abscess if they are closed.[59] When in doubt, wounds should be left open to provide drainage of exudate and allow treatment and assessment until closure or second-intention healing is completed. A thick fibrin layer and variable quantities of exudate can accumulate in open wounds between bandage changes. This may be enough to prevent access of antimicrobial agents to the pathogen, and this should be controlled with enzymatic or debridement dressings. Between bandage changes, topical antiseptic or antibiotic lavage may fail to maintain effective wound concentrations. Various antibiotic ointments, creams, and salves are available that could prolong concentrations of antibiotic in tissues. There is a paucity of information documenting this theory, although benefit has been noted with the use of some of these products.

Not all wounds require treatment with topical antibiotics. As previously discussed, topical antibiotics are most beneficial when used as prophylactic agents in lavage of wounds less than 3 hours old which are to be closed. Topical antibiotics should be used following guidelines similar to those of systemic antibiotics therapy:

1. Recent heavy contamination of tissues
2. Catastrophic infection
3. Immunosuppressed patient
4. Inadequate prophylaxis

Minor contaminants are common in open wounds and can be kept to a minimum with appropriate bandage changes and antiseptic lavage. It is important to avoid the error of relying on topical and/or systemic antibiotic therapy rather than strict aseptic technique and physical debridement. Topical therapy may be harmful by promoting resistance bacteria, superinfections, systemic or local toxicity, or hypersensitivity.

Other Topical Wound Agents

ANTIMICROBIAL OINTMENTS AND CREAMS

Bacitracin, neomycin, and polymyxin are available in a petrolatum base (Neosporin) as a broad-spectrum topical ointment. These antibiotics are poorly absorbed and benefit in preventing contamination and infection in healthy wounds.[54] The efficacy against *Pseudomonas* is poor, which is unfortunate because it is a common pathogen in many chronically infected wounds.[54] The zinc-bacitracin component of this product stimulates reepithelialization. Allergic reactions may occur, and wounds should be monitored during sustained or repeated use of this product.

Topical gentamicin is available as a 0.1% ointment or powder (Garamycin). A gentamicin cream also has been formulated.[52] Gentamicin is an effective agent against many bacteria but is especially useful against gram-negative organisms, including *Pseudomonas aeruginosa, Escherichia coli*, and *Proteus vulgaris*.[54] All preparations of the antibiotic have demonstrated efficacy in controlling wound bacteria.[54] The cream preparation has been shown to decrease wound contraction in dogs.[52]

Nitrofurazone (Furacin) is a broad-spectrum antimicrobial agent available in a polyethylene glycol base solution or powder.[27, 59] Studies in pigs and rats have documented delayed epithelialization with nitrofurazone.[60, 61] In dogs, nitrofurazone, in polyethylene glycol, decreased bacterial contaminants and did not significantly alter wound healing. Allergenic potential of this product has been documented in humans.[62]

Silver sulfadiazine (Silvidene) is available as a 1% water-soluble cream. It is frequently used as an antipseudomonad agent for burn patients, and it has a broad spectrum of activity against other bacteria. In pigs, epithelialization was enhanced when wounds were treated with silver sulfadiazine.[60] It also has been used successfully as a carrier agent for topical growth-factor administration.[63]

An important consideration when using a topical cream or ointment is identification of the carrier or base material. Ease of removal and tissue toxicity are related to the base material used in the product. Polyethylene glycol is a water-soluble base that is innocuous[64] to canine tissues and easily removed from the wound surface. White USP petrolatum and white soft paraffin delay epithelialization and are more difficult to remove.[27, 64, 65] Low-melting-point non-USP petrolatum does not have these adverse effects.[60] Cream-base substances are not standard and have not been evaluated thoroughly, although one formulation has been shown to inhibit wound contraction.[52] Other preparations, including vanishing cream and skin lotion, were shown to enhance epithelialization in partial-thickness skin wounds in pigs; the effects on wound contraction were not studied.[65] Another concern with topical agent bases is the tendency for hydrophilic bases to release their antibiotic slowly, which may reduce concentrations in the wound below effective levels.[52]

Other Agents. Live yeast cell derivative (Preparation-H) is derived from the brewer's yeast, *Saccharomyces cerivisiae*. In humans, it increases wound oxygen consumption, angiogenesis, epithelialization, and collagen synthesis and has been called *wound respiratory factor*.[66, 67] It is available as a water-soluble, over-the-counter hemorrhoid preparation. Subjective reports of its use in selected wounds in dogs have been positive.[68] In a controlled study in horses, exuberant granulation tissue was more frequent in wounds treated with live yeast cell derivative than in controls. Treated wounds took longer to heal, were slower to epithelialize, and healed with less contraction than control wounds. The authors speculated that delays in healing may have resulted, in part, from the effect of the bandage causing more trauma to the exuberant wound site. They did not recommend this treatment for extremities in horses but suggested it may be beneficial on truncal wounds with soft-tissue defects.[68] Further study of this product in animals is warranted.

Occasionally, reports have emerged on the use of honey or sugar pastes in the treatment of chronic, nonhealing, infected wounds.[69, 70] Despite claims of wound debridement, reduction of edema, pronounced *in vivo* antibacterial activity, promotion of granulation and epithelialization, improved wound nutrition, and wound deodorization, use of these products has failed to gain wide acceptance. No clinical veterinary reports are available.

Aloe vera has been touted as a topical agent for burns.[71] In high concentrations, it has antibacterial activity against *P. aeruginosa* and antiprostaglandin activity against thromboxane. Its soothing characteristics have been attributed to a salicylate-like substance. However, because of its anti-inflammatory effects, use in full-thickness wounds has been discouraged.[27]

ANTI-INFLAMMATORY INHIBITORS OF WOUND HEALING

Catabolic steroids administered repetitively in high doses topically or systemically will inhibit wound healing.[72] Epidermal migration, mesenchymal proliferation, and synthesis appear to be inhibited by these agents. Antiprostaglandin agents and vitamin E given in high doses also will inhibit healing. Vitamin A, on the other hand, may reverse some of the detrimental effects of steroids and vitamin E on healing.[72] The effect of anti-inflammatory agents is most pronounced when they are used during the inflammatory stage of healing. The inflammatory process is necessary for the production of mediators that initiate the repair stage. Controlling these effects may be beneficial in wounds with an exaggerated inflammatory response. These effects are utilized prophylactically with corticosteroid administration prior to neurologic surgery. Perhaps there could be beneficial use of these agents in wound healing as well. Anti-inflammatory agents and lathyrogenic agents (β-aminopropionitrile) have been used to modulate the repair phase of healing.[72, 73] Triamcinalone (Panalog) has been shown to reduce exhuberant granulation tissue in horses.[73] Attempts at inhibiting wound contracture and stricture formation met with limited success. Further research is needed to better define the potential role for these agents in wound healing.

ENZYMES

The use of enzymatic agents in debridement of wounds stems from the early use of papain-rich latex taken from the papaw tree (*Carica papaya*) by tropical natives. Papain, pancreatic enzyme preparations, hyaluronidase, trypsin, chymotrypsin, fibrinolysin, deoxyribonuclease, streptodornase (streptococcal deoxyribonuclease), and streptokinase have been investigated for their use on wounds. Proper use of these products dissolves wound exudate, coagulum, and necrotic debris without directly harming living tissue. Bacteria are liberated from these avascular protective havens of proteinaceous and nuclear material, and exposure to cellular and humoral immunity and antimicrobial agents is enhanced.[74]

Trypsin hydrolyzes and extensively degrades many naturally occurring proteins but can cause local inflammation and pyrogenic reactions. It does not require activation, but can be inactivated by serum factors.[74] It has been used successfully to enhance the efficacy of antibiotics in experimentally infected wounds.[43] Papain is another enzyme with wide proteolytic activity. Theoretical advantages include activity over a wide pH range and potential ability to digest collagen. Most enzymes are effective at a neutral pH, whereas papain is effective between pH values of 3 to 9. Collagenolytic action of papain occurs at a low pH. Streptokinase is a derivative of hemolytic streptococcus that activates plasminogen. It is especially effective in lysing fibrin clots. This enzyme is associated with pyogenic reactions and local inflammation. In veterinary medicine, the most commonly available products are trypsin in balsam-of-Peru castor oil (Granulex) and a fibrinolysin–deoxyribonuclease (Elase) combination. One source of deoxyribonuclease is from a streptococcal derivative (streptodornase). This enzyme is capable of liquefying exposed nuclear material but also has been associated with pyogenic and inflammatory reactions. A highly purified enzyme product causes less adverse reactions.

Limitations exist in the use of these agents. Burned skin, necrotic bone, and connective tissue are not digested by currently available enzymes. Most preparations may cause local tissue irritation and should not be used within body cavities. Enzymes must be brought in contact with desired surfaces of the wound for an adequate amount of time to produce the desired effect, and then they must be removed. Repeated use with purified products may be expensive. Despite the number of enzymes available, well-established guidelines and indications for use of these enzymes are lacking.

GROWTH FACTORS

Since the late 1970s, there has been much information published about the function and clinical uses of different biologic modulators or growth factors. These growth factors are cytokines that are released normally during the inflammatory process of wounding and are produced by many cells, including platelets, macrophages, lymphocytes, neutrophils, fibroblasts, and epithelial cells.[63, 75–77] Such factors as epidermal growth factor (EGF), epidermal growth factor–like peptide, platelet-derived growth factor (PDGF), transforming growth factor α and β (TGF-α, TGF-β), nerve growth factor, and basic fibroblast growth factor (bFGF) have been isolated and are being evaluated. Their effects include stimulation of cellular mitogenesis and migration, modulation of gene expression for matrix component, and enzyme production. These agents are effective at nanogram to microgram levels.[63, 75–77] Clinical results have been very promising in animal models and human trials. As yet, however, there are no known clinical reports describing the use of these products in veterinary medicine. This is an exciting area of research that may provide a powerful tool for manipulating wound healing in the future.

WOUND DRESSINGS

Bandages and dressings are important aspects of wound management. There have been numerous technologic advances in biomaterials and it is a constant challenge to determine which material will best suit a wound. Excellent papers are available in the human and veterinary literature to supplement this review.[78, 79]

Bandages are generally composed of three layers. The primary or contact layer may be used to debride tissue, deliver medication, transmit wound exudate, or form an occlusive seal over the wound. Ideally, this layer should provide intimate contact with the wound surface, reduce pain, and keep the wound surface moist. It should not contain substances irritating to the wounded tissues. *The secondary layer is used to absorb or store exudate away from the wound and pad and protect the wound from further injury. The tertiary layer is necessary to protect the underlying layers and wound from external contamination and immobilize the bandage and wound.* Immobilized wounds are more comfortable, heal more rapidly, and produce less scar than mobilized wounds.[79]

The contact layer of the bandage is of prime importance because its composition and physical characteristics directly affect the healing of the underlying tissues. Primary dressings are classified as follows:

1. Adherent
2. Nonadherent
   a. Semiocclusive
   b. Occlusive
      i. Synthetic
      ii. Biologic

The desired functions of the primary layer of a wound dressing vary with the phase of wound healing. Wounds in the inflammatory or debridement phase will often require adherent dressings to remove necrotic tissue that is not amenable to further surgical debridement. Bandage material adheres to wounds when (1) granulation tissue penetrates the interstices of the dressing, (2) fibrinous and capillary invasion entrap the dressing, or (3) proteinaceous exudate and necrotic debris penetrate the dressing and subsequently dry, thus cementing the material to the dressing.[79] The degree of adherence depends on the size of the interstices in the dressing material. Wide-mesh gauze is more appropriate for adherent dressings than fine-mesh gauze.[79] Cut gauze and cotton should be avoided because they may leave strands of dressing material in the wound and lead to a foreign-body reaction.

Adherent gauze dressings may be applied and removed as wet or dry (i.e., dry-to-dry, wet-to-wet, wet-to-dry) depending on the nature of the exudate and degree of desired debridement.[79] Warm, wet gauze is more comfortable to the patient and more effective for dissolving and mobilizing tenacious exudate than dry gauze. Wet gauze also has more rapid capillary action than dry gauze, thus enhancing uptake of sanguinous exudate or transudate and transmitting the material to the secondary layer.[79] Moist bandages are physiologic and do not cause wound injury when properly managed. Sterile saline is the most physiologic wetting agent, and soluble medications, antibiotics, enzymes, and/or antiseptics may be applied with wet gauze. Dry gauze absorbs low-viscosity exudates well and has greater storage capacity than wet gauze. The latter is not useful when an adequate secondary layer is employed in the bandage.

Removal of wet adherent dressings is not painful, but such dressings do not debride tissue well. Warm saline used to rewet a dried dressing will facilitate removal and reduce pain. Complete drying is often not necessary to provide adequate debridement and, in fact, is not desirable in most cases. Gauze dressings may become excessively soaked or clogged in heavily exudative wounds. If, at the time of bandage changes, the gauze is soaked in exudate and tends to slide from the wound, the goals of the adherent dressing are not being met, and bandages should be changed more frequently or the absorptive capacity of the secondary layer should be reevaluated. Bacteria may proliferate in a moist environment, and tissue maceration may occur if the primary layer remains excessively wet.

If no necrotic debris is present or the wound progresses to the repair phase of healing, a nonadherent dressing should be used to protect granulation tissue and migrating epithelium (Fig. 3–1). When these wounds have a large amount of serosanguinous fluid, a semiocclusive dressing is needed to transmit excess wound fluid to the secondary layer and maintain a moist environment conducive to healing.[79, 80] A variety of nonadherent dressings (Telfa, Release) are available commercially. Some have absorptive capacity and a secondary layer (Fig. 3–1A). Others are natural or synthetic fiber meshes impregnated with petrolatum (Xeroform) or polyethylene glycol (Aquaphor) (Fig. 3–1B). These types of dressings also can be made by lightly coating gauze with petrolatum or polyethylene glycol. Petrolatum serves very well for these dressing but can delay epithelialization. Polyethylene glycol is a hydrophilic water-soluble agent that increases the capillary action of the dressing and covers the wound with fluid.[79] Polyethylene glycol may dissolve and require frequent bandage changing. Antibiotic or antiseptic preparations with similar bases also may be used to create semiocclusive dressings. These substances may be applied to sterile gauze immediately before use or may be autoclaved with sponges. The autoclaving technique will impregnate all

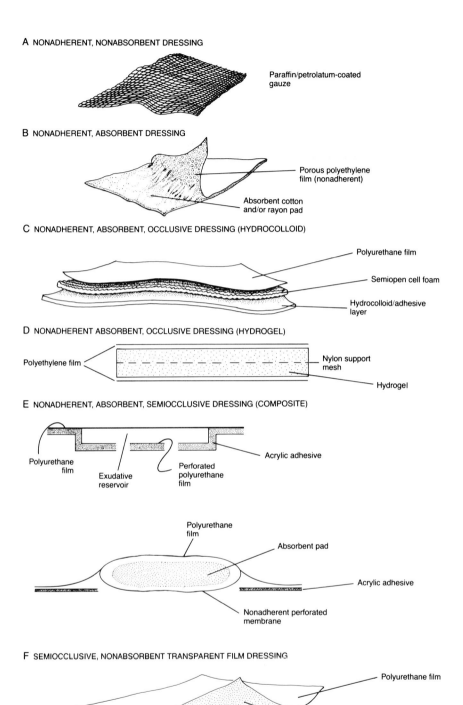

A NONADHERENT, NONABSORBENT DRESSING

Paraffin/petrolatum-coated gauze

B NONADHERENT, ABSORBENT DRESSING

Porous polyethylene film (nonadherent)

Absorbent cotton and/or rayon pad

C NONADHERENT, ABSORBENT, OCCLUSIVE DRESSING (HYDROCOLLOID)

Polyurethane film

Semiopen cell foam

Hydrocolloid/adhesive layer

D NONADHERENT ABSORBENT, OCCLUSIVE DRESSING (HYDROGEL)

Polyethylene film

Nylon support mesh

Hydrogel

E NONADHERENT, ABSORBENT, SEMIOCCLUSIVE DRESSING (COMPOSITE)

Polyurethane film

Exudative reservoir

Perforated polyurethane film

Acrylic adhesive

Polyurethane film

Absorbent pad

Acrylic adhesive

Nonadherent perforated membrane

F SEMIOCCLUSIVE, NONABSORBENT TRANSPARENT FILM DRESSING

Polyurethane film

Ether/acrylic-based adhesive

Figure 3–1. Bandage dressing construction and design. (From Wiseman DM, Rovee DT, Alvanez OM: Wound dressing: Design and use. In Cohen IK, Diegelmann RF, Lindblad WJ (eds): Wound Healing. Philadelphia: WB Saunders, 1992, p 568.)

layers of the sponge, although gauze at the top of the stack tends to be coated lightly, whereas layers at the bottom are heavily coated. Excessive amounts of these coating substances may render the gauze dressing fully occlusive by completely plugging the interstices. Use of this type of occlusive dressing on an exudative wound could lead to excess fluid buildup and tissue maceration.[81] Fine-mesh gauze causes more occlusion, whereas coarse-mesh gauze allows more drainage to occur. Impregnated coarse-mesh gauze may allow some adherence[79] and is indicated for wounds during the transition phase from debridement to repair or in contaminated repair-phase wounds with viscous exudate. In a canine study, petrolatum-containing dressings led to greater contraction of open wounds at 7 days than other types of semiocclusive dressings.[81] There was no difference at 14 and 21 days in contraction, but epithelialization was retarded with petrolatum-containing dressings.

Once a healthy wound in the repair phase with minimal exudate is present, fully occlusive dressings may be used (Fig. 3–2). The primary benefit of occlusive dressings is the ability to accelerate wound epithelialization. Collagen synthesis is also increased under occlusive dressings.[82] Epithelialization can be increased by 50% when this type of dressing is used. The role that oxygen permeability plays in wound healing under occlusive dressings is controversial. Results of studies indicated that high oxygen tension favors rapid epithelialization, while low oxygen tension favors fibroblast growth and angiogenesis.[83, 84] Other studies found similar rates of epithelialization under oxygen-permeable or oxygen-impermeable dressings.[85] At present, it appears that oxygen permeability is not a prerequisite for occlusive dressings to accelerate healing. Another advantage of occlusive dressings is that they require less frequent changing. Monitoring should be performed one to

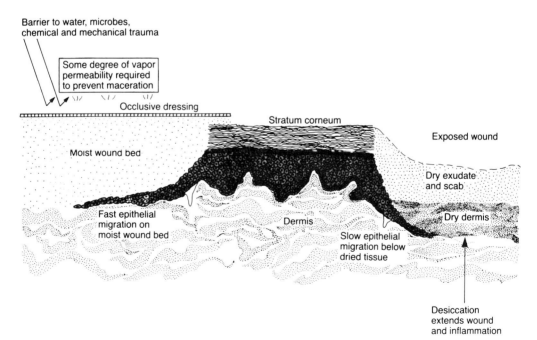

Figure 3–2. Wound healing under an occlusive dressing. (From Wiseman DM, Rovee DT, Alvanez OM: Wound dressing: Design and use. In Cohen IK, Diegelmann RF, Lindblad WJ (eds): Wound Healing. Philadelphia, WB Saunders, 1992, p 565.)

three times daily to guard against slippage, infection, or leakage. Occlusive dressings are available in many different forms with numerous indications. Most of these products were initially designed for human use on smooth skin with good patient compliance. In animals, one of the major problems is maintaining adequate adhesion to surrounding skin. Close shaving of the hair or use of depilatory agents facilitates adhesion.

POLYURETHANE FILMS

These are variable vapor-permeable dressings (Bioclusive) used on partial-thickness dermal injuries or as coverings for hydrogels, hydrophilic pastes, or powders (Fig. 3–1C). They are waterproof, transparent, and reduce pain. Adequate adhesion is difficult on animals. Polyurethane films are contraindicated in infected wounds or wounds with copious drainage.

HYDROCOLLOIDS

These are generally malleable, waterproof dressings (Dermaheal) in the form of a dense dry gel that can easily be cut to size (Fig. 3–1D). Warming the dressings renders them more pliable. Upon contact with the warm, moist wound surface, the hydrocolloid dissolves and produces a sealed moist environment. As wound fluids dissolve the dressing, a blister of fluid forms under the dressing. When this blister becomes excessively large and is in danger of leaking, or if leakage occurs, the dressing should be changed. *Hydrocolloid dressings are indicated for protecting healthy granulating wounds.* They effectively relieve wound pain. Debridement of dense wound coagulum may occur under the dressing through autolysis. These dressings are not transparent, so wound monitoring is difficult, and they should not be used in infection. A tenacious gel may form in the area where the dressing touches intact skin. This aids dressing adhesion but can create difficulty during bandage changes.

HYDROGELS

Hydrogels are expensive dressings (Bio Dres) that are available as a thin composite of the hydrogel adhered to a fine-mesh, thin synthetic sheet (Fig. 3–1E) or as a paste (Fig. 3–1F). They are composed of insoluble hydrophilic polymers that absorb variable amounts of wound fluid (1:1 absorption by weight).[86] They reduce pain and are compatible with topical agents (antibiotics). Hydrogels also may allow some autolytic debridement at the wound surface. The sheets are pliable and easily cut to size. *They are indicated for use on flat granulating surfaces.* They are semitransparent and allow wound monitoring through the dressing. Hydrogels may be used over a noninfected eschar to soften and aid removal. *The gel pastes are indicated for deep defects in the repair phase.* They provide excellent surface contact with the wound. The gel pastes can be retained with a thin film dressing and often require wound lavage for complete removal. *Both forms are contraindicated in infected wounds.*

HYDROPHILIC BEADS, FLAKES, POWDERS, AND PASTES

These polymers rapidly absorb large (30:1, weight:weight) (Copolymer flakes, Debrisan) amounts of wound exudate or transudate and are indicated for use in deep granulating defects (Fig. 3–1F). Flakes and powders may be added in dry form for heavily exudative wounds or may be partially rehydrated into a malleable gel before placement in the wound. These polymers are capable of cleansing wound surface of bacteria and exudate by drawing fluid from the tissues into the polymer. They are easy to use and conform well to the wound surface. They help control odor and are generally less expensive than hydrogels. They may be combined with antimicrobial agents and used on infected wounds. These also require a cover dressing and are best removed with wound lavage.

BIOLOGIC DRESSINGS

Wounds that are closed are more resistant to infection than open wounds during the early stages of healing.[59] Similarly, grafting of infected wounds is an effective means of reducing bacterial numbers.[87] Initial graft adherence is needed to obtain this benefit, and revascularization and graft viability are necessary. This bacterial-reducing effect occurs with allografts and xenografts, as well as autografts. *Grafting should not be attempted on heavily exudative wounds.*[87] Full-thickness grafts will prevent epithelialization under the graft and reduce contraction.[87] In chronic nonhealing infected wounds with minimal exudate, this may be an effective means of controlling wound infection until definitive closure can take place.

Preserved amnionic membrane has been used for the treatment of large skin wounds and burns in humans since the early 1900s. It adheres and conforms to the wound site and reduces pain. It is pliable and improves mobility of the affected area. Amnion acts as an occlusive dressing and stimulates epithelialization and collagen synthesis. Experimental use of amnion on open wounds on the distal aspect of horse limbs yielded promising results.[68] Increased contraction and epithelialization and decreased exuberant granulation tissue resulted in faster, more cosmetic healing than control wounds. Future studies are needed to evaluate this dressing for potential use in small animals.

WOUND THERAPY PRODUCTS

Aquaphor, Beirsdorf, Inc., Norwalk, CT 06854

Bioclusive, Johnson and Johnson, New Brunswick, NJ 08901

Bio Dres, Dermatologics for Veterinary Medicine, Miami, FL 33172

Chlorhexidine (Nolvasan), Fort Dodge Laboratories, Fort Dodge, IA 50501

Copolymer flakes, Summit Hill Laboratories, Navesink, NJ 07752

Debrisan, Johnson and Johnson, New Brunswick, NJ 08901

Dermaheal, E.R. Squibb, Inc., Princeton, NJ 08540

Elase ointment, Parke-Davis, Morris Plains, NJ 07950

Furacin dressing, Norden Laboratories, Lincoln, NE 68501

Garamycin ointment, Schering Corporation, Kenilworth, NJ 07033

Granulex, Beecham Laboratories, Bristol, TN 37620

Neosporin ointment, Burroughs Wellcome Co., Research Triangle Park, NC 27709

Panalog, Solvay Animal Health, Inc., Mendota Heights, MN 55120

Povidone-iodine (Betadine), Purdue Frederick Co., Norwalk, CT 06856

Release—nonadhering dressing, Johnson and Johnson, New Brunswick, NJ 08901

Silvidine creme, Marion Laboratories, Kansas City, MO 64137

Telfa adhesive pads, Kendall Company, Mansfield, MA 02048

Xeroform, Sherwood Medical, St. Louis, MO 63103

REFERENCES

1. Osuna DJ, DeYoung DJ, Walker RL: Comparison of three skin preparation techniques in the dog: 1. Experimental trial. Vet Surg 1990; 19(1):14–19
2. Osuna DJ, DeYoung DJ, Walker RL: Comparison of three skin preparation techniques in the dog: 2. Clinical trial in 100 dogs. Vet Surg 1990; 19(1):20–23
3. Phillips MF, Vasseur PB, Gregory CR: Chlorhexidine diacetate versus pardone-iodine for preoperative preparation of the skin: A prospective randomized comparison in dogs and cats. J Am Anim Hosp Assoc 1991; 27:105–107
4. Swaim SF, Riddell KP, Geiger DL, et al: Evaluation of surgical scrub and antiseptic solutions for surgical preparation of paws. J Am Vet Med Assoc 1991; 198:1941–1945
5. Laufman H: Current use of skin and wound cleansers and antiseptics. Am J Surg 1989; 157:359–365
6. Amber EI, Swaim SF: An update on common wound antiseptics. Aust Vet Pract 1984; 14(1):29–33
7. Branemark PI, Ekhlom R, Albrektsson B, et al: Tissue injury caused by wound disinfectants. J Bone Joint Surg 1963; 49A:48–62
8. Schmidt RM, Rosenkrantz HS: Antimicrobial activity of local anesthetics: Lidocaine and procaine. J Infect Dis 1970; 121:597–607
9. Swaim SF, Henderson RA: Small Animal Wound Management. Philadelphia: Lea & Febiger, 1990; pp 12–13
10. Powell DM, Rodeheaver GT, Foresman PA, et al: Damage to tissues by Emla cream. J Emerg Med 1991; 9:205–209
11. Stevenson TR, Rodeheaver GT, Golden GT, et al: Damage to wounds by use of vasoconstrictors. J Am Coll Emerg Physicians 1975; 4:532.
12. Lozier SM, Pope ER: Effects of four preparations of 0.05% chlorhexidine diacetate on wound healing in the dog. Vet Surg 1992; 2:107–112
13. Edlich RF, Thacker JG, Buchanan L, Rodeheaver GT: Modern concepts of treatment of traumatic wounds. Adv Surg 1979; 13:169–197
14. Rodeheaver GT, Smith SL, Thacker JG, et al: Mechanical cleansing of contaminated wounds with a surfactant. Am J Surg 1975; 129:241–245
15. Ndikuwera J, Winstanley EW: High-pressure pulsatile lavage and high-pressure syringe lavage in the treatment of contaminated wounds in dogs. J Small Anim Pract 1985; 26, 3–15
16. Wheeler CB, Rodeheaver GT, Thacker JG, et al: Side effects of high-pressure irrigation. Surg Gynecol Obstet 1976; 143:775–778
17. Peterson LW: Prophylaxis of wound infection: Studies with particular reference to soaps with irrigation. Arch Surg 1945; 50:177
18. Amber EI, Henderson RA, Swaim SF, Gray BW: A comparison of antimicrobial efficacy and tissue reaction of four antiseptics on canine wounds. Vet Surg 1983; 12(2):63–68
19. Lee AH, Swaim SF, McGuire JA, Hughes KS: Effects of chlorhexidine diacetate, povidone-iodine, and polyhydroxydine on wound healing in dogs. J Am Anim Hosp Assoc 1988; 24:77–84
20. Platt J, Bucknall RA: An experimental evaluation of antiseptic wound irrigation. J Hosp Infec 1984; 5:181–188
21. Sanchez IR, Swaim SF, Nusbaum KE, et al: Chlorhexidine diacetate and povidone-iodine cytotoxicity to canine embryonic fibroblasts and Staphylococcus aureus. Vet Surg 1988; 17(4):182–185
22. Sanchez IR, Swaim SF, Nusbaum KE, et al: Effects of chlorhexidine and povidone-iodine on wound healing in dogs. Vet Surg 1988; 17(6):291–295
23. Lineaweaver W, McCorris S, Soucy D, Howard R: Cellular and bacterial toxicities of topical antimicrobials. Plast Reconstr Surg 1985; 75:394–396
24. Lineaweaver W, Howard R, Soucy D, et al: Topical antimicrobial toxicity. Arch Surg 1985; 120:267–270

25. Edlich RF, Custer J, Madden J, et al: Studies in the contaminated wound: III. Assessment of the effectiveness of irrigation with antiseptic agents. Am J Surg 1969; 118:21–30
26. Zamora JL: Chemical and microbiologic characteristics and toxicity of povidone-iodine solutions. Am J Surg 1986; 151:400–406
27. Swaim SF, Lee AH: Topical wound medications: A review. J Am Vet Med Assoc 1987; 190(12):1588–1593
28. Berkleman RL, Holland BW, Anderson RL: Increased bactericidal activity of dilute solutions of povidone-iodine solution. J Clin Microbiol 1982; 15:635–639
28. Tvedten HW, Till GO: Effect of povidone, povidone-iodine and iodide in locomotion (in vitro) of neutrophils from people rats dogs and cats. Am J Vet Res 1985; 46:1797–1800
30. Viljanto J: Disinfection of surgical wounds without inhibition of normal wound healing. Arch Surg 1980; 115:253–256
31. Prince HN, Nonemaker WS, Norgard RC, Prince DL: Drug resistance studies with topical antiseptics. J Pharm Sci 1978; 67(11):1629–1631
32. Russell AD: Chlorhexidine: Antibacterial action and bacterial resistance. Infection 1986; 14:212–214
33. Rosenberg A, Alatary SB, Peterson AF: Safety and efficacy of the antiseptic chlorhexidine gluconate. Surg Gynecol Obstet 1976; 143:789–792
34. Okano M, Nomura M, Hata S, et al: Anaphylactic symptoms due to chlorhexidine gluconate. Arch Dermatol 1989; 125:50–52
35. Tatnall FM, Leigh IM, Gibson JR: Comparative study of antiseptic toxicity on basal keratinocytes, transformed human keratinocytes and fibroblasts. Skin Pharmacol 1990; 3:157–163
36. Leveen HH, Faik G, Borek B, et al: Chemical acidification of wounds: An adjuvant to healing and the unfavorable action of alkalinity and ammonia. Ann Surg 1982; 178:745–753
37. Gruber RP, Vistnes L, Pardoe R: The effect of commonly used antiseptics on wound healing. Plast Reconstr Surg 1975; 55:472–476
38. Guyton AC: Textbook of Medical Physiology, 7th ed. Philadelphia: WB Saunders, 1986, p 54
39. Rodoman GV, Sultanonv NSH, Khrupalov AA, et al: Prevention of infection of surgical wounds under experimental conditions. Klin Khir 1991;1:16–18
40. Dirschl DR, Wilson FC: Topical antibiotic irrigation in the prophylaxis of infections in orthopedic surgery. Orthop Clin North Am 1991; 22:419–426
41. Scher KS, Peoples JB: Combined use of topical and systemic antibiotics. Am J Surg 1991; 161:422–425
42. Burke JF: The effective period of preventative antibiotic action in experimental incisions and dermal lesions: Role of antibiotics in wound lavage. Surgery 1961; 50:161–184
43. Edlich RF, Smith QT, Edgerton MT: Resistance of the surgical wound to prophylaxis of infection and its mechanisms of development. Am J Surg 1973; 126:583–591
44. Halasz NA: Wound infection and topical antibiotics. Arch Surg 1977; 112:1240–1244
45. Lord JW Jr, Laraja RD, Daliana M, Gordon MT: Prophylactic antibiotic irrigation in gastric, biliary and colonic surgery. Am J Surg 1983; 145:209–212
46. Rosenstein BD, Wilson FC, Funderburk CH: The use of bacitracin irrigation to prevent in postoperative skeletal wounds: An experimental study. J Bone Joint Surg 1989; 71A:427–430
47. Hopson WB, Britt LG, Sherman RT, Ledes CP: The use of topical antibiotics in the control of experimental wound infection. J Surg Res 1968; 8:261–266
48. Scherr DD, Dodd TA: In vitro bacteriological evaluation of the effectiveness of antimicrobial irrigating solutions. J Bone Joint Surg 1976; 58A(1):119–122
49. Seco JL, Ojeda E, Reguilon C, et al: Combined topical and systemic antibiotic prophylaxis in acute appendicitis. Am J Surg 1990; 159:226–230
50. Gingrass RP, Close AS, Ellison EH: The effect of various topical and parenteral agents on the prevention of infection in experimental contaminated wounds. J Trauma 1964; 4:763–783
51. Matushek KJ, Rosin E: Pharmicokinetics of cephazolin applied topically to the surgical wound. Arch Surg 1991; 126:890–893
52. Lee AH, Swaim SF, Yang ST, Wilken LO: Effects of gentamicin solution and cream on the healing of open wounds. Am J Vet Res 1984; 45:1487–1492
53. Waterman NB, Howell RS, Babich M: The effect of nine prophylactic antibiotics on the incidence of wound infection. J Surg Res 1968; 8:261–266
54. Swaim SF, Henderson RA: Small Animal Wound Management. Philadelphia: Lea & Febiger, 1990, pp 47–49
55. Edlich RF, Madden JE, Prusak M, et al: Studies in the management of the contaminated wound: VI. The therapeutic value of gentle scrubbing in prolonging the limited period of effectiveness of antibiotics in contaminated wounds. Am J Surg 1971; 121:668–672
56. Rasmussen JE: Topical antibiotics. J Dermatol Surg Oncol 1976; 2:69–71
57. Ashworth CD, Nelson DR: Antimicrobial potentiation of irrigation solutions containing tris(hydroxymethyl)aminomethane-EDTA. J Am Vet Med Assoc 1990; 197:1513–1514

58. Pearman JW, Bailey M, Harper WE: Comparison of the efficacy of "Trisdine" and kanamycin-colistin bladder installations in reducing bacteruria during intermittent catheterizations of patients with acute spinal cord trauma. Br J Urol 1988; 62:140–144

59. Edlich RF, Rogers W, Kasper G, et al: Studies in the management of the contaminated wound: I. Optimal time for closure of contaminated open wounds. II. Comparison of resistence to infection of open and closed wounds during healing. Am J Surg 1969, 117:323–329

60. Eaglstein WH, Mertz PM: Effect of topical medicaments on the rate of repair of superficial wounds. In Dineen P, Hildick-Smith G (eds): The Surgical Wound. Philadelphia: Lea & Febiger, 1981, pp 150–170

61. Lesiewicz J, Goldsmith LA: Inhibition of rat skin ornithine decarboxylase by nitrofurazone. Arch Dermatol 1980; 116:1225–1226

62. Fischer, AA: The role of topical medications in the management of stasis ulcers. Angiology 1971; 22:206–210

63. Brown GL, Curtsinger L, Jurkiewicz MJ, et al: Stimulation of healing of chronic wounds by epidermal growth factor. Plast Reconstr Surg 1991; 88:189–196

64. Lee AH, Swaim SF, Yang ST, et al: The effects of petrolatum, polyethylene glycol, nitrofurazone, and a hydroactive dressing on open wound healing. J Am Anim Hosp Assoc 1986; 22:443–451

65. Eaglstein WH, Mertz PM: "Inert" vehicles do affect wound healing. J Invest Dermatol 1980; 74:90–91

66. Goodson W III, Hohn DC, Hunt TK, et al: Augmentation of some aspects of wound healing by a "skin respiratory factor." J Surg Res 1976; 21:125–129

67. Kaplan JZ: Acceleration of wound healing by a live yeast cell derivative. Arch Surg 1984; 119:1005–1008

68. Bigbie RB, Schumacher J, Swaim SF, et al: Effects of amnion and live yeast cell derivative on second-intention healing in horses. Am J Vet Res 1991; 52:1376–1382

69. Efem SEE: Clinical observations on the wound healing properties of honey. Br J Surg 1988; 75:679–681

70. Topham JD: Sugar paste in the treatment of pressure sores, burns and wounds. Pharm J 1988; 241:118–119

71. Cera LM, Heggers JP, Robson MC, Hagstrom WJ: The therapeutic efficacy of aloe vera cream (Dermaide Aloe) in thermal injuries: Two case reports. J Am Anim Hosp Assoc 1980; 16:768–772

72. Peacock EE: Collagenolysis and the biology of wound repair. In Peacock EE (ed): Wound Repair. Philadelphia: WB Saunders, 1984, pp 128–133

73. Booth LC: Second-intention healing and delayed closure. In White NA, Moore JN (eds): Current Practice of Equine Surgery. Philadelphia: Lippincott, 1990, pp 123–129

74. Sherry S, Fletcher A: Proteolytic enzymes: A therapeutic evaluation. Clin Pharmacol Ther 1960; 1:202–221

75. Quaglino D, Nanney LB, Kennedy R, Davidson JM: Transforming growth factor β stimulates wound healing and modulates extracellular matrix gene expression in pig skin: I. Excisional wound model. Lab Invest 1990; 63:307–319

76. Brown LB, Nanney LB, Griffen J, et al: Enhancement of wound healing by topical treatment with epidermal growth factor. N Engl J Med 1989; 321:76–79

77. Lawman MJP, Boyle MDP, Gee AP, Young M: Nerve growth factor accelerates the early cellular events associated with wound healing. Exp Molec Pathol 1985; 43:274–281

78. Cuzzell JZ: Choosing a wound dressing: A systematic approach. AACN Clin Iss 1990; 1:567–577

79. Swaim SF, Wilhalf D: The physics physiology and chemistry of bandaging open wounds. Compend Contin Educ Small Anim Pract 1985; 7:146–156

80. Linsky CB, Rovee DT, Dow T: Effects of dressing on wound inflammation and scar tissue. In Dineen P, Hildick-Smith G (eds): The Surgical Wound. Philadelphia: Lea & Febiger, 1981, pp 191–205

81. Lee AH, Swaim SF, McGuire JA, Hughes KS: Effects of nonadherent dressing materials on the healing of open wounds in dogs. J Am Vet Med Assoc 1987; 190:416–422

82. Alvarez OM, Mertz PM, Eaglstein WH: The effect of occlusive dressings on collagen synthesis and re-epithelialization in superficial wounds. J Surg Res 1983; 35:142–148

83. Winter GD: Oxygen and epidermal wound healing: Oxygen transport to tissue. In Silver IA (ed): Advances in Experimental Medicine and Biology. New York: Plenum Press, 1978, pp 673–678

84. Silver IA: Oxygen tension and epithelialization. In Maibach HI, Rovee TD (eds): Epidermal Wound Healing. Chicago: Year Book Medical Publishers, 1972, p 291

85. Berardesca E. Maibach HI: Skin occlusion treatment or drug-like device. Skin Pharmacol 1988; 1:207–215

86. Valdez H: A hydrogel preparation for cleansing and protecting equine wounds. Equine Pract 1980; 2(3):33–36

87. Lees MJ, Fretz PB, Baily JV, Jacobs KA: Principles of grafting. Compend Contin Educ Pract Vet 1989; 11:954–960

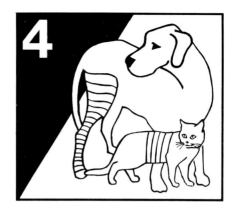

Historically, among physicians, surgeons have demonstrated the greatest interest, and have made the most concerted effort, in developing innovative, comprehensive, and effective methods for providing adequate nutritional support to patients in the widest range of conditions and clinical situations.[1]

NUTRITIONAL SUPPORT OF THE SURGICAL PATIENT

CANDACE E. LAYTON

During the past 20 to 30 years, there has been a significant renewal of interest in the role of nutrition in disease and disease prevention. People are more aware of dietary-affected diseases and diseases are being treated by dietary changes or supplements. Currently, there is an increase in research focused on understanding the persistence of hypermetabolism as a pathologic state and its modulation by specific nutrients. For example, arginine supplementation is associated with increased survival of septic or tumor-bearing animals.[2] Most clinicians are aware of the importance of good nutrition in the management of cases. Yet many patients do not receive adequate or appropriate nutritional support. In fact, many patients suffer nutritional deficiencies because they have been hospitalized. Food is routinely withheld from patients to facilitate diagnostic procedures or surgery. Pain and fear inhibit many patients, especially older ones, from eating. Often one fails to recognize malnutrition in a patient, especially if the patient is obese. Such concerns as the need for sedation or anesthesia in critical patients or surgical implantation of feeding tubes may cause clinicians to be reluctant to instigate enteral feeding.

In human medicine, 50% to 60% of all hospitalized patients suffer from some degree of malnutrition.[3–5] People admitted for elective surgery are expected to lose 5% to 10% of their preadmission weight.[6] Patients who undergo major surgical or medical therapies for significant disease often lose more than 25% of their previous weight.[6]

Weight loss may be the single best predictor of postoperative morbidity and mortality. In several studies in humans and experimental animals, significant weight loss correlated with poor wound healing, decreased immunocompetence, and death.[3, 7–9] The prevalence of malnutrition in veterinary patients is not known.

THE EFFECT OF NUTRITION ON WOUND HEALING

Malnutrition has been associated with poor wound healing. Clinical trials in humans have documented an increased incidence of postoperative wound infection and dehiscence in patients with malnutrition.[3, 5, 10, 11] With regard to wound healing, animals with hypoproteinemia have a prolonged lag phase and delayed onset of the fibroblastic phase.[12, 13] Hypoproteinemic dogs have radiographic signs of poor callus formation during fracture healing.[14]

It is not known if nutritional supplementation can significantly improve wound healing. While a positive response would be expected, not all clinical or experimental studies have supported this assumption. For instance, a study comparing the effects of hyperalimentation on the healing of skin, abdominal wall, and colon in rats suggested that there may be a difference in how malnutrition affects visceral compared with parietal tissue healing. Tensile strength of colonic anastomoses was not as affected by protein malnutrition compared with the tensile strength of the skin and abdominal wounds. It was not until weight loss reached 33% or greater that a significant effect on wound healing was seen. Improved wound healing associated with hyperalimentation was seen only in the abdominal wounds. Visceral wounds were more resistant to the effects of malnutrition and hyperalimentation.[15] Clinical trials in humans have correlated poor wound healing (defined as postoperative wound dehiscence or infection) with malnutrition.[3, 5, 10, 12, 16-18] Measurements associated with malnutrition include decreased plasma proteins (such as albumin, transferrin, and retinol-binding protein), abnormal anthropometric measurements, weight loss, and degree of immunocompetence.

Similar clinical studies have rarely been done in veterinary medicine. A retrospective study reported postoperative complications in 30 hypoalbuminemic dogs undergoing enterotomies.[19] The investigators found no significant abdominal wound dehiscence in the dogs. One dog died of peritonitis following enterotomy dehiscence and one dog with intact enterotomies developed peritonitis.

EFFECT OF NUTRITION ON THE IMMUNE SYSTEM

The relationship of nutrition, infection, and immunity is complex and characterized by conflicting reports from experimental and clinical studies. Malnutrition may be synergistic or antagonistic depending on the situation, degree of malnutrition, type of infection, or species.[20, 21] Infection in a malnourished patient may have more serious results compared with a well-nourished patient. In patients with minimal malnutrition, infection can cause seriously deficient states. Yet, a severe nutritional deficiency may limit the negative effects of infection, especially those involving infectious agents with an obligate dependency on metabolites or enzyme systems of the host.[20, 21]

A complete review of all known nutrient deficiencies and their effects on the immune system is beyond the scope of this chapter. Some specific nutrient deficiencies are mentioned to give a general perspective of the topic.

Protein–Calorie Malnutrition. Malnutrition is associated with absolute decreases in total lymphocyte counts, primarily T-lymphocytes. Cell-mediated immunity is more affected than humoral immunity; there is decreased phagocytosis, opsonification, and complement fixation.[9, 22] The effect on immunoglobulins is not as clear, since elevated, normal, and decreased levels have been reported.[20–22] It also should be noted that while the absolute numbers of immunoglobulins can remain the same, their functional capacity may be altered by malnutrition.[22] Protein–calorie malnutrition has been shown to decrease secretory IgA levels. This could explain why malnourished patients are more at risk for respiratory or digestive tract infections.[20, 22]

Vitamin Deficiencies. Most of the experimental data include the effects of single deficiencies. Classically, vitamin A deficiency has been associated with an increased infection rate. It is not clear if the infection induces a hypovitaminosis or malnutrition results in decreased vitamin A, which exacerbates infection.[9] Other effects of vitamin A deficiency include altered cell-mediated immunity and decreased T-lymphocytes.[22] Nonspecific effects of vitamin A deficiency include increased morbidity and mortality due to diarrheal or respiratory disease.[23, 24] A significant reduction in the mortality rate of malnourished children occurred after regular supplementation of vitamin A.[23]

Vitamin B_6 (pyridoxine) deficiency inhibits nucleic acid synthesis, resulting in decreased cell multiplication, antibody formation, and protein synthesis.[9] Impaired wound healing and an atypical inflammatory response are associated with vitamin C deficiency.[13]

Mineral Deficiencies. Zinc is involved in a number of cellular functions, including protein and nucleic acid metabolism.[25] Poor wound healing and a depressed immune response are associated with zinc deficiency.[9, 13] The relationship of iron to the immune system is not clear. Some studies suggest that an iron deficiency is associated with decreased bactericidal effects of neutrophils and a reduction in T-lymphocytes. Other studies have not supported these findings. Iron supplementation during acute bacterial infections is not recommended, because increasing the serum iron levels enhances bacterial growth.[9] Magnesium deficiency inhibits both primary and secondary immune responses.[9]

PATHOPHYSIOLOGY OF FASTING

There are fundamental differences in the response to fasting by normal patients compared with humans and animals with disease or cancer. An understanding of these differences is important in assessing a patient's nutritive state and in implementing rational therapeutic nutritional protocols.

Fasting in the Nonstressed Patient

In the normal, nonstressed animal or human, the overall response to fasting is to regulate body mechanisms to conserve energy. *The body converts from a glucose-based metabolism to the utilization of fats for energy and spares protein.* As intake decreases, levels of glucose, amino acids, and fatty acids decrease in the portal blood. This, in turn, results in a decrease in insulin, with concurrent increases in glucagon, cortisol, catecholamine, and growth hormone. As blood glucose levels drop, the liver responds by producing glucose. Glucose is produced by the breakdown of glucose stores (glycogenolysis) and the production of new glucose (gluconeogenesis). In the initial days (24 to 48 hours) of fasting, hepatic glycogen stores rapidly deplete. Gluconeogenesis maintains normal blood glucose levels. This is important because red blood cells, white blood cells, the renal medulla, and the central nervous system have an obligate need for glucose as fuel. Other body tissues rapidly adapt by using fatty acids and ketones as energy sources. Amino acids (primarily alanine), lactate, pyruvate, and glycerol are used to make new glucose. Catabolism of body proteins to provide energy results in a negative nitrogen balance. Since the body does not store protein, any loss of protein results in some loss of function. Catabolism of labile protein stores, such as visceral proteins, occurs first, followed by loss of muscle and skeletal protein with prolonged starvation. This differential loss may be the reason why some tissues heal slower than others. Also, since weight loss correlates closely with loss of muscle and fat, patients with significant weight loss have already undergone severe depletion of vital body proteins.

Besides adapting cellular metabolism to a fat-based fuel, the normal body also conserves energy by decreasing resting energy expenditure. This occurs by decreasing basal metabolic rate, loss of cellular mass, and decreasing physical activity. After 7 to 10 days of fasting, the central nervous system adapts to ketones for an energy source, which limits protein catabolism.[26-30]

Fasting in the Stressed Patient

In the stressed patient, the normal response to fasting is inhibited or altered. *A hypermetabolic state occurs with an increased requirement for energy and nutrients for wound healing, the inflammatory response, and immunologic defense.* These patients exhibit a marked negative nitrogen balance in proportion to the severity of the underlying injury.[26] Additionally, these patients continue to have· an obligate demand for glucose, which requires proteins as the primary substrate. The ability to spare protein and utilize fatty acids or ketones is inhibited.[26-30]

Malnutrition and Cancer

Evaluation of the pathophysiology of cancer cachexia is an exciting and controversial area of research. *Weight loss, the hallmark of cachexia, is the result of an imbalance between energy intake and energy expenditure.* Chemotherapy, radiotherapy, and physical obstruction of the gastrointestinal tract by tumor are potential causes of decreased appetite and energy intake.[31, 32] Vomiting, diarrhea, altered taste perception, and depression also contribute to anorexia. Not all patients with weight loss, however, have these signs. Increased energy expenditure could easily account for the weight loss. Unfortunately, measurements of energy expenditure have not been uniform, and hypometabolic, hypermetabolic, and normal rates have been reported.[32, 33]

Several studies suggest that metabolism may be different in a patient with cancer compared with a normal, fasting patient.[31, 32, 34-37] For example, the cancer patient tends to be insulin-resistant and hyperglycemic, with decreased glucose tolerance curves. Tumors cells prefer to metabolize glucose by anaerobic glycolysis and form lactate. Compared with aerobic pathways, this is very inefficient. Glucose, normally metabolized by the host to generate 38 mol of adenosine triphosphate, is now being used by the tumor.[34, 35, 37] Tumor-bearing patients continue to have an obligate demand for proteins because of increased rates of tumor protein synthesis and gluconeogenesis. This failure to adapt occurs even if adequate levels of carbohydrates are available.[31, 35]

Other areas of interest, besides the metabolic derangements associated with cancer, are the effect of nutritional supplementation on cachexia.[32, 38] Will reversing the host's malnutrition increase tumor growth, or will improving the nutritive state allow more patients to complete therapy and increase survival? The answers to these questions, however, are not clear. Experimentally, parenteral nutrition was associated with stimulation of tumor metastasis, although this association has not been documented clinically.[39] Longer survival times, however, also have not been consistently associated with nutritional support.[33, 36]

PATIENT EVALUATION

Assessment of Nutritional Status

The importance of accurate assessment of nutritional status cannot be overlooked. Implementation of appropriate feeding protocols involves expense, expertise, technical support, and a potential for patient morbidity or mortality. The benefits of nutritional support may be improved wound healing, restored immunocompetency, decreased length of hospitalization, less postoperative infections, and a sense of well-being for the patient.

Much evidence exists to correlate malnutrition with increased morbidity and mortality. However, the evidence is not clear that correcting nutritional deficiencies will always be valuable. A recent retrospective study in people suggested that not all patients benefited from parenteral feeding.[40] In fact, a higher rate of complications occurred in patients receiving parenteral feeding compared with patients not nutritionally supported. Most complications were related to catheter-induced problems.[40] This does not mean that parenteral nutrition is contraindicated, but rather that not every patient needs or will benefit from nutritional support. Before giving nutritional supplementation, one should first know if the patient is malnourished or likely to become malnourished during the course of the disease. Also, one needs to assess the response to nutritional therapy and determine if the risks of treatment outweigh the benefits.

Subjective Assessment. Clinical signs such as poor coat condition, dull eyes, decreased mental alertness, lethargy, and loss of muscle mass or fat are often the first clues of malnutrition (Fig. 4–1). These signs also may be present in other disease states, with or without malnutrition. Patients with chronic vomiting, diarrhea, or draining wounds lose large amounts of nutrients. Anorexia lasting more than 3 to 4 days can cause malnutrition. Anticipating anorexia is also important. Animals are routinely held off food prior to diagnostic procedures or surgery. Many drugs, especially steroids and chemotherapeutics, affect the patient's ability to use nutrients and may contribute to increased rates of catabolism. The type of surgical procedure can have an effect on the gastrointestinal tract. For example, patients with major revisions involving the stomach and proximal intestinal tract may not be capable of digesting or assimilating nutrients.

Objective Assessment. In humans, measurements of nutritional status range from simple to complex laboratory techniques. Morbidity, mortality, degree of malnutrition, and response to nutritional protocols correlate with these measurements. There does not appear to be one single, accurate measurement determining nutritional state.[7, 11, 41–45]

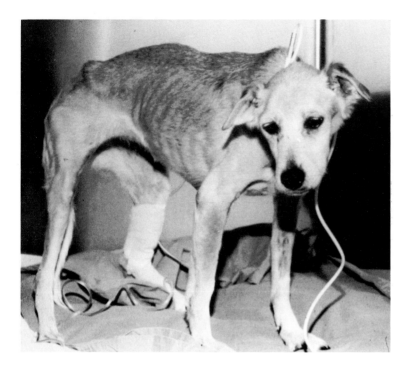

Figure 4–1. Severely malnourished patient being supported by total parenteral nutrition. Note the obvious clinical signs of malnutrition such as loss of body fat and muscle mass and depression.

Anthropometric measurements (such as triceps skin-fold thickness, midarm circumference, weight in relation to height, and creatinine–height index) form the basis of many nutritional assessments in humans.[41, 43–46] These measurements are impractical in veterinary medicine owing to the wide variability of patients.

Laboratory tests for evaluating nutritional status include measurements of total lymphocyte counts, visceral proteins (albumin, transferrin, prealbumin or transthyretin, and retinol-binding protein), and assessment of immunocompetence.[7, 8, 11, 42–44, 46] A patient's response to standardized delayed hypersensitivity skin tests reflects the level of immunocompetence. Anergy, or failure to exhibit a cutaneous response to the injected antigen, correlates with a high incidence of morbidity and mortality in humans.[6, 16, 47, 48] Other diseases, drugs, anesthesia, or surgery, however, can affect immunocompetence regardless of the presence or absence of malnutrition.

Malnutrition depresses total lymphocyte counts and may be an estimation of immune competency. In humans, counts below 800 to 1000/μl reflect an impairment.[6, 47] Ranges of lymphocyte counts in malnourished animals have not been established, and other factors such as drug therapy or disease can cause lymphocytopenia.

Labile protein stores are rapidly exhausted in malnourished humans and animals because of obligate protein catabolism. These labile proteins include visceral proteins and acute-phase proteins such as albumin, transferrin, prealbumin (transthyretin), and retinol-binding protein. Hypoalbuminemia in humans correlates with increased risk of wound dehiscence, postoperative infection, and prolonged hospitalization.[3, 5, 10, 17, 18] Several studies suggest that hypoalbuminemia may be an accurate indicator of malnutrition and a good predictor of morbidity.[3, 5, 10, 17, 18] Problems associated with using albumin as a nutritional marker include nonnutritional causes of hypoalbuminemia such as liver or renal dysfunction. Because of the long half-life of albumin

(8 days), it is not sensitive to early changes associated with refeeding.[49-51] Rapid-turnover proteins, such as retinol-binding protein and transthyretin, may be more sensitive markers of malnutrition and the patient's response to refeeding.[49-54] The significance of these proteins as markers of nutritional status has not been documented in veterinary patients.

Malnutrition affects skeletal muscle function. In humans, stimulation of the ulnar nerve with measurement of the force of contraction of the adductor pollicis correlates highly with malnutrition.[55, 56] Additionally, return to normal function may be recognized before normalization of other nutritional measures such as weight gain.[8, 55]

Weight loss continues to be the hallmark of any nutritional assessment protocol. Moderate or severe weight loss is associated with increased morbidity and mortality in humans and animals.[6, 8, 16, 18] As a single parameter, weight loss may be more accurate in determining malnutrition and in predicting potential outcome. Weight loss greater than 10% is significant and implies that malnutrition exists.

Because of the complex interactions among disease, nutrition, and the immune system, it is difficult to determine accurately the significance and validity of the various measures of nutritional status. Since many of the measurements are cumbersome, impractical, or unknown in the veterinary patient, clinical impression based on historical and physical evidence will continue to be the mainstay of nutritional assessment in the veterinary patient. Studies in humans validate the use of subjective assessment based on clinical impression and history.[7, 17, 41] Guidelines proposed for assessment of nutritional state are summarized in Table 4–1.

FEEDING PROTOCOLS

Enteral versus Parenteral

After establishing a need for nutritional support, decisions can be made about routes of feeding and diets. The clinical status of the patient, experience and motivation of the clinician and support staff, available facilities, and desires of the client provide the basis for these decisions. If the intestinal tract is functional, enteral feeding is preferred. Enteral feeding is less costly, requires less monitoring and technical support, and has less chance for serious morbidity or mortality. Enteral feeding is important to maintain normal intestinal integrity. Structural changes of the intestinal microvilli are seen in starving patients or patients on total parenteral nutrition.[57-59] These structural and functional alterations may allow translocation of intestinal bacteria into the systemic circulation.[60, 61] Humans receiving total parenteral nutrition have decreased secretory IgA and a reduction in intestinal mucosal mass associated with bacterial translocation.[60] Several experimental studies demonstrated the importance of luminal contents (nutrients) in maintaining normal structural and functional intestinal integrity.[58, 60-63] For example, ingested glucose caused a greater insulin response compared to intravenous glucose or glucose given by stomach tube.[7]

Enteral Feeding

Enteral feeding involves the provision of food into the gastrointestinal tract. This can be accomplished by several methods. Selection of an appro-

TABLE 4–1. Guidelines for Nutritional Assessment

Historical evidence

Vomiting
Diarrhea
Chronic draining wounds
Catabolic drugs (steroids, chemotherapeutic drugs)
Anorexia
>1–2 days in young animals
>4–5 days in adults
Anticipated causes
(surgical resection, neurologic problems, postoperative infections or ileus)

Physical examination

Depression
Lack of body fat
Muscle wasting
Dull, dry hair coat
Structural impediments (fractured jaw)
Weight loss
>10% in adult animals
>5% in young animals

Laboratory parameters

Lymphopenia
<1000/μl in dogs
<1500/μl in cats
Hypoalbuminemia, <2.5 mg/dl

priate method is based on patient status, anticipated duration of feeding, the location of functional digestive tract, and technical support. For example, oral tube feedings may be given in tractable patients who you suspect will eat once the gastrointestinal tract is stimulated. A jejunostomy tube may be more appropriate for a patient that has had major revision of the stomach.

Oral Feeding. In some patients with normal function of the mouth and digestive tract, stimulating the appetite may be the only requirement needed to start voluntary eating. Warming a highly palatable food, such as a canned catfood, will intensify the aroma. With animals that will not eat because they are anxious or afraid of their surroundings, hand-feeding the diet in a quiet, reassuring manner may encourage them to eat.

Some animals will tolerate small amounts of food given as bolus feedings. Small balls of food can be placed at the back of the tongue in the pharyngeal area. Closing the mouth and gently rubbing the throat may induce swallowing.

There are several concerns in relying on these techniques for nutrient support. The animal should have a functional digestive tract that will allow it to digest and assimilate the food. Manipulation of the head or mouth for bolus feedings requires a docile animal who tolerates handling. Palatable food with a high caloric density should be used. As most animals will begin to reject force feedings, this technique should not be used for animals requiring long-term (greater than 2 to 3 days) support.

Appetite stimulation has been done both experimentally and clinically using a variety of drugs. Appropriate use of drugs may stimulate normal feeding patterns; however, the underlying cause and treatment of the anorexia should not be overlooked. Even though such animals respond and begin to eat, they rarely consume sufficient calories to correct deficiencies or maintain a positive nitrogen balance. Therefore, selection of a calorie-dense, high-protein, high-fat diet is important.

The benzodiazepine derivatives are effective short-term appetite stimulants in dogs and cats.[64, 65] These drugs work by increasing the activity of a neurotransmitter, γ-aminobutyric acid, which suppresses serotonin. Serotonin inhibits endogenous opiates, resulting in appetite suppression. By blocking the effects of serotonin, the appetite suppression may be reversed. Diazepam (Valium, Hoffman–La Roche, Inc., Nutley, NJ 07110) is an example of a commonly used benzodiazepine given by injection or orally. Intravenous injection has the most effective and predictable response compared with oral administration. Oxazepam (Serax, Wyeth-Ayerst Laboratories, Philadelphia, PA 19101) is another, less commonly used benzodiazepine available only in an oral form. See Table 4–2 for recommended doses.

The benzodiazepine derivatives work best in situations where short-term anorexia is expected. While they can be administered two to three times a day, the drugs may cause depression, sedation, or ataxia. The higher doses are more reliable in stimulating appetite; however, the degree of sedation may contraindicate their use. Another problem with these drugs is their wide variation in response. Dogs seem to be more resistant to the positive effects of diazepam. It also appears that some animals may become resistant to the drugs as additional doses are given. Intravenous administration is more reliable in affecting appetite and initiates a faster response, within minutes. Oral administration may take 20 to 30 minutes before an effect is seen.

Other drugs used for long-term appetite stimulation include corticosteroids and anabolic steroids. Corticosteroids have been used for many years for their nonspecific effect of polyphagia. The benefit of corticosteroids may be overshadowed by negative effects such as increased catabolism or depression of the immune system.

Anabolic steroids also have been used in humans and animals to reverse the catabolic effects of trauma, surgery, or disease.[65, 66] The effectiveness of these drugs has not been evaluated clinically in the dog or cat. Currently, the drug stanozolol (Winstrol-V, Winthrop Veterinary, Sterling Animal Health Products, Division of Sterling Drug, Inc., New York, NY 10016) is the only anabolic steroid approved for use in animals. The U.S. Food and Drug Administration has categorized stanozolol as a schedule III drug. This requires that the drug be secured and careful records of its dispensation be made. As with the other drugs to stimulate appetite, anabolic steroids should not be used in place of appropriate diagnostic and therapeutic procedures to reverse the anorexia.

Oral Tube Feeding. This technique involves placing a feeding tube through the mouth and into the stomach or distal aspect of the esophagus. Before passing the feeding tube, it is measured and marked to the desired level of

TABLE 4–2. Appetite-Stimulating Drugs

DRUG	DOSE	ROUTE	SPECIES	REFERENCE
Diazepam	1–2 mg total	Oral	Cat	Crowe[68]
	0.1–0.2 mg/kg	Oral	Dog	Crowe[68]
	0.05–0.1 mg/kg	IV	Dog/cat	Crowe[68]
	0.2 mg/kg	IV	Dog/cat	Macy and Gasper[65]
Oxazepam	2.5 mg total	Oral	Cat	Macy and Gasper[65]
	0.3–0.4 mg/kg	Oral	Dog	Crowe[68]

insertion. Since the tube will only be in place for the duration of a single feeding, placement into the stomach will not cause a problem with distal esophageal sphincter incompetence. For gastric placement, the tube is measured from the nose to the 12th or 13th rib. To measure for esophageal placement, the tube is marked at the level of the 7th or 8th rib. Alternatively, the tube may be marked at the 13th rib and 75% of this measurement taken. A simple mouth speculum can be made using a roll of adhesive tape (see Fig. 4–2). With the dog's or cat's head held in a neutral position, the feeding tube is passed gently to the back of the throat. By gently bumping the tube against the pharyngeal wall, the animal can be induced to swallow. Many animals object as the tube is initially passed into the mouth but relax as the tube passes into the esophagus. The animal's head should be maintained in a neutral position, since flexing the neck abruptly may allow the tube to pass into the trachea. Small, stiff catheters are likely to be inadvertently passed into the trachea.

Several types of feeding tubes can be used (Table 4–3). Red rubber urinary catheters (Sovereign Feeding Tube and Urethral Catheter, Sherwood Medical Industries, St. Louis, MO 63103, or Bard Urological Catheter, Bard Urological Division, C.R. Bard, Inc., Covington, GA 30209) are inexpensive and commonly available. Silastic (Silastic tubing, Dow Corning Corp., Midland, MI 48640) or polyvinyl (Infant Feeding Tube, Mallinckrodt Critical Care, Division of Mallinckrodt, Inc., Glens Falls, NY 12801) stomach tubes are also available in several sizes. No. 5 French or no. 8 French catheters are best for small patients, whereas a larger-bore catheter is appropriate for large dogs. It is helpful if the catheter has a funneled or graduated end so that a catheter-tip syringe can be used to administer a liquid or blended diet. After placement of the feeding tube, its location should be determined. Ideally, one would expect a dog or cat to cough or choke if the tube was passing into the trachea. This does not always occur, and even the instillation of sterile water (15 to 20 ml) may not elicit a cough. Careful palpation of the neck may reveal the tube within the esophagus. Air also can be blown into the tube and the stomach auscultated for gas bubbles. Specific confirmation requires direct observation of tube passage or radiographic evidence of tube placement in the stomach or esophagus.

Successful use of this technique depends on having a docile yet alert

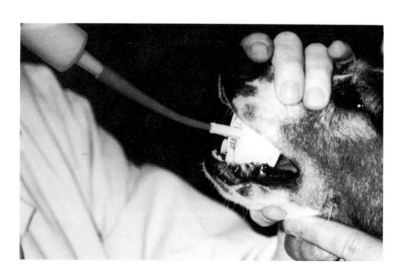

Figure 4–2. Technique of oral tube feeding. A simple mouth speculum has been made using a roll of adhesive tape. Keeping the patient's head in a neutral position will lessen the chances of inadvertently passing the tube into the trachea.

TABLE 4-3. Examples of Enteral Feeding Tubes

Polyurethane enteral feeding tube	Sherwood Medical, St. Louis, MO 63103
Silicone enteral feeding tube with weighted tip	Sherwood Medical, St. Louis, MO 63103
Indwell polyurethane feeding tube	Sherwood Medical, St. Louis, MO 63103
Premature infant feeding tube	Davol, Inc., C.R. Bard, Inc., Cranston, RI 02910
Infant feeding tube	Mallinckrodt Critical Care, Glens Falls, NY 12801
Flexiflo enteral feeding tube	Ross Laboratory, Division of Abbott Laboratories, Columbus, OH 43216
Red rubber feeding catheter	Bard Urological Division, C.R. Bard, Inc., Covington, GA 30209
	Sherwood Medical, St. Louis, MO 63103

patient who will tolerate tube placement. The digestive tract should be normal and able to assimilate food. Complications associated with this technique include endotracheal intubation, vomiting, regurgitation, aspiration pneumonia, pharyngeal trauma, and patient stress. Vomiting may occur if a large volume is delivered too rapidly or if the food is not warm. Endotracheal intubation can be avoided by using a large-bore tube, keeping the head in a neutral position, and critical evaluation of tube placement. If there is any doubt, the tube should be replaced. Aspiration pneumonia may be a problem if a patient vomits or regurgitates and subsequently inhales food particles. This is more likely in debilitated patients or in animals with a depressed gag response (sedation due to drugs or neurologic disorders).

Nasoesophageal, Nasogastric, and Nasoenteral Tubes. Nasal feeding tubes are used frequently in human patients, especially since small, soft plastic or Silastic, weighted catheters are now available. Small, soft catheters increase patient comfort, and people can tolerate nasal intubation for 6 to 8 weeks.[46] Nasal feeding techniques are also used in veterinary medicine. Excellent descriptions of the technique and use in clinical patients have been reported.[27-30, 64, 67-69] Nasal feeding tubes should not be used if the patient is comatose, in lateral recumbency, vomiting persistently, or if functional or structural gastric outflow obstruction exists.

Several sizes and makes of nasal feeding tubes are available, including very small-bore tubes which permit nasal feeding in small dogs and cats (Table 4-3). Polyurethane tubes may be better than polyvinyl tubes because they are softer, more pliable, and cause less irritation to nasal mucosa. Some catheters are available with weighted tips to facilitate passage of the tube into the proximal duodenum. Catheters also may have stylets, which makes insertion of the catheter easier in large dogs.

Nasal feeding tubes may be placed with the animal conscious, sedated, or anesthetized as an adjunctive procedure to the primary surgery. Some animals, especially those which are alert and not debilitated, tend to resist placement of the tube. Sedation may be helpful for these patients to facilitate passage of the tube. Sneezing may be a problem, particularly in dogs, because the animals will sneeze the tube out of the nostril. After selection of an appropriate feeding tube, a few drops of local anesthetic, such as 2% lidocaine, is instilled in the nostril. Some of the commercially available nasal tubes have a hygroscopic polymer that makes the tube slippery when wet. The tube also can be lubricated with 2% lidocaine jelly or a water-soluble jelly. Next, the tube should be measured for placement in the digestive tract.

While the common name used for most nasal feeding tubes is *nasogastric tube*, in animals the tube is often placed in the distal portion of the esophagus to avoid distal sphincter incompetence. For placement in the stomach or esophagus, the tube is measured as was described for orogastric intubation. Because of anatomic differences between the dog and cat, placement of the nasal feeding tube is slightly different for each animal. In the dog, the tube is first directed medially and dorsally over the alar fold and ventrolateral ridge (Fig. 4–3). After passing over this ridge, the tube is directed medially and ventrally into the ventral meatus. If the tube has entered the dorsal meatus, resistance will be felt as the tube hits the ethmoid turbinate at the level of the eye. Backing the tube out and redirecting it medially and ventrally may help. Also, intubation of the other nostril may be more successful. Recently, a modified technique was described to facilitate nasal intubation.[70] After directing the tip of the tube in a caudoventral, medial direction, the external nares are pushed dorsally. This maneuver will open the ventral meatus, allowing easier passage of the feeding tube.[70] Cats lack a ventral ridge, so the tube can be directed medially and ventrally initially. The head should be held in a neutral position. Excessive flexion or extension of the neck may cause the tube to be directed more easily into the trachea. Care should be taken to manipulate the tube gently to avoid nasal hemorrhage.

Correct tube placement is determined by injection of air into the tube. The left paralumbar fossa is auscultated for sounds of air within the stomach or esophagus. Sterile water, 15 to 20 ml, can be injected and the animal observed for coughing. However, not all animals will show a positive response to this test. It is surprising how easily a nasal tube passes into the trachea without the animal showing signs of discomfort or distress. This seems to happen more often with small, stiff tubes or in depressed patients with a reduced gag response. In humans, cannulation of the trachea, even with a cuffed endotracheal tube in place, or insertion into the pleural space has been reported.[71] If any doubt exists about the location of the tube, radiography should be performed.

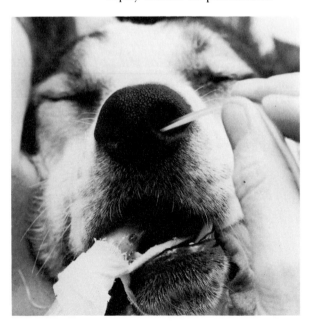

Figure 4–3. To pass the nasogastric tube in a dog, the tube is first directed medially and dorsally over the alar fold and ventrolateral ridge. After passing this ridge, the tube is directed medially and ventrally into the ventral meatus.

The tube can be secured with 3–0 or 4–0 nonabsorbable sutures or superglue. It is important to secure the tube closely to the nostril as it exits from the nose; otherwise, the animal may be able to pull out the catheter (Fig. 4–4). The tube can be positioned on the bridge of the nose, between the ears, or along the side of the face. Tubes that have been placed too close to tactile hairs may bother the animal and stimulate removal of the tube. An Elizabethan collar also may be used to keep the animal from rubbing its nose.

Placement of a nasojejunal catheter is possible using a weighted-tip tube. Problems noted with this procedure include increased cost of the feeding tubes and reverse peristalsis with displacement of the tube into the stomach. In some cases, the tube does not pass through the pylorus.

Advantages of the nasal feeding tube include simplicity, increased patient comfort compared with orogastric feedings, and a relatively long duration of use. Bolus feedings can be given three to four times daily, which makes maintenance easier in a busy practice. Complications are not common but can include vomiting, diarrhea, aspiration pneumonia, rhinitis, and gastroesophageal reflux. Vomiting and diarrhea are most often due to excessive food given rapidly. This can be avoided by small, frequent feedings and warming the food. Feedings also can be administered through an infusion pump. The total caloric requirement can be met, yet the small volumes will be more physiologic. Postoperative vomiting secondary to gastric immotility may be controlled with metoclopramide (Reglan, A.H. Robbins Co., Richmond, VA 23220). This drug is contraindicated if a gastric outflow obstruction exists.

Pharyngostomy Tube. The use of pharyngostomy tubes has been described in veterinary medicine.[72] They may be well tolerated by the animal for several weeks, and often owners can be trained to feed their animal at home. Because large-bore tubes can be placed, it is possible to use a blended diet of canned dog or cat food. The techniques for insertion of a pharyngostomy tube have been reported. [68, 72–77] Several types of feeding tubes can be used. Examples

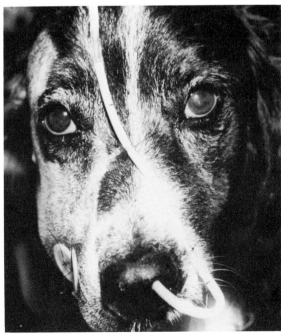

Figure 4–4. It is important to secure the nasogastric tube closely to the nostril as the tube exits from the naris. Otherwise, the patient may be able to remove the tube by rubbing its nose.

of suitable tubes include red rubber feeding catheters and Silastic or silicone tubing. The size of the tube is based on patient size and type of diet to be used. A no. 8 to 12 French is used in small patients, whereas a no. 14 to 20 French may be used in large dogs. Tubes smaller than a no. 8 French can be used but are more likely to kink or be dislodged. Small-bore tubes also require liquid feeding formulas.

In most situations, general anesthesia is needed. A right-handed surgeon may feel more comfortable inserting the tube in the left pharyngeal wall. The rostral, ventrolateral cervical area is clipped, and a surgical scrub is applied. After placing a mouth speculum, the left index finger is passed into the mouth, caudal to the angle of the mandible. The hyoid apparatus is palpated, and a space, termed the *piriform fossa*, will be felt. This space is in the ventral lateral pharyngeal wall between the angle of the jaw and the hyoid apparatus.[73]

A modification of the original pharyngostomy tube placement was reported in 1986.[75] In this retrospective and experimental study, a significant number of complications were associated with pharyngostomy tubes. Major complications were airway obstruction and aspiration pneumonia. Presumably, these complications were induced by cranial placement of the pharyngostomy tube. In anatomic dissections, the tube was seen to course over the larynx, interfering with the epiglottis (Fig. 4–5). *A modified technique was proposed, with placement of the pharyngostomy tube caudal and dorsal to the hyoid apparatus and epiglottis* (Fig. 4–6). *This allows the tube to be inserted more directly into the esophagus, avoiding the epiglottis.*[68, 72, 75]

Regardless of where the tube is placed, the technique of insertion is similar. A small skin incision is made over the bulge created by the surgeon's finger. A hemostat is used to bluntly dissect through the subcutaneous tissue and pharyngeal wall into the oral cavity. It may be necessary to sharply incise the pharyngeal mucosa to complete the ostomy. The end of the feeding tube is grasped and withdrawn through the pharyngeal wall. The opposite end is inserted into the esophagus. As with nasal feeding tubes, the pharyngostomy

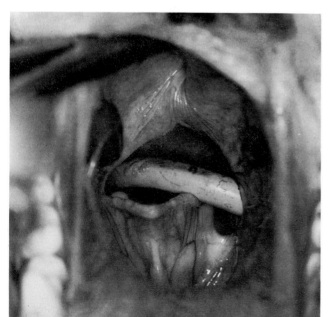

Figure 4–5. Note the interference of the epiglottis by a pharyngostomy tube that has been placed incorrectly.

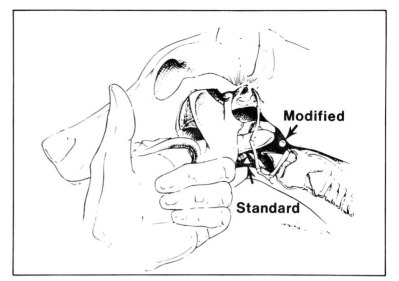

Figure 4–6. Diagram illustrates correct placement for pharyngostomy tube. Triangle indicates standard approach, and circle refers to preferred, modified technique. (From Crowe DT, Downs MO: Pharyngostomy complications in dogs and cats and recommended technical modifications. J Am Anim Hosp Assoc 22:493, 1986. Reprinted with permission.)

tube may be placed to end in the esophagus or stomach. Because of the potential for gastric reflux and esophagitis if the tube is placed into the stomach, midesophageal placement is recommended.[76]

The tube may be secured with a friction suture (Chinese finger trap), tape butterfly, or superglue. A dressing is applied to the exit wound, and the tube is secured to the neck using a light circumferential bandage. The dressing and bandage should be changed frequently, and the skin around the tube site should be cleaned of any exudate.

During the surgical approach, it is possible to damage vital structures such as the hypoglossal nerve, lingual artery, vagosympathetic trunk, external carotid artery, maxillary and lingual facial vein, or mandibular salivary gland and lymph node. These structures can be avoided by careful palpation and observation. By applying enough force to displace the lateral pharyngeal wall, vessels and nerves will roll out of the way. It is also important that blunt dissection be performed instead of using a scalpel blade.

Pharyngostomy tubes are suited for patients that require bypass of the oral cavity and have a normal esophagus and gastrointestinal tract. Because the tube may interfere with normal esophageal healing, it is not recommended for use in patients with esophageal lesions. Minor complications include mild stridor, coughing, vomiting, regurgitation, esophagitis, pharyngitis, tube displacement or obstruction, and wound infection. Aspiration pneumonia and upper airway obstruction are serious and potentially life-threatening complications. Problems such as vomiting or regurgitation can be avoided by proper patient selection and feeding small boluses of food at frequent intervals. Because anorectic patients have small stomach volumes and may have delayed gastric emptying, volumes of 5 to 20 ml/kg per feeding are recommended. If the tube has been placed into the stomach, aspiration of fluid and food indicates that the next feeding should not be given. Once the animal's gastrointestinal tract has become accustomed to the feeding, larger volumes may be infused (50 to 75 ml/kg). Using relatively small, pliable tubes may decrease pharyngitis and esophagitis.[74] Kinking may be a problem with the softer tubes. The tubes must be capped between use and flushed with 15 to 20 ml of warm water before and after feeding to prevent clogging. Some animals, especially cats, are good at dislodging the tube by manipulating it with their tongue. Animals can also regurgitate the tube. Usually the tube is easily replaced, although it is possible that the animal can damage the tube by chewing. Wound infection is not a common clinical problem. Good nursing care will eliminate many complications.

To remove the tube, the patient may need to be sedated. After flushing the tube, it is removed from the esophagus. The tube is cut flush with the skin, and the rest pulled into the oral cavity. Alternatively, the tube can be capped and withdrawn quickly from the outside. There is a chance that contamination of the ostomy site may occur with this technique. The incision is allowed to heal by second intention, which occurs in a few days.

Some clinicians believe that pharyngostomy is not as useful as other enteral feeding techniques. The potential for serious complications is greater compared with other, less invasive techniques such as nasal feeding tubes. Percutaneous gastrostomy tube feeding involves a similar anesthetic protocol with less chance of complications. These tubes are also tolerated for longer periods of time. The main difference between pharyngostomy and percutaneous gastrostomy is that the gastrostomy technique requires an endoscope for placement.

Gastrostomy Feeding Tubes. Gastrostomy feeding tubes can be placed through a keyhole celiotomy in the left flank.[29, 78] A gastrostomy tube also may be placed following an abdominal exploratory by a ventral midline approach. The technique of tube gastrostomy has been well described for providing postoperative nutrition and gastric decompression and to stimulate adhesion of the stomach to the abdominal wall to prevent recurrence of gastric torsion.[27, 29, 68, 69, 72, 79] A balloon-tipped urethral catheter (Bardex Foley catheter, Bard Urological Division, C.R. Bard, Inc., Covington, GA 30209) is inserted through a purse-string suture placed in the antral area of the stomach. The balloon is inflated to help secure the tube in the stomach. Additional sutures are placed to secure the stomach to the abdominal wall. Relatively large catheters can be used, which makes it easier to infuse blended pet foods. In small dogs and cats, a no. 12 French to no. 18 French catheter may be used. Larger sizes can be used in big dogs weighing over 30 kg. The main advantage of this technique is that large tubes can be placed and are well tolerated by the patient. The tubes can be used for several weeks, and owners can continue home feedings. A disadvantage of the surgically placed gastrostomy tube is that it requires general anesthesia and a surgical approach to insert the tube. Because of the stab incision into the stomach, there is a potential for leakage around the tube. This can be minimized by placing a double purse-string suture around the catheter, creating a seromuscular tunnel with an inverting suture pattern, or placing the omentum around the gastrostomy site (Fig. 4–7). Impaired wound healing and compromise of the gastrostomy site may occur in hypoalbuminemic patients.

Percutaneous Endoscopic Gastrostomy. A technique for percutaneous endoscopic gastrostomy (PEG) has been described in the human[80] and veterinary medical literature.[30, 81–83] This technique utilizes an endoscope to place the gastrostomy feeding tube. Indications for using a gastrostomy tube include anticipated long duration of tube feeding and a normal gastrointestinal tract. Patients with persistent vomiting, delayed gastric outflow, or lower esophageal sphincter incompetence are not good candidates for the technique. Animals with megaesophagus or esophageal reflux or comatose patients are more likely to experience vomiting and aspiration.

While commercial PEG catheter kits designed for endoscopic placement

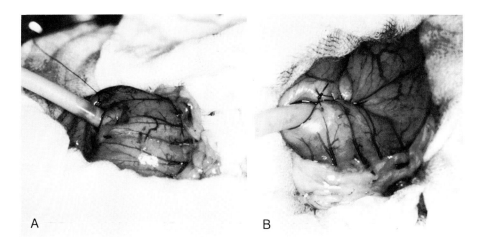

Figure 4–7. *A,* A purse-string suture has been placed and the Foley catheter directed through a stab incision. *B,* By placing an inverting pattern such as a Lembert, the stomach can be folded around the catheter to prevent leakage.

in people can be used effectively in animals, urologic catheters are less expensive and practical. Mushroom catheters such as the Pezzer and the Malecott urologic catheters (Bardex Urologic Catheter, Bard Urological Division, C.R. Bard, Inc., Covington, GA 30209) have been described in the veterinary literature.[82] More problems may occur with the Malecott catheter because the open bulb on the end tends to collapse easily (Fig. 4–8). Because this catheter can be readily removed by the patient (even with an inner flange), its use cannot be recommended.

Typically, nos. 14 to 18 French catheters work well in all sizes of dogs and cats. The patient is placed in right lateral recumbency. A small area (8–12 cm²) caudal to the 13th rib and centered midway between the paravertebral epaxial musculature and the ventral midline is prepared for surgery. A mouth speculum is placed, and the endoscope is passed into the stomach. The stomach is insufflated, taking care not to excessively inflate the stomach. Severe distention can compromise venous return and cardiac output. By darkening the room, the endoscope light can be seen through the abdominal wall. An assistant gently ballots the inflated stomach caudal to the last rib.

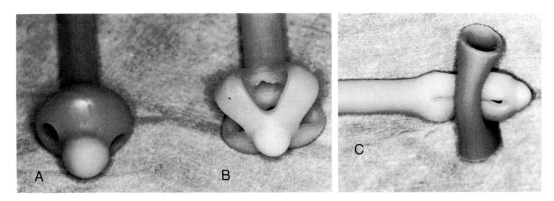

Figure 4–8. *A,* Pezzer urologic catheter. *B,* Malecott urologic catheter. *C,* Note collapse of the Malecott catheter, which allows it to be easily pulled through the flange.

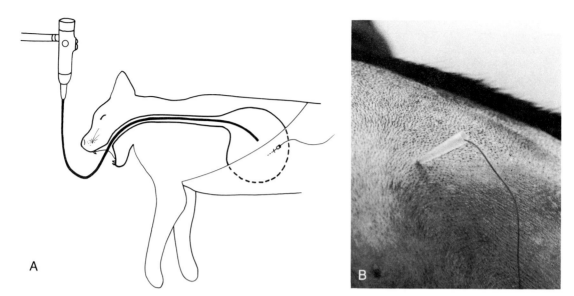

Figure 4–9. *A*, Line drawing illustrating placement of the endoscope within the stomach. The over-the-needle catheter or pipette is inserted into the distended stomach, and strong suture is threaded through the catheter into the stomach. (Drawing courtesy of Dr. David Williams and artist Mal Rooks Hoover.) *B*, Note suture material exiting from the catheter inserted into the gas-distended stomach. Placing a fingertip over the catheter during subsequent manipulations may be needed to keep the stomach from deflating.

This can be observed by the endoscope operator to provide a landmark for insertion of the catheter.

Next, a small incision is made in the skin with a scalpel blade, and an 18-gauge over-the-needle catheter (Argyle Medicut intravenous catheter, Sherwood Medical Industries, Inc., St. Louis, MO 63103) is inserted into the stomach (Fig. 4–9). Once the needle and stylet are seen through the scope, the stylet is withdrawn. Large gauge or size suture, such as 1–0 mersilene or nylon, is threaded through the catheter into the lumen of the stomach. The suture is grasped by endoscopic biopsy or grasping forceps. The length of the suture should reach from the caudal aspect of the abdomen to outside the mouth. After the suture is grasped, it is slowly withdrawn through the esophagus and out of the mouth (Fig. 4–10). Once the suture end is outside the patient, the intravenous catheter is removed from the abdominal wall and stomach. In the original description of this technique, the intravenous catheter was used as an introducer for the urologic catheter. Since the original catheter has been modified recently, a disposable pipette (MLA pipette tip, Medical Laboratory Automation, Inc., Pleasantville, NY) can be used in its place.[83]

The next part of the PEG is securing the feeding tube to the catheter or pipette tip. The tip of the Pezzer catheter can be cut to prevent plugging. Two V-shaped cuts are made in the distal end at 180 degrees from each other. This allows the end of the feeding tube to be collapsed so that it will fit more tightly into the flared end of the intravenous catheter or pipette. The end of the suture exiting from the mouth is passed in a retrograde manner through the pipette tip (or IV catheter) from the smaller lumen to exit through the larger lumen. A 15- or 16-gauge hypodermic needle is passed through the modified end of the mushroom catheter. The suture is threaded through the hypodermic needle, and the needle is removed, leaving

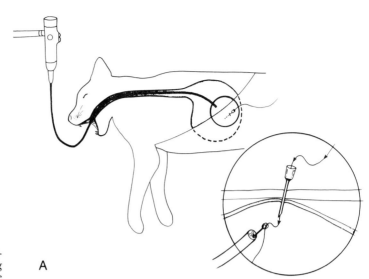

A

Figure 4–10. *A*, The suture is visualized through the scope, and grasping or biopsy forceps are used to snare the suture end. (Drawing courtesy of Dr. David Williams and artist Mal Rooks Hoover.) *B*, After the suture is grasped by the forceps, both the suture and the endoscope are carefully withdrawn from the digestive tract.

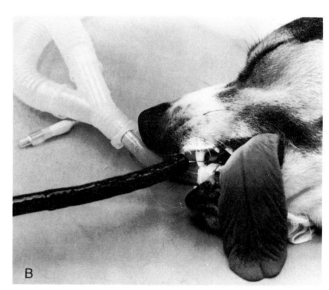

B

the suture transfixing the end of the catheter. A square knot is firmly tied, securing the suture through the pipette to the mushroom catheter. The modified end of the catheter is fitted into the flared end of the pipette. The combined pipette and mushroom catheter are lubricated with a water-soluble jelly (Fig. 4–11).

The assistant begins to apply traction to the suture emerging from the lateral abdominal wall. The pipette acts as a dilator, to gently spread the tissues to accommodate the larger mushroom catheter. Firm counterpressure can be placed by the assistant's hand on the abdominal wall and around the exit site (Fig. 4–12). With large-sized tubes, it may be necessary to bluntly dissect the tissues with a hemostat or increase the size of the skin incision. After the distal end of the mushroom catheter has been retracted, the endoscope is passed into the stomach again to observe positioning of the tube. The tip of the catheter should be resting gently against the stomach. The stomach should be deflated prior to removal of the endoscope.

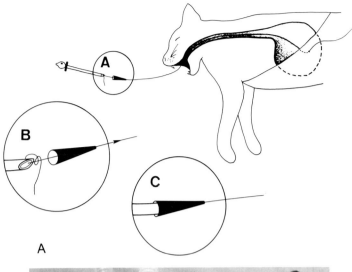

Figure 4–11. *A*, The end of the urologic catheter is modified by cutting the flared end (which can subsequently be used to make an internal flange). It also helps to obliquely cut the catheter end or notch the tip to facilitate insertion into the catheter or pipette. The suture is passed through the venous catheter or pipette from the narrow end to exit out the wider opening. Next, the suture is passed through the urologic catheter and tied securely with square knots. (Drawing courtesy of Dr. David Williams and artist Mal Rooks Hoover.) *B*, The completed catheter ensemble illustrating position of the internal flange behind the mushroom tip (*arrow*) and wedging of the urologic catheter into the dilator or pipette.

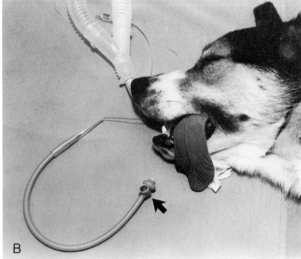

The catheter may be secured with a friction suture, or an outer flange can be constructed. A light dressing is applied around the ostomy site, and a bandage is used to secure the tube. Often the bandage can be very minimal, just enough to keep the feeding tube out of the way. An Elizabethan collar also can be used if needed.

Ideally, the tube should be left in place a minimum of 3 to 5 days to stimulate formation of adhesions. In debilitated, hypoproteinemic patients, the tube should be left in place for at least 5 to 7 days. Complications such as leakage and peritonitis have not been a problem. Two techniques can be used to remove the tube. In the first, the tube is simply withdrawn from the stomach through the abdominal wall. Gentle counterpressure against the abdomen may help in removal. An alternative technique, which may be less stressful for the patient, is to gently apply traction to the tube. The tip is cut off at its base and forced into the stomach lumen with a cotton-tipped applicator or a pair of hemostats (Fig. 4–13). In small dogs or cats, the tip can be retrieved with the endoscope. In larger dogs, the catheter tip passes through the digestive tract. The gastrostomy site is cleaned and allowed to heal by second intention.

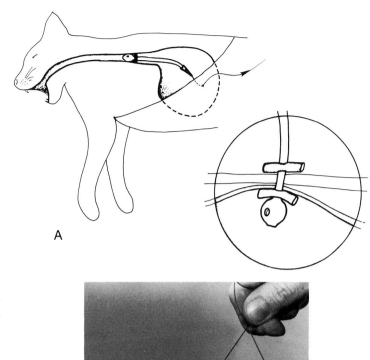

Figure 4–12. *A*, Line drawing illustrating retraction of the suture from the abdominal wall and final position of the mushroom catheter and flange against the stomach wall. (Drawing courtesy of Dr. David Williams and artist Mal Rooks Hoover.) *B*, Retraction of suture through the abdominal wall. Often a small incision in the skin or subcutaneous tissue may be needed to help the larger catheter exit through the abdominal wall.

Controversy exists regarding the use of a flange for PEG. In several descriptions of the technique, a 4-cm length of tubing from the distal end of the mushroom catheter is removed. This segment is cut into two pieces, and stab incisions are made through the longitudinal portion of the tube. One of these segments is threaded onto the mushroom catheter until it rests just behind the mushroom tip. The other tube segment is used in a similar manner as an outside flange. Problems have arisen with these flanges. While they may be helpful in securing the gastrostomy tube, they may cause pressure necrosis of the stomach or abdominal wall if placed too tightly. Another problem occurs with the inner flange when the PEG is removed. In dogs larger than 15 kg, the flange and tip should pass through the intestinal tract. With small dogs and cats, there is a potential for intestinal obstruction, and the flange and tip should be retrieved with the endoscope. Because of this problem, the mushroom catheter has been used without the flange. Major problems have not been noted, unless the Malecott catheter was used (LJ DeBowes, personal communication).

Complications related to PEG are minimal. Minor problems include peristomal infection, accidental tube removal, gastric bleeding and subsequent melena, vomiting and diarrhea. Major complications include peritonitis, perforation of the bowel, aspiration pneumonia, and laceration of the spleen. Vomiting is the most common problem and is generally related to overfeed-

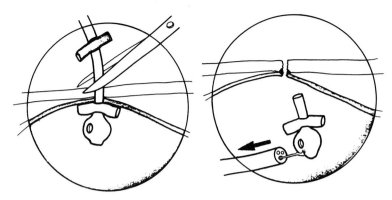

Figure 4–13. Line drawing illustrating one technique of tube removal. Gentle retraction is placed on the tube, and the tube is cut flush with the abdominal wall. Using a forceps or cotton-tipped applicator, the end of the mushroom catheter is pushed into the stomach. Once the mushroom tip and flange are in the stomach, it can be removed with an endoscope or, in large dogs, the tip and flange will pass through the GI tract. (Drawing courtesy of Dr. David Williams and artist Mal Rooks Hoover.)

ing. Aspiration of the tube should be done in patients who have delayed gastric emptying. If a large volume of fluid is in the stomach, the next feeding should not be given. Aspiration pneumonia is most often a problem in patients with pharyngeal or esophageal dysfunction.

Enteral Feeding Tubes. Enteral feeding is accomplished by inserting a tube or catheter directly into the intestinal segment or by threading a catheter into the proximal bowel through a gastrostomy tube. Feeding tubes also may be placed through the nose to end in the duodenum or jejunum. In humans, the technique of feeding directly into the intestinal tract was first reported in 1858.[84]

The technique of tube or needle catheter jejunostomy has been well described in the veterinary literature.[27, 29, 68, 69, 72, 85, 86] Several types of catheters or tubes may be used, depending on the technique. A small-gauge (no. 5–6 French) polyvinyl or polyurethane feeding tube (such as that used for a nasogastric tube) works well. A 14- or 16-gauge through-the-needle intravenous catheter (Brinton L-Cath Tracheal Wash Catheter, Animal Health Care Products, Luther Medical Products, Inc., Santa Ana, CA 92705 or Venocath-16 Venisystems, Abbott Ireland, Ltd, Sligo, Republic of Ireland) also can be used effectively, but the length may be too short for large patients. Catheter length should be at least 45 cm, because 20 to 30 cm is threaded aborally into the intestinal tract. Shorter lengths are likely to be dislodged.

Enteral feeding techniques are indicated in patients who have a functional intestinal tract but may be unable to eat or assimilate food from other routes. Parenteral techniques can be used in these malnourished patients but are contraindicated if the intestinal tract is still functional. The primary disadvantage of enteral feeding is the need for a surgical approach.

Examples of patients in which enteral feeding tubes have been used include those with major revision of the stomach or proximal intestinal tract. Patients with extensive resection of liver, pancreas, or spleen also may be candidates. The technique is also applicable in patients with extensive malnutrition due to cancer cachexia and when postoperative problems are expected to exacerbate anorexia.

Placement of the enterostomy tube or needle catheter enterostomy is similar. An appropriate segment of bowel is selected. This may be the distal portion of the duodenum or proximal segment of jejunum. Care must be taken not to traumatize the pancreas if the duodenum is selected. The enterostomy tube or catheter is first introduced through the ventral lateral abdominal wall at the level of insertion into the bowel. A large-gauge needle

(12- to 14-gauge) can be used as a guide. The hypodermic needle is inserted through the abdominal wall from the serosal surface to the skin. The catheter or feeding tube is inserted through the needle, and the needle is withdrawn, leaving the end of the catheter within the abdomen. The next step is insertion of the tube or catheter into the intestinal segment. A purse-string suture of 3–0 to 4–0 absorbable material is made in the antimesenteric border of the bowel. A small puncture is made into the lumen, and the enteral feeding tube is passed aborally for 20 to 30 cm. The purse-string suture is tightened to seal the intestine around the tube. To further prevent leakage, the enterostomy site is sutured to the abdominal wall. In debilitated patients with poor wound healing, a nonabsorbable suture (polypropylene) or synthetic absorbable suture (polydioxanone, polyglyconate) should be used. Sutures should penetrate the submucosa of the intestine for security.

If a needle catheter enterostomy is used, the insertion can be modified. The 14-gauge hypodermic needle is used to introduce the catheter into the bowel. Alternatively, the needle from the intravenous catheter is disengaged from the catheter and used as a guide. An advantage of this technique is that the ostomy site can be kept very small, thus decreasing the chance for leakage. In one method, the needle is inserted on the antimesenteric border into the lumen. The needle is directed orally to emerge from the bowel. By angling the needle through the bowel wall, it is possible to create a short seromuscular tunnel for the catheter. After the tip of the needle penetrates outside the intestinal lumen, the catheter is inserted into the needle. Both the needle and the catheter are withdrawn as a unit until they are within the lumen (Fig. 4–14). The needle is removed, leaving the catheter inside the intestine. The catheter is advanced aborally for several centimeters, and a purse-string suture is tied to secure the catheter. The first puncture made by the needle is oversewn with a simple interrupted or cruciate suture. The ostomy site is sutured to the abdominal wall as described before (Fig. 4–15). Other methods have been described to protect the catheter from leakage. These involve inversion of the small intestine around the catheter with concentric purse-string sutures or a seromuscular tunnel. In most cases, this

Figure 4–14. *A,* One technique for placement of a needle catheter jejunostomy tube. The tip of the large-gauge needle has been directed orally and obliquely through the intestinal wall. *B,* After emerging from the intestinal wall, the jejunostomy catheter is inserted into the needle lumen. The needle and catheter are withdrawn into the intestinal lumen. At that point the catheter is separated from the needle, the needle withdrawn from the bowel, and the catheter passed aborally for 20 to 30 cm.

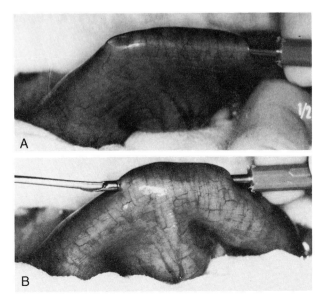

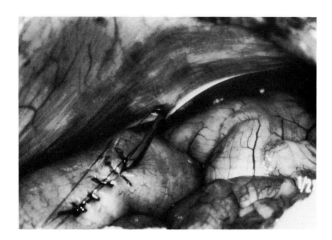

Figure 4–15. The jejunostomy catheter is secured to the abdominal wall in a similar fashion to the gastrostomy tube. An inverting Lembert pattern can be placed on the antimesenteric border to protect the site from leakage. This technique can compromise lumen diameter in very small patients. Interrupted sutures are placed around the ostomy site to secure the intestine to the abdominal wall.

is not necessary because leakage is rarely a problem even if the catheter is introduced directly into the lumen. Inversion of the intestine in small dogs or cats may cause intestinal obstruction. If the tube or catheter used does not have a flared end or a Luer-Lock hub, it can be inserted directly into the intestinal lumen using the hypodermic needle as a guide. After the catheter has been passed aborally, the hypodermic needle is withdrawn from the catheter. The end of the catheter is then directed through the abdominal wall using the needle as a guide. The enterostomy tube or catheter is secured to the skin with a friction (Chinese finger trap) suture. A sterile dressing with an antibiotic ointment is applied, and the catheter is incorporated into an abdominal bandage. The end of the catheter is capped with an intravenous catheter plug or a three-way stopcock to prevent influx of air or leakage of intestinal contents. Premature removal of the tube by the patient is prevented by applying an Elizabethan collar or aluminum sidebar brace. In debilitated patients, an abdominal bandage may be sufficient.

It is important to flush the enteral catheter if bolus feedings are given. Small-volume feedings given at frequent intervals (four to six times a day) can be used in some patients. Vomiting and diarrhea are commonly seen with this technique, especially if a high osmolar or a monomeric diet is fed. In most patients, fewer complications are seen if a constant infusion is performed by gravity drip sets or infusion pumps.

As gastrointestinal function returns to normal, the patient is encouraged to begin eating. The enteral feeding is slowly discontinued over a 24- to 48-hour period. Because of the constant glucose infusion, insulin levels tend to remain elevated. Abruptly stopping the feeding may cause a rebound hypoglycemia before the body can compensate for the immediate reduction of glucose. The enteral feeding tube or catheter is removed by simply cutting the retention suture and pulling the catheter out. The stoma is allowed to heal by second intention.

CALCULATION OF NUTRIENT NEEDS

Once the decisions have been made for supportive alimentation and route of feeding, the next question—how much to feed—arises. It is common to underestimate the amount of calories actually being consumed or given to the patient. For example, 5% dextrose solution is often used to provide calories for anorectic animals. Using one method to calculate the hospitalized energy requirements of a 10-kg dog, one needs to feed approximately 500 kcal/day = [30(wt kg) + 70] × 1.35.[30] One liter of 5% dextrose has 170 kcal. To supply the energy requirements of a 10-kg dog, it would take approximately 3 L, which is five times the maintenance water requirement of 600 ml/day (60 ml/kg × wt kg/24 h).

Because these animals are in a state of hypermetabolism and are relatively glucose intolerant, protein also must be supplied. Exogenous protein is used to replace protein deficiencies and also as an energy source.

To be effective at minimizing losses and correcting deficits, measurements or estimation of energy and protein needs should be made. In humans, accurate measurements can be made to determine patient energy expenditures. Because these techniques are not available or impractical in the veterinary patient, estimation of energy and protein needs has been extrapolated from experimental and human data. Some controversy exists regarding the validity of formulas used to calculate energy requirements. Confusion also remains about definition of terms.[87] The goal of this discussion is to provide a simple technique that can be easily used in a clinical setting. The following terminology and formulas are given as guidelines to provide a basis for determining food volume. Adjustments can be made based on clinical experience and patient response.

Basal Metabolic Rate

Basal metabolic rate (BMR) refers to the minimum energy expended by a subject at complete rest, 10 to 12 hours after digestion, and in a thermoneutral environment. Body surface area affects the basal metabolic rate because much energy is lost as heat from the body surface. As body weight decreases, the body surface area becomes proportionally greater, resulting in higher basal metabolic rates for small animals. *Basal energy expenditure (BEE)* or *basal energy requirement (BER)* are other terms often used instead of basal metabolic rate.[30, 87]

Maintenance Energy Requirement

Maintenance energy requirement (MER) is energy required by a moderately active adult animal in its own thermoneutral environment. The MER for dogs is about two times the BER. Because of the more sedentary nature of cats, their MER is 1.4 times the BER.[30]

Animals hospitalized for diagnostic tests, medical therapy, or surgery are usually inactive and often anorectic. Therefore, they tend to require fewer calories for maintenance compared with the normal animal in a nonhospital environment. There are, however, increased caloric needs for animals who are stressed, diseased, or recuperating from surgery. These increased caloric needs are proportional to the severity of the illness or injury.[46] Because the lack of physical exercise offsets the increased caloric needs due to disease or stress, caloric requirements for hospitalized animal patients rarely exceed maintenance energy requirements. Only in cases of severe sepsis or major burns will the caloric needs reach two times the BER.

In humans, many of these hospital-related situations have been investigated. Energy expenditures were calculated from techniques such as indirect calorimetry or measurement of oxygen uptake and carbon dioxide production.[87, 88] From these studies, factors were proposed to allow estimation of caloric needs based on the patient's basal metabolic rate (or BER) and the hospital setting. These same factors can be used effectively in the veterinary hospital to calculate an illness energy requirement (IER = hospital factor × BER). Refer to Table 4–4 for a listing of commonly used factors.

Exogenous protein should be given to replace protein losses and serve as an energy source. Protein continues to be utilized for energy even if sufficient calories are supplied by carbohydrate sources. This is due to a failure of normal physiologic mechanisms to limit protein degradation. A calorie–nitrogen ratio of 150:1 fosters nitrogen sparing. Dogs should receive 5.0 to 7.5 gm of protein per 100 kcal of calculated energy needs. For cats, 6 to 9 gm of protein per 100 kcal is appropriate. In patients with renal or hepatic insufficiency, the protein level should be 3 gm/100 kcal or less in dogs and 4 gm/100 kcal in cats.[29] In situations of severe protein loss such as peritonitis or burn injuries, the amount of protein needed may be even greater. Other authors recommend a level of exogenous protein of 24% to 48% of metabolizable energy for hospitalized patients.[87] Diets that are high in the branched-chain amino acids valine, leucine, and isoleucine are recommended because these amino acids are preferentially metabolized with surgical stress or trauma.[89]

Supplementation with vitamins and minerals depends on losses and food source. Enteral diets, especially those formulated from pet foods or for dogs and cats specifically, generally have adequate vitamin and mineral content. Polymeric or meal-replacement diets formulated for humans have been used effectively in veterinary patients. These diets, however, may not be balanced for animal needs, particularly if used for extended periods of time. Excessive amounts of zinc may be loss through the urinary tract in patients sustaining significant trauma or on total parenteral nutrition. Zinc may be supplemented at the dose of 1 mg/kg of body weight. There also may be an increased loss and an increased demand for the B-complex vitamins. These vitamins are important as coenzyme precursors and coenzymes, and supplementation may be beneficial.

Food Dose

After calculating the energy and protein needs of the patient, a food dose can be determined. The total calories needed per day are divided by the food caloric density to find a volume of food per 24 hours. That volume is given either as bolus feeding or by infusion. Following is an example for a 10-kg dog with multiple pelvic fractures.

TABLE 4–4. Estimation of Patient Energy Requirements

CONDITION	ADJUSTMENT FACTOR
Cage rest	1.25 × BER*
Postoperative	1.25 to 1.35 × BER
Trauma	1.35 to 1.5 × BER
Cancer	1.35 to 1.5 × BER
Sepsis	1.5 to 1.7 × BER
Major burn	1.7 to 2.0 × BER

*BER = basal energy requirement
= 30(wt kg) + 70 = kcal/day for dogs greater than 2 kg
= 70(wt kg$^{0.75}$) = kcal/day for any size dog or cat[30]

1. BER = (30 × 10 kg) + 70 = 370 kcal/day.
2. IER = 1.35 (factor for trauma) × 370 = 500 kcal/day.
3. Food source has an energy density of 1.5 kcal/ml, so 500 kcal/1.5 kcal/ml = 333.3 ml/day of food.

Feeding frequency is based on the type of diet and patient tolerance. Initially, one-fourth to one-third of the calculated calories is given on day 1. Over the next 2 to 5 days, this amount is gradually increased to full levels. Lower osmolar diets, such as those with an osmolarity of 200 to 350 mOsm/kg, are usually well tolerated and can be fed full strength. Hyperosmolar diets should be diluted and gradually reconstituted to full strength over several days. In most patients, small, frequent feedings are better than a few bolus feedings. A normal dog or cat can handle 50 to 90 ml/kg volume feedings. In a patient that has been anorectic for a number of days, small volumes (10 to 20 ml per feeding) every 1 to 2 hours may be more appropriate. Critically ill animals, especially those being fed by enterostomy tubes, often do better with continuous-drip compared with bolus feedings.

The most common side effect of enteral feeding techniques is vomiting and diarrhea. These effects are due to large-volume feeding and hyperosmolar diets. Diluting the diet with water and feeding a small volume at frequent intervals may be needed to stop the vomiting and diarrhea. Metaclopramide may be given at the dose of 0.2 to 0.5 mg/kg SC every 6 to 8 hours to improve gastrointestinal emptying.

DIETS

There are many products designed for enteral feeding in humans. Many of these products have been used successfully in small animal patients. Long-term use of these diets has not been critically evaluated and could conceivably result in nutritional deficiencies. A liquid diet formulated for dogs and cats is commercially available under the trade name Clinicare (Clinicare Care for dogs or cats, PetAg, Inc., Hampshire, IL 60140). A renal formulation with a lower protein content is also available (Renal Care Canine or Feline Liquid Diet, PetAg, Inc., Hampshire, IL 60140). Blended dog or cat food also may be administered through enteral feeding tubes. Recently, a diet formulated for nutritional management of catabolic patients with malnutrition has been released (Hill's Prescription Diet a/d, Hill's Pet Products, Topeka, KS 66601). This diet has a high protein, high fat, and low carbohydrate content in an energy-dense palatable form. The diet can be fed directly or blended with water for use in enteral feeding tubes.

Nutritional Concerns

Nutritional requirements vary according to species. Unlike dogs and humans, cats require the amino acid taurine, free fatty acids linoleate and arachidonic acid, and vitamins A and niacin.[27, 89] Most human products are based on soy and casein as a protein source and use corn oil as a source of fatty acids. These diets are not appropriate for cats because soy and casein are deficient in taurine and corn oil does not contain sufficient arachidonic acid.[89] To supplement these diets for use in cats, egg yolk can be added.[27]

Arginine may be an essential amino acid in dogs and cats. Deficiencies are rare but can occur if casein is used as the sole source of protein.[89] Examples of diets based on casein include Nutramigen (Nutramigamin, Mead Johnson Nutritional Division, Bristol-Myers Co., Evansville, IN 47721) and Portagen (Portagen, Mead Johnson Nutritional Division, Bristol-Myers Co., Evansville, IN 47721).

Classification of Enteral Diets

Three general categories of enteral diets are described. Meal replacement or polymeric diets contain complex carbohydrates, intact or partially digested proteins, and fats. These diets require digestion, although some products are tolerated by jejunostomy patients. A clinical trial in humans showed no difference in gastrointestinal function between people fed a polymeric diet compared with those fed an elemental diet.[90] The osmolarity of polymeric diets is approximately 300 to 350 mOsm/L.

Elemental or monomeric diets contain amino acids, peptides, oligosaccharides, monosaccharides, and medium-chain triglycerides. These diets require minimal digestion and are infused into the intestinal tract. One disadvantage of these diets, besides a higher cost, is that they are more hyperosmolar, 600 to 800 mOsm/L. Because of the increase in osmolarity, the diets should be introduced gradually. Slow continuous infusion is better than bolus feedings. Diluting the diet to half strength is also recommended during the initial days of administration. Dietary supplements or feeding modules is the third category of diets. These products are composed of single nutrients that can be used to supplement meal-replacement diets or to formulate diets for specific patient needs.

Feeding Recommendations

Small tubes are more comfortable for patients; however, small tubes can become obstructed. Blended canned dog or cat food will pass through a no. 8 French or larger feeding tube. This mixture should be strained because small particles easily clog the tube. For tubes smaller than no. 8 French, a liquid diet is required.

Feeding tube care is critical with all enteral tubes. To prevent clogging, the tube needs to be flushed on a regular basis and after every feeding. Between feedings, the tube should be capped to prevent leakage of contents and to keep air from entering the digestive tract.

Diarrhea may be prevented by slowly conditioning the bowel to the diet. Initially, quarter to half strength solutions are infused during the first 24 hours. If the patient tolerates the feeding, the concentration is gradually increased. In some patients, it may take several days of gradually increasing the rate and concentration until the total caloric needs can be met. Polymeric diets, such as Ensure Plus (Ross Laboratories, Division of Abbott Laboratories, Columbus, OH 43216), Osmolite (Ross Laboratories, Columbus OH 43216), and Clinicare for dogs and cats, also can be given through an enterostomy tube. These formulations require some digestion but have a lower osmolality due to the higher molecular-weight forms of the carbohydrates and proteins. The most common problem is diarrhea, which can be avoided by infusing half-strength solutions. The concentration and rate should be increased gradually over the next 3 to 4 days. Protein content of these diets can be increased by adding ProMod Protein Supplement (Ross Laboratories, Division of Abbott Laboratories, Columbus, OH 43216).

Ideally, using a blended dog or cat food is the easiest, least expensive, and most physiologic for many small animal patients. Homemade diets of baby food, eggs, and corn syrup also can be effectively used. See Table 4–5 for recipes.

Summary

Early instigation of enteral feeding may limit postoperative complications and improve the patient's quality of life. Accurate assessment of malnutrition is essential to permit selection of patients who can benefit from nutritional support. Anticipating anorexia in patients will facilitate placement of appropriate feeding tubes without requiring a second delivery of anesthesia.

PARENTERAL NUTRITION

Parenteral nutrition has been used in humans since 1967 and is rapidly gaining favor in veterinary medicine. Comprehensive reviews of parenteral nutritional support have been reported.[91, 92]

Total parenteral nutrition (TPN) is the administration of essential nutrients intravenously. Because of the high osmolarity and volume of solutions, infusion is usually into a large central vein such as the vena cava. Peripheral veins may be used if the solution is not highly osmolar. Partial parenteral nutrition (PPN), which is often given through a peripheral vein, supplies part of the patient nutrient requirements. The remainder of the nutrients can be given enterally, which prevents a negative nitrogen or energy balance and maintains intestinal integrity.

Patient Selection

Instigation of TPN requires technical support and appropriate facilities. The solutions are relatively expensive, and there is a risk of introducing infection

TABLE 4–5. Blended Enteral Diets

Recipe 1[30]

1. ½ can of Prescription Diet Feline p/d*
   ¾ cup of water (170 ml)
2. Mix for at least 60 seconds in a blender at high speed. Mixture should be strained.
3. Metabolizable energy = 0.8 kcal/ml
4. By adding 1 tablespoon (15 ml) of corn oil, the metabolizable energy can be increased to about 1 kcal/ml

Recipe 2[89]

1. 1 jar strained meat baby food (100 gm)
   1 whole cooked egg
   1 tablespoon (15 ml) corn oil
   1 tablespoon (15 ml) corn syrup
   100 ml of water
2. Mix well in a blender at high speed.
3. Metabolizable energy = 1 kcal/ml

*Feline p/d, Hill's Pet Products, Topeka, KS

during the admixing of the solution or its administration. Besides sepsis, other metabolic complications such as hyperglycemia can occur. For these reasons, patients being considered for TPN should be assessed carefully. If the digestive tract is functioning, then parenteral nutrition is not warranted. Clinical trials in people suggest that not all patients benefit from TPN.[93, 94] There is an increased incidence of infection, usually catheter-induced, in TPN patients.[93] Patients with less severe malnutrition did not benefit as much as those more severely malnourished. Humans and animals sustained on total TPN develop gastrointestinal atrophy with a risk of subsequent bacterial translocation.[95] Feeding some nutrients enterally will reverse the atrophy.[96]

Patients selected for TPN should meet the following criteria: (1) they should be significantly malnourished using objective and subjective measurements, and (2) they should not be able to digest or assimilate sufficient nutrients given via the enteral route. In humans, TNP has been given in a variety of clinical situations, including short-bowel syndrome, cancer cachexia, intestinal obstruction, massive intestinal resection, acute renal failure, pancreatitis, respiratory distress syndrome, and neonatal care.

Calculation of Nutrient Requirements

Calculation of energy and protein requirements is similar to that for enteral feeding protocols. In cats, calories from the protein should be included in the total calories fed; otherwise, overfeeding may be a problem.[96] Protein requirements are calculated as described previously. In animals that are experiencing severe protein loss, such as with open peritoneal drainage, higher levels of protein should be used. Patients with renal or hepatic insufficiency should have their protein levels decreased. Parenteral feeding solutions include glucose, amino acids, lipids, and electrolytes. By including lipids in the solution, the osmolarity can be greatly reduced, and calorie needs can be met using less volumes. Lipids also provide a source of essential fatty acids. In most diet formulations, 40% to 60% of the nonprotein calories are provided by the lipid source. Following are examples of a diet formulation for a 10-kg dog that has recently undergone major surgery.[92]

1. BER = (30 × 10 kg) + 70 = 370 kcal/day of metabolizable energy.
2. IER = 1.5 × BER = 1.5 × 370 = 550 kcal/day.
3. Protein requirement = 5 to 7.5 gm protein/100 kcal
   = 6 × 5.5 = 33 gm protein.
4. TPN volume calculations: Protein supplied by 8.5% amino acid solution = 85 mg/ml. Need 33 gm or 3300 mg protein divided by 85 mg/ml = 39 ml of 8.5% amino acid solution. A 50% dextrose solution provides 1.7 kcal/ml. Dextrose is to provide for 40% to 60% of total kcal/day. 50% of 550 kcal = 275 kcal. 275 kcal divided by 1.7 kcal/ml = 162 ml/day 50% dextrose. A 20% lipid solution provides for 2 kcal/ml. Lipids supply balance of calories not met by glucose. 275 kcal divided by 2 kcal/ml = 137.5 ml of 20% lipid solution.

Total volume of TPN solution is 39 ml of amino acid solution plus 162 ml of 50% dextrose solution plus 137.5 ml of 20% lipid solution, or 338.5 ml over 24 hours. Maintenance water requirement is 60 ml/kg per day, or 600 ml. The volume of TPN can be subtracted from the required water measurement and additional water and electrolytes can be given through a separate peripheral catheter.

Calculations of nutrient requirements in cats is similar. One exception is that the calories supplied by the calculated protein needed is subtracted from the total calories needed per day. Following in an example for a 4-kg cat following major surgery.

1. BER = (30 × 4 kg) + 70 = 190 kcal/day metabolizable energy.
2. IER = 1.4 × BER = 1.4 × 190 = 266 kcal/day.
3. Protein requirements of 6 to 9 gm/100 kcal. 2.6 × 9 gm = 23 gm protein. 4 kcal/gm protein = 4 × 23 gm = 92 kcal.
4. Calculation of TPN volume requirements: An 8.5% amino acid solution supplies 85 mg/ml. Need 23 gm or 2300 mg protein. 2300 mg divided by 85 mg/ml = 27 ml of 8.5% amino acid solution. A 50 % dextrose solution supplies 1.7 kcal/ml. Need 40% to 60% of nonprotein calories (266 − 92 = 174 kcal). 50% × 174 kcal = 87 kcal from dextrose. 87 kcal divided by 1.7 kcal/ml = 51 ml of 50% dextrose solution. A 20% lipid solution supplies 2 kcal/ml. Need balance of nonprotein calories not supplied by dextrose. 87 kcal divided by 2 kcal/ml = 43.5 ml of 20% lipid solution.

Total volume of TPN solution is 27 ml of 8.5% amino acid solution plus 51 ml of 50% dextrose plus 43.5 ml of 20% lipid solution, or 121.5 ml TPN. Maintenance water requirement for a 4-kg cat is 60 ml/kg per day = 240 ml.

A multivitamin preparation can be added to the TPN solution. Vitamin K should be given by injection because it is not compatible with the TPN solution. In cats, it is important to add taurine if TPN administration exceeds 1 week. Trace minerals are generally not added unless the duration of TPN is greater than 1 to 2 weeks. The TPN solution is deficient in iron, copper, zinc, calcium, phosphorus, magnesium, iodine, and selenium.

Compounding

Initially, TPN solutions were compounded under strictly sterile conditions using a laminar-flow hood. Often the lipid solution was given through a separate catheter or a Y-infusion set. Recently, the trend has been to mix all three ingredients together in a single delivery bag. Mixing can be done using three-lead transfer sets with vented filters (an All-in-One Bag with a three-lead transfer set, Clintec Nutrition Co., Baxter Healthcare Corp., Deerfield, IL 60015). Ideally, mixing should be done under a laminar-flow hood, but other clean areas can be used. All injection ports should be swabbed with 70% isopropyl alcohol before using. Air should not be injected into the bottles or bags to facilitate withdrawal. The lipid and glucose solutions are not compatible and should not be mixed directly. Glucose and amino acids are added, then lipids. The TPN solution should be made up daily, and solution not used within 24 hours should be discarded.

Generally, 50% dextrose solutions are used for TPN. The lipid emulsions contain soybean or safflower oil, egg yolk phospholipids, and glycerol and are available in 10% and 20% formulations (Intralipid Emulsion 10% or 20%, Clintec Nutrition Co., Baxter Healthcare Corp., Deerfield, IL 60015-0760). Amino acid solutions are available in several concentrations with or without electrolytes (Travasol 10% or 8% with or without electrolytes, Clintec Nutrition Co., Baxter Healthcare Corp., Deerfield, IL 60015-0760).

Administration

The most serious consequence of TPN is sepsis. Absolute attention must be paid to observing strict asepsis during compounding and delivery of the TPN solution. The TPN catheter is placed in a central vein such as the cranial vena cava. The patient may require sedation or light anesthesia to ensure that sterile techniques can be maintained. The area is clipped and surgically prepared. The catheter is placed using sterile technique, including draping, gloves, caps, and masks. TPN catheters with multiple ports are available but tend to be expensive. A single-lumen polyurethane catheter (L-Cath, Luther Medical Products, Inc., Santa Ana, CA 92705) can be used effectively. The catheter can be placed percutaneously (preferred) or by cutdown to the vein. After inserting the catheter, a sterile bandage is placed. This bandage should be changed every day and the catheter site inspected for signs of redness or swelling. The TPN catheter is "dedicated" only for administration of the TPN solution. Because of the risk of introducing sepsis, the catheter is never used for giving antibiotics or drugs or for withdrawing blood samples.

It is useful to cover the intravenous administration set connections in a disinfectant-soaked gauze wrapped with tape. The administration sets should be changed every 2 days.

Rate of administration is based on the volume of TPN given over a 24-hour period. Only half the calculated volume of glucose is given during the first 24 hours. If hyperglycemia does not occur, the volume of glucose is increased. Ideally, infusion pumps are better for the continuous administration of TPN. The patient also should be closely monitored, and 24-hour care is required. TPN can be given over a shorter time period such as 12 to 15 hours. However, there is more potential for hyperglycemia and rebound hypoglycemia. Using lipid solutions to supply part of the calories may decrease this risk and also allow use of a peripheral vein.

The TPN administration should not be discontinued abruptly. Typically, the patient is gradually weaned from parenteral feeding by gradually increasing the amount of calories supplied enterally and decreasing the volume of TPN over several hours.

Complications

Complications associated with TPN range from minimal to life-threatening. Patients should be monitored carefully and vital signs assessed at least twice a day. The patient should be weighed daily, because a sudden increase or decrease in weight is indicative of changes in fluid volume. Urinalysis or blood glucose evaluation should be performed three to four times a day because hyperglycemia is a common problem. Electrolytes should be measured at least every other day.

Complications can include sepsis, acid–base and electrolyte imbalances, renal or hepatic compromise, thrombophlebitis, and catheter-related problems. The most common complications are generally related to catheter care, such as breaks in asepsis, catheter occlusion, and difficulty in recatheterizing patients. Patients that develop a fever or leukocytosis should be carefully assessed for a catheter-induced infection. The bandage should be changed and the site inspected. If redness, heat, or swelling is present, the catheter is aseptically removed and the tip cultured. If the insertion site looks normal, blood can be withdrawn from the TPN catheter and cultured. Often a peripheral blood sample is cultured for comparison. If there is a positive culture, the catheter should be removed and the patient treated with appropriate antibiotics. Once the temperature returns to normal, the TPN catheter can be replaced.

Hyperglycemia and glucosuria are also commonly seen but rarely cause significant problems for the patient. If glucosuria is greater than 500 mg/dl on the first day of administration, half the calculated glucose requirement is continued. If glucosuria persists, the volume of glucose can be further decreased and more calories provided by lipid. Regular insulin can be added to the TPN solution at the rate of 10 units. This is adjusted by monitoring blood and urine glucose.

Hypokalemia may be a problem and should be monitored closely. Standard rates of potassium supplementation can be used, and the rate should not exceed 0.5 mEq/kg per hour. Hyperlipidemia is a problem in some animals. Persistent increases in serum triglycerides indicate that the amount of lipid should be decreased and the deficit made up by additional dextrose. Intravenous fat infusion in dogs does not stimulate exocrine pancreatic function.[97]

Summary

Parenteral nutrition can be a safe and effective procedure for appropriate patients. Meticulous attention to maintaining complete asepsis in mixing and administering the TPN solution will limit the risk of sepsis. TPN is expensive, but in select patients, it may reduce patient morbidity or mortality associated with malnutrition.

REFERENCES

1. Dudrick SJ: Past, present, and future of nutritional support. Surg Clin North Am 1991; 71:439–448
2. Cerra FB: Nutrient modulation of inflammatory and immune function. Am J Surg 1991; 161:230–234
3. Mullen JL, Gertner MH, Buzby GP, et al: Implications of malnutrition in the surgical patient. Arch Surg 1979; 114:121–125
4. Bistrian BR, Blackburn GL, Hallowell E, Heddle R: Protein status of general surgical patients. JAMA 1974; 230:858–860
5. Reinhardt GF, Myscofski JW, Wilkens DB et al: Incidence and mortality of hypoalbuminemic patients in hospitalized veterans. J Parent Ent Nutr 1980; 4:357–359
6. Herndon DN: Nutritional assessment in surgical patients. In Yarborough MF, Curreri PW (eds): Surgical Nutrition. New York: Churchill Livingstone, 1981, pp 1–11
7. Detsky AS, Baker JP, Mendelson RA, et al: Evaluating the accuracy of nutritional assessment techniques applied to hospitalized patients: Methodology and comparisons. J Parent Ent Nutr 1984; 8:153–159
8. Meguid MM, Campos AC, Hammond WG: Nutritional support in surgical practice, part 1. Am J Surg 1990; 159:345–358
9. Alexander JW, Stinnett JD: Changes in immunologic function. In Kinney JM, Jeejeebhoy KN, Hill L, Owen OE (eds): Nutrition and Metabolism in Patient Care. Philadelphia: WB Saunders, 1988, pp 535–549
10. Ching N, Grossi CE, Angers J, et al: The outcome of surgical treatment as related to the response of the serum albumin level to nutritional support. Surg Gynecol Obstet 1980; 151:199–202
11. Seltzer MH, Bastidas JA, Cooper DM, et al: Instant nutritional assessment. J Parent Ent Nutr 1979; 3:157–159
12. Haydock DA, Hill GL: Impaired wound healing in surgical patients with varying degrees of malnutrition. J Parent Ent Nutr 1986; 10:550–554
13. Peacock EE Jr: Wound Repair, 3d ed. Philadelphia: WB Saunders, 1984, p 102
14. Rhoads JE, Kasinskas W: The influence of hypoproteinemia on the formation of callus in experimental fracture. Surgery 1942; 11:38–44

15. Irvin TT: Effects of malnutrition and hyperalimentation on wound healing. Surg Gynecol Obstet 1978; 146:33–37
16. Halliday AW, Benjamin IS, Blumgart LH: Nutritional risk factors in major hepatobiliary surgery. J Parent Ent Nutr 1988; 12:43–48
17. Detsky AS, Baker JP, O'Rourke K, et al: Predicting nutrition-associated complications for patients undergoing gastrointestinal surgery. J Parent Ent Nutr 1987; 11:440–446
18. Mughal MM, Meguid MM: The effect of nutritional status on morbidity after elective surgery for benign gastrointestinal disease. J Parent Ent Nutr 1987; 11:140–143
19. Harvey HJ: Complications of small intestinal biopsy in hypoalbuminemic dogs. Vet Surg 1990; 19:289–292
20. Sheffy BE, Williams AJ: Nutrition and the immune response. J Am Vet Med Assoc 1982; 180:1073–1076
21. Sheffy BE: Nutrition, infection, and immunity. Compend Contin Educ Pract Vet 1985; 7:990–997
22. Gross RL, Newberne PM: Role of nutrition in immunologic function. Physiol Rev 1980; 60:188–302
23. Rahmathullah L, Underwood BA, Thulasiraj RD, et al: Reduced mortality among children in southern India receiving a small weekly dose of vitamin A. N Engl J Med 1990; 323:929–935
24. Keusch GT: Vitamin A supplements—Too good not to be true. N Engl J Med 1990; 323:985–986
25. Shenkin A, Fell GS: Mineral and vitamin requirements in parenteral nutrition. In Karran SJ, Alberti KGMM (eds): Practical Nutritional Support. Kent, England: Pittman Medical, 1980, pp 68–80
26. Alberti KGMM: Metabolic pathways—Hormone–metabolite interrelations. In Karran SJ, Alberti KGMM (eds): Practical Nutritional Support. Kent, England, Pitman Medical, 1980, pp 5–19
27. Allen TA: Specialized nutritional support. In Ettinger SJ (ed): Textbook of Veterinary Internal Medicine, 3rd ed. Philadelphia: WB Saunders, 1989, pp 450–455
28. Crowe DT Jr: Enteral nutrition for critically ill or injured patients, part 1. Compend Contin Educ Pract Vet 1986; 8:603–613
29. Wheeler SL, McGuire BH: Enteral nutritional support. In Kirk RW, Bonagura JD (eds): Current Veterinary Therapy X. Philadelphia: WB Saunders, 1989, pp 30–37
30. Lewis LD, Morris ML Jr, Hand MS: Anorexia, inanition, and critical care nutrition. In Lewis LD, Morris ML Jr, Hand MS (eds): Small Animal Clinical Nutrition III. Topeka, Kansas: Mark Morris Associates, 1987, pp 1–43
31. Copeland EM III, Dudrick SJ, Daly JM, Ota DM: Nutritional changes in neoplasia. In Kinney JM, Jeejeebhoy KN, Hill GL, Owen OE (eds): Nutrition and Metabolism in Patient Care. Philadelphia: WB Saunders, 1988, pp 515–534
32. Fearon KCH, Carter DC: Cancer cachexia. Ann Surg 1988; 208:1–5
33. Bozzett F, Pagnoni AM, Del Vecchio M: Excessive caloric expenditure as a cause of malnutrition in patients with cancer. Surg Gynecol Obstet 1980; 150:229–234
34. Heber D, Byerley LO, Chi J, et al: Pathophysiology of malnutrition in the adult cancer patient. Cancer 1986; 58:1867–1873
35. Vail DM, Ogilvie GK, Wheeler SL: Metabolic alterations in patients with cancer cachexia. Compend Contin Educ Pract Vet 1990; 12:381–386
36. Silberman H: Hyperalimentation in patients with cancer. Surg Gynecol Obstet 1980; 150:755–757
37. Vail DM, Ogilvie GK, Wheeler SL, et al: Alterations in carbohydrate metabolism in canine lymphoma. J Vet Int Med 1990; 4:8–11
38. Buzby GP, Mullen JL, Stein TP, et al: Host–tumor interaction and nutrient supply. Cancer 1980; 45:2940–2948
39. Torosian MH, Donoway RB: Total parenteral nutrition and tumor metastasis. Surgery 1991; 109:597–601
40. Perioperative total parenteral nutrition in surgical patients. N Engl J Med 1991; 325:525–532
41. Baker JP, Detsky AS, Wesson DE, et al: Nutritional assessment: A comparison of clinical judgment and objective measurements. N Engl J Med 1982; 306:969–972
42. Pettigrew RA, Charlesworth PM, Farmilo RW, Hill GL: Assessment of nutritional depletion and immune competence: A comparison of clinical examination and objective measurements. J Parent Ent Nutr 1984; 8:21–24
43. Goode AW: The scientific basis of nutritional assessment. Br J Anaesth 1981; 53:161–167
44. Young GA, Hill GL: Assessment of protein–calorie malnutrition in surgical patients from plasma proteins and anthropometric measurements. Am J Clin Nutr 1978; 31:429–435
45. Gray GE, Gray LK: Anthropometric measurements and their interpretation: Principles, practices, and problems. J Am Diet Assoc 1980; 77:534–539
46. Canizaro PC: Methods of nutritional support in the surgical patient. In Yarborough MF, Curreri PW (eds): Surgical Nutrition. New York: Churchill Livingstone, 1981, pp 13–37

47. Grant JP, Custer PB, Thurlow J: Current techniques of nutritional assessment. Surg Clin North Am 1981; 61:437–463
48. Buzby GP, Mullen JL, Matthews DC, et al: Prognostic nutritional index in gastrointestinal surgery. Am J Surg 1980; 139:160–167
49. Ingenbleek Y, Van Den Schrieck HG, DeNayer P, De Visscher M: Albumin, transferrin and the thyroxine-binding prealbumin/retinol-binding protein (TBPA-RBP) complex in assessment of malnutrition. Clin Chim Acta 1975; 63:61–67
50. Bernstein LH: New markers of nutritional status. Am Clin Lab 1989; 8:20–23
51. Shetty PS, Watrasiewicz KE, Jung RT, James WPT: Rapid-turnover transport proteins: An index of subclinical protein–energy malnutrition. Lancet 1979; 2:230–232
52. Helms RA, Dickerson RN, Ebbert ML, et al: Retinol-binding protein and prealbumin: Useful measures of protein repletion in critically ill, malnourished infants. J Pediatr Gastroenterol Nutr 1986; 5:586–592
53. Raubenstine DA, Ballantine TVN, Greecher CP, Webb SL: Neonatal serum protein levels as indicators of nutritional status: Normal values and correlation with anthropometric data. J Pediatr Gastroenterol Nutr 1990; 10:53–61
54. Giacoia GP, Watson S, West K: Rapid turnover transport proteins, plasma albumin, and growth in low birth weight infants. J Parent Ent Nutr 1984; 8:367–370
55. Russell DMcR, Prendergast PJ, Darby PL, et al: A comparison between muscle function and body composition in anorexia nervosa: The effect of refeeding. Am J Clin Nutr 1983; 38:229–237
56. Meguid MM, Curtas S, Chen M, Nole E: Adductor pollicis muscle tests to detect and correct subclinical malnutrition in pre-operative cancer patients. (abstract) Am J Nutr 1987; 45:843
57. Duque E, Lotero H, Bolanos O, Mayoral LG: Enteropathy in adult protein malnutrition: Ultrastructural findings. Am J Clin Nutr 1975; 28:914–924
58. Feldman EJ, Dowling RH, McNaughton J, Peters TJ: Effects of oral versus intravenous nutrition on intestinal adaptation after small bowel resection in the dog. Gastroenterology 1976; 70:712–719
59. Lippert AC, Faulkner JE, Evans T, Mullaney TP: Total parenteral nutrition in clinically normal cats. J Am Vet Med Assoc 1989; 194:669–676
60. Burke DJ, Alverdy JC, Aoys E, Moss GS: Glutamine-supplemented total parenteral nutrition improves gut immune function. Arch Surg 1989; 124:1396–1399
61. Alverdy J, Chi HS, Sheldon GF: The effect of parenteral nutrition on gastrointestinal immunity: The importance of enteral stimulation. Ann Surg 1985; 202:681–684
62. Lo CW, Walker WA: Changes in the gastrointestinal tract during enteral or parenteral feeding. Nutr Rev 1989; 47:193–198
63. McArdle AH, Palmason C, Morency I, Brown RA: A rationale for enteral feeding as the preferable route for hyperalimentation. Surgery 1981; 90:616–623
64. Macy DW, Ralston SL: Cause and control of decreased appetite. In Kirk RW (ed): Current Veterinary Therapy X. Philadelphia: WB Saunders, 1989, pp 18–24
65. Macy DW, Gasper PW: Diazepam-induced eating in anorexic cats. J Am Anim Hosp Assoc 1985; 21:17–20
66. Dennis JS: Anabolic steroids: Their potential in small animals. Compend Contin Educ Pract Vet 1990; 12:1403–1410
67. Crowe DT Jr: Clinical use of an indwelling nasogastric tube for enteral nutrition and fluid therapy in the dog and cat. J Am Anim Hosp Assoc 1986; 22:677–682
68. Crowe DT Jr: Nutrition in critical patients: Administering the support therapies. Pet Pract 1989; 152–180
69. Stone EA: Alimentation. In Gourley IM, Vasseur PB (eds): General Small Animal Surgery. Philadelphia: WB Saunders, 1985, pp 1051–1057
70. Abood SK, Buffington CA: Improved nasogastric intubation technique for administration of nutritional support in dogs. J Am Vet Med Assoc 1991; 199:577–579
71. Valentine RJ, Turner WW: Pleural complications of nasoenteric feeding tubes. J Parent Ent Nutr 1985; 9:605–607
72. Crowe DT Jr: Enteral nutrition for critically ill or injured patients, part II. Compend Contin Educ Pract Vet 1986; 8:719–732
73. Bohning RH Jr, DeHoff WD, McElhinney A, Hofstra PC: Pharyngostomy for maintenance of the anorectic animal. J Am Vet Med Assoc 1970; 156:611–615
74. Lantz GC: Pharyngostomy tube installation for the administration of nutritional and fluid requirements. Compend Contin Educ Pract Vet 1981; 3:135–142
75. Crowe DT Jr, Downs MO: Pharyngostomy complications in dogs and cats and recommended technical modifications: Experimental and clinical investigations. J Am Anim Hosp Assoc 1986; 22:493–503
76. Lantz GC, Cantwell HD, VanVleet JF, et al: Pharyngostomy tube induced esophagitis in the dog: An experimental study. J Am Anim Hosp Assoc 1983; 19:207–212
77. Fox SM: Placing a pharygostomy tube for enteral feeding. Vet Med 1987; 82:903–906
78. Hand MS, Crane SW, Buffington CA: Surgical nutrition. In Betts CW, Crane SW (eds):

Manual of Small Animal Surgical Therapeutics. New York: Churchill Livingstone: 1986, pp 91-115

79. Crane SW: Placement and maintenance of a temporary feeding tube gastrostomy in the dog and cat. J Am Anim Hosp Assoc 1980; 11:770–776
80. Gauderer MWL, Ponsky JL: A simplified technique for constructing a tube feeding gastrostomy. Surg Gynecol Obstet 1981; 152:83–85
81. Bright RM: Percutaneous tube gastrostomy with and without endoscopy. Abstract, Proc Am Acad Vet Intern Med 1986; 1:265–269
82. Mathews KA, Binnington AG: Percutaneous incisionless placement of a gastrostomy tube utilizing a gastroscope: Preliminary observation. J Am Anim Hosp Assoc 1986; 22:601–610
83. Armstrong PJ, Hardie EM: Percutaneous endoscopic gastrostomy. Vet Med Rep 1989; 1:404–410
84. Ryan JA Jr: Jejunal feeding. In Kinney JM, Jeejeebhoy KN, Hill GL, Owen OE (eds): Nutrition and Metabolism in Patient Care. Philadelphia: WB Saunders, 1988, pp 757–777
85. Goring RL, Goldman A, Kaufman KJ, et al: Needle catheter duodenostomy: A technique for duodenal alimentation of birds. J Am Vet Med Assoc 1986; 189:1017–1019
86. Orton CE: Enteral hyperalimentation administered via needle catheter-jejunostomy as an adjunct to cranial abdominal surgery in dogs and cats. J Am Vet Med Assoc 1986; 188:1406–1411
87. Kronfeld DS: Protein and energy estimates for hospitalized dogs and cats. Purina Int Nutr Sym 1990; 5–11
88. Smith LC, Mullen JL: Nutritional assessment and indications for nutritional support. Surg Clin North Am 1991; 71:449–457
89. Crowe DT Jr: Tube feeding diets for nutritional support of the critically ill or injured patient . J Vet Emerg Crit Care 1985; 1:8–18
90. Jones BJM, Lees R, Andrews J, Frost P, Silk DBA: Comparison of an elemental and polymeric enteral diet in patients with normal gastrointestinal function. Gut 1983; 24:78–84
91. Armstrong PJ, Lippert AC: Selected aspects of enteral and parenteral nutrition support. Sem Vet Med Surg 1988; 3:216–226
92. Lippert AC, Armstrong PJ: Parenteral nutritional support. In Kirk RW (ed): Current Veterinary Therapy X. Philadelphia: WB Saunders, 1989, pp 25–30
93. Detsky AS: Parenteral nutrition–Is it helpful? N Engl J Med 1991; 325:573–575
94. Goodgame JT Jr: A critical assessment of the indications for total parenteral nutrition. Surg Gynecol Obstet 1980; 151:433–441
95. Alverdy JC, Aoys E, Moss GS: Total parenteral nutrition promotes bacterial translocation from the gut. Surgery 1988; 104:185–190.
96. Lippert AC, Faulkner JE, Evans AT, Mullaney TP: Total parenteral nutrition in clinically normal cats. J Am Vet Med Assoc 1989; 194:669–676
97. Burns GP, Stein TA: Pancreatic enzyme secretion during intravenous fat infusion. J Parent Ent Nutr 1987; 11:60–62

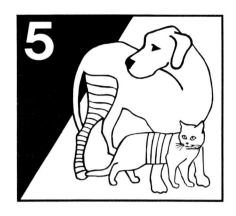

THE EFFECTS OF CHEMOTHERAPY AND RADIATION ON WOUND HEALING

ELIZABETH J. LAING

Surgery is used in cancer patients to establish a diagnosis, for staging, or as the primary mode of treatment for many localized solid-tissue tumors. Because cancer patients are often debilitated or immunosuppressed, surgery may be required to treat secondary infections or disease-related complications, as well as other traumatic injuries associated with everyday life.[1]

Wound healing in these patients may be affected for several reasons. The amount of tumor burden, with its associated metabolic changes, may alter the host's healing response. Adjuvant chemotherapy and radiation therapy also may affect the healing wound. This chapter reviews the potential problems associated with surgery in the cancer patient, and the effect of chemotherapy and radiation on wound healing.

WOUND HEALING IN THE CANCER PATIENT

Metabolic Effects

Wound healing may be impaired in the cancer patient as a result of primary disease or the patient's overall condition. Most cancer patients are older animals with some compromised organ function. Food intake and absorption may be reduced due to mechanical or functional disturbances, or as a result of cancer-induced anorexia. The chemical mechanism for cancer-induced anorexia has not been identified, but it may involve altered tryptophan metabolism, taste perception, and hypothalamic function.[1] Nutrients also may be lost through vomiting, diarrhea, proteinuria, hemorrhage, and open or draining wounds.

Cancer cachexia is a paraneoplastic syndrome that has a profound effect on the nutritional and metabolic status of the patient.[2] It is defined as a state of severe malnutrition and wasting despite adequate caloric intake. The pathogenesis involves a complex series of alterations in carbohydrate, protein, and fat metabolism. Glucose is the preferred substrate for energy production by tumor cells. However, the inefficient metabolism of glucose by tumor cells requires large amounts of glucose to meet energy demands. The increased rate of glucose turnover, coupled with glucose intolerance and less efficient utilization of glucose, contributes to the increased energy expenditure observed in many cancer patients.[3] Protein requirements may be increased as a result of increased protein use by the growing tumor and increased protein metabolism by the host. Cachectic cancer patients do not alter their metabolism to use fats as a primary energy source, as do other malnourished patients. This results in breakdown of protein from body stores, primarily skeletal muscle, to provide amino acid precursors for hepatic gluconeogenesis. Less protein is thus available to the host for collagen synthesis and cellular, hormonal, and immune functions. Altered metabolism of vitamins and minerals, especially vitamin A, zinc, and selenium, also may occur.[1,3]

Normally, wound healing is a preferred biologic process that provides for energy and substrate mobilization despite other metabolic abnormalities. In the cancer patient, wound healing has competition from another preferred biologic process, that of carcinogenesis. Wound-healing impairments have been demonstrated in tumor-bearing experimental animals.[1] A decreased supply of energy and protein substrates, coupled with impaired macrophage function and altered immune status, may lead to an increased complication rate in cancer patients undergoing surgery.

Severe caloric and protein depletions, defined as a loss of 15% to 20% of body weight, are recognized inhibitors of wound healing.[4] Recent clinical studies in human surgical patients suggest that protein–energy malnutrition also may impair wound healing before any measurable changes in body fat and protein stores occur. In patients undergoing elective gastrointestinal resection, Windsor and colleagues[5] found no correlation between the nutritional status (determined by changes in weight, total-body fat and protein, and plasma protein values) and the rate of wound healing. However, in patients with a 50% reduction in food intake for 1 week prior to surgery, the rate of wound healing was significantly less than in control patients with a normal food intake preoperatively. Supplemental nutrition in these patients restored the healing response to normal within a short time before there was significant or measurable restoration of fat and protein stores.[5] It is postulated that preoperative protein supplementation increases the patient's labile protein reserves, thus providing a biologic advantage in the face of depleted total-body reserves.

Specific Tumor Effects

The histologic type of tumor may influence the rate of wound healing or development of postoperative complications. Certain tumors are known to complicate wound healing; the most common of these in veterinary medicine is the cutaneous mast-cell tumor. Mast cells contain biologically active compounds such as proteolytic enzymes, histamine, and other vasoactive amines that participate in the inflammatory response. These compounds, if released during surgical manipulation of the tumor, bind to H1 and H2 histamine receptors of macrophages and suppress normal fibroplasia.[6] Delayed healing, with the tendency for wound dehiscence, may result. In theory, both H1 and H2 antihistamines may prevent delayed healing associated with mast-cell tumor excision, but this has not been examined clinically.

Thrombocytopenia, with the risk of increased hemorrhage at surgery, is a potential complication associated with a variety of neoplasms. This paraneoplastic disorder has been associated with malignant lymphoma, mammary adenocarcinoma, nasal adenocarcinoma, mast-cell tumor, hemangiosarcoma, and fibrosarcoma. The overall incidence of thrombocytopenia in tumor-bearing dogs has been estimated to be as high as 36%.[7] Mechanisms associated with decreased platelet numbers in cancer patients include decreased bone marrow production, sequestration of platelets in capillaries, increased platelet destruction, and increased platelet consumption, as in disseminated intravascular coagulation (DIC). DIC is most often seen with tumors involving the spleen or bone marrow and is diagnosed by thrombocytopenia, prolonged clotting times, decreased fibrinogen levels, and increased fibrinogen degradation products. Administration of intravenous fluids and heparin may be of therapeutic value in these cases. In most cases of tumor-associated thrombocytopenia, platelet numbers return to normal values following elimination of the tumor.

Tumor Recurrence

Local tumor recurrence can cause delayed or incomplete healing following cancer surgery. Tumor recurrence is most often the result of incomplete tumor excision and neoplastic invasion of the surgical margins.[8] Tumor growth follows the path of least resistance, extending along vascular structures and tissue planes. Surgical wounds and biopsy tracts create well-vascularized tissue planes, thus producing an ideal setting for local spread of residual tumor within the surgical site and through the healing incision.[9]

Another cause for local tumor recurrence is tumor seeding. *Seeding* is defined as the exfoliation and mechanical spread of tumor cells into the surgical wound and bloodstream, resulting in cell growth and gross tumor formation.[10] Unlike incomplete excision, in which the tumor regrowth begins from cells remaining at the surgical margins, neoplastic cells are deposited in the wound as a result of surgical or invasive diagnostic manipulation. The occurrence of tumor seeding depends on the cell biology of the seeded tumor, available blood supply and waste transport in the local environment, and number of cells seeded. Tumor seeding has been described in veterinary medicine after incisional biopsies and major excisional procedures and usually occurred at the primary incision site.[9] The median time from surgery to tumor recurrence was 6 weeks, ranging from 2 to 30 weeks. Aggressive carcinomas, particularly of the urinary tract, were the most common tumor seeded.

A third mechanism for tumor recurrence following surgical excision is inflammatory oncotaxis. This syndrome is characterized by a predisposition of neoplastic cells to deposit and grow in sites of inflammation.[9] Following surgical manipulation of a tumor, secondary tumors of the same histologic type can appear at distal sites of injury. In addition, implantation and growth of circulating tumor cells may result in recurrence at the site of primary excision.[8] Inflammation may result in increased delivery and entrapment of circulating tumor cells at the site of injury. However, since tumor cells form metastases at selective sites, tumor delivery itself is not sufficient for tumor development.[8] The extent of trauma or inflammation, as well as the number of tumor cells presented to the site, greatly influences the success rate of tumor-cell lodgment and growth. The frequency of tumor formation is greatest when tumor cells are presented to wounds in the early stages of healing. As wounds heal, they are less susceptible to tumor-cell growth. Surgical manipulation of tumors has not been shown to increase the incidence of tumor metastasis to nontraumatized organs.[8]

Surgical Guidelines

In most cases, surgical procedures are well tolerated by the cancer patient if appropriate diagnostic protocols and supportive care are provided. Preoperative evaluation should include a complete physical examination and assessment of the patient's overall health status. Ancillary diagnostics may include a complete blood count, clotting profile, renal and liver function tests, serum electrolyte levels, electrocardiogram, and radiographs of the affected area and common metastatic sites. The clinician should be aware of the various paraneoplastic syndromes associated with a given tumor type so that the appropriate diagnostic and therapeutic measures may be instituted.[11]

For malnourished patients, supplemental nutrition prior to surgery will help restore the wound-healing response to normal and may decrease the risk of postoperative complications. Animals most at risk for nutritional complications are those with severe weight loss (more than 20% of their body weight), hypoalbuminemia, partial or complete anorexia, or gastrointestinal dysfunction for more than 5 days.[2] Because of the profound metabolic alterations in cancer patients, 30% to 50% of nonprotein calories supplied each day should be from fat. Adequate protein intake is essential to meet the patient's increased demand. Vitamin and mineral supplementation is also recommended.[5]

Since most cancer patients are older and may have compromised organ function, a thorough consideration must be given to the anesthetic regimen. Local infiltrative anesthesia for superficial lesions should be avoided because it may distort tumor architecture (complicating histologic interpretation) and tumor margins and potentiate metastasis. In these cases, epidural or regional blocks may be preferred.[12]

During surgery, strict aseptic technique, gentle tissue handling, and attention to hemostasis will minimize postoperative complications. If the tumor has a vascular pedicle, the venous and arterial blood supply should be ligated early to avoid dissemination of tumor cells and control hemorrhage. Wide surgical excision is essential. The extent of excision should include a minimum margin of 1 cm of normal tissue in all planes and previous biopsy tracts. Invasive, inflamed tumors or those types known to be highly malignant will require wider margins. Tumors should never be "shelled out," since malignant tumors are often surrounded by a pseudocapsule of compressed tumor cells.[13] Nonreactive, nonabsorbable suture material, such as nylon or polypropylene, should be used for wound closure when excising inflamed or infected tumors or in cases where delayed wound healing is anticipated.

To reduce the likelihood of tumor seeding, avoid manipulation of the tumor in surgery and during the preoperative preparations. If, during excision, surgical equipment is contaminated by contact with the tumor, gloves and instruments should be changed and the wound flushed with sterile saline. When tumors are removed from the abdominal or thoracic cavity, the wound margins should be protected with impervious draping material to minimize the risk of seeding the skin margins with tumor cells.[11, 12]

Only lymph nodes clinically affected with tumor should be excised. If regional lymph nodes are to be removed, *en bloc* resection is recommended (removal of tumor, lymph node, and intervening lymphatics). This will remove any malignant cells remaining within lymphatic channels. Normal lymph nodes should not be removed because they may act as a mechanical filter and immunologic barrier.[12, 13]

Following surgical excision, the excised tissue should be submitted for histologic diagnosis. It is essential that the tissue submitted be representative of the lesion, well-fixed, and submitted with an accurate history.[13] Tissue that is necrotic, ulcerated, or too superficial may result in an inaccurate histologic evaluation. If the mass is large, several small, representative samples should be submitted. Often the junction between normal and neoplastic tissue is used to evaluate the differences in tissue type and invasiveness. The biopsy sample should be less than 1 cm thick and fixed in $10\times$ volume of 10% neutral buffered formalin. After fixation for 24 hours, the sample may be placed in an equal volume of formalin for mailing. If a malignancy is suspected, the surgical margins should be labeled with suture material and the pathologist asked to check the extent of excision. Incomplete excision may require further surgery and/or adjuvant therapy.

EFFECT OF CHEMOTHERAPY ON WOUND HEALING

Chemotherapy is combined with surgery to treat locally invasive, nonresectable, or potentially metastatic tumors. The goal of surgery is to decrease the patient's tumor burden to subclinical levels so that residual tumor cells are more sensitive to chemotherapy.[11] By the time a tumor is clinically detectable (approximately 1 cm^3 in size), 90% of tumor cells have stopped dividing and are relatively resistant to chemotherapy. For this reason, cytoreductive surgery is used to decrease the overall tumor burden, ideally to microscopic levels, and to remove drug-resistant cells. The remaining tumor cells then shift into a more active growth phase with the potential for increased sensitivity to chemotherapy.[14] In addition, the reduced tumor volume may stimulate the host's immune system by removing circulating immune complexes and other tumor-associated immunosuppressants.[15] Experimental studies have confirmed that, in terms of tumor-cell kinetics, antineoplastic agents are most beneficial when given at or near the time of surgery.[4, 15] Because surgical wounds have a high percentage of dividing cells, they are also susceptible to growth inhibition by these agents.

Indirect Effects

Antineoplastic drugs may affect wound healing by direct inhibition at the cellular level or indirect alteration of the nutritional or immune status of the patient.[16] In the latter case, prolonged or repeated episodes of chemotherapy-induced anorexia may result in weight loss and decreased nitrogen balance. Certain chemotherapeutic drugs may damage the gastrointestinal tract and interfere with nutrient absorption, thus decreasing the amount of substrate available for collagen synthesis. The net effect is decreased collagen production and delayed fibroplasia.[1, 17]

The cellular part of the immune system plays an important role in wound healing. Immunosuppression has a wide range of effects, including altered availability of certain cell substrates and impaired cell function such as inhibition of cell migration, proliferation, and protein synthesis. Despite these effects, most wounds in immunosuppressed patients heal without complications if good surgical practices are followed. However, if infection or dehiscence should occur, these patients may not have the reserves necessary to overcome postoperative complications.[18]

Direct Cellular Effects

Antineoplastic chemotherapy may affect all phases of wound healing.[1, 11] The inflammatory phase begins immediately after injury with local vasodilation and increased vascular permeability mediated by proteolytic enzymes, kinins, and prostaglandins released from injured cells. Neutrophils and macrophages phagocytize cellular debris and bacteria. Macrophages also stimulate fibroblast proliferation and neovascularization. Chemotherapy-induced bone marrow suppression may result in thrombocytopenia and neutropenia. Theoretically, fewer cells will then be available for phagocytosis, thereby prolonging the inflammatory phase and increasing the risk of infection. However, in the uncontaminated wound, the tissue macrophage is sufficient for phagocytosis, and wound healing can proceed despite anemia, neutropenia, or lymphopenia.[17, 19] If, however, the wound becomes contaminated with sufficient bacteria (approximately 10^6 organisms per gram of tissue), neutropenia may result in an increased rate of wound infection and delayed healing.[20] In addition to bone marrow suppression, other deleterious effects of chemotherapy at this stage include altered vascular permeability and platelet aggregation and stabilization of lysosomal membranes. These may all serve to prolong the inflammatory response.[17, 21]

Because of the high rate of cell division, the proliferative phase of wound healing is most susceptible to inhibition by antineoplastic agents.[22] Fibroblast proliferation, neovascularization, and epithelial-cell migration begin 3 to 5 days after injury and last about 2 weeks. Any drug that inhibits DNA replication, RNA production, or protein synthesis may inhibit fibroplasia and neovascularization, resulting in decreased collagen formation. *Epithelialization and wound contraction also may be affected. It is this phase of healing that is most often affected by cancer cachexia and chemotherapy-induced malnutrition.*[17]

Wounds reach their maximum collagen content 8 weeks after surgery, but wound strength continues to increase during the following months because of realignment and cross-linking of collagen fibers. *This maturation phase of healing may be disrupted by any drug that interferes with collagen metabolism.*[11]

Antineoplastic drugs are classified according to their mechanism of action into alkylating agents, antibiotics, mitotic inhibitors, antimetabolites, hormones, and miscellaneous agents. The effect of these agents on wound healing reflects their underlying mechanisms of action and the time of administration.

ALKYLATING AGENTS

The alkylating agents include mechlorethamine hydrochloride (nitrogen mustard), cyclophosphamide, chlorambucil, melphalan, dacarbazine, and busulfan. These agents inhibit cell division by inserting an alkyl radical for a hydrogen ion, resulting in DNA cross-linkage, inhibition of DNA synthesis, and immunosuppression.[23] They may affect cells in any phase of the cell cycle but are most toxic to those cells undergoing DNA synthesis. Experimentally, alkylating agents display a dose-dependent effect on the proliferative phase of wound healing by decreasing wound strength, inhibiting wound contraction, and decreasing collagen production. This effect is greatest when these agents are given in the immediate postoperative period. If administration is delayed 4 days after surgery, the impact on the healing wound is less severe.[19, 24]

Of these agents, cyclophosphamide is the drug most commonly used in veterinary medicine. In addition to the effect on cells in the proliferative phase, cyclophosphamide has the unique effect of producing immunosuppression and decreasing neovascularization.[17] It may indirectly promote wound infection as a result of bone marrow suppression and the resulting neutropenia. Large doses also will delay scar maturation.[11]

ANTIMETABOLITES

The antimetabolites include methotrexate, 5-fluorouracil, cytosine arabinoside, and 6-mercaptopurine. These agents interfere with DNA synthesis by substituting abnormal molecules for normal nucleotides, thereby causing misreading of the genetic code. Methotrexate and 6-mercaptopurine also inhibit RNA and protein synthesis. In both clinical and experimental studies, these agents have demonstrated a dose-dependent effect on the proliferative phase of wound healing.[17, 19] Complications occurred most frequently in patients with weight loss and nutritional deficiencies or when the drug was administered during the first 5 days after surgery. These effects were minimized by either giving the drug 5 days prior to surgery or delaying chemotherapy 10 to 14 days after surgery. In the case of methotrexate, the effect was entirely reversed with simultaneous folic acid administration.[10, 25]

MITOTIC INHIBITORS

Vincristine sulfate, vinblastine sulfate, and etoposide are mitotic inhibitors used in veterinary medicine. These agents bind to the intracellular microtubular system, preventing cell division. Experimentally, administration of vincristine sulfate on the day of surgery caused a transient delay in wound healing, and this effect was gone by the seventh day after surgery.[19] Impairment at this early stage of healing carries little clinical significance because collagen production has not yet begun. These agents appear to have little effect on later stages of wound healing in either experimental or clinical studies.[19, 25]

ANTITUMOR ANTIBIOTICS

The antitumor antibiotics include doxorubicin hydrochloride, bleomycin sulfate, actinomycin, and mitomycin. These agents are natural products of soil fungi and prevent DNA, RNA, and protein synthesis by a variety of mechanisms. They may interfere with the proliferative phase of wound healing by decreasing overall wound strength secondary to inhibition of cellular proliferation and protein synthesis. They also may indirectly promote wound infection as a result of bone marrow suppression and the resulting neutropenia.[17]

Of these agents, doxorubicin has been studied most extensively. As with cyclophosphamide, the effect of doxorubicin on wound healing was most profound when it was given during the first few days following surgery. In mice, doxorubicin impairment of wound healing was found to be related to the degree of weight loss, which, in turn, depended on the dose. Apparently, the initial effect on the healing wound is due, in part, to a short-term nutritional deficit perhaps brought on by drug-induced anorexia and gastrointestinal dysfunction. Later effects are due to inhibition of cellular proliferation and protein synthesis.[16, 26]

When doxorubicin is combined with radiation therapy, there is an additive impairment on wound healing with decreased production of wound collagen and decreased wound breaking strength. Systemic doxorubicin chemotherapy may produce ulceration in areas previously treated with radiation. This radiation "recall effect" suggests that irradiated fibroblasts have permanently impaired synthetic or proliferative function. When these tissues are exposed to doxorubicin, they are unable to maintain their integrity, and chronic ulcerations develop. A similar effect has been demonstrated with actinomycin D.[27]

CORTICOSTEROID HORMONES

Corticosteroids are the most commonly used antitumor hormones in veterinary medicine. Steroids interfere with wound healing by altering the initial anti-inflammatory response to injury. Specific mechanisms include stabilization of intracellular lysosomal membranes, mobilization of neutrophils with decreased local phagocytosis, and inhibition of DNA synthesis.[28] Inhibition of phagocytosis and intracellular killing, coupled with impaired cellular and humoral immune response, also may increase susceptibility to infection.[29] The chemical structure of the compound also may affect the resultant susceptibility to infection. Sodium phosphate and acetate compounds are more likely to be associated with increased risk of infection than sodium succinate compounds.[29, 30]

Corticosteroids may delay later phases of healing by inhibiting fibroblast proliferation and granuloma formation, delaying collagen synthesis and epithelialization, and decreasing the rate of wound contraction. Steroids also may influence healing by inducing mild anorexia or protein depletion. Finally, steroids may delay wound maturation by inhibiting collagenase activity.[29]

The effect of corticosteroids on wound healing will vary with the dose and route of treatment. Systemic treatment requires a higher dose than local treatment to produce the same adverse effect.[17, 29] The type of steroid also will determine the effect on wound healing. In experimental studies, dexamethasone appeared to have less effect on tensile strength than hydrocortisone or methylprednisolone acetate.[29] However, when compared with an equipotent anti-inflammatory dose of methylprednisolone sodium succinate, dexamethasone caused a significant dose-dependent delay in wound healing. The effect of the different compounds on wound healing has been attributed to differing effects on cellular processes, such as collagen synthesis and cellular uptake of amino acids and collagenase activity, rather than differing anti-inflammatory effects due to cell population changes or altered protein or carbohydrate metabolism. In other words, steroid-induced inhibition of wound healing is not solely a result of inhibition of inflammation during the early phase of wound healing.[29, 31]

Clinically, only prolonged or high-dose corticosteroid therapy started prior to surgery causes a significant delay in wound healing. This effect is enhanced by mild starvation or protein depletion. DL-Methionine, which is converted to cysteine in the body, can be used to supplement the diet of protein-deficient animals undergoing surgery and, in part, mitigate this effect. Once the inflammatory phase is established, usually within 3 days of injury, corticosteroid therapy has little effect on subsequent healing.[29, 31]

If prolonged or high-dose preoperative corticosteroid therapy is necessary, vitamin A or zinc supplementation may be used to mitigate the adverse effects of steroids on wound healing. Vitamin A counters the effect of steroids on lysosomal membranes by acting as a membrane labilizer, enhancing the early inflammatory reaction. It also may increase the accumulation of reparative collagen by modulating collagenase activity, stimulate epithelial-cell and fibroblast differentiation, and stimulate immune responsiveness.[32] Systemic vitamin A supplementation is most effective in the vitamin A–deficient patient; the benefit of treating nondeficient patients is less clear. Experimentally, vitamin A therapy is less effective in animals that have undergone significant weight loss in association with steroid therapy.[33] Large doses of vitamin A carry a risk of associated toxicity, such as headache, blurred vision, nausea and vomiting, calcification of tendons and ligaments, periosteal new bone formation, neuritis, and skin hyperpigmentation. Topical application of vitamin A should be avoided because it may inhibit wound healing.[33]

Prolonged corticosteroid therapy results in decreased serum zinc levels.[34] Zinc is a cofactor in at least 18 metalloenzyme systems used in protein synthesis. Zinc deficiency causes incomplete epithelialization and decreased rate of gain of wound strength. Clinically, delayed wound healing and cutaneous ulceration may result. In serum zinc–deficient animals, zinc supplementation will increase fibroblast and epithelial proliferation. Clinical improvement occurs in 12 to 14 days. Zinc supplementation has shown little effect on wound healing in nondeficient experimental animals.[28]

Other agents that have shown some promise in countering corticosteroid-induced healing include anabolic steroids, growth hormone, and specific growth factors, such as platelet-derived growth factor. Tetrachlorodecaoxy-gen–anion complex, an inorganic agent, has been shown to antagonize corticosteroid-induced inhibition of wound contraction. These agents offer potential new therapeutic modalities for the treatment of corticosteroid-induced healing impairment.[1, 35]

Medical Guidelines

Most of the available information on the effect of chemotherapy on wound healing comes from experimental animal studies. These finding may not necessarily correlate with clinical findings for several reasons.[14] Experimental tumor models are often selected for their rapid rate of growth and response to therapy. This response may not be representative of spontaneous tumors in clinical patients. Experimental studies on wound healing measure defined parameters, such as wound tensile strength and collagen content, to determine the impact of drug on the rate of healing. Minor changes in these parameters would not be detected in a clinical setting. In fact, in most clinical situations, 15% of ultimate tensile strength may be sufficient to resist normal wound stress.[30] Finally, interpretation of both experimental and clinical results may be complicated by the additive effects of tumor burden and nutritional status on wound healing.[25, 36]

The experimental work on wound healing and chemotherapy has shown these agents to have a diverse range of measurable effects on different phases of the healing process. However, comparison of early individual studies revealed varied and often contradictory results. Cohen and colleagues[37] and other researchers were instrumental in documenting that the time of administration, treatment schedule, dose level, differential organ sensitivity, and time of evaluation were all experimental variables that would influence the results. For example, drugs that primarily affect the inflammatory phase of healing would be expected to show early wound-healing changes, whereas test results taken 2 to 3 weeks after surgery may be normal. Drugs affecting cell division and protein synthesis would be more likely to show a delayed effect. Drugs that cause bone marrow suppression with secondary pancytopenia are most likely to interfere with healing when given a week or so prior to surgery, since pancytopenia usually develops 7 to 10 days after administration.[17] The toxicities of these agents on the various organ systems are summarized in Table 5–1.

In most experimental studies using therapeutic dosage regimens, antineoplastic agents generally do not have a significant impact on wound healing.[21, 26] The vinca alkaloids have the fewest adverse effects on wound healing. Doxorubicin and the antimetabolites, on the other hand, are most often associated with subsequent wound complications. High-dose or long-term corticosteroid therapy also may delay wound healing. Little information is available on the effect of combinations of chemotherapeutic agents, but in general these combinations would be potentially more toxic than individual agents.

In considering perioperative chemotherapy in the clinical setting, the following treatment guidelines are proposed.[4, 11, 21] Cytoreductive surgery should remove at least 90% of tumor cell, meaning virtually all visible tumor

TABLE 5–1. Organ System Toxicities of Common Antineoplastic Agents in Animals

DRUG	BONE MARROW	SKIN AND MUCOSA	GI TRACT	LIVER	KIDNEY	URINARY BLADDER	HEART	LUNGS	NERVOUS SYSTEM	IMMUNE SYSTEM
Alkylating Agents										
Cyclophosphamide	X		X			X				X
Chlorambucil	X		X							
Nitrogen mustard	X		X							
Busulfan	X		X					X		
Antimetabolites										
Methotrexate	X	X	X	X	X					
6-Mercaptopurine	X		X	X						
5-Fluorouracil	X	X	X						(Cats only)	
Cytosine arabinoside	X		X							
Mitotic Inhibitors										
Vincristine			X						X	
Vinblastine	X		X							
Antibiotics										
Doxorubicin	X		X		(Cats only)		X			
Bleomycin								X		
Hormones										
Prednisone			X							X

Source: From Rosenthal RC: Chemotherapy. In Withrow SJ, MacEwen EG (eds): Clinical Veterinary Oncology. Philadelphia: Lippincott, 1989, with permission.

mass, to alter cell kinetic and immune parameters. Less complete excision may benefit the patient in terms of function or cosmetics but is unlikely to alter the tumor response to adjuvant chemotherapy. Conscientious attention to aseptic technique, hemostasis, and gentle tissue handling is essential to minimize the risk of postoperative complications. The surgeon should close the incision in the most secure manner and leave skin sutures in place for 14 to 21 days. Nutritional supplementation should be considered in malnourished patients to maximize their nutritional status and correct any vitamin, mineral, and substrate imbalances. Following surgery, the animal should be monitored closely until the risk of serious complications is minimal.

The clinician should expect that the benefit of perioperative chemotherapy outweighs the risk to the patient and the expense to the owner. Drug selection should be based on a demonstrated effect for that particular tumor type in veterinary or human clinical trials. In the latter case, the clinician should be familiar with species variations in terms of dosage, administration, and toxicity. The patient should be monitored closely for therapy-related complications. The facilities for supportive care, such as fresh blood transfusions, should be available if complications occur.

The ideal time to start chemotherapy must be decided on an individual basis, with the benefits of immediate chemotherapy weighed against the risk of wound complications. *In tumors with a slow doubling time, a delay of 1 or 2 weeks following surgery is unlikely to have an adverse effect on patient survival. In more rapidly growing tumors, earlier therapy may be warranted.* The adverse effects of these agents on wound healing usually occur within a week or two of administration. For this reason, the best time to start chemotherapy is after the period of risk for serious postoperative complications has passed. *For simple procedures, such as lymph node biopsies, this may mean that treatment can be started later the same day. For large tumor resections, a delay of 7 to 10 days may be more prudent.*[21]

Extravasation Injuries

In addition to systemic effects, many antineoplastic chemotherapeutics can produce local wound problems at the site of injection if they are inadvertently administered perivascularly. The amount of tissue damage is determined by the type, rate, and amount of agent and the nature of the tissue into which the drug is administered. High-risk areas are those with poor blood supply, low-grade blood flow, fragile veins, poor lymphatic drainage, and previously irradiated areas.[17, 38] Vesicant (Latin *vesica,* "blister") drugs, such as doxorubicin and vincristine, are most irritating because of their affinity for intracellular binding and secondary tissue necrosis. Alkylating agents and antimetabolites are associated with fewer injuries because they generally are not active when infiltrated into subcutaneous tissues. They may produce tissue irritation but rarely tissue necrosis.[1]

Following perivascular infusion, pain may be the only initial sign of injury. Later, superficial and then deep ulcerations may develop as a result of progressive tissue damage.[1, 39] Tissue ulceration occurs secondary to vascular obliteration and collagen necrobiosis, with little inflammation. Increased systemic levels of drug may further affect healing secondary to the vesicant effect.

Because of the potentially devastating effect of perivascular infusion of vesicant agents, the clinician should take extra care in their administration.

Extravasation of a highly concentrated solution will produce a greater local tissue reaction than a diluted dose. However, excessive dilution will prolong infusion times, which increases the risk of extravasation. Therefore, vesicant drugs should be mixed in the appropriate dilution and given over the shortest period of time consistent with the patient's venous capacity and tolerance.

These drugs should be administered using an indwelling or butterfly catheter placed in a superficial vein some distance from joints or neurovascular bundles. After catheterization, a small volume of normal saline is injected to test vein integrity and flow, as well as extravasation. If extravasation is observed, another vein is selected. The drug is given during a minimum 3-minute time interval. The recommended infusion rates for specific agents are listed in Table 5–2. Administration is discontinued immediately at the first sign of pain or discomfort. Following drug administration, the catheter is flushed with an appropriate volume of sterile saline prior to removal.

Many different treatments have been used on extravasation injuries in an attempt to prevent secondary tissue necrosis and ulceration. Current treatment philosophy in human medicine favors a conservative approach. The initial treatment is to remove the IV line immediately and apply ice to the area to retard the locally destructive effect of the vesicant. This treatment is continued for 15 minutes, four times daily for 3 days.[39] For most extravasation injuries, no further treatment is required. However, if erythema and blistering appear, the patient is at risk of tissue ulceration.

Treatment of extravasation ulcers requires aggressive surgical intervention because the ulcers do not respond to routine wound debridement by forming granulation tissue.[1] The entire affected area should be surgically excised to prevent residual drug from spreading from dying cells to adjacent viable

TABLE 5–2. Intravenous Infusion Rates for Various Antineoplastic Agents

DRUG	BRAND NAME (MANUFACTURER)	RECOMMENDED DILUENT	ADMINISTRATION RATE	VESICANT
Bleomycin	Blenoxane (Bristol Myers)	Normal saline or sterile water	Not available	No
Cyclophosphamide	Cytoxan (Mead Johnson)	Sterile or bacteriostatic water	Not available	No
Doxorubicin	Adriamycin (Adria Laboratories)	Normal saline to provide 2 mg/ml	10–15 minutes	Yes
5-Fluorouracil	Fluorouracil (Roche Laboratories)	Normal saline	3–5 minutes	No
Mitomycin	Mutamycin (Bristol Myers)	Normal saline or sterile water to provide 0.5 mg/ml	3–5 minutes per 20 ml	Yes
Nitrogen mustard	Mustargen (Merck Sharp & Dohme)	Normal saline to provide 1 mg/ml	2–3 minutes	Yes
Vinblastine	Velban (Eli Lilly)	Normal saline to provide 1 mg/ml	2–3 minutes	Yes
Vincristine	Oncovin (Eli Lilly)	Normal saline to provide 0.5 mg/ml	1–2 minutes	Yes

Source: Data compiled from refs. 38 and 47.

ones. Following excision, the area should be covered by a reconstructive skin flap or graft.

EFECT OF RADIATION ON WOUND HEALING

Surgery and radiation therapy may be combined sequentially or performed simultaneously, depending on the objectives of therapy. In all cases, the goal of combined therapy is to extend treatment to subclinical disease outside the surgical margins and improve the radioresponsiveness of tumors too large to be controlled by radiation alone. The use of adjuvant radiation therapy also may permit less radical surgical excision, thus minimizing cosmetic, anatomic, or functional loss to the patient.[40]

Biologic Effects

The effects of radiation are randomly induced in both normal and neoplastic cells in the treated area, and it is only with higher doses over a period of time that the majority of tumor cells may be killed or rendered sterile. The likelihood of damage to normal cells also increases.[1] Cells that divide quickly are affected by radiation sooner than cells that divide slowly. For this reason, healing wounds are susceptible to inhibition from adjuvant radiation therapy. In addition, wounds made in previously irradiated tissue also may have healing impairment.

The biologic effects of radiation therapy result from damage to cellular DNA. Radiation interacts with biologic tissues by generating free·radicals that damage DNA and associated proteins. This results in cell death at the time of cell division.[41] A major determinant of the type of damage is the type of radiation energy delivered. Negatively charged electrons can only penetrate the skin for approximately 1 cm, whereas photons and neutrons have the ability to penetrate more deeply.[1] The injuries caused by radiation are dose-dependent and affect only exposed tissues. Healing at distant sites is unaffected unless significant weight loss has occurred.[27]

Immediately following irradiation, an acute inflammatory reaction occurs. The skin may become moist and erythematous or dry and scaly. As these initial changes resolve, chronic epithelial and dermal changes consistent with radiation injury may be seen.[42] Cellular changes and alteration of the ground substance result in thinning and flattening of the dermis and epidermis. Other chronic changes include pigmentation, woody induration, telangiectasia, and decreased normal adnexal structures.[27, 43, 44] If the germinal epithelial cells are undamaged, most of these changes will resolve. However, if the epithelial cells fail to repopulate, the end result may be an atrophied dermis incapable of nourishing the epidermis and prone to chronic ulceration.

Ulceration and poor skin healing following radiation therapy have been attributed to tissue ischemia caused by progressive obliterative endarteritis of the microvasculature. The resulting decrease in blood flow contributes to poor healing following radiation, but it is clearly not the only cause. Recent experimental work has suggested that ionizing radiation has a direct effect on fibroblast proliferation and that fibroblasts can be permanently damaged by radiation. This·suggests that ionizing irradiation may have a direct inhibitory effect on wound healing.[27, 42]

Manifestation of this effect is influenced by other complicating factors such as prior surgery, trauma, and infection. Radiation therapy can affect all phases of wound healing. The impact on healing will vary with the anatomic site, surgical technique, and dose/time/scheduling factors of radiation therapy.

Preoperative Irradiation

Radiation is given prior to surgery to decrease the risk of metastasis during surgical manipulation of the tumor by sterilizing the tumor periphery. It also may decrease tumor size, thereby allowing less radical surgery to be performed. Finally, it may improve the outcome of subsequent surgery by removing nonresectable portions of the tumor. Surgery is then performed to remove the central, less radiosensitive tumor cells.

Preoperative radiation should be considered in animals with "fixed" tumors (i.e., tumors attached to deeper tissues), since fixation is usually the result of grossly infiltrating tumor. These infiltrating cells are often mitotically active, well oxygenated, and thus most sensitive to radiation therapy. It is generally recommended that preoperative radiation therapy encompass both primary lesion and regional lymph nodes.[45]

The healing of irradiated tissue is significantly impaired. Decreased blood supply and fibrosis may limit the delivery of platelets and inflammatory cells to the wound. This delay will decrease the quantity of factors available for stimulation of chemotaxis, mitogenesis, and collagen synthesis. The lack of inflammatory cells also may permit bacteria to proliferate more readily. The end result is slower wound healing with a higher risk of wound infection and other postoperative complications.[1]

Preoperative radiotherapy usually precedes surgery by 3 to 4 weeks. This delay allows normal tissues to recover from radiation damage before surgery yet avoids the later wound complications resulting from tissue fibrosis.[40] Experimental studies have revealed that wounds created later than 6 weeks after radiation have an increased incidence of complications due to delayed effects of radiation, such as fibrosis and tissue hypoxia.[22, 41] The optimal timing of preoperative radiation has yet to be evaluated in a prospective, randomized clinical trial.

Postoperative Irradiation

Radiation therapy is given after surgery to control local or regional tumor present in subclinical amounts beyond the margins of surgical resection or to treat nonresectable tissues after cytoreductive surgery. In the latter instance, cytoreductive surgery is performed first to improve the therapeutic response to radiation. The dose of radiation required to kill an aggregate of tumor cells increases with the number of cells. Because the radiation dose is limited by toxicity to normal tissue, radiotherapy alone often fails to control large tumor masses. By decreasing the tumor volume, cytoreductive surgery increases the probability that radiotherapy can control the remaining tumor cells. Another advantage of postoperative radiation is that information acquired at the time of surgery will assist in defining the extent of the disease and allow better planning of radiation therapy.[40, 45]

Radiation may be more effective postoperatively because there are fewer tumor cells to kill and because increased radiation may be more safely delivered to the area. Clinically, postoperative irradiation is associated with a lower complication rate compared with preoperative irradiation, at least in human medicine.[10] The disadvantage of postoperative radiation is that the tissues may be more fibrotic, less oxygenated, and thus less responsive to radiation.

Radiation therapy has maximal effect on wound healing when given within 2 weeks of surgery. Decreased infiltration of leukocytes may result in an increased incidence of wound infection. Decreased and delayed fibroblast proliferation also may delay healing. Some authors suggest that radiotherapy should be delayed until wound healing is completed, usually 2 to 3 weeks after surgery.[41, 46] Longer delays are associated with increased scar-tissue formation and secondary local hypoxia, which may interfere with subsequent irradiation. Longer delays also may allow tumor cells to repopulate, leading to decreased likelihood of residual tumor control by radiation.[40]

Radiation Guidelines

Both preoperative and postoperative radiation therapy may interfere with wound healing, but in most instances the clinical effect will not be detrimental and healing will occur. The following guidelines are recommended to minimize the risk of complications following combined surgery and radiation therapy.

When surgery is performed as a prelude to radiation therapy, the surgeon should mark the lines of excision, tumor margins, and residual cancer with metallic clips, sutures, or skin tattoos. A detailed description of the surgical findings should be included in the operative report to aid in radiation planning.[45] Standard principles of oncologic surgery should be followed to minimize tumor-cell exfoliation and scar-tissue formation. Theoretically, any reduction in the total number of tumor cells may increase the chance for tumor control. However, surgical excision has the greatest beneficial adjuvant value when it reduces residual disease to a subclinical level. Gross tumor remaining after surgery is likely to contain viable but hypoxic tumor cells. Hypoxic cells are two to three times more radioresistant than fully oxygenated cells. In addition, incomplete or sloppy excision may have a detrimental effect on the patient owing to manipulation of tumor with exfoliation of cells and decreased radiation tolerance as a result of tissue trauma. For surgery to have a meaningful benefit on future radiation therapy, only small foci of cells should be left behind.[40, 46]

When surgery is to be performed in previously irradiated tissue, it is best to wait until the initial inflammation has subsided but before secondary fibrosis becomes dense.[1] The surgical procedure should be planned in anticipation of decreased tensile strength and delayed wound healing. Irradiated tissue is fibrotic and unyielding, and it is prone to dehiscence if it is sutured under tension. Any systemic deficiency that might inhibit wound healing, such as protein–caloric malnutrition, should be corrected before treatment, if at all possible.

If dehiscence or ulceration occurs, the affected area should be debrided to remove all necrotic tissues.[43, 44] With the newer techniques using higher-voltage machines, radiation injury may extend into the deeper tissues. Debridement must include these tissues. If surgical debridement is incomplete, mechanical debridement with wet-to-wet dressings can be used. Wound desiccation should be avoided. Primary or reconstructive closure should immediately follow debridement.[42] Simple debridement of radiation wounds without subsequent closure should be avoided because these wounds are prone to further necrosis and ulceration. If a skin graft is needed, a split-thickness graft is preferred to a full-thickness graft because it requires less blood supply from the graft bed. Flaps or grafts created in irradiated skin are prone to infection and poor healing and should be avoided. The risk of graft failure following high-energy radiation is great because of damage to deeper tissues. In this case, a pedicled or axial-pattern skin flap, with its abundant blood supply, is recommended to provide coverage of the compromised tissue.

REFERENCES

1. Lawrence WT: Wound healing in the cancer patient: Effects of the disease and its treatment. In Moossa AR, Schimpff SC, Robson MC (eds): Comprehensive Textbook of Oncology. Baltimore: Williams & Wilkins, 1990, pp 1697–1705
2. Stone EA: Nutritional therapy in cancer patients. Proc Am Coll Vet Surg Forum, 1983; 1:31–35
3. Herber D, Byerly LO: Pathophysiology of malnutrition in the adult cancer patient. Cancer 1986; 58:1867–1873
4. Gundez N, Fisher B, Saffen EA: Effects of surgical removal on the growth and kinetics of residual tumor. Cancer Res 1979; 39:3861–3865
5. Windsor JA, Knight GS, Hill GL: Wound healing response in surgical patients: Recent food intake is more important than nutritional status. Br J Surg 1988; 75:135–137
6. Macy DW: Canine and feline mast cell tumors: Biologic behavior, diagnosis, and therapy. Semin Vet Med Surg (Small Animal) 1986; 1:72–83
7. Ogilvie GK: Paraneoplastic syndromes. In Withrow SJ, MacEwen EG (eds): Clinical Veterinary Oncology. Philadelphia: Lippincott, 1989, pp 29–40
8. Murthy SM, Goldschmidt RA, Rao LN, et al: The influence of surgical trauma on experimental metastasis. Cancer 1989; 64:2035–2044
9. Gilson SD, Stone EA: Surgically induced tumor seeding in eight dogs and two cats. J Am Vet Med Assoc 1990; 196:1811–1815
10. Ariyan S, Kraft RL, Goldberg NH: An experimental model to determine the effects of adjuvant therapy on the incidence of postoperative wound infection: Evaluating preoperative chemotherapy. Plast Reconstr Surg 1980; 65:338–345
11. Laing EJ: The effect of antineoplastic agents on wound healing: Guidelines for the combined use of surgery and chemotherapy. Compend Contin Educ Pract Vet 1989; 11:136–143
12. Harvey HJ: General principles of veterinary oncologic surgery. J Am Anim Hosp Assoc 1976; 12:335–339
13. Withrow SJ: Surgical oncology: Old and new ideas. Semin Vet Med Surg (Small Animal) 1986; 1:17–20
14. Spiegel RJ, Muggia FM: Cancer chemotherapy. In Kahn SB (ed): Concepts of Cancer Medicine. New York: Grune & Stratton, 1983, pp 337–351
15. Fisher B, Gundez N, Saffen EA: Influence of the interval between primary tumor removal and chemotherapy on kinetics and growth of metastasis. Cancer Res 1983; 43:1488–1492
16. Greenhalgh DG, Gamelli RL: Do nutritional alterations contribute to Adriamycin-induced impaired wound healing? J Surg Res 1988; 45:261–265
17. Ferguson MK: The effect of antineoplastic agents on wound healing. Surg Gynecol Obstet 1982; 154:421–429
18. Barbul A: Immune aspects of wound repair. Clin Plast Surg 1990; 17:433–442
19. Schaumberg RC, Devereux DF, Brennan MF: The effect of chemotherapeutic agents on wound healing. Int Adv Surg Oncol 1981; 4:15–58
20. Braunschweiger PG, Ting HL, Schiffer LM: Role of corticosteroids in the control of cell proliferation in residual tumor after surgical cytoreduction. Cancer Res 1983; 43:5801–5807
21. Graves G, Cunningham P, Raaf JH: Effect of chemotherapy on the healing of surgical wounds. Clin Bull 1980; 10:144–149
22. Newcombe JF: Effect of intraarterial nitrogen mustard infusion on wound healing in rabbits: Formation of granulation tissue and wound contraction. Ann Surg 1966; 163:319
23. Stanton ME, Legendre AM: Effects of cyclophosphamide in dogs and cats. J Am Vet Med Assoc 1986; 188:1319–1322
24. Desprez JD, Kiehn CL: The effects of Cytoxan (cyclophosphamide) on wound healing. Plast Reconstr Surg 1960; 26:301
25. Falcone RE, Nappi JF: Chemotherapy and wound healing. Surg Clin North Am 1984; 64:779–794

26. Devereux DF, Kent H, Brown MF: Time-dependent effect of Adriamycin and x-ray therapy on wound healing in the rat. Cancer 1980; 45:2805–2810
27. Shamberger R: Effect of chemotherapy and radiotherapy on wound healing: Experimental studies. Recent Results Cancer Res 1985; 98:17–34
28. Trevisani MF, Ricci MA, Tolland JT, Beck WC: Effect of vitamin A and zinc on wound healing in steroid-treated mice. Curr Surg 1987; 1:390–393
29. Goforth P, Guidas CJ: Effect of steroids on wound healing: A review of the literature. J Foot Surg 1980; 19:22–28
30. Madden JW, Anem AJ: Wound healing: Biologic and clinical features. In Sabiston DC (ed): Textbook of Surgery. Philadelphia: WB Saunders, 1981, pp 265–286
31. Dostal GH, Gamelli RL: The differential effect of corticosteroids on wound disruption strength in mice. Arch Surg 1990; 125:636–640
32. Weinzweig J, Levenson SM, Rettura G, et al: Supplemental vitamin A prevents the tumor-induced defect in wound healing. Ann Surg 1990; 211:269–276
33. Golan J, Mitelman S, Baruchin A, Ben-Hur N: Vitamin A and corticosteroid interaction in wound healing in rats. Isr J Med Sci 1980; 16:572–575
34. Ruberg RL: The role of nutrition in wound healing. Surg Clin North Am 1984; 64:705–714
35. Hatz RA, Kelley SF, Ehrlich HP. The tetrachlorodecaoxygen complex reverses the effect of cortisone on wound healing. Plast Reconstr Surg 1989; 84:956–959
36. Bland KL, Palin WE, von Fruanhofer JA, et al: Experimental and clinical observations on the effect of cytotoxic chemotherapeutic drugs on wound healing. Ann Surg 1984; 199:782–790
37. Cohen SC, Gabelnick HL, Honhson RK, et al: Effects of antineoplastic agents on wound healing in mice. Surgery 1975; 78:238–244
38. Ignoffo RJ, Friedman MA: Therapy of local toxicities caused by extravasation of cancer chemotherapeutic drugs. Cancer Treat Rev 1980; 7:17–27
39. Larsen DL: Alterations in wound healing secondary to infusion injuries. Clin Plast Surg 1990; 17:509–517
40. McLeod DA, Thrall DE: The combination of surgery and radiation in the treatment of cancer: A review. Vet Surg 1989; 18:1–6
41. McEntee MC, Page RL: Effect of radiation and chemotherapy on wound healing. Vet Cancer Soc Newsletter 1988; 12:4–5
42. Miller SH, Rudolph R: Healing in the irradiated wound. Clin Plast Surg 1990; 17:503–508
43. Luce EA: The irradiated wound. Surg Clin North Am 1984; 64:821–829
44. Reinsch JF, Puckett CL: Management of radiation wounds. Surg Clin North Am 1984; 64:795–802
45. Moss WT: The integration of irradiation and surgery as the treatment for selected cases. Int J Radiat Oncol Biol Phys 1982; 10:1373–1378
46. Fletcher GH: Basic principles of the combination of irradiation and surgery. Int J Radiat Oncol Biol Phys 1979; 5:2091–2096
47. Rosenthal RC: Chemotherapy. In Withrow SJ, MacEwen EG (eds): Clinical Veterinary Oncology. Philadelphia: Lippincott, 1989, pp 63–78

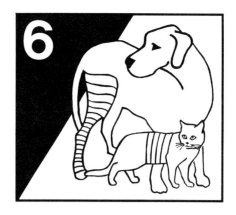

PATHOPHYSIOLOGY AND TREATMENT OF THERMAL BURNS

ERIC R. POPE
JOHN T. PAYNE

Severe thermal burns are treated infrequently in veterinary medicine. As a result, much of the information concerning care and treatment must be extrapolated from the human literature. A great deal can be learned from experimental studies using animal models. Thermal burns in small animals may result from building fires (Fig. 6–1), scalding injuries from hot water or grease (Fig. 6–2A), hot semiliquid/semisolid substances such as tar, direct contact with hot metals such as radiators, stoves, and automobile exhaust pipes, and iatrogenic burns caused by placing anesthetized or debilitated animals on heating pads for prolonged periods (Fig. 6–3A) or by improper use of heat lamps (Fig. 6–4) and hair dryers.

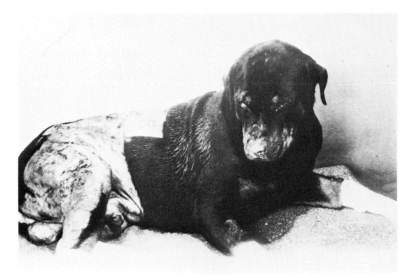

Figure 6–1. Extensive partial-thickness burns on a dog trapped in a burning building. Burns involved the head, forelimbs, and areas where the hair has been clipped.

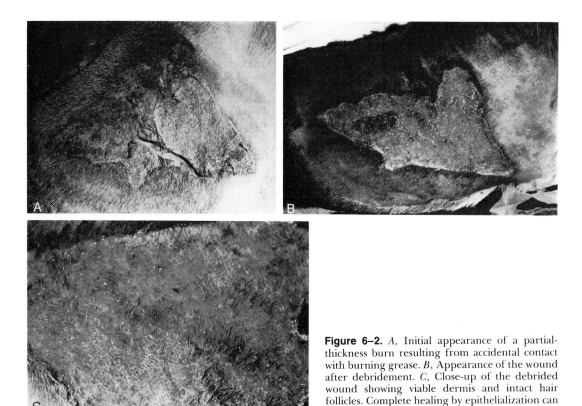

Figure 6–2. *A*, Initial appearance of a partial-thickness burn resulting from accidental contact with burning grease. *B*, Appearance of the wound after debridement. *C*, Close-up of the debrided wound showing viable dermis and intact hair follicles. Complete healing by epithelialization can be expected.

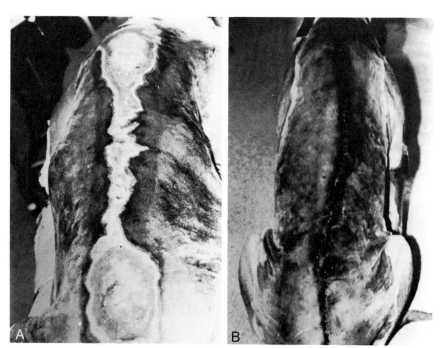

Figure 6–3. *A*, Large full-thickness burn on the dorsal midline resulting from a malfunctioning heating pad. *B*, Appearance after fascial excision and advancement of the surrounding skin to close the defect.

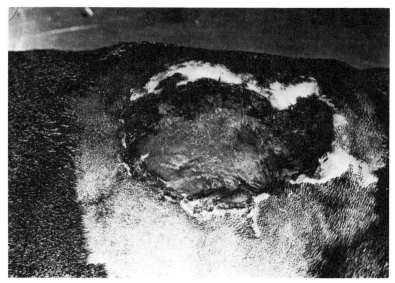

Figure 6–4. Full-thickness burn caused by a heat lamp. The eschar is beginning to spontaneously separate. Excision of the eschar and wound debridement are indicated.

CLASSIFICATION OF BURNS

Historically, burns have been classified as first-, second-, or third-degree based on the depth of injury.[1, 2] In some systems, a fourth category is added to denote extension of the injury into subcutaneous tissue, fascia, muscle, or bone.[1, 3] Because of differences in the skin between humans and animals, burns in animals are more appropriately classified as partial-thickness or full-thickness. Partial-thickness burns can be further divided as superficial or deep. Full-thickness burns include the full thickness of the skin and underlying structures.

In small animals, partial-thickness burns involving less than 15% of the total body surface area (TBSA) require minimal supportive therapy and local wound treatment.[4] Deep partial-thickness and full-thickness burns involving greater than 15% TBSA usually require emergency supportive therapy, extensive wound management, and reconstructive surgery.[4] Some reports[5–7] indicate that healthy animals with larger and more severe burns can survive with minimal supportive treatment because of the effectiveness of the normal compensatory mechanisms. Early and aggressive treatment, however, would be expected to decrease morbidity and mortality when other complicating injuries such as smoke inhalation are present. Considering the high morbidity and mortality, enormous expense, and suffering of the animal, euthanasia should be considered in patients with full-thickness burns covering greater than 50% TBSA. The location of the burn also should be considered because it may be best to euthanize a veterinary patient with severe burns of the face or external genitalia, or one in which a reasonable return to function cannot be expected.

PATHOPHYSIOLOGY OF THE BURN WOUND

Burns occur when heat energy is applied to tissue at a rate faster than it can be absorbed and dissipated. The severity of a thermal burn is influenced by the (1) temperature of the heat source, (2) duration of contact, and (3) and heat conductance characteristics of the contacted tissue.[1, 8] As with most wounds, a transition area separates completely devitalized tissue from uninjured healthy tissue. In the innermost zone closest to the heat source, excessive heat causes denaturation of cellular proteins and coagulation of blood within vessels, resulting in an area of complete necrosis *(zone of destruction or coagulation).*[3, 8, 9] Adjacent to this irreversibly damaged tissue is an area of injured tissue characterized by reduced blood flow and intravascular sludging *(zone of stasis).* The injuries in this area can be reversible. In the tissue furthest from the heat source, blood flow is increased, tissue damage is minimal, and complete healing usually occurs *(zone of hyperemia).*

Some vessels in the zone of stasis are completely thrombosed as a result of the burn, whereas others are patent but have damaged endothelial cells; this condition leads to platelet aggregation and thrombus formation.[10] Thromboxane A_2, one of the vasoactive metabolites of arachidonic acid released from injured tissue, is a potent vasoconstrictor and platelet aggregator responsible for the development of progressive dermal ischemia during the first 24 to 48 hours after burning.[10-12] Progressive dermal ischemia is an important factor in the conversion of partial-thickness burns into full-thickness injuries. Specific thromboxane synthetase blockers such as dipyridamole have been used to inhibit platelet adherence selectively, thereby preventing red blood cells (RBCs) and white blood cells (WBCs) from sticking to vessel walls. These compounds also cause vasodilation, but they do not interfere with the formation of other desirable prostaglandins such as prostacyclin.[10] Aspirin and corticosteroids, which affect other sites in the synthetic pathway, have not been shown to be more effective and can produce detrimental side effects.[10] Tissue trauma during wound treatments, edema formation, desiccation, and bacterial invasion also influence progression of the tissue damage.[8]

Hypovolemic shock and shock-induced renal failure were the leading cause of death in human burn patients in the 1940s.[13, 14] Hypovolemic shock is caused primarily by massive fluid shifts and vascular changes. Aggressive fluid replacement markedly decreases mortality but also can lead to massive edema formation in burned tissue and later throughout the body. Three processes contribute to the fluid shifts: (1) an increase in microvascular fluid flux, both local and generalized, (2) generalized impairment of the cell membrane, and (3) an increase in osmotic pressure of burn tissue, leading to further fluid accumulation.[13-15]

As in other injuries, thermal burns cause an immediate but transient decrease in blood flow to the damaged tissue. This is followed by pronounced arteriolar vasodilation in the microcirculation that remains.[13, 14] Capillaries and venules become highly permeable, allowing the movement of large volumes of fluid, electrolytes, and proteins from the vascular to the extracellular space.[8, 14] The protein concentration of the edema fluid in dogs is identical to that of plasma and contains proportionately as much globulin as albumin.[16]

Vascular damage due to direct thermal injury and the release of vasoactive substances such as histamine, leukotrienes, prostaglandins, and oxygen radicals from damaged tissue results in the formation of large gaps between endothelial cells. This allows movement of fluid and molecules with molecular weights of up to 150,000 from the vascular to the intersitial space.[14] Chemical mediators act primarily in venules and cause swelling and contraction of endothelial cells, whereas increased capillary permeability is primarily caused by direct heat injury to the endothelial cells.[15] The basement membrane usually remains intact, even in areas where endothelial cells are completely missing.[15] The formation of endothelial cell gaps is important in the disruption of the semipermeable membrane function of vessels; it is a primary determinant in the development of vascular thrombosis. A question still to be answered is why the major fluid loss is limited to the first few hours when endothelial gaps can persist for days or longer.

Some restriction of protein movement into the interstitial space occurs despite the large gaps between endothelial cells, and the basement membrane and interstitial matrix may play a major role in this control of fluid and protein flux.[15] The interstitium (including the basement membrane) consists of a complex network of hyaluronic acid fibers, a gel matrix of proteoglycans and glycosaminoglycans, and high concentrations of fibronectin, which serves as an intercellular cement.[15, 17] There is evidence that oxygen radicals, generated primarily in the extracellular space of the burned tissue, cause fragmentation of the interstitial hyaluronic acid fibers, which allows increased movement of protein into the interstitial space.[15] Three radicals are produced (superoxide anion, hydrogen peroxide, and hydroxyl ion), but the hydroxyl ion is the most damaging to tissues. Oxygen radicals are the only mediators that alter the basement membrane and the interstitium.[15] They are highly reactive and short-lived unless conditions favor their continued generation. Partially ischemic tissue generates more free radicals than totally ischemic tissue because there is a continuous, though much reduced, supply of oxygen.[17] Few free radicals are generated in totally ischemic or well-vascularized tissue.[17] A number of substances, including cholesterol, glutathione, and antioxidative enzymes such as superoxide dismutase and catalase, are naturally occurring free-radical scavengers.[18] This is an important concept because it helps to explain the temporal discrepancy in massive edema formation, which is generally confined to the first 24 to 36 hours, and reestablishment of the endothelial cell junctions, which may take days or weeks.[15]

Edema can also occur in nonburned tissue during fluid resuscitation. A generalized increase in vascular permeability owing to histamine release from damaged tissue is only transient and of relatively little significance.[14] Increased vascular permeability in the burned tissue allows large quantities of protein to enter the extracellular space at a rate that rapidly exceeds the ability of the lymphatic system to return the protein to general circulation. As the protein-rich fluid becomes trapped in the extracellular space, severe hypoproteinemia develops. Hypoproteinemia is further magnified during fluid resuscitation, and this results in generalized edema that is caused in two ways.[14, 15] A decrease in the plasma oncotic pressure causes an imbalance of the Starling forces and results in the movement of fluid out of the vascular tree and into the interstitial space. Also, in soft tissues an increase in the ease of water transport from the vascular to the interstitial space is caused by interstitial protein depletion,[14, 15] which seems to loosen the interstitial matrix and favor outward movement of fluid, even without an alteration in the balance of the Starling forces. Burn tissue also sequesters sodium, possibly by its increased binding to altered collagen, and the osmotic pressure generated by extracellular sodium pulls additional water from the circulation.

A generalized alteration of cell transmembrane potentials is a third process influencing fluid shifts, particularly in muscle.[13–15] Profound hypovolemia results in poor tissue perfusion, and impaired delivery of oxygen and nutrients leads to a reduction in cell membrane adenosine triphosphatase (ATPase). The potentials in cell membranes decrease from -90 to -70 to -80 mV, which cause a shift of extracellular sodium and, passively, water into the cell. Without fluid replacement, cell membrane potentials continue to fall until cell membrane function ceases at -60 mV.[16] Adequate volume replacement improves delivery of oxygen and nutrients to the tissues to reestablish cell membrane potentials. Cell membrane potentials are generally reestablished 24 to 36 hours after injury.[13–15]

Protein is lost into the extracellular space at its highest rate during the first 8 to 12 hours after injury. For example, as much as 50% of a human's total plasma volume can be lost from the vascular space within 2 to 3 hours following a burn injury of 40% TBSA or greater.[19] This rate decreases substantially by 18 to 24 hours if adequate perfusion is maintained.[15] Nevertheless, during the first 4 days after the patient suffers a moderate-sized burn, twice the normal plasma pool of albumin can be lost from the circulation.[8] Partial-thickness burns of 20% TBSA in dogs can result in a loss of 28% of the plasma volume during the first 6 hours after burning.[7]

INHALATION INJURY

Inhalation injury can occur alone or in conjunction with cutaneous burns. In humans, inhalation injuries occur in approximately one-third of all major burn victims and result in a significant increase in mortality.[20] Three problems are associated with inhalation injury: thermal burns of the upper airway, carbon monoxide poisoning, and smoke inhalation.[20–22]

Direct thermal injury is most frequently restricted to the upper airway because air conducts heat poorly and the airway itself dissipates heat effectively.[20] As an example, hot air entering the canine larynx at 270°C in one study cooled to 50°C while still in the trachea.[23] In the oropharynx and larynx, however, thermal injury causes progressive edema, leading to upper airway obstruction[21, 24] during the first 24 hours after injury. If respiratory distress and/or stridor develop in the first few hours after injury, upper airway injury should be suspected, especially if the fire occurred in a closed space. If the thermal injury extends further down the airway to the distal trachea and primary bronchi, bronchospasm and bronchorrhea can develop.[25] The clinical signs of such injury include wheezing and productive cough.

Carbon monoxide is generated during a fire as a result of the imperfect combustion of wood,[26] and, in humans, it is the most immmediate life-threatening disorder in the early hours after burn injury.[20, 21, 27] Because of its great binding affinity for hemoglobin (210 to 240 times that of oxygen), carbon monoxide displaces oxygen from hemoglobin and causes hypoxemia.[27] It also shifts the oxygen–hemoglobin dissociation curve to the left, further reducing oxygen delivery to the tissues. Carbon monoxide levels as high as 8% have been measured in experimental house fires,[26] and carboxyhemoglobin levels of 50% to 70% developed within 10 minutes in rats breathing air containing 1% carbon monoxide.[26] (Carboxyhemoglobin levels above 60% are usually fatal.[20]) With carbon monoxide levels of this magnitude, tissue hypoxia occurs in all end organs, and cardiac arrythmias are the most common cause of death.[27]

In addition to its direct effects, carbon monoxide also favors the development of pulmonary injury by depressing the normally reflexive decrease in breathing that occurs when heated air is inhaled.[26] The exact mechanism for this effect is unclear, but it may be related to (1) reduced consciousness interfering with the animal's ability to react to the heat by suppressing respiration, (2) suppression of tracheal secretion production secondary to hypoxia, or (3) hyperventilation induced by hypoxia.[26] Deep breathing or hyperventilation associated with carbon monoxide poisoning allows heated air that would normally be restricted to the upper airways to reach the pulmonary parenchyma. Inhalation of toxic substances is also enhanced in this condition.

There are many toxic by-products of combustion. For example, there are over 250 in pure pine smoke.[20] Polyvinyl chloride (PVC) polymers, which are widely used in insulation and plastic materials, release at least 75 toxic products, of which the most prominent are carbon monoxide and hydrogen chloride gas.[22, 24] Upper and lower airways also can be injured by other toxic gases and carbon particles coated with irritants such as aldehydes (the most toxic being acrolein), ketones, and organic acids.[20–22]

Concentrations of the various toxic products vary tremendously, but the response seen in the respiratory tract is similar. Diffuse tracheobronchial mucosal injury and pulmonary edema develop concurrently in sheep by 8 to 12 hours after smoke inhalation.[28, 29] Within 12 to 72 hours, necrosis and sloughing of the epithelial lining can be easily seen in the trachea and larger bronchi.[29] Partial or complete obstruction of the affected airways is caused by mucous plugs and shedding of the necrotic epithelial lining. Regeneration of damaged epithelium occurs by proliferation and migration of epithelial cells from surviving cells in the basal lamina and mucous glands.[29]

Within minutes, changes can be seen in the pulmonary parenchyma that produce signs of the adult respiratory distress syndrome.[30] Reduced surfactant levels and damage to pulmonary endothelium favor the development of interstitial and intraalveolar edema,[30, 31] and the end result is a marked decrease in lung compliance. In dogs, inactivation of pulmonary surfactant rapidly leads to the development of atelectasis.[31]

Following inhalation injury, a marked redistribution of blood flow results in a tenfold increase in bronchial blood flow.[22] This increased bronchial blood flow contributes to hypoxemia by augmenting venous admixture. Alterations in the bronchial vascular permeability cause interstitial and pulmonary edema, especially in patients with concomitant cutaneous burns who require vigorous fluid therapy.[31]

Bacterial pneumonia is a common sequela to inhalation injury and is now the major cause of death in patients with concurrent cutaneous burns who survive the initial resuscitative efforts.[21, 22] Bacterial invasion occurs by aerogenous or hematogenous routes. Necrotic tissue in the airway is an ideal culture medium for bacterial growth. Alteration of the normal mucociliary transport mechanism, impairment of pulmonary macrophage function, and systemic immunosuppression predispose the burn patient with inhalation injury to the development of pneumonia.[22, 32]

SYSTEMIC EFFECTS OF THERMAL BURNS

Cardiac Abnormalities

Cardiac output decreases soon after injury, even before major fluid shifts leading to hypovolemia occur. Scalding burns of 50% TBSA in dogs can cause a 40% to 50% decrease in cardiac output within minutes.[33] During the first hours, a further decrease of 10% to 20% can occur. Without adequate therapy, cardiac output continues to decline slowly until death occurs. A combination of peripheral vascular responses and direct myocardial effects causes this decrease in cardiac output. For example, peripheral vascular resistance doubles within minutes in dogs with 50% TBSA burns and remains high unless adequate fluid therapy is instituted.[34] Because of these peripheral responses, blood pressure is frequently normal despite reduced cardiac output. The increased resistance is due primarily to vasoconstriction caused by catecholamine release, although increased blood viscosity also plays a role.[34] In untreated dogs, blood viscosity rises two- to threefold within hours after burning,[34] and the increased viscosity (primarily due to the increased hematocrit) results in aggregation of red cells in postcapillary venules, impeding blood flow.

Following full-thickness burns covering 35% TBSA in dogs, direct myocardial depression caused decreases in left ventricular pressure and coronary blood flow.[34] The depressed contractility was attributed to hypoxia resulting from decreased oxygen uptake and altered carbohydrate metabolism. Nevertheless, controversy still surrounds the importance of the myocardial depressant factor in the development of cardiac dysfunction.[35, 36]

Hypovolemia secondary to fluid shifts is a primary cause of the continuing decreased cardiac output,[36] but cardiac output improves with fluid resuscitation. In dogs, a combination of crystalloid and protein is more effective than crystalloids alone in increasing cardiac output.[34] The use of protein (plasma), however, during the first 8 to 12 hours after injury, when vascular permeability is still altered, contributes to edema formation. Peripheral vasodilators reduce peripheral resistance and increase cardiac output in dogs,[19, 34] but they should not be administered until volume replacement has been achieved.

With restoration of the plasma volume by 48 hours after burning, peripheral vascular resistance decreases and a hypermetabolic or recovery phase begins. Cardiac output rises to one and one-half to three times normal and remains elevated until the wounds are closed.[37] Blood flow to all organs and tissues increases.

Anemia

Many factors contribute to the development of anemia in severely burned patients. Temperatures greater than 65°C lyse RBCs almost immediately.[34] Lower temperatures induce morphologic and physiologic changes that may not result in lysis until several hours later. In dogs, 50% TBSA burns caused by a 30-second scalding injury resulted in an 8% decrease in red cell volume by 6 hours.[38] Decreases in red cell mass are usually clinically inapparent, however, because the fluid shifts maintain the hematocrit at or above normal levels.[34, 36]

Thermal injury induces morphologic changes in red cells that result in their early removal from the circulation. Early morphologic changes include roughening of the cell membrane and the formation of buds that split off to form microcytes,[34, 39] and the membrane-damaged cells crenate, fragment, or become spheroid.[34] Spherocytes show increased osmotic fragility and are less deformable, making them more likely to be entrapped in capillaries. In dogs, most damaged red cells are removed from the circulation by the reticuloendothelial (RE) cells in the spleen, but RE cells in the liver also aid in this function.[34] Younger RBCs are more susceptible to injury, so there is an overall decrease in life span of the remaining RBC population.[36, 39]

In addition to direct heat injury, one or more plasma factors also can damage RBCs.[34, 40] Labeled RBCs from normal donors transfused into burned humans and experimental animals have a significantly reduced life span,[34, 40] whereas RBCs from burned patients transfused into normal volunteers exhibit a normal life span.[40] Alterations in plasma lipid constituents appear to be an important factor because RBCs transfused into burned patients undergo characteristic membrane changes and exhibit diminished survival while administration of plasma containing normal lipid constituents in normal quantities restores RBC survival time to normal.[41] A number of substances such as catecholamines, prostaglandins, and norepinephrine affect RBC survival through membrane-induced changes.[42]

Bone marrow suppression and inhibition of erythropoiesis also contribute to the anemia.[36] Impaired hematopoiesis persists until the burn wound is closed.[35] The anemia is normocytic and normochromic and accompanied by low serum iron level and iron-binding capacity similar to the anemia seen with chronic disease.[43] Plasma taken from burned patients 3 to 4 weeks after injury inhibits RBC colony growth.[43] Erythropoietin levels are variable, but even when they are elevated, erythropoiesis is not increased.[45] The plasma inhibitory substance and the cause of the diminished erythropoietin response have not been identified.

Multiple wound debridements and the harvesting of skin grafts frequently result in significant blood loss.[34, 36] It is essential to accurately monitor the amount of blood loss. Acute hemolytic anemia can occur following multiple blood transfusions or as a reaction to topical medications.[36] Wound infection and gastric ulceration also contribute to anemia.

Electrolyte Abnormalities

As previously discussed, alteration of cell membrane potentials and the affinity of sodium for denatured collagen in the burn wound cause a shift of sodium and water from the vascular space to the interstitial and intracellular spaces. Since volume replacement during the initial resuscitation is usually accomplished with isotonic crystalloid solutions containing sodium,[1, 37] hyponatremia is generally not seen clinically.[37]

If hypertonic saline solutions are used as the resuscitation fluid, however, hypernatremia can develop.[13, 36] Excessive sodium causes a significant hyperosmolar state and can produce central nervous system damage. Hypernatremia also can result from inadequate replacement of water lost by evaporation from the burn wound.[37]

Hyperkalemia is common in the early postburn period because the damaged RBCs and tissue release intracellular potassium into the circulation.[36, 37] This hyperkalemia is transient, and usually there are no clinical signs if renal function is maintained by adequate fluid resuscitation. Metabolic acidosis induces compensatory mechanisms, however, that can aggravate the elevation in serum potassium.

Hypokalemia is sometimes seen in the postresuscitation period as a result of the diuresis induced by the fluid therapy and later as a result of mobilization and excretion of burn wound edema fluid.[37] Potassium should be added to replacement fluids to maintain normal serum potassium levels.

In addition, hypokalemia can be accentuated if alkalosis develops secondary to hyperventilation as a result of respiratory distress.[36]

Hypophosphatemia is also common in humans with extensive burns.[36, 37] The clinical consequence of acute hypophosphatemia have not been clearly defined, but it can cause abnormalities in RBC and platelet function and reduce the phagocytic activity of WBCs.[36] Moreover, respiratory failure and abnormal brain cell function also have been reported.[36]

Hypocalcemia is caused by sequestration of calcium in burn tissue, presumably from saponification of fat in the subcutaneous tissue.[36] The measured serum calcium level also can be decreased early on because of loss from the circulation of calcium bound to albumin.

Renal Function

Aggressive fluid therapy to combat hypovolemia in early postburn period has markedly reduced the incidence of acute renal failure. Failure to provide adequate fluid volume or a delay in instituting therapy results in decreased renal blood flow, reduction in the glomerular filtration rate, and renal tubular necrosis.[37, 45] Severe burns that cause extensive intravascular hemolysis or muscle injury increase the risk of acute renal failure.[45] The increased free hemoglobin and/or myoglobin load in the face of reduced urine output results in acute tubular necrosis, which has a high mortality.[45] Renal failure also can occur later in the course of treatment as a result of septic shock, and if the circulation is not restored, acute ischemic tubular damage can occur.[45]

Hepatic Function

Hepatic hypoperfusion results from the reduced cardiac output, increased blood viscosity, and splanchnic vasoconstriction seen with hypovolemic shock. Hepatic blood flow in dogs decreases by 50% within 30 minutes of burning and drops an additional 25% during the next hour.[34] Prominent histologic changes include cellular swelling, vacuolization and centrilobular necrosis of hepatocytes, and congestion of sinusoids and central veins.[36] Other causes of liver dysfunction include administration of cholestatic drugs, blood transfusion, anesthetic agents, and burn toxin.[36] Fifty-eight percent of human burn patients develop clinical and/or laboratory evidence of liver dysfunction within the first week postburn.[46] Liver enzyme elevations can be detected within 24 hours of injury. Ninety percent of the patients who develop jaundice die.

Immune System

Infection is the primary cause of death in 75% of thermal injury fatalities.[47, 48] Alterations in the normal host defense mechanisms play a major role in the increased susceptibility to infection of burned patients. In general, experimental animals and humans with 40% or less TBSA burns show a transient depression of the immune response over the first several days after injury. Subsequently, the immune response returns to normal.[34] More extensive burns cause a more severe depression of the immune response that persists for a longer period of time.[34]

Most facets of the immune system are affected by thermal injury.[47, 49] Host defense mechanisms can be broadly classified into three categories: (1) external barrier provided by the intact skin and mucosa, (2) nonspecific defense system, and (3) specific immune system.[47] Thermal injury destroys the skin barrier, allowing bacterial colonization. Continued bacterial proliferation results in burn wound infection, and this can progress to septicemia. Depletion of nonspecific humoral factors, such as complement, impairs neutrophil chemotaxis.[47, 49] In addition, complement is one of the major nonspecific humoral opsonins.[49] Fibronectin is also a primary opsonin for substances removed by the RE system, and decreased levels reduce recognition and phagocytosis of circulating debris and bacteria.[49] Secondary decreases in the fibronectin levels of convalescent burn patients have been associated with an increased risk of developing sepsis.[49]

Increased vascular permeability and aggressive fluid therapy can lead to marked losses of immunoglobulins, particularly IgG and IgA.[47] In humans, depletion of IgG, which is the most important opsonic antibody for gram-positive and gram-negative bacteria, has been correlated prognostically with the development of septic complications.[47] Cell-mediated immune responses are also depressed in major burns, as evidenced by the delayed rejection of allografts in human burn patients.[47] In addition, decreased T-helper cell activity and increased T-suppressor cell activity also impair the immune response.

Other factors affecting the function of the immune system include nutritional status, production of immunosuppressive factors in burned skin, the presence of necrotic tissue, and the need for multiple anesthesias and surgeries.[47, 49] Early wound debridement and careful attention to nutritional needs have been shown to improve the immune response in humans.[49]

Gastroduodenal Ulceration

A gastric or duodenal ulcer in a burned patient is called a *Curling's ulcer*. The incidence in humans is estimated to be between 10% and 25%,[36, 50] but the incidence in animals is unknown. Mucosal ischemia as a result of altered submucosal blood flow has been implicated as the primary factor in ulcer development in the immediate postburn period.[50]

Hematemesis, melena, or the demonstration of occult blood in the stool should alert the clinician to the possibility of ulceration. Since more specific clinical signs are often absent, endoscopy has been recommended as the procedure of choice for diagnosing ulceration in humans.[50] This procedure would typically require general anesthesia in small animal patients. Antacids and/or histamine H2-receptor antagonists are often administered prophylactically to human burn patients,[36, 50] and therefore, the use of histamine H2-receptor antagonists in veterinary patients also would seem prudent. The buffering effect of early enteral feeding is another important step in preventing ulceration.[36]

Multiple-Organ-Failure Syndrome

Multiple-organ-failure (MOF) syndrome is the simultaneous failure of two or more of the organ systems.[36, 51] The lung, kidney, liver, heart, and blood-clotting system are most commonly involved. Humans with inhalation injury or a "complicated-shock phase" were at increased risk for developing MOF syndrome.[51] Overall mortality in patients with MOF syndrome was 76.9%, compared with 1.5% in those without MOF syndrome. The mortality rate increased as the number of organ failures increased. Because of high incidence of septicemia in patients with MOF syndrome, it is speculated that bacteremia or toxemia may be the final common pathway in the development of MOF syndrome.[51]

Burn Toxins

At least three types of "toxins" have been isolated from burn patients. Myocardial depressant factor (MDF) or a similar "toxin" has been isolated from the sera of burned patients.[34] MDF has a small molecular weight (8000) and it causes a marked decrease in cardiac contractility and alterations in the electrocardiogram indicative of decreased cardiac output and ischemia of cardiac muscle.[34] In addition, MDF also decreases blood pressure and impairs respiratory function. The sera of convalescent burned patients neutralizes the effects of this "toxin."[34]

Another burn "toxin" comes from the skin. It has a relatively large molecular weight (300,000) and is believed to be a polymer of naturally occurring compounds in the skin,[36] being composed of 40% lipid and 60% protein. It appears that a high-temperature flame burn is necessary to convert the nontoxic precursors into the "toxic" polymer. The apoprotein is responsible for the "toxic" activity, but the specific effects of the "toxin" are less clear, since various studies have shown different activities.[36]

Bacteremia and toxemia can occur secondary to the adverse effects of "burn shock" on the protective mechanisms in the gastrointestinal tract that normally limit their absorption and dissemination. As mentioned earlier, the RE system of the liver and spleen, which is primarily responsible for the neutralization of endotoxin, is impaired in the burned patient. Endotoxemia also can occur later in the postburn period as a result of sepsis associated with burn wound infection.[36, 52]

TREATMENT OF THERMAL BURNS

Initial Assessment of the Burned Patient

When a burned patient is presented to the veterinarian, a brief history should be obtained. It is important to ascertain whether the burn took place in an enclosed area and if other injuries are likely (e.g., animals with friction burns from being hit by a car). Inhalation injury is common with fires in enclosed areas (e.g., house fires).

The next step is to perform a thorough physical examination, with emphasis on body systems likely to be affected by the burn. It is essential to recognize signs of burn shock (i.e., pale mucous membranes, prolonged capillary refill time, tachycardia). *Burn shock is frequent in severe burns and should be a treatment priority.* If thermal injury of the upper airway or pulmonary parenchyma is suspected, close monitoring is necessary, and aggressive treatment should be instituted if respiratory distress develops. Finally, the wounds must be assessed and decisions made as to the practicality of treatment.

Since fluid recommendations are generally given based on percent total body surface area (TBSA) of the burn, it is useful to calculate or estimate the area of the burn. The wound can be measured and its area calculated and divided by the TBSA obtained from a weight-conversion chart, or the area can be estimated using the rule of nines.[19] In this method, each forelimb equals 9% TBSA, each hindlimb equals 18% TBSA, the head and neck equal 9% TBSA, and the dorsal and ventral trunk (thorax and abdomen) equal 18% TBSA apiece.

Fluid Resuscitation in the Burned Patient

Fluid resuscitation is critical. The burned patient must be monitored carefully during fluid resuscitation because of the rapid rate at which fluids are given. The usual clinical parameters of shock, such as heart rate, capillary refill time, and mucous membrane color, should be monitored and kept within normal limits if possible. Additionally, urine output should be maintained at 0.5 to 1 ml/kg/h.[53] Body weight should be recorded daily after fluid shifts have stabilized to help assess hydration status and monitor nutritional status. Serum electrolytes also should be monitored because burn patients tend to lose electrolytes in the burn transudate/exudate. It is also important to monitor the complete blood count, since it gives an indication of hydration status, bearing in mind that many burn patients suffer RBC loss as a result of hemolysis and protein loss from transudation. Additionally, thrombocytopenia is present in some burn patients.[53]

Many types of fluids that have been evaluated for the treatment of burn patients. In the first 24 hours after a burn, isotonic crystalloids (lactated Ringer's solution) are usually given at a rate of 4 ml/kg body weight/% TBSA burned.[14] Because of the increased vascular permeability, there is little advantage to giving the more expensive colloid solutions in the first 24 hours.[14] Isotonic crystalloids closely resemble normal intersitial fluid and thus replace the water and sodium lost from the burn wound. Since the majority of the fluid is lost in the early postburn period, approximately half the total volume is given in the first 8 hours, and the rest is delivered over the next 16 hours.[14] The time period begins at the time of the burn, not at the time of initiation of fluid therapy. The guideline given here is an approximation, and adjustments need to be made based on urine output and other physiologic parameters.

Hypertonic saline solutions have been used in the treatment of hypovolemic shock. Hyperosmotic solutions cause expansion of the vascular space by borrowing water from the intracellular space. The advantage in burned patients is that less total fluid is given, and this may limit edema in the burn wound.[14] Hypertonic saline solutions also have the advantage of increasing cardiac output. When using these solutions, it is recommended that the serum sodium concentration not exceed 160 mEq/L.[14]

Significant protein losses accompany the fluid shifts in severe burn injury. Protein colloid solutions may be needed as part of the fluid resuscitation to prevent severe hypoproteinemia. Fresh-frozen plasma or albumin solutions are the most common protein colloids used. If possible, protein solutions should be avoided during the first 8 to 12 postburn hours unless hypoproteinemia becomes life-threatening, because proteins administered during the first hours after injury are likely to be lost into the burn wound and aggravate edema formation. Attempts to restore plasma volume with protein solutions before 8 to 12 hours are ineffective and uneconomical. The amount of required protein varies and can be monitored with laboratory data. *Preventing significant hypoproteinemia is an important step in limiting edema in nonburned tissues.*

Nonprotein colloid solutions such as dextran 70, dextran 40, or hetastarch also have been used in resuscitating burned patients. These high-molecular-weight polysaccharide solutions are osmotically active and are excreted at variable rates through the kidneys. The lower-molecular-weight solutions are more osmotically active and have a shorter half-life. Approximately 40% of dextran 70 is excreted through the kidneys in the first 24 hours.[14] It appears that the greatest use for the dextran solutions is combined with saline in the early postburn period. The use of nonprotein colloids in the early postburn period results in improved survival and less edema formation,[14, 53] but once fluid resuscitation is complete, protein-containing solutions may be needed to treat the existing protein deficit. Fluid volume requirements also may increase to maintain vascular stability.[14]

Anemia is a frequent complication of severe burns. Red blood cell mass should be monitored by hematocrit and hemoglobin determinations and transfusion therapy with packed RBCs or whole blood as indicated.

Treatment of Smoke Inhalation Injury

Inhalation injury may be obvious in the severely affected animal or it may be insidious. Indirect evidence of inhalation injury includes facial burns, singed vibrissae, bronchorrhea, and sooty sputum.[22] These signs should heighten the clinician's suspicion of inhalation injury, although they are not pathognomonic. Conversely, the absence of these signs does not rule out inhalation injury. Blood gas measurements in the early postburn period may show an elevated level of carboxyhemoglobin, indicating carbon monoxide poisoning. Thoracic radiography is not helpful in the early postburn period because abnormalities usually are not apparent until fluid resuscitation is initiated. Changes in chest radiographs include pulmonary edema, atelectasis, and pneumonia, and they are usually not seen until after the clinician has instituted treatment for inhalation injury. Fiberoptic bronchoscopy is the most readily available and accurate method for diagnosing inhalation injury of the upper respiratory tract.[22] Typical findings include mucosal edema, inflammation, and necrosis, but soot and charring of the airways may be seen in severe cases.[22] Lower respiratory tract injury can be detected by xenon-133 lung scanning,[22] a technique that is relatively accurate but requires specialized equipment and licensing. Pulmonary function tests such as spirometry and tidal breathing flow–volume loop also help to detect inhalation injury, but they also require specialized equipment that is not often readily available in private practice.

The initial therapy in all animals suspected of having an inhalation injury is administration of 100% oxygen. Oxygen combats the asphyxiants in smoke and improves the generally poor oxygenation of patients with inhalation injury. Administration of 100% oxygen decreases the half-life of carbon monoxide from 250 minutes to less than 50 minutes.[22] In humans with severe carbon monoxide poisoning (carboxyhemoglobin levels > 30%), hyperbaric oxygen therapy is recommended at 2.5 atm for 90 minutes.[54] Hyperbaric oxygen therapy can dramatically decrease the half-life of carbon monoxide, but it is generally not available for veterinary patients. In addition, patients in the hyperbaric oxygen chamber are not readily accessible for monitoring. Veterinary patients with mild smoke inhalation or simple carbon monoxide poisoning can be treated solely with routine supplemental oxygen therapy.

Aggressive airway management is essential in patients with more severe inhalation injury. Patients with severe inhalation injury frequently have severe edema of the retropharyngeal area or will develop pulmonary edema. Consequently, tracheostomy is indicated in patients with upper airway swelling or severe tracheobronchial secretions. Tracheostomy bypasses the retropharynx and the larynx and provides access for suctioning of tracheal secretions. Lastly, tracheostomy allows mechanical ventilation of the conscious veterinary patient.

In patients with severe inhalation injury that have a low arterial oxygen tension or oxygen saturation while breathing 100% oxygen, mechanical ventilatory support is indicated. Continuous positive airway pressure (CPAP) or positive end-expiratory pressure (PEEP) improve oxygenation by combating atelectasis and poor lung compliance resulting from surfactant abnormalities.[22] It has been shown that CPAP decreases intrapulmonary shunting and edema in dogs with experimentally induced inhalation injury.[22] The inspired air should be humidified and an aerosolized bronchodilator should be used during ventilatory support to decrease mucous production and loosen tracheal and pulmonary secretions.[22] Meticulous pulmonary cleansing must be performed at frequent intervals to clear the tracheobronchial tree of excess secretions.

Antibiotics are indicated for the treatment of inhalation injury only when bronchopneumonia is documented. Prophylactic antibiotics are of no benefit and are potentially harmful because they may result in infections with resistant strains of bacteria.[22] Since bronchopneumonia is common, however, the clinician must remain vigilant and treat pneumonia aggressively when it occurs.

Corticosteroids have been evaluated as an adjunctive therapy for inhalation injury because they are known to reduce inflammation in certain diseases. In experimental animal models, though, corticosteroid administration has had mixed results, but the majority of studies demonstrate no beneficial or detrimental effects (e.g., increased mortality, increased infection rates).[22] Currently, there is little support for the use of corticosteroids for inhalation injury.

Inhalation injury is relatively uncommon in animal patients. Clearly, when inhalation injury accompanies a severe cutaneous burn, mortality is very high. The poor prognosis and high cost of treating of severe burns with accompanying inhalation injury should be thoroughly discussed with the client prior to instituting therapy.

Treatment of the Burn Wound

The burn wound is not static and must be continually reassessed. Applying cold water to the burn is excellent first aid because it may limit the loss of tissue in the zone of stasis and dilute chemical irritants, and these effects may be beneficial even after a short delay. However, the patient should be monitored closely to avoid inducing hypothermia, particularly when large burns are present. The veterinary surgeon should make a decision on how to manage the wound as soon as possible. Burn wound management options include complete excision of the wound with primary closure; complete excision of the wound with immediate application of auto-, allo-, or xenografts; debridement of the wound with second-intention healing; and debridement of the wound with delayed grafting.[8]

TOPICAL MEDICATIONS

With adequate fluid resuscitation, burn patients rarely die from burn shock. Survival past the initial 24 hours depends on appropriate management of the burn wound, respiratory injury, and infection. During treatment of hypovolemia and inhalation injury, bacterial colonization of the burn wound should be prevented to avoid infection and the potential for death from sepsis. *The two most important principles in preventing sepsis are use of topical antibacterial agents and early wound closure.* When treating the burn wound, the veterinary surgeon must decide whether or not to remove the eschar. Eschar can provide a covering for the wound that prevents drying of the underlying tissues, but bacteria colonizing this avascular tissue are protected from the immune system and systematically administered antibiotics. Gram-positive cocci colonize an untreated burn wound within 24 hours, and within 3 to 5 days dense colonization with gram-negative bacteria, typically *Pseudomonas* spp., results.[55] If the superficial colonization is left untreated, the bacteria invade deeper tissues and potentiate systemic sepsis. Topical antibacterial agents have decreased the mortality rate from infection by 50% in humans.[55]

The ideal topical medication should have a broad antimicrobial spectrum, with effectiveness against bacteria typically found in burn wounds, such as *Staphylococcus, Streptococcus,* and *Pseudomonas* spp.[55] It should penetrate the eschar without being systemically absorbed, should not cause local or systemic toxicity, and should not promote the development of resistant strains of bacteria.[55] Topical medications should be soothing and comfortable for the patient and cost-effective. Topical wound medications can delay colonization of wounds, decrease the bacterial density in a wound, and control infections by different types of bacteria.[55] The most commonly used topical antibacterial agents are silver sulfadiazine, silver nitrate solution (0.5%), cerium nitrate–silver sulfadiazine, and mafenide.

Silver sulfadiazine is the most widely used topical antibacterial agent in human and veterinary medicine. It is made by reacting silver nitrate with sodium sulfadiazine[55] and is marketed commercially as a 1% water-soluble creme that is active against most of the bacteria commonly found in burn wounds. Silver sulfadiazine gradually dissociates in the wound, releasing ionic silver and sulfadiazine groups.[55] Both the parent compound and the dissociated groups have antibacterial properties. Ionic silver is a potent antiseptic, even in minute amounts and has multiple sites of action. Ionic silver binds to bacterial DNA, preventing replication. Sulfadiazine acts by inhibiting the *para*-aminobenzoic acid necessary for bacterial metabolic pathways.[55] The parent compound acts by inhibiting bacterial cell wall formation.[55] Silver sulfadiazine is painless upon application and does not stain like silver nitrate. It delays bacterial colonization of the wound for 10 to 14 days. As with other topical agents, however, its effectiveness decreases when burn wound size exceeds 50% to 60% TBSA.[55] Silver sulfadiazine penetrates the eschar better than silver nitrate but not as well as mafenide. Systemic absorption is minimal; blood levels in humans have been shown to be between 1.5 and 4 mg/dl.[55] Systemic toxic reactions include crystalluria and methemoglobinuria but are rare.[55] Transient leukopenia is common, but it usually resolves even with continued use of the drug.[55] Bacterial resistance to silver sulfadiazine occurs but is relatively uncommon.[55]

Silver nitrate solution is an antiseptic that has been used for many years on burn patients. A 0.5% concentration of silver nitrate is not histotoxic and is a potent antimicrobial agent effective against most of the bacteria encountered in burn wounds. Bacteria rarely develop resistance to silver.[55] Like silver sulfadiazine, silver nitrate solution is an effective prophylactic agent, but it loses effectiveness in wounds exceeding 50% to 60% TBSA.[12] Silver is minimally absorbed from the burn wound, and toxic reactions are rare. Electrolyte imbalances occur commonly as a result of leaching of sodium and potassium into the wound in response to the application of a hypotonic solution.[55] Some bacteria can reduce nitrate to nitrite, which, when absorbed, may lead to methemoglobinemia. Typical signs of methemoglobinemia are cyanosis and a brownish discoloration of the blood. If these signs occur, the silver nitrate must be discontinued. Since silver nitrate does not penetrate the eschar as well as silver sulfadiazine, treatment in patients with established infections is inappropriate. Silver nitrate is applied as a wet dressing that must be kept moist to avoid increasing the concentration of silver nitrate solution to toxic levels. Application is not painful, but nearly all materials that come in contact with silver nitrate will be stained brown or black. The problems associated with managing wet dressings as well as the staining limit the usefulness of this compound in veterinary medicine. Silver nitrate solution is relatively inexpensive to use.

Cerium nitrate–silver sulfadiazine creme has been used experimentally in this country.[55] Cerium is bactericidal, nontoxic, and enhances the effectiveness of silver sulfadiazine. No differences in mortality rates with use of this compound and silver sulfadiazine have been demonstrated; however, bacterial concentrations in the burn wound are lower with the addition of cerium nitrate.[55] This compound is not available currently in the United States, but it is more effective than other agents in treating burns exceeding 50% to 60% TBSA.[55]

Mafenide is a compound of essentially historical interest. When first introduced, mafenide led to a dramatic decrease in the rate of wound sepsis, but subsequent experience with this drug has demonstrated unacceptable side effects.[55] Because mafenide is rapidly absorbed through the burn wound, it must be reapplied every 12 hours to maintain adequate tissue levels. It is a potent carbonic anhydrase inhibitor that can lead to severe hypochloremic metabolic acidosis.[55] Mafenide also causes severe pain on application. Because of its superior tissue penetration, mafenide is used primarily in wounds with established infections. It is used only until the infection is controlled, and the patient's acid–base should be monitored carefully during treatment.

Chlorhexidine solution (0.05%) is a common veterinary antiseptic that has been shown to decrease bacterial numbers in canine wounds and to accelerate healing of infected wounds.[56] Chlorhexidine binds to the stratum corneum, leading to a prolonged residual antibacterial effect,[57] and has the additional advantage of being effective in the presence of organic debris. Chlorhexidine is very safe, causes few toxic reactions, and is painless to apply. Chlorhexidine is also available as a 1% ointment; however, this product is recommended for superficial wounds only and is probably inappropriate for use in most burns.

Povidone-iodine (PVI) solution (1%) and ointment also have been used in the treatment of burn wounds. PVI is less effective in controlling infection in canine wounds than chlorhexidine because it is inactivated by organic debris and has no prolonged residual effect.[57] In addition, PVI is very hyperosmolar and can cause hyponatremia and metabolic acidosis when used to treat large burn wounds.[57, 58] It is probably preferable to use chlorhexidine when both solutions are available.

Other topical agents may be used occasionally when a wound with a resistant bacteria is being treated. Such topical medications as gentamicin, neomycin, polymyxin B, nitrofurazone, and bacitracin are used occasionally, but systemic absorption of these compounds may lead to serious toxicity. These compounds should be used only when wound bacteria are documented by culture and sensitivity tests to be resistant to safer topical agents.

WOUND DEBRIDEMENT

Early excision of the burned tissue reduces the risk of infection and hopefully allows immediate closure of the wound with skin flaps or grafts. Partial-thickness wounds are debrided by epluchage or tangential excision.[8, 59] *Epluchage involves daily debridement of loose necrotic tissue using sharp dissection or mechanically with dry sterile sponges.*[8] It is performed following whirlpool therapy, which helps loosen necrotic tissue. More extensive debridement can be performed once or twice weekly using sharp dissection or small, guarded skin-graft knives.[8] This technique of debridement results in minimal hemorrhage and spares as much viable tissue as possible (see Fig. 6–2B and C). Since hair is a good insulator, burn wounds in animals often have intermixed areas of partial- and full-thickness injury. Piecemeal removal of tissue in this manner minimizes the amount of tissue excised, but it may take 2 to 3 weeks before the wound is suitable for grafting and longer if the wound is allowed to heal by second-intention healing. This type of debridement is indicated in veterinary patients with partial-thickness burns that have a great potential for reepithelialization.

Tangential excision is the sequential excision of thin layers of tissue until viable dermis or subcutaneous tissue is reached. It is usually performed during the first few days after burning using guarded skin-grafting knives.[8] In large burns, tangential excision is potentially better than full-thickness excision because viable tissue in areas of partial-thickness injury can be preserved and allowed to heal by second intention.

Enzymatic debridement is another technique that has been used to treat burns in animals and humans. A satisfactory enzymatic debriding agent should remove necrotic tissue while sparing living tissue, not affect skin-graft "take," not cause significant blood loss, and not increase wound sepsis.[60] Widely conflicting results regarding the efficacy of enzymatic debridement have been seen, but it is clear that enzymatic agents are often ineffective in removing large quantities of necrotic tissue.[60] However, enzymatic agents can be used in conjunction with epluchage to conserve as much tissue as possible in partial-thickness wounds.

Complete excision may be the most practical and easiest form of debridement in many veterinary patients with deep partial-thickness and full-thickness burns. Blood loss is minimal, and the depth of excision is easy to control. If all devitalized tissue is excised and infection is not present, wound closure is performed by simple advancement of tissue or by skin flaps (see Fig. 6–3B). If infection is present or skin grafting is necessary, the wound should be managed open until healthy granulation tissue forms.

WOUND MANAGEMENT

To avoid further tissue loss once the burn eschar has been removed, desiccation of the underlying tissue must be prevented. This can be accomplished by the use of appropriate bandaging materials, biologic dressings, skin substitutes, or skin grafts (auto-, allo-, or xenografts). If the wound is in an appropriate location and of appropriate size, healing by contraction and epithelialization may only be required. It is important to note, however, that bandaging techniques can either help or hinder wound healing.

Bandages typically consist of a primary or contact layer, a secondary layer, and a tertiary layer. The primary layer touches the wound surface and should conform well to its contours. This layer should be permeable to oxygen and allow drainage to pass through into the secondary dressing. It also should protect the wound from environmental contamination. In the early postburn period, when the wound still contains necrotic tissue, adherent bandages are preferred because they mechanically debride the wound by carrying loose debris into the bandage as fluid is drawn into the bandage by capillary action. In addition, as the dressing dries, tissue on the surface of the wound adheres to the dressing and is removed when the bandage is changed.

Wet-to-dry dressings are the most common type of adherent dressing used in veterinary medicine. They maintain a moist, physiologic environment that minimizes further tissue loss.[61] Wet dressings also help dilute and absorb viscous exudates. An antibacterial agent should be added to the wetting agent until healthy granulation tissue is present because bacteria tend to flourish in moist environments.

After debridement is complete and granulation tissue forms, the contact layer of the bandage should be changed to a nonadherent material. Since nonadherent bandages do not stick to the wound surface, such bandages do not disturb granulation tissue and delicate migrating epithelial cells. Most of the nonadherent dressings used in veterinary medicine are semiocclusive; that is, they keep the wound surface moist but allow excess fluid to pass from the wound into the secondary layer of the bandage. Telfa pads (The Kendall Co, Boston, MA) and gauze that has been lightly impregnated with petrolatum are examples of semiocclusive bandages. Petrolatum is nontoxic and very effective in preventing adherence, but it may delay epithelialization of the wound.[61]

The primary function of the secondary bandage layer is to absorb and hold exudates and transudates removed from the surface of the wound by the primary dressing. The secondary layer also provides support for and immobilization of the wound, thereby increasing patient comfort. Bacteria present in the wound produce a variety of toxins and enzymes that inhibit healing, and these bacteria and toxins are also removed as the fluid is lifted away from the wound surface by the primary dressing and passes into the secondary dressing. All adherent and semiocclusive dressings used on burn patients should be covered with an absorbent layer.

The final layer of the bandage, the tertiary layer, should help make the primary and secondary layers conform comfortably to the patient and prevent the bandage from slipping and thus exposing the wound to the environment. There are many adhesive and cohesive materials that work well, but it is essential to apply this layer properly in the burned patient so that exposure of the wound to the environment does not occur.

CLOSURE OF THE OPEN WOUND

Once debridement is complete and healthy granulation tissue is present, wound closure should be performed as soon as possible. Although even large wounds on the dog or cat may heal by contraction and epithelialization, this is a relatively slow process and may lead to interference with normal function as a result of wound contracture. Large wounds, wounds on the limbs, and wounds over the flexion surface of a joint should be closed with skin grafts or flaps, if possible.

Skin flaps and skin grafts are the techniques of choice used to close large wounds in the dog and cat when second-intention healing is undesirable. Dogs and cats have an abundance of relatively loosely attached skin that can be mobilized to close large wounds. Most wounds on the trunk and proximal aspects of the extremities can be closed by simple undermining and skin advancement or by skin flaps. Skin grafts are used most commonly to reconstruct defects on the distal aspects of the extremities but are occasionally used when an extensive burn is treated.[62]

If simple closure is not possible, the excision should be carefully planned so that random skin flaps and regional axial-pattern skin flaps can be used to their greatest advantage. In some cases, more than one axial-pattern or random skin flap may be necessary to completely close a wound. To this end, multiple axial-pattern flaps have been described for use in the dog and cat along with their surgical landmarks[63] (see Table 6–1). The advantages of early wound excision and closure are reduction of healing time and minimal costs. The major disadvantages are that not all wounds are closable because of a lack of donor tissue and closure of infected wounds is inappropriate.

Skin grafts are usually applied to healthy granulation beds in burned animals. Healthy granulation tissue is smooth and pink and bleeds easily. If the granulation tissue surface is rough, it can be smoothed by excision with a razor blade or scalpel to allow more even bed–graft contact. Chronic granulation tissue has a grayish yellow color because it consists of proportionately more collagen and less blood vessels than fresh granulation tissue. The decreased vascularity and infected superficial layers make chronic granulation tissue an undesirable graft bed, so chronic granulation tissue should be excised to its base and a fresh bed allowed to form before a graft is applied.

Full-thickness skin grafts consisting of the entire epidermis and dermis are preferred because they function like normal skin. Split-thickness grafts consist of the epidermis and only a portion of the dermis. In general, split-thickness grafts do not regrow hair as well as full-thickness grafts and, depending on the thickness, may be more susceptible to trauma. Full-thickness meshed grafts have a high success rate and certain advantages over other grafting techniques. They are prepared by cutting staggered rows of parallel slits in the graft. Mesh grafts allow excess fluid to drain from under the graft, conform well to uneven surfaces, and can be expanded to cover large areas. The slits can be cut in the graft using a scalpel blade or a commercially available dermatome. The Mesh Skin Graft Expander (Padgett Instruments, Kansas City, MO) is the dermatome used most commonly in veterinary medicine. It provides a maximum expansion ratio of 3:1. Since this instrument was designed for meshing split-thickness grafts in humans, the blades may not be high enough to mesh full-thickness skin in animals, but a mesher with higher blades can be specially ordered from the company.

TABLE 6–1. Axial-Pattern Flaps

ARTERY	REFERENCE INCISIONS	POTENTIAL USE
Cervical cutaneous branch of the omocervical artery	*Caudal incision:* spine of scapula in a dorsal direction *Cranial incision:* parallel to the caudal incision equal to the distance between the scapular spine and cranial scapular edge (Cranial shoulder depression) *Flap length:* variable; contralateral scapulohumeral joint	Facial defects Ear reconstruction Cervical defects Shoulder defects Axillary defects
Thoracodorsal artery	*Cranial incision:* spine of the scapula in a dorsal direction *Caudal incision:* parallel to the cranial incision equal to the distance between the scapular spine and caudal scapular edge (caudal shoulder depression) *Flap length:* variable; can survive ventral to contralateral scapulohumeral joint	Thoracic defects Shoulder defects Forelimb defects Axillary defects
Deep circumflex iliac artery	*Caudal incision:* midway between edge of wing of ilium and greater trochanter *Cranial incision:* parallel to caudal incision equal to distance between the caudal incision and cranial edge of ilial wing *Flap length:* dorsal to contralateral flank fold	Thoracic defects Lateral abdominal wall defects Flank defects Lateral/medial thigh defects Defects over the greater trochanter
Caudal superficial epigastric artery	*Medial incision:* abdominal midline; in the male dog the base of the prepuce is included in the midline incision to preserve the epigastric vasculature *Lateral incision:* parallel to medial incision at an equal distance from the mammary glands *Flap length:* variable; may safely include last four mammary glands	Flank defects Inner thigh defects Stifle area defects Perineal area defects Preputial area defects
Genicular artery	*Base of flap:* 1 cm proximal to the patella and 1.5 cm distal to tibial tuberosity (laterally) *Flap borders:* extend caudodorsally parallel to the femoral shaft; flap terminates at the base of the greater trochanter	Lateral or medial aspect of the lower limb from the stifle to the tibiotarsal joint

Source: Adapted with permission from Pavletic MM: Skin grafting techniques, in Bojrab MJ (ed): Current Techniques in Small Animal Surgery, 3d ed. Philadelphia: Lea & Febiger, 1990, p 472.

Split-thickness skin grafts are used occasionally in dogs when donor sites are limited and the burn wound is extensive.[64] Split-thickness grafts are classified as thin (0.008 in thick), intermediate (0.010–0.015 in thick), or thick (0.015–0.025 in thick).[64] The recipient bed is prepared in the same way as for full-thickness grafts. Split-thickness grafts can be harvested with a free-hand graft knife, a safety razor, or a scalpel, but these instruments are technically difficult to use (free-hand knives) or severely limit graft size (razors). Larger grafts can be harvested using drum or oscillating electric and pneumatic dermatomes. However, these instruments are very expensive, and the cost is hard to justify unless large numbers of grafts are being performed. Thin and intermediate-thickness grafts have poor hair growth because most of the follicles are retained in the donor site. Thin grafts may be susceptible to trauma, but intermediate and thick grafts should have acceptable durability. In one study, five patients treated with split-thickness grafts healed satisfactorily, and the durability of the skin was acceptable.[64]

Postoperatively, a nonadherent pad impregnated with antibiotic ointment is placed over the graft, and a pressure bandage is applied[62] to prevent movement of the graft and maintain close graft–bed adherence. Generally, this bandage should be left in place for 48 hours prior to changing to allow a good fibrin seal to form under the graft. Then the bandage is carefully changed and the site is inspected for hematoma or seroma formation. The graft will appear pale white to bluish or bluish black for 3 to 4 days after surgery, but the color will change to pink as the circulation is reestablished. The bandage is left in place for 10 to 14 days and can be removed when healing is advanced and hair growth is returning.

Skin graft survival depends on many factors, most of which the surgeon can control. With careful attention to technique and good postoperative management, 90% to 100% graft survival is usual.[62] To achieve a high percentage graft "take," the surgeon must ensure good contact between the recipient bed and the graft, properly immobilize the graft, and prevent hematoma/seroma formation and infection under the graft. Good contact between the graft and recipient bed is necessary for early revascularization. Hematomas and seromas under the graft prevent proper contact and decrease the chances of inosculation and vascular ingrowth prior to graft necrosis. It is essential, therefore, that the graft be immobilized on the recipient bed by the proper use of bandages, because graft movement shears off ingrowing blood vessels, resulting in graft necrosis. Bacterial infection is detrimental to grafts in two ways: bacteria dissolve the fibrinous adhesion of the graft to the recipient bed, and their presence causes exudate production, which lifts the graft off the recipient bed.

Burns in excess of 50% TBSA are rarely treated in veterinary medicine. Skin flaps and autogenous skin grafts can be used to cover less extensive wounds. If treatment of larger burns is attempted, there may be inadequate donor sites for harvesting full- or split-thickness grafts. Allografts, xenografts, skin substitutes, and cultured epidermal sheets are all used for temporary or permanent coverage of wounds in humans in the absence of adequate autograft donor sites,[65] and these techniques also could be used in animals. Allograft skin can be obtained from cadaver donors and stored in fresh, frozen, and lyophilized forms. Fresh, viable allograft is preferred because it adheres to the wound for a longer period of time and has greater bacteriostatic activity than nonviable lyophilized or frozen allograft.[66] Allograft skin adheres to the wound bed and revascularizes like autografts. Normal subjects reject allografts in approximately 1 week; however, in the immunosuppressed burn patient, allografts may remain viable for many weeks.[65] Allografts are rarely used in small animal patients, but they can be used to provide temporary covering of burn wounds when other materials are unavailable.

Frozen porcine xenografts are available commercially and are used in humans for temporary coverage of burn wounds. These grafts contain no viable cells, but they do adhere to the wound bed and undergo fibrovascular ingrowth. They undergo early proteolysis and degradation and never "take" like autografts and allografts.[65] Xenografts do not control bacterial infection as well as allografts, so they are sometimes soaked in silver nitrate solution to add bacteriostatic qualities to the graft.[65] These grafts are relatively expensive and are not generally used in small animal patients.

Skin substitutes are synthetic composite materials designed to temporarily or permanently replace skin. Biobrane (Woodruff Laboratories, Santa Ana, CA) is a commonly used skin substitute composed of a layer of knitted nylon fabric and a layer of ultrathin silicon.[65] Both layers have porcine collagen molecules covalently bonded to their surfaces to increase adherence to the wound bed.[66] Biobrane has a high permeability to fluids and medications and adheres to the wound bed well. It also stretches and has excellent flexibility, which allows it to conform well to the wound. These "artificial skin" products can be used as a temporary covering for burn wounds and are less expensive than maintaining cadaver skin banks. Some skin substitutes can be used to generate a neodermis, after which the silicone layer is peeled off to expose a layer of newly generated dermal tissue on which ultrathin cutaneous autografts are laid.[65] The neodermis also can be used as a base for *in vitro* cultured epithelial cells in severe cases.

Culture-derived epidermal sheets have been used to cover extensive burn wounds in humans. In this technique, a small cutaneous biopsy specimen is removed, minced, trypsinized, and cultured in tissue-culture medium.[65] The cells are subcultured many times until enough epidermal cells are present to cover the entire wound. These cultured cells are able to provide permanent closure of very large wounds with an epidermis six to eight cells thick. However, such grafts are fragile and difficult to work with, and they require a minimum of 3 weeks to prepare.[65] Cultured epidermal sheets work best when applied to dermis or to neodermis obtained through the use of skin substitute material. They will adhere to fascia, but when used in the absence of dermis, they lead to considerable scarring. Culture-derived epidermal sheets have not been used in veterinary patients and would likely be prohibitively expensive.

SUMMARY

When treating the burned patient, the first priority is to administer first aid and prevent shock so that tissue loss can be minimized. The next priority is to prevent septic complications by using good wound-management practices and topical antimicrobials. Wound debridement and wound closure by local movement of skin, skin flaps, or skin grafts should be performed as soon as possible.

REFERENCES

1. Baxter CR, Waeckerie JF: Emergency treatment of burn injury. Ann Emerg Med 1988; 17:1305–1315
2. Bayley EW: Wound healing in the patient with burns. Nurs Clin North Am 1990; 25:205–222

3. Wachtel TL: Major burns. Postgrad Med 1989; 85:178–196
4. Davis LE: Thermal burns, in Swaim SF (ed): Surgery of the Traumatized Skin: Management and Reconstruction in the Dog and Cat. Philadelphia: WB Saunders, 1980, pp 214–233
5. Fox SM, Goring RL, Peyton LC et al: Management of thermal burns. Compend Contin Educ Pract Vet 1986; 8:439–444
6. Probst CW, Peyton LC, Raymond LB: The surgical management of a large thermal burn in a dog. J Am Anim Hosp Assoc 1984; 20:45–49
7. Salzberg AM, Evans EI: Blood volumes in normal and burned dogs. Ann Surg 1950; 132:746–759
8. Achauer BM, Martinez SE: Burn wound pathophysiology and care. Crit Care Clin 1985; 1:47–58
9. Jackson D: The diagnosis of the depth of burning. Br J Surg 1953; 40:588–596
10. Robson MC, DelBeccaro EJ, Heggers JP, et al: Increasing dermal perfusion after burning by decreasing thromboxane production. J Trauma 1980; 20:722–725
11. DelBeccaro EJ, Robson MC, Heggers JP, et al: The use of specific thromboxane inhibitors to preserve the dermal microcirculation after burning. Surgery 1980; 87:137–141
12. Robson MC, Heggers JP: Pathophysiology of the burn wound, in Carvajal HF, Parks DH (eds.): Burns in Children: Pediatric Burn Management. Chicago: Year Book Medical Publishers, 1988, pp 27–32
13. Demling RH: Fluid and electrolyte management. Crit Care Clin 1985; 1:27–45
14. Demling RH: Fluid replacement in burned patients. Surg Clin North Am 1987; 67:15–30
15. Demling RH: Pathophysiology of burn injury, in Richardson JD, Polk HC, Flint LM (eds): Trauma: Clinical Care and Pathophysiology. Chicago: Year Book Medical Publishers, 1987, pp 121–166
16. Baxter CR: Fluid volume and electrolyte changes of the early postburn period. Clin Plast Surg 1974; 1:693–709
17. Angel MF, Ramasastry SS, Swartz WM, et al: Free radical: Basic concepts concerning their chemistry, pathophysiology, and relevance to plastic surgery. Plast Reconstr Surg 1987; 79:990–997
18. Rochat MC: An introduction to reperfusion injury. Compend Contin Educ Pract Vet 1991; 13:923–930
19. Fox SM: Management of thermal burns, part I. Compend Contin Educ Pract Vet 1985; 7:631–639
20. Heimbach DM, Waeckerie JF: Inhalation injuries. Ann Emerg Med 1988; 17:1316–1320
21. Cahalane M, Demling RH: Early respiratory abnormalities from smoke inhalation. JAMA 1984; 251:771–773
22. Haponik EF, Summer WR: Respiratory complications in burned patients: Pathogenesis and spectrum of inhalation injury. J Crit Care 1987; 2:49–74
23. Moritz AR, Henriques FC, McLean R: The effect of inhaled heat on the air passages and lungs. Am J Pathol 1945; 21:311–331
24. Herndon DN, Thompson PB, Traber DL: Pulmonary injury in burned patients. Crit Care Clin 1985; 1:79–97
25. Moylan JA: Inhalation injury a primary determinant of survival following major burns. J Burn Care Rehabil 1981; 2:78–84
26. Watanabe K, Makino K: The role of carbon monoxide poisoning in the production of inhalation burns. Ann Plast Surg 1985; 14:284–295
27. Strongin J, Hales CA: Pulmonary disorders in the burn patient, in Martyn JAJ (ed): Acute Management of the Burned Patient. Philadelphia: WB Saunders, 1990, pp 25–45
28. Herndon DN, Traber DL, Niehaus GD, et al: The pathophysiology of smoke inhalation injury in a sheep model. J Trauma 1984; 24:1044–1051
29. Linares HA, Herndon DN, Traber DL: Sequence of events in experimental smoke inhalation. J Burn Care Rehabil 1989; 10:27–37
30. Horovitz JH: Heat and smoke injuries of the airway, in Carvajal HF, Parks DH (eds): Burns in Children: Pediatric Burn Management. Chicago: Year Book Medical Publishers, 1988, pp 255–262
31. Nieman GF, Clark WR, Wax SD, et al: The effect of smoke inhalation on pulmonary surfactant. Ann Surg 1980; 191:171–181
32. Shirani KZ, Pruitt BA, Mason AD: The influence of inhalation injury and pneumonia on burn mortality. Ann Surg 1987; 205:82–87
33. Moncrief JA: Effect of various fluid regimens and pharmacological agents on the circulatory hemodynamics of the immediate post burn period. Ann Surg 1966; 164:723–752
34. Davies JWL: Physiological Responses to Burning Injury. New York: Academic Press, 1982
35. Demling RH: Pathophysiological changes after cutaneous burns and approach to initial resuscitation, in Martyn JAJ (ed): Acute Management of the Burned Patient. Philadelphia: WB Saunders, 1990, pp 12–24
36. Shinozowa Y, Aikawa N: Complications of burn injury, in Martyn JAJ (ed): Acute Management of the Burned Patient. Philadelphia: WB Saunders, 1990, pp 159–179
37. Pruitt BA: Fluid and electrolyte replacement in the burned patient. Surg Clin North Am 1978; 58:1291–1312

38. Raker JW, Rovit RL: The acute red blood cell destruction following severe thermal trauma in dogs. Surg Gynecol Obstet 1954; 98:169–176

39. Baar S, Arrowsmith DJ: Thermal damage to red cells. J Clin Pathol 1970; 23:572–576

40. Loebl EC, Marvin JA, Curreri PW, et al: Erythrocyte survival following thermal injury. J Surg Res 1974; 16:96–101

41. Harris RL, Cottman GL, Johnston JM, et al: The pathogenesis of abnormal erythrocyte morphology in burns. J Trauma 1981; 21:13–21

42. Baar S: Mechanism of delayed red cell destruction after thermal trauma: Experimental in vitro scanning electron microscope study. Br J Exp Pathol 1974; 55:187–193

43. Wallner SF, Vautrin RM, Buerk C, et al: The anemia of thermal injury: Studies of erythropoiesis in vitro. J Trauma 1982; 22:774–780

44. Andes WA, Rogers PW, Beason JW, et al: The erythropoietin response to the anemia of thermal injury. J Lab Clin Med 1976; 88:584–592

45. Herrin JT: Renal function in burn patients, in Martyn JAJ (ed): Acute Management of the Burned Patient. Philadelphia: WB Saunders, 1990, pp 239–255

46. Czaja AJ, Rizzo TA, Smith WR, et al: Acute liver disease after cutaneous thermal injury. J Trauma 1975; 15:887–894

47. Moran K, Munster AM: Alterations of the host defense mechanism in burned patients. Surg Clin North Am 1987; 67:47–56

48. Seligman M, Martyn J: Burn wound infections, in Martyn JAJ (ed): Acute Management of the Burned Patient. Philadelphia: WB Saunders, 1990, pp 288–305

49. Deitch EA: Immunologic considerations in the burned child, in Carvajal HF, Parks DH (eds): Burns in Children: Pediatric Burn Management. Chicago: Year Book Medical Publishers, 1988, pp 195–212

50. Fuchs GJ, Gleason WA: Gastrointestinal complications in burned children, in Carvajal HF, Parks DH (eds): Burns in Children: Pediatric Burn Management. Chicago: Year Book Medical Publishers, 1988, pp 273–279

51. Aikawa N, Yamamoto S: Clinical analysis of multiple organ failure in burned patients. Burns 1987; 13:103–109

52. Howerton EE, Kolmen SN: The intestinal tract as a portal of entry of pseudomonas in burned rats. J Trauma 1972; 12:335–340

53. Demling RH: Fluid resuscitation after major burns. JAMA 1983; 250:1438–1440

54. Wiseman DH, Grossman AR: Hyperbaric oxygen in the treatment of burns. Crit Care Clin North Am 1985; 1:129–145

55. Monafo WW, Freedman B: Topical therapy for burns. Surg Clin North Am 1987; 67:133–145

56. Sanchez IR, Swaim SF, Nusbaum KE, et al: Effects of chlorhexidine diacetate and povidone-iodine on wound healing in dogs. Vet Surg 1988; 17:291–295

57. Swaim SF, Lee AH: Topical wound medications: A review. J Am Vet Med Assoc 1987; 190:1588–1593

58. Scoggin C, McClellen JR, Cary JM: Hypernaetremia and acidosis in association with topical treatment of burns (letter). Lancet 1977; 1:959

59. Punch JD, Smith DJ, Robson MC: Hospital care of major burns. Postgrad Med 1989; 85:205–215

60. Makepeace AR: Enzymatic debridement of burns: A review. Burns 1983; 9:153–157

61. Swaim SF, Wilhalf D: The physics, physiology, and chemistry of bandaging open wounds. Compend Contin Educ Pract Vet 1985; 7:146–156

62. Pope ER: Skin grafting in small animal surgery: I. The normal healing process. Compend Contin Educ Pract Vet 1988; 10:915–923

63. Pavletic MM: Skin grafting techniques, in Bojrab MJ (ed): Current Techniques in Small Animal Surgery, 3d ed. Philadelphia: Lea & Febiger, 1990, pp 460–477

64. Probst CW, Peyton LC, Bingham HG, et al: Split thickness skin grafting in the dog. J Am Anim Hosp Assoc 1983; 19:555–568

65. Waymack JP, Pruitt BA: Burn wound care. Adv Surg 1990; 23:261–290

66. Zapata-Sirvent R, Hansbrough JF, Carroll W, et al: Comparison of Biobrane and scarlet red dressings for treatment of donor sites. Arch Surg 1985; 120:743–745

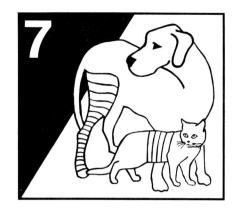

REPAIR OF INJURED PERIPHERAL NERVES, TENDONS, AND MUSCLES

CHERYL R. KILLINGSWORTH

PERIPHERAL NERVE INJURIES

Anatomy

The axial part of the nervous system is called the *central nervous system* and consists of the brain and spinal cord. The *peripheral nervous system* is represented by ganglia, nerves that emerge bilaterally from the brain (cranial nerves) and spinal cord (spinal nerves), and afferent and efferent nerve endings. The peripheral nervous system carries information back and forth between the effector organs and the central nervous system. An understanding of the anatomy and pathophysiology of peripheral nerves is necessary to correctly diagnose and treat peripheral nerve injuries.

An isolated nerve identified by dissection is completely surrounded by fibrous connective tissue. The external epineurium surrounds the nerve, and the internal epineurium separates the bundles of fascicles (Fig. 7–1). Bundles of nerve fibers (axons) called *fascicles* or *funiculi* lie within the epineurium and make up the peripheral nerve. Normal epineurium is quite resilient and may retract when cut or may slide in a preputial fashion over the ends of the nerve fibers. From a surgical standpoint, sutures placed in epineurium may permit retraction and gap formation between underlying nerve fibers. Sutures placed too far from the cut edge may cause telescoping of nerve bundles and inversion of the epineurium into the suture line. In this case, the epineurium may become an unwanted barrier to regenerating axons.

A fairly prominent connective-tissue sheath, termed the *perineurium*, surrounds each fascicle of nerve fibers. The perineurium separates the fascicles and functions to protect and maintain the nerve fiber under tension. Nerve fibers run slightly undulating courses inside the funiculi so that when nerve trunks are stretched, the nerve fibers do not share the load until stretching reaches the point where these undulations are eliminated.

Within a fascicle, a delicate sheath of loose vascular connective tissue

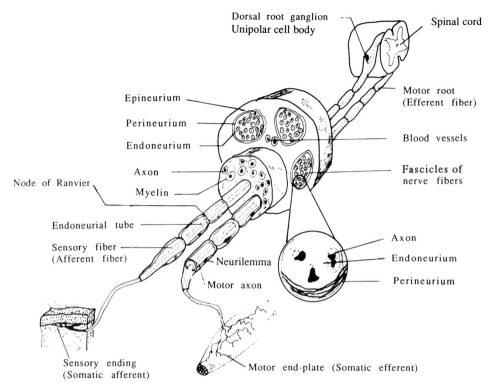

Figure 7–1. Schematic representation of the anatomy of a peripheral nerve. (From Cormack DH [ed]: Ham's Histology, 9th ed. Philadelphia: Lippincott, 1987, p 374; and Jabalay ME: In Evarts CM (ed): Surgery of the Musculoskeletal System, vol 1. Edinburgh: Churchill Livingstone, 1983, p 1:111.)

termed the *endoneurium* envelops each individual nerve fiber. The integrity of the endoneurium is essential to normal function. Small peripheral nerves may have only perineurium and endoneurium and lack an epineurium, whereas the nerve fascicles in large peripheral nerves are bound together by inward extensions of the epineurium. Depending on the specific nerve and the level of examination, the epineurium, perineurium, and endoneurium constitute from 30% to 75% of the cross-sectional area of most nerves. The fascicles and epineurium are important anatomic structures in peripheral nerve surgery, with the fascicle being the smallest unit that can be surgically repaired. Although it is not possible to directly manipulate nerve fibers and endoneurium, the ultimate goal is to align them accurately and with the least amount of trauma in order for the normal process of regeneration to occur.

Each peripheral nerve is composed of two types of fascicles. *Simple fascicles* contain motor or sensory fibers and serve a single cutaneous area or a particular muscle. *Compound fascicles* contain axons from several sources in varying combinations and proportions, allowing for integration of different fascicles that distribute to innervate specific anatomic regions. Because of this plexus formation, partial function of a nerve may remain in cases of injury. However, because fascicle anatomy changes every 0.5 to 15 mm, fascicle alignment may not be possible during surgical repair if a section of the nerve is lost.[1]

Obviously, the nerves in a mature German shepherd are larger than the corresponding nerves in a 6-week-old puppy. Although sizes of the bundles vary among nerves of different caliber, the types of fibers are rather consistent. Peripheral nerves contain varying proportions of motor (efferent), sensory (afferent), and sympathetic (postganglionic) axons. Motor nerve fibers originate in the anterior horn neurons of the spinal cord and terminate in the neuromuscular endings of skeletal muscle. Sensory nerve fibers have been divided into cutaneous and deep groups on the basis of the distribution of their endings.[2] Cutaneous sensory fibers travel in the cutaneous nerves, terminate in skin and tissues superficial to the deep fascia, and carry information regarding the sensations of touch, pressure, pain, warmth, and cold (general somatic, afferent, exteroceptive). The deep sensory fibers travel in the muscular and deep branches of the main nerve trunks and terminate in muscles, tendons, articular and periarticular structures, connective tissue, and bone. These fibers mediate sensations of pressure, pain, temperature, and stretch (general somatic, afferent, proprioceptive). Sympathetic fibers pass to the vessels, piloerector muscles, and glandular structures of the skin by way of the cutaneous nerves and to deeper structures by way of deep branches of the main nerve trunks. Fusion of the dorsal and ventral spinal roots results in a combination of both sensory and motor fibers. *Therefore, the long portion of most peripheral nerves is mixed (both sensory and motor), whereas the sensory and motor components tend to be separated at each end of the nerve (see Fig. 7–1). Trauma to a mixed nerve can cause a motor deficiency (paresis or paralysis) and a sensory loss (hyperesthesia or anesthesia).*

Axons, which are extensions of the nerve-cell body, are conducting components of the nerve and may be myelinated or nonmyelinated. Processes from Schwann cells wrap concentrically around an axon to form the myelin sheath (Fig. 7–2). When present, the myelin sheath begins near the cell body (soma) and ends just before the axon synapses onto other neurons, muscle fibers, and additional tissues. The myelin sheath insulates axons from one another and also limits current flow across the neurilemma (synonyms: axon membrane, Schwann's membrane). Current travels along the membrane effectively only at nodes of Ranvier, which are gaps that occur every 1 to 2 mm in the myelin sheath. There is rapid conduction of the nerve action potential from node to node in a saltatory, or "jumping," fashion. Conduction in myelinated nerve fibers may be up to 50 times faster than in the fastest nonmyelinated axons.[3]

The functions of Schwann cells are complex and not completely understood. In addition to forming a mechanical matrix in which the neurons are embedded, electrically insulating axons from one another, and increasing

Figure 7–2. Processes from Schwann cells wrap concentrically around an axon to form the myelin sheath. The myelin sheath functions to insulate axons and limit current flow across the neurilemma. (From Cormack DH (ed): Ham's Histology, 9th ed. Philadelphia: Lippincott, 1987, p 375.)

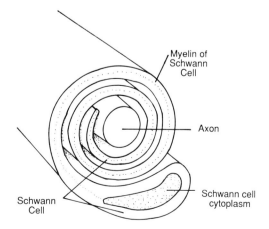

Myelin of Schwann Cell

Axon

Schwann cell cytoplasm

Schwann Cell

the speed of nerve conduction, Schwann cells appear to be phagocytic. After nerve injury, these cells ingest clumps of degenerating axon, fragments of myelin, and other debris.[4] Using perfusion studies, three plexuses of vessels with abundant anastomoses have been demonstrated in the epineurium, perineurium, and endoneurium of peripheral nerves.[5] The adventitial tissue that surrounds the nerve and contains collateral vessels is called *mesoneurium.* Considerable dissection outside or within a nerve trunk can be performed without affecting the blood supply. However, studies investigating the effect of stretch in rabbit sciatic nerve demonstrated that as little as 8% elongation compromised and 15% elongation stopped intraneural blood flow.[5, 6] While the percent of elongation may vary among mammals, the effect of stretch on nerve blood supply is probably similar in most cases. *These data suggest that tension should be avoided in nerve repair because of its effect on blood supply and to avoid physical disruption and functional loss.*

Pathophysiology of Nerve Injuries and Repair

Peripheral nerve injuries are generally due to contusion, stretch or compression with or without disruption, and laceration. From a repair standpoint, these injuries may be divided into those causing a focal injury, such as lacerations from a piece of glass, knife, or bone fragments; those causing localized injury but imparting force to adjacent areas, such as a gunshot or bite wound; and those causing damage to long segments of the nerve, such as stretch after dislocation of a limb or compression from swelling under a rigid cast.

The most common indication for peripheral nerve surgery in the dog is radial nerve damage secondary to humeral fractures.[7] Severely comminuted femoral fractures can result in sciatic nerve damage that also may require nerve repair. In addition, the sciatic nerve can be damaged secondary to injection of a drug near the nerve, pelvic fractures, or cutting the nerve near the proximal end of the femur during coxofemoral surgery.[8] Automobile accidents can result in brachial plexus avulsion or injury to the pelvis or tail with sacral nerve-root avulsion. Neurologic damage also may occur after orthopedic or soft-tissue surgeries. Peripheral nerve damage may be detected with vertebral fractures and luxations or intervertebral disk extrusions. Finally, primary neoplasms such as schwannomas or neurofibromas or metastatic tumors can cause peripheral nerve dysfunction.

Nerve injuries may be classified from first degree (least severe) to fifth degree (most severe) based on the structural damage.[9] Three specific terms also have been used to classify nerve injuries: *neuropraxia, axonotmesis,* and *neurotmesis* (Table 7–1). Any combination of these three types of nerve injuries can occur. Neuropraxia is a comparatively mild injury caused by moderate compression, slight stretching, or tissue damage due to missiles, ischemia, injections, lacerations, or surgical intervention near a nerve trunk. Anatomic continuity is preserved, but there is selective demyelination of large nerve fibers that typically results in complete motor paralysis with very little muscle atrophy and partial to complete sparing of sensory and autonomic function. Electrical conductivity of the nerve distal to the lesion is preserved. Surgical repair is not necessary, and recovery is rapid (days or weeks).

Axonotmesis generally offers a favorable prognosis.[11] The axons and neurilemma may be broken, but the stroma of the nerve, which includes the

TABLE 7–1. Characteristics of Peripheral Nerve Injuries

	NEUROPRAXIA	AXONOTMESIS	NEUROTMESIS
Pathologic			
Anatomic countinuity	Preserved	Preserved	May be lost
Essential damage	Selective demyelination of larger fibers; no degeneration of axons	Nerve fibers interrupted, Schwann sheaths preserved	Complete disorganization
Clinical			
Motor paralysis	Complete	Complete	Complete
Muscle atrophy	Very little	Progressive	Progressive
Sensory paralysis	Usually much sparing	Complete	Complete
Autonomic paralysis	Usually much sparing	Complete	Complete
Electrical Phenomena			
Reaction of degeneration	Absent	Present	Present
Nerve conduction distal to the lesion	Preserved	Absent	Absent
Motor-unit action potentials	Absent	Absent	Absent
Fibrillation	Occasionally detectable	Present	Absent
Recovery			
Surgical repair	Not necessary	Not necessary	Essential
Rate of recovery	Rapid; days or weeks	1–2 mm a day	1–2 mm a day after repair
March of recovery	No order	According to order of innervation	According to order of innervation
Quality	Perfect	Perfect	Always imperfect

Source: From Seddon H (ed): Surgical Disorders of the Peripheral Nerves. Edinburgh: Churchill Livingston, 1975, p 33.

endoneurial tubes, endoneurium, perineurium, and epineurium, is usually intact. In mild crush injuries, the architecture of the nerve is preserved, whereas in nerves that are severely crushed, tears are produced in the supporting tissues. The intact stroma acts as a guide, and axonal misdirection is minimized during regeneration. Therefore, the rate and quality of nerve recovery are usually quite good. Axonotmesis may be caused by compression, temporary ischemia, injections, fractures, and temperature extremes. There is complete motor, sensory, and/or autonomic paralysis and progressive muscle atrophy. Surgical repair is not necessary. Regeneration averages 1 mm per day or approximately 1 inch per month. However, if the insult is prolonged or severe, axonal deterioration may progress to neurotmesis, which may not be reversible.

Neurotmesis is a more severe injury. There is extensive disorganization within the nerve or complete transection, which precludes recovery without surgical repair. From the time of injury, there is complete motor, sensory, and autonomic paralysis and progressive muscle atrophy. The entire nerve segment distal to the injury undergoes degeneration of the myelin and axons (Wallerian degeneration). Unless the nerve is repaired and regrowth of the axons occurs, the connective-tissue elements of the distal segment continually shrink. There is gradual loss of electrical conductivity in the distal portion of the nerve over a period of several days. Degeneration in the proximal nerve stump is not as extensive as in the distal stump. This has been called *traumatic degeneration* and extends to the second or third node of Ranvier from the point of severance.

It can be difficult for the veterinarian to determine whether or not to repair a partially transected nerve. A sharp object, such as glass or the fragments from a bone fracture, may cut through part of a nerve, with the remainder being minimally affected structurally or functionally. The severed portion of the nerve behaves like a nerve that has been completely transected. The proximal segment can produce a neuroma, and the distal cut segment swells as a result of proliferation of fibroblasts and Schwann cells. If a high-velocity missile has nicked the nerve, the portion of the nerve that is intact is likely to suffer more damage. Axonotmesis may occur in the intact segment of the nerve, or with marked intraneural disruption, ensuing collagenization may preclude spontaneous regeneration. In summary, the damage may be much greater than is suggested by the gross appearance. The decision to resect and suture a partially severed nerve in hope of obtaining a better regeneration is generally based on the nature of the wound. Satisfactory regeneration can occur across a small gap without suturing.

After nerve transection, connective-tissue proliferation begins almost immediately and is clinically visible by 4 to 5 days. *Therefore, if peripheral nerve repair is attempted at this time or later, the nerve ends will probably require freshening by recutting before they can be sutured.* The process of Wallerian degeneration in the distal segment is more insidious. Gradual absorption of axoplasm results in a structure consisting primarily of proliferating Schwann cells, fibroblasts, and empty endoneurial tubes, with a diameter reduced by 50% or more. Although it was previously believed that axons regenerating in the distal segment of nerve entered old endoneurial tubes after Wallerian degeneration rendered them empty, newer evidence indicates that only a very few regenerating axons use old neural tubes.[12] Most axons move along new interfaces and form a new tube as they regenerate.

At about 10 to 20 days after neurotmesis, axonal sprouting begins.[13] If scar tissue blocks the entrance into the distal nerve segment, these sprouts will form a painful neuroma. A traumatic neuroma is an unorganized nodular mass of nerve fibers and Schwann cells produced by hyperplasia of nerve fibers and supporting structures after accidental or surgical sectioning of the nerve. Neuromas have been consistently reported in the dog after experimental nerve transections.[14] However, there is little clinical evidence of painful postoperative neuroma formation in the dog compared with other species such as the horse and humans.[15] If the nerve has been repaired, the average rate of regeneration will be the same as with axonotmesis. However, initially, there is a delay until regeneration crosses the anastomosis. Then regrowth may occur as fast as 3 mm per day. There is an additional delay with the formation of new connections with the muscle and sensory organs.

Several factors can affect the rate and success of nerve regeneration.[10, 13, 16] The type of nerve is important. *Motor or sensory nerves recover better than mixed nerves.* For example, recovery is better in the radial and musculocutaneous nerves than in the median nerve, and the tibial division of the sciatic nerve recovers better than the peroneal division. There is no possibility of successful function if a motor fiber is attached to a sensory fiber, or vice versa.[17] Correct alignment of fascicles is a major objective of nerve repair, especially in a mixed nerve.

Clinically, younger animals seem to have a faster and more complete recovery than older animals.[18, 19] It is not proven whether this is the result of faster or better rates of axonal regeneration. There is a faster rate of degeneration in the nerve fiber distal to the site of injury in the young, and this may permit faster or more satisfactory axonal regrowth. Compensation and adaptation of the young also may favor overcoming incomplete or even complete absence of nerve function. This may be due to a greater capacity for sensory reeducation and adaptation in substituting or modifying muscle or limb function.

The level of the nerve injury and the duration of denervation also affect recovery. The more proximal the level of axonal interruption, the greater is the distance required for axonal regrowth to the end organ, and the greater is the time required for reestablishing function in that end organ. If several months are required for regenerating axons to reach a denervated muscle, significant muscle atrophy may occur, and muscle function may not be regained. Other factors that affect prognosis for recovery are the type of nerve injury, the severity of injuries to other tissues such as bone, muscles, tendons, and blood vessels, and the nature and timing of surgical treatment.

Diagnosis

Evaluation of peripheral nerve injuries is similar in principle to evaluation of central nervous system injuries. It is essential to thoroughly evaluate the sensory and motor nerves thought to be injured. A standardized approach to neurologic examination allows subtle changes to be detected more readily. By performing serial examinations, recognition of progressive neurologic deficit or improvement can be detected. Comparison of later examinations with the initial one is important in determining the prognosis and the mode of therapy. Peripheral nerve injuries often occur with extensive trauma, so it may be necessary to reexamine for neurologic deficits after injuries to other body systems receive attention or conditions stabilize.

Accurate knowledge of the anatomy and function of the nerve suspected of injury is critical to competent evaluation. During initial examination or treatment, the veterinarian should not hesitate to consult an anatomy book and review the anatomic relations and the motor and sensory function of the involved nerves (Fig. 7–3). Heat, pain, cold, and electrical stimuli can be used to supply a noxious stimulus for sensory evaluation of peripheral nerves.[20] Similarly, motor function may be evaluated by observing gait, testing upper and lower motor neuron reflexes, and looking for asymmetry in muscle mass and tone. Responses to these stimuli may aid in locating damaged peripheral nerves. A pinprick test over the regions shown in Figures 7–4 and 7–5 helps to reveal the pattern of peripheral nerve dysfunction in the limbs of most animals. More noxious stimulation or repeated evaluation may be required to evaluate sensory function in stoic animals or animals with trauma to multiple body systems.

Electrodiagnostic testing can be important in evaluation of peripheral nerve injury but is not always available to the veterinarian. Electromyography (EMG) determines electrical activity in striated muscle motor units. A *motor unit* consists of the motor nerve and all the muscle fibers innervated by that nerve.[4] With direct or indirect electrical stimulation, the EMG can demonstrate quantitative or qualitative changes in electrical activity of the motor units at rest or during voluntary or reflex activation.[20] Denervation or early reinnervation of affected muscle groups can be monitored. Sensory and

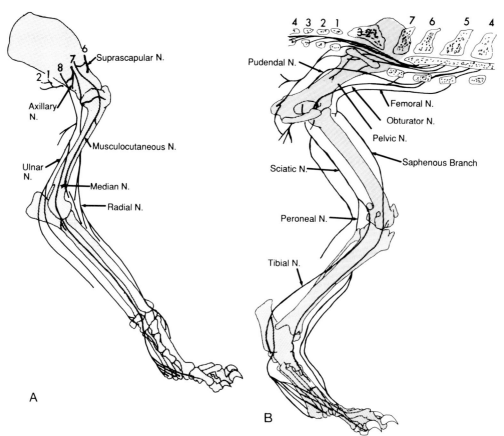

Figure 7–3. Medial views of the thoracic limb *(A)* and the pelvic limb *(B)* indicating the course and distribution of the major nerves. (From Hoerlein BF: In Hoerlein BF (ed): Canine Neurology: Diagnosis and Treatment, 3d ed. Philadelphia: WB Saunders, 1978, pp 234, 240.)

motor nerve conduction velocities and nerve terminal conduction time also can be evaluated with EMG testing.[21] In some settings, motor nerve conduction velocity (evoked nerve potentials) can be used to detect early functional recovery.

Specific techniques for electrodiagnostic testing in veterinary medicine have been described.[21–23] Briefly, one of the common EMG techniques requires placement of three small percutaneous needle electrodes over the region to be tested.[20, 24] The first electrode serves as the ground. A recording electrode is placed into the striated muscle belly that is to be tested. The difference in the electrical potential between the recording and a third reference electrode reflects relative changes in electrical activity within the muscle. From the recording electrode, the signal travels to a preamplifier and then to an amplifier unit. The signal can be displayed to the examiner through audio and oscilloscopic display. A permanent record can be made with magnetic tape or photographic or paper recordings. Normally, a brief burst of electrical activity occurs with electrode insertion (insertion potentials). Electrical silence should follow, except during voluntary muscle contraction or passive limb movement.[21] Peripheral nerve injury can result in denervation to a muscle group. Five to 7 days after nerve damage, spontaneous electrical activity can be detected due to loss of neural influence. This activity will be detectable until (1) an approximately normal pattern of activity occurs with

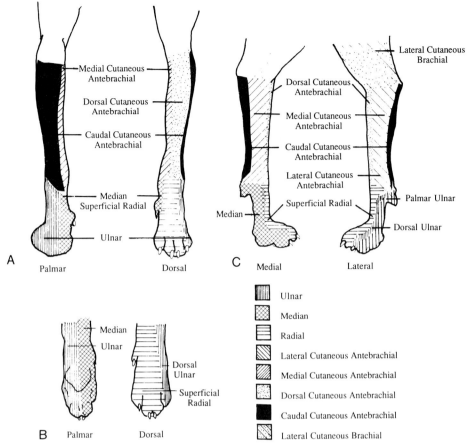

Figure 7–4. Cutaneous sensory innervation in the thoracic limb representing palmar and dorsal views *(A, B)* and medial and lateral views *(C)*. (From Hoerlein BF: In Hoerlein BF (ed): Canine Neurology: Diagnosis and Treatment, 3d ed. Philadelphia: WB Saunders, 1978, p 235.)

nerve regeneration or (2) electrical quiescence develops because of denervation and muscle fibrosis.

Principles of Peripheral Nerve Repair

Whether nerve repair should be performed as soon as possible or delayed until soft-tissue healing has occurred has been fiercely debated in human surgery. For many years, delayed nerve repair was favored.[25] Increased interest in primary repair at the time of injury has arisen because of expanded knowledge of microanatomy, construction of microsurgical instruments, creation of fine suture materials, an understanding of the factors involved in nerve repair and healing, and current methods for elimination of wound infection.[19, 25] Experimental studies of evoked electrical potentials, peripheral muscle response, and histologic patterns in the nerves of monkeys strongly suggest that, when possible, best results will be obtained if a transected nerve is repaired immediately.[12] *Immediate repair* refers to repair during the first stage of wound healing, which is the inflammatory stage, which lasts about 3 days. *Therefore, neurorrhaphy, or the suturing of a cut nerve, should occur ideally before connective-tissue proliferation is clinically evident at approximately day 4.*

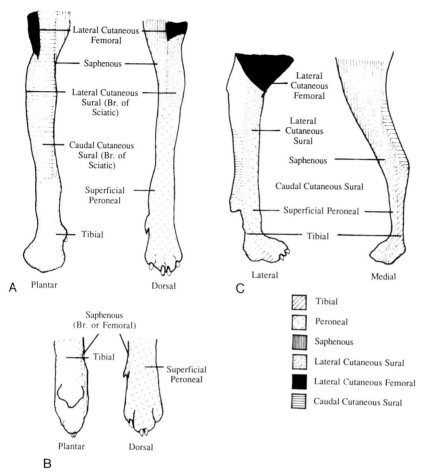

Figure 7–5. Cutaneous sensory innervation in the pelvic limb representing plantar and dorsal views *(A, B)* and medial and lateral views *(C)*. (From Hoerlein BF: In Hoerlein BF (ed): Canine Neurology: Diagnosis and Treatment, 3d ed. Philadelphia: WB Saunders, 1978, pp 240–241.)

The circumstances surrounding nerve injury help to determine the timing for surgical repair.[19, 25] The advantages of primary repair are that structures are easier to identify and mobilize prior to scar formation, nerve ends have not retracted as much as they will in subsequent weeks, and the greatest time is allowed for regeneration before irreversible muscle atrophy occurs. The disadvantages are that emergency conditions may make peripheral nerve evaluation difficult and may not be ideal for careful operation, damage to the nerve may be more extensive than is initially apparent, and the epineurium and perineurium are delicate and difficult to suture at this stage.

With *secondary repair,* 3 to 8 weeks after injury, optimal operating room conditions can be arranged, the extent of damage to the nerve can be better assessed and the correct amount removed, and the epineurium and perineurium are stronger and will hold sutures better. In addition, there is no lag time for Wallerian degeneration, so regenerating axons in the peripheral segment can penetrate the repair site before there is scar formation. Even with secondary nerve repair, initial exploration may be required to debride and treat the wound. The ends of the nerve can be tagged and loosely approximated with wire so that they can be found during secondary repair.[25]

Otherwise, the normal elasticity of the nerve will cause the ends to retract, and they will become fixed in the contracted state because of fibrous connective-tissue formation. Placing a temporary suture may make the difference between direct suturing of the nerve at a later date or having to insert a nerve graft to close the gap.

There are six reasons for exploratory surgery after peripheral nerve injury: (1) to visualize the extent and severity of a lesion, (2) to establish an accurate diagnosis when clinical diagnostic methods have been inconclusive or contradictory, (3) to establish a prognosis, (4) to avoid long delays associated with possible spontaneous recovery in severe cases such as pelvic fractures and sciatic nerve damage, (5) when improvement with conservative treatment has ceased prior to adequate functional recovery, and (6) to treat painful lesions such as sciatic injury secondary to intramedullary pin placement for stabilizing femoral fractures.[9, 15, 20]

In general, suspected nerve injuries should be explored and primary repair performed within 3 days after nerve transection, when possible. A damaged nerve must be considered within the context of total injuries. Overall wound management is the prime consideration and always takes precedence over the nerve injury.

Instrumentation. Auxiliary lighting and magnification are extremely important ancillary aids to peripheral nerve surgery. Operating microscopes with magnification ranges of $10\times$ to $25\times$ are becoming more common in veterinary teaching institutions, but a $4\times$ to $6\times$ loupe can be a useful alternative. Ultimately, the skill of the surgeon determines the outcome rather than the power of the magnifying device or the instruments. Because the nerve is already injured, the surgeon must avoid crushing, stretching, and adding foreign material, including lint from surgical linens or gauze and suture material, which might further injure the nerve. Preferably, instruments should be cleaned in an ultrasonic cleaning apparatus with detergent-free solution that is 20% acetone by volume.[8] Instruments should be packed in metal containers without linen to decrease the possibility of foreign-body reaction at the suture site.

The initial surgical approach can be made with general surgical instruments. Ophthalmic and microsurgical instruments can be used for peripheral nerve repair. Ophthalmic instruments are generally satisfactory for use in veterinary medicine and are less expensive. Instruments that may be helpful include mouse-tooth Adson forceps, two pairs of jeweler's forceps, 4-in strabismus scissors, 4-in iris scissors, and an ophthalmic needle holder.[26] Disposable supplies include wooden tongue depressors, double-edge razor blades or scalpel blades, and lint-free sponges (Weck-Cel, Edward Weck Co, New York, N.Y., and Gelfoam, Upjohn Co, Kalamazoo, Mich). The suture material should be monofilament, have a low coefficient of friction, and be nonreactive. Nylon or polypropylene 5–0 to 7–0 suture with a swaged-on tapered or slightly cutting needle is satisfactory for most repairs. Noninflammatory, absorbable suture of similar size that retains adequate tensile strength, such as monofilament polyglycolic acid or polydioxone suture, is a good alternative.[24, 27] Fascicular repair may require 8–0 to 10–0 suture. High frictional resistance, large knots, and excessive tissue reaction make natural absorbable suture such as catgut inappropriate.

Because every suture creates fibrous tissue reaction,[12] various types of "biologic glue" have been used.[28, 29] Theoretical advantages of a sutureless method for nerve repair include more uniform approximation, improved hemostasis, less tissue handling and consequent trauma, and less potential for granuloma formation. These techniques have demonstrated mixed results. Poor results have generally been attributed to inadequate tensile strength of the anastomosis. For biologic glues to become clinically useful in nerve repair, investigations need to be directed toward examining the immunologic responses to substances such as thrombin, evaluating the effects of fibrinolysis inhibitors on the healing process, and improving the bonding strength of these glues.

General Surgical Techniques. After routine exposure of the nerve, tissue surrounding the nerve is dissected to allow mobilization of the cut ends of the nerve. This dissection removes mesoneurium, which contains collateral vessels. Hemostasis is critical because blood in the surgical field may promote scar formation at the nerve suture site. Standard cautery should be avoided around nerves, if possible. A bipolar coagulator with a jeweler's forceps or lint-free sponges soaked in a 1:100,000 epinephrine solution may be used to stop persistent bleeding.[17, 26] Approximately 6 to 8 cm of mesoneurium can be removed to facilitate nerve repair.[20, 30] A 1-cm gap may be overcome by mobilizing the nerve trunk for approximately 4 to 5 cm in each direction to gain 0.5 cm at each end.[17] The nerve should be handled gently to minimize any additional fascicular damage. The epineurium or mesoneurium can be grasped gently with fine forceps. Sutures placed through the epineurium also may provide traction and landmarks for alignment if anastomosis is performed. If the nerve trunk is intact, the response to stimulation with microelectrodes can aid in localizing the level of nerve injury.

Visual inspection for induration or neuroma formation also may determine if resection and anastomosis of the nerve is required. Finding a neuroma indicates axonotmesis or neurotmesis. The shape, location, and consistency of the neuroma assist in deciding the best surgical therapy. A neuroma of soft consistency suggests a chance for spontaneous healing.[2, 8] If fibrosis has occurred, the neuroma will be firm, suggesting that there is a decreased chance of spontaneous regeneration of axons across the neuroma and into the distal nerve segment.

The location of the neuroma also may determine whether excision and neurorrhaphy are required. A neuroma that is considered bulbous or dumbbell-shaped and which extends across the diameter of the nerve suggests widespread neurotmesis. Similarly, a laterally located neuroma that spans greater than 50% of the nerve trunk has a poor prognosis for spontaneous recovery. Trial section of the neuroma at the time of exploration may be necessary to determine if surgical resection is required. Internal neurolysis by longitudinal incision through the epineurium allows examination of individual nerve fascicles and removal of excess fibrous tissue. Dissection of individual fascicles within the nerve trunk can be technically difficult.[2] A neuroma also can be examined by using a transverse method of trial section.[20] A transverse incision is made at the largest part of the neuroma and is deepened 0.5 mm at a time until normal nerve tissue is visualized. If over 50% of the diameter of the nerve trunk is involved, resection and anastomosis of the nerve are necessary. Resection requires removal of 1-mm serial transverse sections on the proximal and distal nerve segments until normal tissue is seen (Fig. 7–6). Epineurial marking sutures can be placed proximal and distal to the resection site to later aid in alignment of fascicles. Nerve ends should be sectioned with a sharp blade, with the least amount of pressure, and while the nerve is free of any longitudinal tension.[12] Prior to

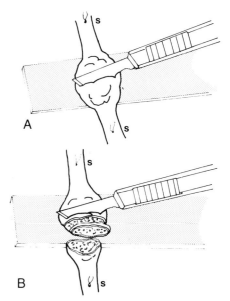

Figure 7–6. Resection of a neuroma. *A,* The nerve may be placed over a wooden tongue blade and held with a proximal traction suture to avoid retraction of the nerve stump. *B,* Serial transverse sections of 1 mm are removed from the proximal and distal nerve segment until normal tissue is detected. Epineurial marking sutures *(S)* can be placed proximal and distal to the resection site to aid in later alignment of fascicles. (From Swaim SF: In Bojrab MJ (ed): Current Techniques in Small Animal Surgery, vol 1. Philadelphia: Lea & Febiger, 1975, p 11; and Swaim SF: In Hoerlein BF (ed): Canine Neurology: Diagnosis and Treatment, 3d ed. Philadelphia: WB Saunders, 1978, p 306.)

resection, the nerve may be placed over a wooden tongue blade and held with a proximal traction suture to avoid retraction of the nerve stump. Repeated cuts, sawing motion, excessive pressure from a dull knife, and sectioning under tension can cause fraying of epineurium and distortion of the nerve fascicles. This makes accurate approximation of the nerve ends difficult. Fragmented epineurium can turn in and block the flow of axoplasm. Visual examination of the proximal nerve segment during neuroma resection should reveal a mushroom-shaped bulge of fascicles from the cut surface with immediate retraction of the epineurium.[12] If the proximal surface appears homogeneous, without identifiable fascicles, sections should be taken more proximally. The assumption is that if the epineurium and perineurium are rigidly fixed by new collagen deposition, then axons will be passing through a scarred and somewhat constricted channel, which further decreases the chance of successful repair. Wide excision should be avoided to prevent undue tension on the suture line. It has been shown experimentally that there is measurable tension on the nerve ends with simple transection and anastomosis.[17] Tension is present without resection because of the natural elasticity of the nerve; therefore, gap length should be minimized.

Several characteristics of the nerve also result in a high incidence of neuroma formation at the site of nerve suture. The size of the neuroma that forms after surgery often approximates the neuroma that is present on the proximal stump before operation.[2] Dissimilar fascicular patterns at the nerve ends, widely separated fascicles, and large amounts of epineurial tissue favor the entry of regenerating axons into the interfascicular epineurial tissue and re-formation of the bulb. Resection and anastomosis of the nerve do not eliminate postoperative neuroma formation.

Nerve Anastomosis. The simplest surgical technique is end-to-end anastomosis. The nerve trunk is sutured by placement of sutures in the epineurium or by placement of a single suture through the center of the nerve trunk.[8, 20] Adequate realignment of the cut ends of the nerve is critical for return of function. Most commonly, simple interrupted sutures are placed through the epineurium only. The epineurium can be grasped with fine forceps and sutures placed about 0.5 to 1.0 mm from the cut edge. The suture begins on the external surface of the epineurium and exits subepineurially (Fig. 7–7). The least number of sutures is used so that inflammation secondary to the suture is minimized. Four equidistant sutures generally provide adequate alignment for healing, but the number of sutures depends on the diameter of the nerve.[8, 12] Preplacement of sutures and tying all at once help to ensure equal tension around the suture line. Two sutures are initially placed 180 degrees apart to maintain alignment of nerve ends. One or more sutures are then placed in the upper part of the nerve. The nerve trunk is gently rotated to facilitate placement of sutures on the underside of the nerve. Care should be taken not to invert the epineurium, which would produce a mechanical barrier to the nerve fascicles. Ideally, sutures should not incorporate nerve fascicles. In a large nerve trunk, it may be necessary to place one or two sutures in the internal epineurium that surrounds and separates nerve bundles (see Fig. 7–1). These sutures can align nerve bundles and hold the nerve trunk more securely. If fascicular ends are carefully abutted with no tension, a plasma bond forms to hold them together.[17] There is a bulge of axoplasm on the freshly cut ends of nerve bundles, and these ends seem to have a natural affinity for each other.

Small severed nerves in the dog and cat can be apposed using the monosuture technique (Fig. 7–8). Square bow knots incorporating a 3-mm^2 fascial or silicone pad are placed at each end of one intraneural suture. The suture is passed through the pad three times so that a loop and strand of suture can be used to tie a square knot. The anastomosis begins about 8 mm from the cut edge and is directed to the center of the nerve trunk. The suture is redirected to follow the central longitudinal axis of the nerve. The suture crosses the anastomotic site, enters the other nerve end, and passes centrally about 8 mm. The suture exits the nerve trunk at the opposite site of the initial suture placement, forming a Z pattern (see Fig. 7–8). Double-armed suture material also can be used, inserting a needle in the center of each nerve stump and then completing the suture pattern described above. Larger nerves also can be repaired with a 6–0 monosuture through the

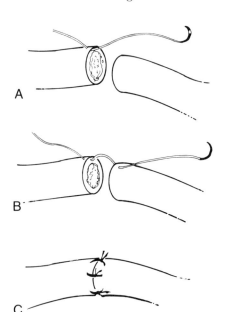

Figure 7–7. End-to-end anastomosis using simple interrupted sutures. The suture is placed only in the external epineurium to avoid damaging nerve fibers. (From Raffe MR: Peripheral nerve injuries in the dog (part II). Comp Contin Educ Pract Vet 1979; 1:274.)

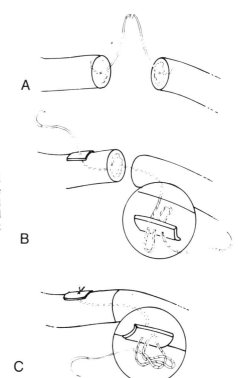

Figure 7–8. The monosuture technique. *A,* The suture is placed through the center of the nerve to aid alignment. *B, C,* Square bow knots incorporating a 3-mm² fascial or silicone pad are placed at each end of the intraneural suture. (From Raffe MR: Peripheral nerve injuries in the dog (part II). Comp Contin Educ Pract Vet 1979; 1:274.)

center of the nerve. Three of more 6–0 sutures are also placed in the epineurium. The advantage of the monosuture technique is the minimal foreign-body reaction caused by one suture; therefore, less postoperative neuroma formation occurs.[19] The monosuture technique is technically difficult even with the help of magnification. Complications include stump rotation, iatrogenic trauma during manipulation, and instability if the suture is not carefully centered in the nerve ends.

Nerve anastomosis by apposing internal epineurium surrounding nerve fascicles with 10–0 suture has been described (Fig. 7–9). The anchor funicular suture is another suture pattern that is intermediate between the epineurial suture and the fascicular suture techniques. Two or three 5–0 to 7–0 interrupted horizontal mattress sutures are placed in the epineurium (Fig. 7–10). If major nerve fascicles are not well aligned, 10–0 sutures can be placed in the internal epineurium. Both methods of repair require

Figure 7–9. Nerve anastomosis by apposing internal epineurium surrounding nerve fascicles with 10-0 suture. Magnification, such as an operating microscope, is required. (From Grabb WC, Bement SL, Koepke GH, Green RA: Comparison of methods of peripheral nerve suturing in monkeys. Plast Reconstr Surg 46:32, 1970; and Swaim SF: In Hoerlein BF (ed): Canine Neurology: Diagnosis and Treatment, 3d ed. Philadelphia: WB Saunders, 1978, p 309.)

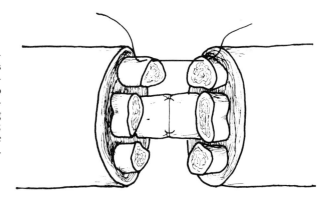

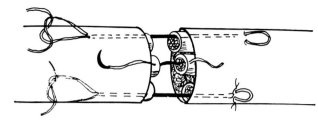

Figure 7–10. Nerve anastomosis using the anchor funicular technique, which uses both fascicular sutures and epineurial anchor sutures. Excellent surgical technique and magnification are necessary when this suture pattern is employed. (From Swaim SF: In Hoerlein BF (ed): Canine Neurology: Diagnosis and Treatment, 3d ed. Philadelphia: WB Saunders, 1978, p 309.)

excellent surgical technique and magnification. In addition, no matter how well executed, suturing produces local reaction and edema formation. This reaction may distort the stroma and alter the pattern of axon regeneration.[31]

Nerve Grafts. Mobilization of nerve ends and flexion or extension of associated joints have been the mainstay in overcoming nerve gaps.[17] Nerve stumps can be stretched to a limited extent to overcome voids. However, any degree of stretching of the nerve may decrease the possibility of healing.[12, 20] By careful tissue dissection, enough length usually can be obtained to overcome a gap of 2 to 3 cm.[20] Efforts to overcome gaps greater than 3 cm may result in breakdown at the suture line due to compromise of the blood supply to the nerve and excessive tension.

Extensive injuries may result in loss of a section of nerve, which makes anastomosis impossible without extreme tension on the nerve. Methods to overcome irreducible nerve gaps include bone resection to shorten a limb, direct neurotization of muscles, extensive surgical dissection and anatomic relocation of the nerve, tubulization, and nerve pedicle flaps.[12, 15] Various forms of nerve grafts also have been used to repair nerve gaps. The graft provides a passage for regenerating axons to reach the distal stump. The primary advantage of nerve grafting is the ability to obtain an absolutely tension-free nerve union. Nonetheless, nerve grafting is a salvage procedure that should only be used when unacceptable tension is required to appose the two ends of a nerve.[17] The long gap in a scarred bed, necessity for successful graft vascularization, problems of correct graft alignment with the nerve ends, and the presence of two suture lines with two scar interfaces can lessen the possibility of a successful outcome. In addition, many autograft failures are due to inadequate training of the surgeon and improper instrumentation. Nerve-grafting procedures tend to be lengthy and require careful attention to hemostasis, frequent wound irrigation, and gentle tissue handling.

From the standpoint of veterinary medicine, fresh autografts from the patient remain the most practical. Free-graft donor sites in small animals include the median nerve of the front leg and the lateral cutaneous nerve in the hindlimb. To maximize the possibility of successful grafting, several principles should be observed. The diameter of the graft and that of the nerve trunk should be similar. Incomplete axonal regrowth can occur because of an insufficient number of endoneurial tubes in a narrow graft. In addition, the graft should be 15% to 25% longer than the gap. This length releases tension on the suture lines and allows for graft shrinkage.[8]

Protecting the Anastomotic Site. Ingrowth of connective tissue can be a major complication after nerve repair. Therefore, many different biologic and synthetic materials have been used to ensheathe the suture line. A Millipore membrane, plasma clot, or Silastic tubing can be used as a nerve cuff. The cuff must be placed onto a nerve stump before anastomosis. The epineurium is gently grasped, and the cuff is slipped onto the nerve stump using a small hemostat or a jeweler's forceps (Fig. 7–11). After anastomosis, a single suture through the epineurium at each end of the cuff helps to anchor and prevent twisting of the cuff.

The cuff needs to be of adequate length and diameter to provide protection of the suture line yet not constrict the nerve. The cuff should be about 8 to 10 mm in length. Longer cuffs can inhibit collateral circulation. The internal cross-sectional area of the cuff should be two to three times greater than the nerve to allow for postoperative swelling without constriction. A cuff that is too large may allow connective tissue to grow under the cuff and block axonal regeneration.

Postoperative Care. Immobilizing the limb in a splint or cast for at least 2 weeks can relieve stress on the repaired nerve. Bandaging longer than 2 weeks may be necessary with nerve grafting because two anastomotic sites must be crossed by the regenerating axons.[24] It is important to avoid muscle atrophy and to maintain normal limb positioning during the healing period. Passive movement of the limb should occur between 2 and 5 weeks. Proper nutrition; slow, controlled exercise; massage; and the application of moist and dry heat can help maintain good condition of the joints, muscles, tendons, and skin of an affected limb.[15] Ideally, full range of motion should be obtained 5 weeks after surgery.

It is also important that prior to nerve regeneration the limb be protected from further injury by padded bandages and splints. Self-mutilation of the denervated limb can occur with early stages of axon regeneration and reinnervation of sensory-deprived areas. An Elizabethan collar, muzzling, or a side brace may be required to protect the limb.

Repeated clinical examination and electrodiagnostic testing will help evaluate the healing process. As previously mentioned, evoked nerve potentials can be used to detect early functional recovery and assess axon–end organ

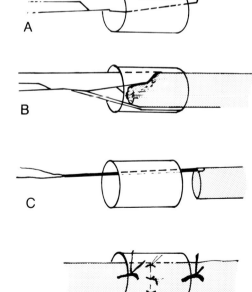

Figure 7–11. Techniques for passing a nerve cuff *(A)* using hemostats *(B)* or a traction suture that is placed in the epineurium *(C)*. The cuff is placed over the anastomotic site and anchored at both ends *(D)*. The cuff should not be longer than 8 to 10 mm. (From Swaim SF: In Hoerlein BF (ed): Canine Neurology: Diagnosis and Treatment, 3d ed. Philadelphia: WB Saunders, 1978, p 311; and Raffe MR: Peripheral nerve injuries in the dog (part II). Comp Contin Educ Pract Vet 1979; 1:276.)

8-10mm

reinnervation. The time of functional recovery can range from 3 to 6 months depending on the lesion.[20] Completely normal function will probably not be regained, but the goal is to obtain sufficient function for daily activity.

TENDON INJURIES

Anatomy and Pathophysiology

Skeletal muscles are connected to cartilage or bone by direct attachment, aponeurosis, or tendon. A tendon exists where a muscle exerts its forces of contraction across a joint or if the point of insertion is distant to the muscle. The major difference between a tendon and a ligament is their function. *Ligaments* attach one bone to another, whereas *tendons* attach muscle to bone. Tendons tend to be less flexible than ligaments and, like ligaments, possess minimal elasticity. Therefore, tendons can be stretched to a limited degree before they rupture. Mature tendons are composed primarily of closely packed longitudinal bundles of type I collagen fibers, which have tremendous strength. These fibers are generally oriented parallel to the long axis of the tendon. There are intermittent rows of highly compressed fibrocytes (tenocytes) that produce the collagen. A connective-tissue sheath, or *epitenon,* on the surface of the tendon is continuous with the endotenon and with loose areolar tissue called the *paratenon.* The *endotenon* is composed of type III collagen fibers of smaller diameter than type I collagen. The endotenon is composed of looser connective tissue that permeates the tendon, separating the tendon fascicles and providing a pathway for nerves and vessels. The paratenon and the epitenon contain both elastic fibers and irregularly arranged collagen fibers. This arrangement of paratenon, epitenon, and endotenon provides minimal resistance to movement of the tendon through tissues and needs to be preserved for tendon gliding function.

Tendons may be enclosed within tendon sheaths, or *synovial sheaths,* at locations where they would otherwise rub against bone or some other friction-generating surface. In addition, cartilaginous or osseous sesamoid bones may lie adjacent to tendons and act to protect tendons at sites where they bend around a bone surface. The inner layer (visceral layer) of the tendon sheath encloses the tendon and is firmly attached to it. The outer layer (parietal layer) is attached to periosteum and other surrounding tissues. Friction-reducing synovial fluid fills the space between the inner and outer layers of the tendon sheath. The *mesotendon* connects the inner and outer layers of the tendon sheath and provides an important pathway for nerves and blood vessels that supply the tendon tissue within the sheath.

The nerve supply of tendons is almost exclusively afferent. Specialized afferent receptors exist in tendons near the musculotendinous junction. The sparse blood supply to tendons originates primarily from adjacent muscle, paratenon tissue, and synovial sheaths. Small arterioles from muscle run longitudinally in the endotenon accompanied by veins and lymphatics. These blood vessels anastomose in the mesotendon with vessels from the paratenon or synovial sheaths.

The most commonly injured tendons in small animals are located in the lower limbs. The tendons that are most likely to be damaged include superficial and deep flexors and extensors of the forepaw, calcanean tendon, triceps tendon, and quadriceps tendon.[33, 34] The majority of these injuries, particularly to flexor tendons, are caused by sharp objects that lacerate the tendons during normal activity. Tendon lacerations also may occur in combination with fractures. The calcanean tendon can be severed after automobile accidents, fights, or extreme flexion of the hock. Rupture of the musculotendinous junction or avulsion of a tendon from its insertion onto bone is usually due to trauma. Extensor injuries are associated more commonly with mechanical injury. Intrinsic degradation can predispose a tendon to rupture without an associated laceration. Conditions reported to weaken tendons in humans include hyperparathyroidism, systemic lupus erythematosus, rheumatoid arthritis, hyperbetalipoproteinemia, and hemangioendothelioma.[35] Chronically administered systemic corticosteroids and injections of corticosteroids into a tendon also may predispose the tendon to rupture.[33, 36] Other abnormal conditions generally associated with flexor tendons include contracted tendons or excessively long tendons. Loss of function in any tendon may occur after atrophic contracture of the corresponding muscle or as a result of binding scars.

Principles of Tendon Repair

Besides nervous tissues, tendons and other dense collagenous tissues are the only soft tissues that require several weeks to heal primarily.[37] There are also two other critically important aspects of tendon healing. The first is the enormous tensile strength required between tendon ends, and the second is that healed tendon must glide through scar tissue.[38] The problems of tendon repair would be decreased if the wound between two tendon ends could be managed independently of the wound of overlying skin or underlying bone. However, tendon injuries generally include damaged fat, blood vessels, dermis, and sometimes bone or cartilage, which complicate tendon healing. Most of the cells of mature tendons are relatively inactive fibrocytes, which have minimal ability to divide or synthesize fibrous protein in amounts necessary to develop strong union between tendon ends. *Although some new collagen is synthesized by cells in the tendon, most tendon healing is the result of extrinsic cell synthesis and deposition of collagen.*[12] After tendon injury, the increase of different cell types is due primarily to an influx of multipotential cells migrating into the wound. Inflammatory cells are also delivered by the intrinsic blood supply. Studies performed in chicken flexor tendons have shown that epitenon cells proliferate 3 days after injury, whereas fibrocytes do not begin producing collagen until 14 to 21 days after injury.[39] From 3 to 5 weeks, the entire repair site and the adjacent tendon are hypercellular with collagen-synthesizing cells. These cells may originate from the epitenon, endotenon, or tendon sheath. Studies of chicken flexor tendons suggest that the epitenon is a major source of these cells.[39]

During the lag phase of 4 to 6 days in healing after tendon injury, wound strength does not increase substantially. Nonetheless, in a properly coapted wound, some strength develops in the first 24 hours after injury due to formation of fibrin clot in the wound. Additional strength is also produced by regenerating capillaries and newly formed ground substance, which is derived from serum glycoprotein that leaks into the wound from the circulation. Strength increases significantly from 4 to 6 days to reach an early maximum strength at 14 to 16 days. During this phase of wound healing, there is a rapid period of fibroplasia and collagen production. Hydroxyproline, a measure of collagen concentration, increases rapidly beginning at day

4, with highest rates of formation between days 5 and 12, a decreased rate of synthesis between days 12 and 21, and a markedly lower rate from days 21 to 60.[38] Long-term remodeling of the collagen matrix follows with a subsequent increase in tensile strength; however, original strength rarely is restored.[40] Reestablishment of tendon strength after injury requires cross-linking of newly synthesized collagen to the original type I collagen fiber. Cells involved in tendon healing have the ability to produce type I and type III collagen. Thus, if increased amounts of type III collagen are produced, type I collagen cross-linking could be delayed. Studies of equine tendon scars indicate increased amounts of type III compared with type I collagen, which cannot provide sufficient mechanical support and could account for frequent reinjury.[41] Other studies completed in rabbits suggest that collagen types detected in healing flexor tendons are similar to those in normal tendons obtained from the same animal.[42] These investigators concluded that if adjacent tissues and adhesions are not included in the analysis of the repair sites and normal tendon type I and type III collagen ratios are known for the animal model, changes in total collagen content of healing tendons can be directly related to type I collagen turnover. Furthermore, the return of mechanical strength to an injured tendon may be more directly related to reestablishment of cross-links between newly synthesized collagen bundles and preexisting healthy collagen matrix rather than collagen type.

Morphologically, it appears that newly synthesized scar tissue remodels according to the architecture of tissue in juxtaposition.[12] New connective tissue growing between two tendon ends and in contact with the cut surface of tendon remodels to look almost exactly like the tendon it joins. Similarly, a tendon that is damaged by rough handling or injured along its external longitudinal surface by laceration so that the interior of the tendon is exposed tends to develop restrictive scar tissue on the outer surface that resembles normal tendon. Because of a paucity of histologic studies on gliding tendons after injury, it is less certain if nonrestricting adhesions remodel to resemble normal paratenon. However, if these theories hold true, it would appear that mature connective tissues may exert an inductive influence on newly made connective tissue in which secondary remodeling can be influenced by ensuring that newly synthesized fibrous tissue comes in contact only with the type of tissue one would like the scar to ultimately resemble.[12]

When tendon ends are left unrepaired in a connective-tissue bed, the ends become atrophied and rounded. With scar formation, remodeling occurs so that longitudinally oriented tissue joins the tendon ends. In actuality, new tendon has not sprouted similar to a regenerating peripheral nerve. The tendon-like tissue between the tendon ends is organized fibrous tissue that joins with the connective tissue surrounding the tendon and tendon bundles. With further secondary remodeling, the longitudinally oriented fibrils become thicker and stronger. Collagen fibrils that are not between the tendon ends obtain a transverse orientation such that a type of tendon sheath or paratenon is formed. Ultimately, a highly efficient re-formation, not regeneration, of a tendon has occurred, with, however, minimal gliding function. Besides lacking gliding function, this "healed" tendon may be too long and lack supporting function. Some contraction of the re-formed tendon will occur with further scar maturation. The supporting function may be better preserved if the tendon ends are sutured together or held together by an external splint that holds the leg in flexion. The scar can then join the tendon ends without tendon lengthening, or the scar can join the tendon stump to adjacent bone or other structures to maintain support.

Primary versus Secondary Tendon Repair. Conditions must be ideal to maintain gliding function after primary repair. Requirements include a clean laceration, minimal contamination, excellent facilities, and an experienced surgeon. These factors are rarely present in veterinary medicine. *In animals, the basic objective is to maintain supporting function, whereas gliding function is of secondary importance.* Primary repair may be attempted within 4 hours of injury.[43] If the wound is very well debrided, the time to primary repair may be extended slightly. Primary repair should not be attempted if the severed tendon overlies a fracture or if there are severe contusions or contamination that could result in lower tissue vitality. Rarely, the quadriceps femoris tendon will rupture transversely just proximal to the patella in the dog and cat. In these cases, best results seem to follow when repair occurs within 48 hours of injury.[33] Generally, the tendon injury should be treated open or closed and the affected joint stabilized with an external device to reduce tension on the tendon. If the wound is initially debrided, tendon ends may be tagged with suture material to aid in identification of the tendon stumps when definitive repair is planned.

Secondary tendon repair is necessary in animals when primary repair fails or was not attempted. It should be performed between 2 and 4 weeks after the initial wound is healed. Secondary repair provides good supporting function, but gliding function is almost always lost. A longitudinal incision over the planned site of tendon repair provides suitable exposure but also can increase the possibility of a binding scar that further inhibits gliding function. Alternatively, an incision transverse to the longitudinal axis of the tendon may be used if exposure is adequate. A longitudinal skin incision, parallel but at some distance to the tendon, may be a better option. The incision can be extended perpendicularly through the underlying soft tissue. As the injured tendon is approached, it should be grasped only with forceps or skin hooks in an area to be removed or where an adhesion is desirable. At the time of secondary repair, tendon ends are generally found embedded in scar tissue. Tendon stumps should be mobilized with the connecting scar tissue, and the ends should be brought together so that tendon length can be restored. It may not be possible to appose the original tendon stumps because of overall shortening of the muscle and tendon tissue. In this instance, the re-formed tendon tissue may be left long, folded, and sutured to the desired length. However, better results may be obtained if the re-formed tendon tissue can be incorporated into the repair by severing transversely and accurately suturing the new tissue to obtain the appropriate tendon length. Sturdy repair can be further achieved by securing the tendon stump to new tendon tissue, to adjacent firm structures, or both. It is important to remember that the primary goal of tendon repair in veterinary medicine is restoration of tendon length for support.

The ideal tendon suture is nonreactive, has high tensile strength, and has knot stability. The suture material should be nonabsorbable or slowly absorbable, such as polydioxanone or polyglycolic acid suture. The size of the material varies with the size of the animal and the function of the tendon. The largest suture that will pass atraumatically through the tendon should be used. The pattern should be simple, contain a minimum of suture material, and not strangulate the tissue.[44] Hemostasis is also critical to successful tendon repair. Uncontrolled bleeding may lead to additional trauma to the tendon and surrounding tissue because of overzealous sponging. Hemostasis may be best accomplished by proper use of tourniquets and meticulous use of electrocoagulation. Saline and suction should be employed to avoid drying of the tissue and to allow adequate visualization of the surgical field.

Suture Patterns Used in Tendon Repair. If the tendon injury is relatively fresh without fixed retraction of the ends, primary end-to-end tenorrhaphy is the repair of choice. Digital extensor tendon lacerations seldom require repair because of the many anastomoses after branching from the main tendon. If repair is necessary, hyperextension of the paw helps to identify the cut ends. Frayed or degenerated tags of the injured tendon should be excised, and a horizontal mattress or figure-of-eight suture should be used to appose the ends (Fig. 7–12). Lacerations of the superficial and deep digital flexor tendons should be repaired when one or more of the digits is flattened and the claw and digital pad are elevated with weight-bearing. Tenorrhaphy of the digital flexor tendon is less complicated when the laceration occurs in the metacarpal or metatarsal area. Surgery in the digital area is more difficult because of the presence of synovial sheaths, annular ligaments, and digital pads. In addition, surgery in the digital area is more demanding because of the small size of the tendons. Chronic digital tendon tears may be very difficult to repair because of retraction of the tendon ends and scar formation. Visualization of the surgical field is improved by use of a tourniquet. The suture pattern employed is largely determined by the size of the torn tendon. Tenorrhaphy failure and adhesion formation may follow surgical repair; thus the prognosis for return of normal posture of the digits is guarded.

A number of suture patterns have been used to repair larger injured tendons. The Bunnell pattern has been used extensively for tendon repair because of its mechanical strength.[45] This pattern has lost some favor because of reported interruption of intrinsic blood flow in tendons.[46] Localized areas of ischemia are produced that result in decreased suture-holding strength. In addition, the Bunnell pattern may cause buckling of the tendon ends as

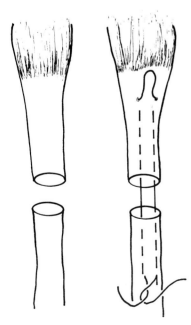

Figure 7–12. Repair of an extensor tendon with a simple horizontal mattress suture. (From Whittick WG (ed): Canine Orthopedics. Philadelphia: Lea & Febiger, 1974, p 124.)

the suture is tightened, resulting in gaps that can weaken the repair and induce adhesion formation. The locking-loop, or modified Kessler, pattern has been reported to minimize adhesion formation in the gliding tendons of the human hand.[47, 48] It also has been used with good results in veterinary medicine.[49–51] A minimum amount of suture material is needed for tendon holding with the locking-loop pattern. Thus, with complete ruptures of the calcanean tendon, a separate locking-loop suture can be placed in each of the three components of the tendon. The locking-loop suture pattern is applied as shown in Figure 7–13. When possible, the transverse and longitudinal elements of the suture pattern should be placed at different levels in the tendon, with the transverse component crossing just superficial to the longitudinal component. When flexible, smooth suture material such as polypropylene or monofilament nylon is used, the configuration allows the loops to tighten on the tendon fibers. The suture may begin in either the proximal or distal tendon stump. If the tendon suture is placed so that the suture patterns in the proximal and distal stumps are mirror images of each other, the tendon ends will be well apposed with minimal buckling. The paratenon is sutured with fine, nonreactive sutures in a simple interrupted or simple continuous pattern.

The three-loop pulley pattern may provide even greater tensile strength and resistance to gap formation than the locking-loop pattern.[52, 53] In treating injuries such as rupture of the canine triceps or calcaneus tendons, the primary goal is to provide adequate tensile strength to prevent distraction during weight-bearing rather than to prevent adhesions. Success depends largely on the maintenance of close apposition of the severed ends, particularly during the first 2 weeks of healing, when the strength of the anastomosis relies on the suture.

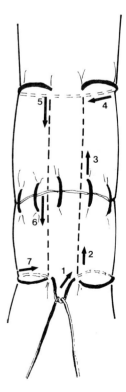

Figure 7–13. Locking-loop suture pattern. The numbers correspond to the order of needle penetration, and the arrows represent the direction. The paratenon is closed with simple interrupted or simple continuous suture pattern. (From Aron DN: A "new" tendon stitch. J Am Anim Hosp Assoc 1981; 17:588.)

The three-loop pulley pattern consists of a continuous pattern comprising three suture loops each of which is oriented approximately 120 degrees from the other two loops (Fig. 7–14). The first loop is made with needle passes one and two placed in a near-far pattern. The second loop is made 120 degrees from the first loop with needle passes three and four oriented midway between the near and far sites. The third loop is started 120 degrees from each of the other two loops with needle passes five and six situated in a far-near pattern. As tension is applied to the tendon or ligament, the suture material glides through the tissue in a pulley fashion so that an equal tensile load is supported by each of the three loops. This redistribution of tension is maximized if each loop is tightened prior to tying the knot. The suture pattern can be tightened more easily if monofilament suture is used, but a braided suture material may be preferred because of its superior tensile strength.[49, 52] Failure of both the three-loop pulley pattern and the locking-loop pattern depends on the size of the structure being sutured and the suture material.[52] With smaller structures such as collateral ligaments in the dog, both patterns fail most commonly because the suture pulls free from the tissue. In larger structures such as the triceps tendon, the strength of both suture patterns depends primarily on the strength of the suture material.

Neglected tears and failed tenorrhaphies result in retraction of the ruptured tendon stumps and formation of extensive scar tissue. Chronic ruptures of tendons such as the calcanean may not be amenable to repair by end-to-end anastomosis. A number of surgical procedures have been described for repairing chronic tendon tears and bridging tendon gaps, including transfer of the deep digital flexor tendon, fasciae latae transplantation, V-Y tendinous flaps, and the use of carbon fiber implants.[33, 54–56] Inconsistent results are reported with a more conservative doubling-over technique used to shorten the tendon without removing redundant scar tissue.[33] A better method of reestablishing the muscle-tendon segment after a failed tenorrhaphy or a

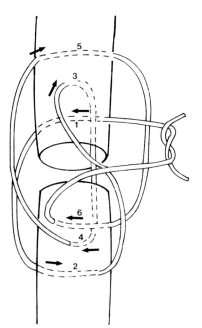

Figure 7–14. Three-loop pulley suture pattern. The first loop is made with needle passes 1 and 2 placed in a near-far pattern. The second loop is placed approximately 120 degrees from the first loop, with passes 3 and 4 located midway between the near and far positions. The third loop is placed about 120 degrees from the other two loops, with passes 5 and 6 placed in a far-near pattern. (From Berg JR, Egger EL: In vitro comparison of the three loop pulley and locking loop suture patterns for repair of canine weightbearing tendons and collateral ligaments. Vet Surg 1986; 15:108.)

neglected tendon rupture may be to remove the excessive scar tissue, followed by repair with one of the above-mentioned techniques.

Tendon Avulsions from Bone and Musculotendinous Tears. The common calcanean tendon can avulse from the tuber calcaneus, or less commonly, the triceps tendon will avulse from the olecranon. If the avulsed bone fragment is large enough, it may be reattached with the tendon using the tension-band technique. If there is no bone or a very small avulsed bone fragment, one or more locking-loop sutures are placed in the tendon to be reattached. The tendon can then be fixed to the bone by passing the ends of the suture through separately drilled holes in the bone and tying them over the distal cortex.[57]

For ruptures of the musculotendinous junction, one of the suture patterns described previously, such as Bunnell or locking-loop pattern, is placed in the tendon stump. A bed for the tendon is created in the muscle, and the suture ends are passed through a polypropylene or Silastic button to anchor the suture to the muscle.[33] The junction between the tendon and muscle may be reinforced with simple interrupted or mattress sutures (Fig. 7–15).

Tendon Lengthening. The condition termed *tendon contracture* can occur as a result of contraction of the muscular attachment of the tendon after trauma and is not due to contraction of the tendon itself. Surgical intervention may be necessary if the contracture is severe, as can be seen in contracture of the flexor tendons of the paw. Tenotomy, in which the tendon is divided and allowed to retract, is the simplest method for lengthening the tendon. Tenotomy within a tendon sheath is contraindicated because the tendon and tendon sheath contain few cells with the potential to synthesize new collagen.[12] Cells for regeneration are externally derived, as discussed previously.

After tenotomy, the ensuing gap will fill with scar tissue that will function as a tendon if the tendon ends retract less than 3 cm. However, if the gap is greater than 3 cm, the resulting union will be weak because the scar is thin and lacks the tensile strength of a normal tendon. A common technique to lengthen a tendon in which the potential gap is greater than 3 cm is the Z tenotomy (Fig. 7–16). A longitudinal cut equal to the distance needed to lengthen the tendon is made in the center of the tendon. A transverse cut is made at each end of the incision on opposite sides of the tendon, creating an elongated Z pattern. The ends of the tendon are sutured. An alternative

Figure 7–15. Technique for repair of musculotendinous rupture using a polypropylene or Silastic button to anchor the suture to the muscle. (From Aron DN: In Bojrab MJ, Birchard SJ, Tomlinson JL (eds): Current Techniques in Small Animal Surgery, 3d ed. Philadelphia: Lea & Febiger, 1990, p 553.)

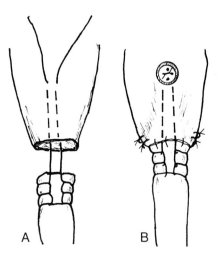

A   B

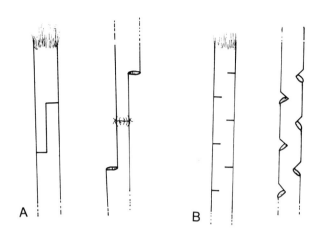

Figure 7–16. Techniques for tendon lengthening using the Z tenotomy *(A)* or the accordion technique *(B)*. One of these techniques can be used when the potential tendon gap after transection is greater than 3 cm. (From Newton CD: In Harvey CE, Newton CD, Schwartz A (eds): Small Animal Surgery. Philadelphia: Lippincott, 1990, p 550.)

is the accordion method of tendon lengthening (see Fig. 7–16). A series of cuts is made on opposite sides of the tendon to allow the tendon to lengthen.

Postoperative Care After Tenorrhaphy. One of the most important aspects of tendon repair is management of the sutured tendon to produce maximal strength and minimal adhesions. Many types of barriers have been used to prevent the formation of adhesions between healing tendon and the surrounding tissue. Barriers have included fetal membranes, scar tissue, blood vessels, and synthetic materials such as Millipore membrane.[38] However, barriers may act to limit the migration of fibroblasts and white cells that are necessary for tendon healing. Collateral blood flow in addition to the longitudinally oriented vessels of the tendon is also necessary to maintain the healing tendon. Therefore, isolation of a tendon not only can prevent healing by inhibiting the migration of collagen forming cells into the site of injury but also can impair revascularization and produce necrosis of a portion of the tendon. *Consequently, rather than placing a barrier between the tendon and surrounding tissue, reduction of scar tissue to the absolute minimum is the most important factor in promoting an active gliding mechanism after tendon healing.* Less scar tissue will develop if there is minimal trauma to the tissue, minimal hematoma and abscess formation, and rest to promote optimal healing. "Breaking down" adhesions produces further inflammation and scar tissue. A healed tendon with satisfactory gliding function is characterized not by the absence of adhesions, but by the presence of adhesions that have been the source of fibroblasts and blood vessels and which have adequate length to allow tendon gliding. Within limits, the amount of scar tissue surrounding a tendon does not seem to be as critical as the physical characteristics of the scar tissue. Examination of nonrestrictive scar tissue suggests that, at some time, reduction in lateral cross-linking or friction between subunits permits longitudinal slipping so that elongation of the entire adhesion occurs. It would seem that repaired tendons either glide or fail to glide because circumferential adhesions elongate or fail to elongate.[12] *Therefore, current techniques of physical therapy based on the concept of breaking or stretching adhesions, as well as various surgical techniques aimed at preventing adhesions, may not be valid.* There is considerable evidence to show that adhesions are part of normal wound healing, and blood vessels intermingled with fibrous elements are needed for nourishment of the tendon.

Optimal healing occurs with a 3-week period of immobilization after surgery. During this time period, the tendon ends revascularize, healing progresses, and minimal scar tissue forms around the tendon. The peritendinous scar tissue remodels when motion is resumed after 3 weeks. The purpose of postoperative movement is to encourage secondary remodeling of scar tissue rather than to rupture adhesions. After the 3-week period of immobilization, the sutured tendon is not strong enough to permit active motion and full weight-bearing. The tendon should be supported by less restrictive external splintage for a minimum of 3 additional weeks. An important caveat in veterinary medicine is that the time of absolute immobilization is based on the nature of the patient and the injury. A human finger tendon may be strong enough to resist rupture when gentle movement is begun after 3 weeks of immobilization, but premature mobilization of tendons such as the triceps or common calcanean tendon in a large dog can result in destabilization. Unrestricted muscle contraction can cause dehiscence of a tendon anastomosis 5 weeks or longer after surgery.[33] However, prolonged immobilization after tendon repair can result in muscle atrophy, infection, skin necrosis, atrophy and ulceration of joint cartilage, joint stiffness, and osteoarthritis.[58] In addition, there is no significant increase in tensile strength with continued immobilization at 5 weeks compared with 3 weeks. Nonetheless, if motion is allowed after 3 weeks of immobilization, the tensile strength at 5 weeks is three times greater than at 3 weeks.[59]

Transarticular external skeletal fixation can be employed to immobilize ruptures of the common calcanean tendon and triceps tendon for 4 to 6 weeks. For the triceps tendon, the elbow joint can be held in extension, and for the calcanean tendon, an external fixation device can be applied to maintain the hock in 160 degrees of plantarflexion.[33] External skeletal fixators are particularly useful when open wounds require management. If a cast is applied to maintain immobilization after calcanean tendon repair, it should be placed above a stifle joint positioned in 140 degrees of flexion with the hock plantarflexed to 160 degrees. When the external fixator is removed after the initial period of immobilization, the triceps tendon should be immobilized in a coaptation splint that ends above the elbow. The splint should maintain the foreleg in a functional walking position and be reinforced with aluminum rods or laterally placed yuka board, plaster, or fiberglass slabs. A coaptation splint with cranial or craniolateral reinforcement is used to protect repair of the common calcanean tendon. The splint ends below the stifle, and the hock is maintained at an angle for walking. The coaptation splint can be removed after 4 weeks. A soft wrap is used to prevent unrestricted weight-bearing and extreme joint flexion for approximately 4 more weeks. Normal activity is gradually established within 4 to 8 weeks after removal of the padded wrap.

SKELETAL MUSCLE INJURIES

Anatomy and Pathophysiology

A single muscle cell is termed a *muscle fiber*. Each muscle fiber is a cylinder, with a diameter of 10 to 100 μm and a length that may reach 300,000 μm or approximately 1 ft.[60] In some instances, skeletal muscle fibers span the entire length of the muscle, but in other cases they are not as long as the muscle and their pull is transmitted by the endomysial connective tissue.[60] There are several hundred slender, oval nuclei within every fiber. In addition, satellite cell nuclei lie alongside skeletal muscle fibers, enclosed within the same basement membrane. They make up 4% to 10% of the nuclei and play an important role in muscle fiber regeneration.[38] Satellite cells appear to persist throughout adult life as a stem-cell population that serves as a potential source of myoblasts capable of fusing to form new muscle fibers.[60] After muscle trauma, an attempt is made to regenerate new muscle fibers to replace damaged or necrotic fibers. This seems to be the only recourse in skeletal muscles, because nuclei that have become incorporated into skeletal muscle fibers do not divide. Furthermore, loss of muscle function due to injury is compensated primarily by hypertrophy of the undamaged muscle fibers and, to a lesser degree, by regeneration of new fibers.[60] Successful regeneration depends on preservation of the endomysial connective-tissue framework because this serves as an essential scaffolding during the repair process.

The term *muscle* refers to a number of muscle fibers bound together by connective tissue (Fig. 7–17). The relation between a single muscle fiber (cell) and a muscle is similar to that between a single nerve fiber (axon) and a nerve composed of many axons. The entire muscle is enclosed by a sheath of dense ordinary connective tissue called the *epimysium* (Fig. 7–18). Blood vessels, lymphatics, and nerves enter or leave the interior of the muscle from the epimysium by way of fibrous partitions that extend into the muscle and surround the bundles of muscle fibers. These partitions form the *perimysium*. Continuous with the perimysium, sheets of delicate connective tissue extend between each muscle fiber and comprise the *endomysium*. The endomysium contains many capillaries and nerve fibers that supply the muscle fibers.[60]

Skeletal muscle cells, like cardiac muscle, are classified as striated because of a highly organized arrangement of subcellular structures (see Fig. 7–17).

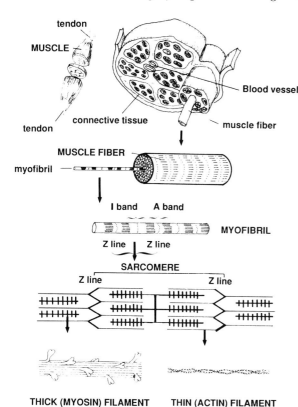

Figure 7–17. Levels of structural organization in a skeletal muscle. (From Vander AJ, Sherman JH, Luciano DS (eds): Human Physiology: The Mechanisms of Body Function, 4th ed. New York: McGraw-Hill, 1985, p 257.)

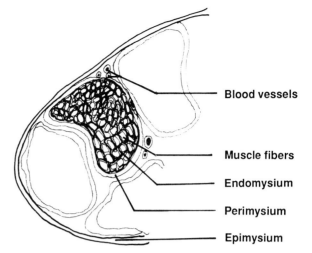

Figure 7–18. Diagram of connective-tissue components of skeletal muscle. Epimysium encloses the entire muscle, perimysium surrounds each bundle of fibers, and endomysium lies between the individual muscle fibers. (From Cormack DH (ed): Ham's Histology, 9th ed. Philadelphia: Lippincott, 1987, p 389.)

- Blood vessels
- Muscle fibers
- Endomysium
- Perimysium
- Epimysium

A series of transverse light and dark bands form a regular pattern along each fiber. Although the pattern appears to be continuous across the cytoplasm of a single fiber, the bands are actually confined to a number of cylindrical elements, known as *myofibrils*, that are 1 to 2 μm in diameter (see Fig. 7–17). Myofibrils occupy about 80% of the fiber volume and vary in number from several hundred to several thousand per fiber, depending on the fiber's diameter. Each myofibril consists of smaller filaments that are arranged in a repeating pattern along the length of the fibril. One unit of this repeating pattern is termed a *sarcomere* ("little muscle"). Each sarcomere contains two types of filaments. Thick filaments are 12 to 18 nm in diameter and are composed primarily of the contractile protein myosin. Thin filaments are 5 to 8 nm in diameter and contain tropomyosin and troponin in addition to the contractile protein actin.

Skeletal muscle cells are effectors that generate force, produce movement, and are responsible for voluntary actions that range from vocalization to running. The output of a muscle depends on the size of the muscle cells and their parallel anatomic arrangement. Increasing the diameter of a fiber by synthesis of new myofibrils (hypertrophy) will increase the force-generating capacity of a cell. The formation of more cells (hyperplasia) also increases tissue force output. *However, differentiated skeletal muscle has only a limited capacity to form new cells.* The musculoskeletal system is arranged so that most gravitational loads are sustained by the skeleton and ligaments. Skeletal muscle cells are normally relaxed and are recruited to generate force and movement.

The cell bodies of motor nerves to skeletal muscle are in the ventral horn of the spinal cord. The axon exits via the ventral root and reaches the muscle through a mixed peripheral nerve, which contains both sensory and motor fibers. The motor nerves branch in the muscle, with each terminal innervating a single muscle cell in mammals. A *motor unit* consists of the motor nerve and all the muscle fibers innervated by that nerve. The motor unit, not the individual cell, is the functional contractile unit because all cells within a motor unit contract synchronously when the motor nerve fires.[4]

Two types of muscle fibers have been defined based on the speed of contraction and biochemical characteristics. *Type I fibers* are also known as *red fibers* or *slow-twitch fibers* and are capable of sustained or weight-bearing action. *Type II fibers,* or *fast-twitch fibers,* are paler (*white fibers*) and are capable of sudden action.[4, 38] All fibers in one motor unit are of the same type; however, the two fiber types are intermingled within a muscle, and the predominance of one over the other depends on the function of the whole muscle.

Skeletal muscle is subject to degeneration and necrosis due to infection, trauma, or ischemia.[61] The repair process is similar to that in other tissues. The debris is removed by mononuclear cells and macrophages. Then, during repair, two processes compete: the regeneration of disrupted muscle from surrounding normal muscle fibers and the ingrowth of granulation tissue and production of a connective-tissue scar. Such scarring may inhibit the complete regeneration of muscle fibers by excessive formation of granulation tissue. Collagen is considered to be necessary for muscle regeneration, forming a sheath around fusing myoblasts,[62] but when a large volume of muscle is devitalized by major trauma, proliferation of fibroblasts can rapidly lead to the formation of excessive scar tissue. This scar tissue may form a dense mechanical barrier to regenerating muscle fibers. In the early stages of muscle repair, synthesis of type III collagen increases even before any mature fibroblasts can be detected, the source believed to be primitive multipotential cells. As repair progresses, there is a return to a marked predominance of type I collagen. After approximately 6 weeks, the area grossly and microscopically appears normal except for occasional small areas of fibrosis.[63] *This sequence of events suggests that damaged muscle should be protected for a minimum of 6 weeks before allowing unrestricted activity.* Re-rupture after muscle injury commonly results from overvigorous activity after prolonged immobilization. Restricted exercise can help avoid the severe disuse atrophy associated with complete immobilization.

Types of Muscle Injury and Treatment

Muscle can be injured by direct trauma, such as a forceful blow, gunshot wound, fracture, or dislocation, or indirect trauma, which stretches and tears the muscle fibers. The usual cause of closed muscle rupture is powerful active contraction of a flexor motor unit at the same time that forced passive extension occurs.[12] Damage to muscle results in tearing and disruption of the muscle fibers, connective tissue, and blood and lymph vessels. Muscle–tendon injuries can occur at any point from the origin to the insertion of the muscle. When a closed injury is restricted to a few muscle fibers and the supporting connective tissue, it is termed a *pull, tear,* or *strain.* Strain is more specifically defined as damage to some part of a muscle–tendon unit, which may involve injury to the muscle, tendon, or associated attachment sites.[64] The point of damage commonly occurs at the weakest link of the muscle–tendon unit at the time of injury. Strains can be chronic and multiple or acute and singular in nature and can vary in their severity from mild to complete rupture. Milder forms tend to produce minimal changes in gait and are often overlooked except in animals such as the racing greyhound, in which a slight decrease in speed can be detected.[56] The affected muscles can be located by deep palpation of the muscle and tendon. Digital pressure tends to cause pain in the dog.

Greyhounds in training and racing acquire a substantial number of closed traumatic injuries to muscles and tendons.[65] Other chronic muscle disorders, including fibrotic myopathy and contracture of the quadriceps, infraspinatus, and gracilis muscles, are diagnosed in breeds other than greyhounds. These disorders can be secondary to trauma, but they may not be detected immediately after the injury.[66–68] The etiology of muscle tears is uncertain. In greyhounds, conformation of the dog and the specific forefoot leading in galloping are of prime importance. In addition, the faster dogs appear to be more prone to injury.[69] The gracilis is the most frequently damaged muscle in the greyhound. Acute injury to the gracilis has also been termed "dropped muscle," presumably because of the bulge that often develops on the inner aspect of the thigh secondary to tearing of muscle fibers and hemorrhage. In one study of 40 greyhounds, the gracilis in the right hind leg was affected in 31 dogs, the left in 8, and bilateral gracilis injury occurred in 1 dog.[65] Muscle tears also may involve the sartorius, quadriceps, adductor, gastrocnemius, and semimembranosus, and rarely, the pectineus may be torn from its insertion into the femur. Damage to blood vessels results in hematoma formation. The clot will remain friable for 2 to 3 days. During this period, vigorous massage or ultrasonic therapy can cause further hemorrhage. The hematoma resolves through absorption and fibrosis, which can cause some degree of scarring and adhesions.

Pain may be the predominant sign associated with muscle injury. Pain is caused by swelling that can be due to a space-occupying hematoma. Nonetheless, lameness at walk may be slight even when the muscle is severely damaged. Detectable lameness and associated discomfort can go unnoticed until the second or third day after injury.[64] This delay is believed to be due to some form of biochemical injury that requires a finite period of time to reach maximal effect. In addition, a variable amount of subcutaneous bruising and edema may be present in the affected limb.[65] Treatment is aimed at preventing hematoma formation and promoting rapid resolution of a hematoma, if present. With detection of acute muscle injury, pressure should be applied to the area with a padded elastic bandage. Cold compresses should be applied to diminish blood flow and thus decrease hemorrhage into the area. Finally, rest is critical to rapid, comparatively uncomplicated recovery. Treatment tactics can change within 24 to 48 hours, when surgical or additional nonsurgical therapy may be required. Proposed nonsurgical approaches include massage, ultrasonic therapy, and administration of corticosteroids and various topical agents.[69]

Ruptures that are incomplete usually do not require operative repair unless a palpable gap between muscle ends is present. Complete separation of muscle ends with total loss of function generally is an indication for surgical repair, and the sooner the muscle ends can be coapted, the better is the prognosis.[12] Because muscle is quite friable, a tension suture technique is preferable.[70] The suture tension can be spread over a larger area of the muscle by using a button, Silastic tubing, or similar material.

Delay of definitive treatment allows extensive fibrous protein synthesis in and around muscle ends. Late repair involves complete excision of all new connective tissue so that muscle units can be extended and fresh, unscarred muscle can be coapted with unscarred muscle on the other side of the wound. Just as scar tissue elsewhere in the body is subject to remodeling after physical stress and strain, fibrous scar between muscle fragments can elongate such that serious loss of power may occur. One of the most important steps in primary or secondary muscle repair is to carefully excise scar tissue or damaged muscle. *The biologic key to healing of muscles is the ability of muscle to regenerate if it is not strangled by extensive fibrous tissue.* Healing between muscle ends by fibrous protein synthesis is not as desirable as regeneration of myofibrils. Careful excision of old scar in secondary repair and precise debridement of damaged muscle so that fibrous tissue replacement will not occur offer the best chance of maximal muscle regeneration and minimal fibrous protein synthesis after an acute injury.

Muscle trauma secondary to automobile accidents or gunshot wounds requires different treatment strategies. Control of external bleeding is accomplished by direct pressure and bandaging. Open wounds are covered with sterile dressing to avoid further contamination during the initial period of patient management. Early, vigorous treatment of open wounds in the muscle is necessary to prevent contamination from becoming an established infection.

REFERENCES

1. Sunderland S: Factors influencing the course of regeneration and the quality of the recovery after nerve suture. Brain 1952; 75:19–54
2. Sunderland S: Nerves and Nerve Injuries. Baltimore: Williams & Wilkins, 1968
3. Ganong WF: Excitable tissue: Nerve. In Ganong WF (ed): Review of Medical Physiology, 12th ed. Los Altos, Calif: Lange Medical Publications, 1985, pp 32–44
4. Berne RM, Levy MN: Physiology, 2d ed. St. Louis: Mosby, 1988
5. Lundborg G: Intraneural microvascular pathophysiology as related to ischemia and nerve injury. In Daniel RK, Terzis JK (eds): Reconstructive Microsurgery. Boston: Little, Brown, 1977, pp 334–341
6. Lundborg G, Rydevik B: Effect of stretching the tibial nerve of the rabbit: A preliminary study of the intraneural circulation and the barrier function of the perineum. J Bone Joint Surg 1973; 55:390–401
7. Knecht CD, St. Clair LE: The radial-brachial paralysis syndrome in the dog. J Am Vet Med Assoc 1969; 154:653–656
8. Swaim SF: Peripheral nerve surgery in the dog. J Am Vet Med Assoc 1972; 161:905–911
9. Sunderland S: A classification of peripheral nerve injuries producing loss of function. Brain 1951; 74:491–516
10. Sedon HJ: Surgical Disorders of the Peripheral Nerves, 2d ed. London: Churchill Livingstone, 1975
11. Tyndall DA, Gregg JM, Hanker JS: Evaluation of peripheral nerve regeneration following crushing or transection injuries. J Oral Maxillofac Surg 1984; 42A:314–318
12. Peacock EE: Wound Repair, 3d ed. Philadelphia: WB Saunders, 1984
13. Ducker TG, Kempe LG, Hayes GJ: The metabolic background for peripheral nerve surgery. J Neurosurg 1969; 30:270–280
14. Poth EJ, Fernandez EB, Drager GA: Prevention of formation of end-bulb neuromata. Proc Soc Exp Biol Med 1945; 60:200–207
15. Swaim SF: Peripheral nerve surgery. In Hoerlein BF (ed): Canine Neurology. Philadelphia: WB Saunders, 1978, pp 296–318
16. Nulsen FE, Kline DG: Acute injuries of peripheral nerves. In Youmans JR (ed): Neurological Surgery, vol 2. Philadelphia: WB Saunders, 1973, pp 1089–1140
17. Jabaley ME: Peripheral nerve injuries. In Evarts CM (ed): Surgery of the Musculoskeletal System, vol 1. New York: Churchill Livingstone, 1983, pp 107–144
18. Brown PW: Factors influencing the success of the surgical repair of peripheral nerves. Surg Clin North Am 1972; 52:1137–1155
19. Snyder CC, Leonard LG: Peripheral nerve surgery. In Gourley IM, Vasseur PB (eds): General Small Animal Surgery. Philadelphia: Lippincott, 1985, pp 917–925
20. Raffe MR: Principles of peripheral nerve repair and regeneration. In Newton CD, Nunamaker DM (eds): Textbook of Small Animal Orthopaedics. Philadelphia: Lippincott, 1985, pp 791–832
21. Bowen JM: Peripheral nerve electrodiagnostics, electromyography and nerve conduction velocity. In Hoerlein BF (ed): Canine Neurology. Philadelphia: WB Saunders, 1978, pp 254–279
22. Griffiths IR, Duncan ID: The use of electromyography and nerve conduction studies in the evaluation of lower motor neuron disease or injury. J Small Anim Pract 1978; 19:329–340
23. Duncan ID: Peripheral nerve disease in the dog and cat. Vet Clin North Am 1980; 10:177–211

24. Shores A: Peripheral nervous system. In Bojrab MJ, Birchard SJ, Tomlinson JL (eds): Current Techniques in Small Animal Surgery, 3d ed. Philadelphia: Lea & Febiger, 1990, pp 50–62
25. Wilkins RH: Peripheral nerve injuries. In Sabiston DC (ed): Davis-Christopher Textbook of Surgery: The Biological Basis of Modern Surgical Practice, 12th ed. Philadelphia: WB Saunders, 1981, pp 1502–1504
26. Raffe MR: Peripheral nerve injuries in the dog (part II). Compend Contin Educ Pract Vet 1979; 1:269–276
27. Bratton BR, Kline DG, Hudson AR, Coleman WT: Use of monofilament polyglycolic acid suture for experimental peripheral nerve repair. J Surg Res 1981; 31:482–489
28. Freeman BS: Adhesive anastomosis techniques for fine nerves: Experimental and clinical techniques. Am J Surg 1964; 108:529–532
29. Braun RM: Comparative studies of neurorrhaphy and sutureless peripheral nerve repair. Surg Gynecol Obstet 1966; 122:15–18
30. Smith JW: Factors influencing nerve repair: I. Blood supply of peripheral nerves. Arch Surg 1966; 93:335–341
31. Eppley BL, Doucet MJ, Winkelmann T, Delfino, JJ: Effect of different surgical repair modalities on regeneration of the rabbit mandibular nerve. J Oral Maxillofac Surg 1989; 42:267–274
32. Butler HC: Surgery of tendinous injuries and muscle injuries. In Newton CD, Nunamaker DM (eds): Textbook of Small Animal Orthopaedics. Philadelphia: Lippincott, 1985, pp 835–842
33. Aron DN: Tendons. In Bojrab MJ, Birchard SJ, Tomlinson JL (eds): Current Techniques in Small Animal Surgery, 3d ed. Philadelphia: Lea & Febiger, 1990, pp 549–561
34. Newton CD: Orthopedic basic sciences. In Harvey CE, Newton CD, Schwartz A (eds): Small Animal Surgery. Philadelphia: Lippincott, 1990, pp 533–559
35. Justis EJ Jr: Affections of muscles, tendons, and associated structures. In Edmonson AS, Crenshaw AH (eds): Campbell's Operative Orthopaedics, 6th ed. St. Louis: Mosby, 1980, pp 1379–1417
36. Davies JV, Clayton Jones DG: Triceps tendon rupture in the dog following corticosteroid injection. J Small Anim Pract 1982; 23:779–787
37. O'Donoghue DH: Treatment of Injuries to Athletes, 4th ed. Philadelphia: WB Saunders, 1984, pp 593–595
38. Johnston DE: Tendons, skeletal muscles, and ligaments in health and disease. In Newton CD, Nunamaker DM (eds): Textbook of Small Animal Orthopaedics. Philadelphia: Lippincott, 1985, pp 65–76
39. Garner WL, McDonald JA, Koo M, et al: Identification of the collagen-producing cells in healing flexor tendons. Plast Reconstr Surg 1989; 83:875–879
40. Hirsch G: Tensile properties during tendon healing. Acta Orthop Scand 1974; 153(suppl): 7–79
41. Williams IF, Heaton A, McCullagh KG: Cell morphology and collagen types in equine tendon scar. Res Vet Sci 1980; 28:302–310
42. Stein LE, Pijanowski GJ, Johnson AL: Collagen types in healing rabbit tendons: A biochemical assessment. Vet Surg 1985; 14:149–152
43. Bunnell S: Primary repair of severed tendons. Am J Surg 1940; 47:502–516
44. Mason ML: Primary and secondary tendon suture. Surg Gynecol Obstet 1940; 70:392–402
45. Ketchum LD, Martin NL, Kappel OA: Experimental evaluation of factors affecting the strength of tendon repairs. Plast Reconstr Surg 1977; 59:708–719
46. Stein LE, Pijanowski GJ, Johnson AL: A histological evaluation of rabbit tendons sutured using the Bunnell pattern. Vet Surg 1985; 14:145–148
47. Kessler I, Nissim F: Primary repair without immobilization of flexor tendon division within the digital sheath: an experimental and clinical study. Acta Orthop Scand 1969; 40:587–601
48. Pennington DG: The locking-loop tendon suture. Plast Reconst Surg 1979; 63:648–652
49. Aron DN: A "new" tendon stitch. J Am Anim Hosp Assoc 1981; 17:587–591
50. Earley TD: Tendon disorders. In Bojrab MJ (ed): Pathophysiology in Small Animal Surgery. Philadelphia: Lea & Febiger, 1981, pp 851–866
51. Tomlinson J, Moore R: Locking loop tendon suture use in repair of five calcanean tendons. Vet Surg 1982; 11:105–109
52. Berg RJ, Egger EL: In vitro comparison of the three loop pulley and locking loop suture patterns for repair of canine weightbearing tendons and collateral ligaments. Vet Surg 1986; 15:107–110
53. Jann HW, Stein LE, Good JK: Strength characteristics and failure modes of locking-loop and three-loop pulley suture patterns in equine tendons. Vet Surg 1990; 19:28–33
54. Braden TD: Fascia lata transplant for repair of chronic Achilles tendon defects. J Am Anim Hosp Assoc 1976; 12:800–805
55. Vaughn LC, Edwards GB: The use of carbon fibers (Grafil) for tendon repair in animals. Vet Rec 1978; 102:287–288

56. Malnati GA: Deep digital flexor tendon transposition for rupture of the calcanean tendon in a dog. J Am Anim Hosp Assoc 1981; 17:451–454
57. Brinker WO, Piermattei DC, Flo GL: Handbook of Small Animal Orthopedics and Fracture Healing, 2d ed. Philadelphia: WB Saunders, 1990
58. Enwemeka CS, Speilholz NI, Nelson AJ: The effect of early functional activities on experimentally tenotomized Achilles tendons in rats. Am J Phys Med Rehabil 1988; 67:264–269
59. Mason ML, Allen H: The rate of healing of tendons: An experimental study of tensile strength. Ann Surg 1941; 113:424–459
60. Cormack DH: Ham's Histology, 9th ed. Philadelphia: Lippincott, 1987
61. Saunders JH, Sissons HA: Effect of denervation on regeneration of skeletal muscle after injury. J Bone Joint Surg 1953; 35B:113–124
62. Allbrook D: Muscle regeneration. Physiotherapy 1973; 59:240–247
63. Turek SL: Diseases of muscle. In Turek SL (ed): Orthopaedics: Principles and Their Application, vol 1, 4th ed. Philadelphia: Lippincott, 1984
64. Farrow CS: Sprain, strain, and contusion. Vet Clin North Am 1978; 8(2):169–182
65. Vaughan LC: Gracilis muscle injury in greyhounds. J Small Anim Pract 1969; 10:363–375
66. Moore RW, Rouse GP, Piermattei DL, Ferguson RH: Fibrotic myopathy of the semitendinosus muscle in four dogs. Vet Surg 1981; 10:169–174
67. Bennett RA: Contracture of the infraspinatus muscle in dogs: A review of 12 cases. J Am Anim Hosp Assoc 1985; 22:481–487
68. Carberry CA, Gilmore DR: Infraspinatus muscle contracture associated with trauma in a dog. J Am Vet Med Assoc 1986; 188:533–534
69. Davis PE: The diagnosis and treatment of muscle injuries in the racing greyhound. Aust Vet J 1967; 43:519–523
70. Reinke JD, Kus SP: Achilles mechanism injury in the dog. Compend Contin Educ Pract Vet 1982; 4:639–645

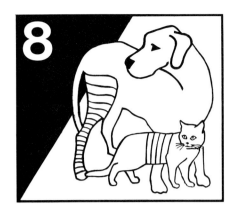

HEALING OF BONE FRACTURES

KARL H. KRAUS

Although intramedullary pinning was described as early as the age of the Aztecs, little improvement was made in promoting bone healing until the 20th century. It was not until medical scientists began to critically examine mechanisms of bone healing that better therapies could be developed. A veterinary orthopedic surgeon, therefore, must first know the mechanisms of bone healing before selecting the most appropriate coaptation device or surgical fixation.

In analyzing fractures, the surgeon should use a routine approach based on the principles of fracture mechanics and bone healing. First, the mechanics of the injury should be evaluated to ascertain which types of forces caused the fracture. Next, the secondary forces acting on the fracture segments should be assessed so that they can be neutralized by the therapy. The type of therapy chosen is also based on the type of bone healing (primary or secondary) best suited to the patient and fracture. An appropriate fracture fixation technique is based on the effects of the stabilization device on bone healing and vascular supply.

FRACTURE BIOPHYSICS

Bone as a Material

A bone fractures when a force greater than its tolerance is applied to it. Bone, as a material, can absorb great amounts of force associated with normal activity, such as running, and is less able to tolerate a nonphysiologic force, such as bending. Bone is not totally rigid and deforms due to forces placed on it. When mild deforming forces are released from bone, it resumes its original shape. This is called *elastic deformation*. Great forces will deform bone to a point at which it cannot resume its original shape and will remain bent. This is called *plastic deformation*. Even greater forces will result in failure of bone and cause a fracture. The relationship between force and bone is described in graphic form as a *force–deformation curve* (Fig. 8–1). Another term for this graph is a *stress–strain curve*, where the force applied to bone is stress and the deformation is strain.

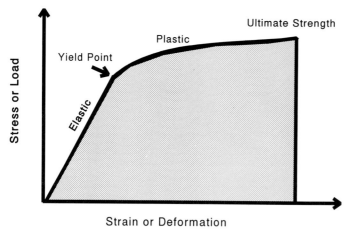

Stress or Load

Strain or Deformation

Absorbed Energy

Figure 8–1. An "ideal" stress–strain curve.

The elastic phase of the force–deformation curve is generally linear. That is, increased forces result in equivalent degrees of deformation. The stiffer the material, the greater is the slope of this line. The area under this curve relates to the total energy absorbed by bone. If force is released during the elastic phase of this curve, bone pushes back into its original shape, thus releasing much of the energy imparted to it (like a spring). If the force to bone in increased, the bone bends to a point where it will not fully resume its original shape. This is called the *yield point*. After this point, the bone will remain deformed. Energy imparted to bone will be absorbed and not released. Further deformation will lead to failure, i.e., fracture.

The force–deformation curve is a general engineering description of bone as a material. Every bone is a complex structure with an assembly of components each having different material properties.[1] For example, the metaphysis of the humerus will have different material properties than the diaphysis. The principle of the force–deformation curve is most helpful if the heterogeneous nature of bone is kept in mind.

The material properties of bone tend to be different depending on the rate at which force is applied to bone. If a force is applied rapidly, bone will behave with greater stiffness and higher ultimate strength. A material with this load rate–dependent property is referred to as *viscoelastic*. This characteristic is important because bone will tend to absorb more energy if it is loaded quickly. Fractures of bone loaded quickly tend to be comminuted.

In terms of material properties, bone is very heterogeneous. A single bone is composed of both cortical and cancellous bone, with porosity ranging from 3% to 90%.[2] The material properties of cortical and cancellous bone are different and reflect their general biomechanical purposes. The metaphysis is composed mostly of cancellous bone. When a large compressive force is applied, the fine trabeculae will collapse. The wide metaphysis, though early to deform, will continue to deform without complete failure. Thus, the elastic part of the force–deformation curve is short while the plastic part is prolonged (Fig. 8–2). This material property is suited to absorbing forces across joints and preventing direct damage to cartilage.

The diaphysis, on the other hand, is composed of cortical bone. In this region, great forces are needed to deform the bone. Since the bone is rigid yet brittle, there is little plasticity to cortical bone (Fig. 8–3). Once enough

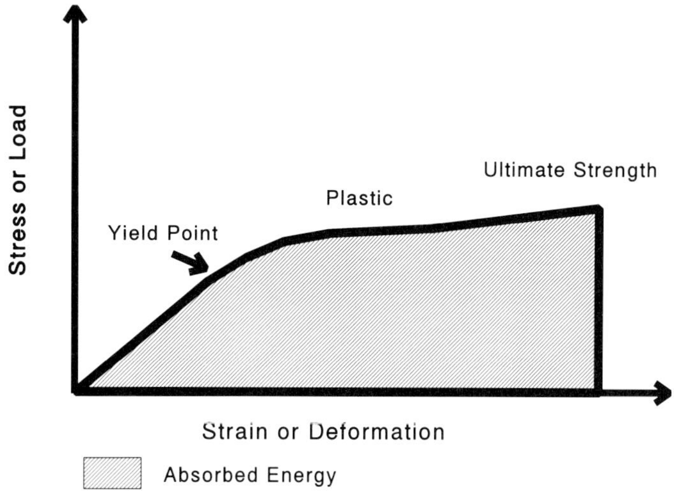

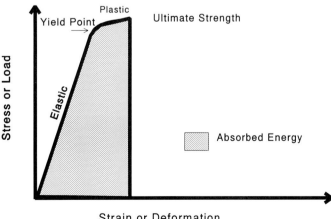

Figure 8–2. Stress–strain curve for can-cellous bone. The slope of the elastic region of the curve is reduced, and a long plastic phase relates to collapse of bone trabeculae.

strain occurs, the diaphysis breaks. This property provides inflexible levers for movement.

A final material consideration is the strength of bone if a force is applied in a physiologic direction and weakness if a force is applied in an abnormal direction. A material with strength related to load direction is called *aniso-tropic*. For example, a tibia can tolerate large stresses if an axial force is applied and much less stress if a bending force is applied.

Fracture Mechanics

A bone can be loaded in all directions of three-dimensional space. These forces are compression, distraction, shear, bending, and torsion.[3, 4] Because of the complex shape of bone, most fractures result from two or more of these forces. When analyzing a fracture, a surgeon must consider which forces caused the fracture and, more importantly, how normal physiologic forces will affect the fracture lines.

COMPRESSION

Two opposing forces acting on a material along a single axis is *compression* (Fig. 8–4). For homogeneous materials, this force results in a shortening of

Figure 8–3. Stress–strain curve for cor-tical bone. The slope of the elastic re-gion of the curve is increased due to cortical bone rigidity. The plastic phase of the curve is very short, which indi-cates that cortical bone cannot be de-formed easily before failing.

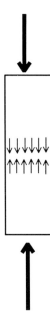

Figure 8–4. A compressive force applied to a material and subsequent internal forces. A compressive force leads to buckling of the material.

the material and failure by buckling. Purely compressive forces infrequently cause fracture in animals because bone is very strong against this normal physiologic type of load. Strength against compression is directly related to a bone's mineral content. The greater the mineral content per unit volume, the greater is the bone's strength against compression.

Fractures caused by external forces are usually the result of other types of loads for two reasons. First, bones have complex shapes. External forces are infrequently aligned to cause pure compression. Rather, since bones are curved, bending or shear forces are usually present. In addition, loads placed on bone are usually not a single type of load, but a combination. Since bone is strong against compressive forces, other types of loads in complex loading, will cause failure before compression.

Since bone is strong against compression, fractures caused by purely compressive forces are usually the result of great forces that are absorbed by the elastic phase of the stress–strain curve. Much of the energy contained at the time of fracture is released into adjacent tissue by disruption of the structure of the bone. Frequently, fracture caused by purely compressive forces are highly comminuted. An example of a fracture caused by compression would be a burst fracture of a vertebra.

DISTRACTION

Tension, the opposite of compression, is the result of opposite forces pulling bone apart (Fig. 8–5). Unlike compression, the opposing force comes not from the strength of bone's mineral component, but from the arrangement and properties of collagen. An example would be the avulsion of a malleolus in a tarsal luxation as the collateral ligament pulls a bone fragment from the tibia or fibula. Tensile forces generally result in failure perpendicular to the distracting forces. These forces are generally not physiologic, and bone is weaker against these forces. Fractures resulting from distraction tend to be simple.

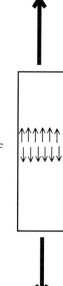

Figure 8–5. A distractive force applied to a material and subsequent internal forces. A distractive force leads to transverse separation of bone.

SHEAR

A *shear* force occurs when forces in opposite directions and different planes act on a material (Fig. 8–6). The opposing force is the resistance of constituents of the material to slide across each other. The bone fails and fractures when bonds between the constituent parts fail, as in distraction. A frequent example of a shear fracture is a capitular (condylar) fracture of the distal humerus. Shear forces are also generally not physiologic, and therefore, fractures easily occur secondary to these forces. The resulting fracture is usually simple.

BENDING

Bending, classically described in the four-point bending model, results in distractive and compressive forces acting simultaneously on the material (Fig. 8–7). Since bending and distractive forces are opposite, the plane within the material between bending and distractive forces must contain no forces and is called the *neutral plane*. The opposing forces are the material's (bone) strength against compression (great) and the bonding of its constituent parts (weak). The bone will fail first on the aspect that is subjected to tension. The fracture line will progress across the bone transversely or slightly obliquely.

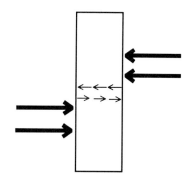

Figure 8–6. A shearing force applied to a material and subsequent internal forces. Shearing causes the components of the material to slide against each other.

Neutral Plane

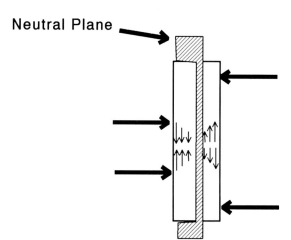

Figure 8–7. Bending applied by a four-point model and resulting compressive and distractive internal forces. Between the compressive and distractive forces is the neutral plane.

Since many long bones have some bend, forces acting from each end of the bone result in bending forces along with compressive forces. The greatest distractive force is found on the convex aspect of the curved bone, and the greatest compressive force is on the concave aspect. In these cases, the combination of bending forces with compressive forces results in transverse or oblique fractures and comminution of the concave aspect with "butterfly" fragments or small comminutions (Fig. 8–8).

TORSION

Torsion occurs when rotating forces in opposite directions and different planes act on a material (Fig. 8–9). The opposing forces tend to be complex and depend on the geometry of the material. Shear and distractive forces are the major constituent forces; thus, opposing forces are the bonding substances of bone. Since strong torsional forces are not generally encountered in physiologic motion and an angled distal limb easily acts as a rotational

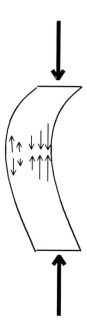

Figure 8–8. Forces applied to each end of a curved object result in internal forces much like the four-point bending model. Compressive forces occur on the concave surface, and distractive forces occur on the convex surface. Increased compressive force on the concave surface will lead to comminution or a "butterfly" fragment when a bone fractures because of this load.

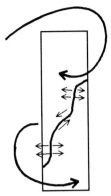

Figure 8–9. A rotational force applied to a material and subsequent internal forces. Resulting internal forces are mainly shearing and distraction forces.

lever arm, fractures due to torsion are common. In bone, torsional loads usually result in spiral oblique fractures.

COMPLEX FRACTURES

Fractures are often comminuted due to complex loads and rapid rates of loading. Complex loads are due to the angles of the load and complex geometry of the bones. Additionally, the heterogeneous nature of bone as a material allows for different areas of bone to be strong or weak in response to the different stresses. Forces will tend to concentrate and propagate along weak areas of bone.

As noted earlier with regard to the viscoelastic property of bone, high rates of loading lead to bone acting rigidly and with greater ultimate strength. Higher energies are needed to fracture bone when the load is applied quickly. Since the bone is absorbing greater energies before failure, greater energies are released. The consequence is more comminution. Highly comminuted fractures result from external forces of high energy that are transferred through soft tissue to bone. Alternatively, energy absorbed by bone is, to some degree, transferred to soft tissue. In either regard, highly comminuted fractures reflect severe soft-tissue damage.

Counteracting Internal Forces

Abnormal forces result in fracture, and repair of fractures relies on opposing physiologic forces acting on the fracture fragments to prevent interfragmentary motion. Physiologic forces are those acting on bone by gravity while standing and in motion, and those acting on bone by muscles. Both geometry in relation to gravity *and* muscle pull should be considered in fracture fixation. Fixation devices that counteract these forces should be used and each fracture line should be evaluated.

For example, a common fracture is a midshaft transverse fracture of the femur with a small comminution or "butterfly" piece. This fracture is caused by a bending force, with compression as an additional component force. In terms of only geometry and gravitational forces, bending and compression would act on this fracture. Bending is a combination of compressive and distractive forces. Due to the presence of the femoral neck, the femur can be considered curved with a convex aspect under tension and a concave side under compression. Since bone is normally strong under compression, the tensile force must be counteracted. This could be achieved with an intramedullary rod. Unfortunately, this repair for such a fracture is often insufficient because it neglects the effects of the strong internal and external rotating muscles of the coxofemoral joint. These forces can be opposed with addition of a type I two- or four-pin external fixator.

BONE HEALING

Composition of Bone

Bone can be considered, in physical terms, as a complex material with properties that interact with applied forces. It is, however, also biologically dynamic and capable of almost perfect repair. It is constantly changing in response to stresses and physiologic needs.

Bone is comprised of organic material (35%) and mineral (65%).[5] The organic material includes cells and matrix material. Bone cells include osteocytes, osteoblasts, and osteoclasts, which constitute a very small portion of bone composition. Osteocytes are mature osteoblasts. They are relatively quiescent, yet play an important role in calcium homeostasis. Osteoblasts are metabolically active cells responsible for bone production. Their role and activity are essential for bone healing. The third type of cell is the osteoclast, which is a multinucleated cell responsible for bone, cartilage, and osteoid resorption. Organic bone matrix is type I collagen and interstitial substance, which is principally glycosaminoglycans.[6]

The inorganic constituent of bone forms in a specific relationship to collagen fibrils. The inorganic component of bone is hydroxyapatite $[Ca_{10}(PO_4)_6(OH)_2]$. It is this crystal that provides bone rigidity.[7] Decreasing the mineral content of bone results in bone becoming more elastic and less able to absorb compressive loads. Hydroxyapatite crystals are oriented parallel to the long axis of the collagen fibril. As the crystal grows, it maintains its bond to the collagen fiber and assumes the same 640-Å periodicity. It is the orientation of collagen fibrils and the associated hydroxyapatite that give bone its unique physical properties. The long interconnected collagen fibrils provide resistance to tensile forces, and the strong crystal provides resistance to compressive forces. Orientation and composition of these bone constituents are responsible for the anisotropic and heterotopic property of bones.

In general terms, bone can be cancellous or cortical. Cancellous bone is very porous and consists of thin trabeculae filled with blood and hematopoietic cells. Cortical bone is arranged in a specific manner called a *haversian system* (Fig. 8–10). In this system, small vascular channels are surrounded by layers of bone called *lamellae*. The haversian canals run parallel to the long axis of the bone. Within these canals are nutrient vessels, lymphatics, and nerves. These channels connect with each other and with endosteal and periosteal vessels by means of transverse canals called *Volkmann's canals*. Osteocytes are located in lacunae within the lamella. Very fine pores called *canaliculi* perpendicularly connect haversian canals to lacunae. These channels provide perfusion of osteocytes with noncellular plasma nutrients.

Bone is supplied with blood from three sources: the principal nutrient artery, the proximal and distal metaphyseal arteries, and the periosteal arterioles[8, 9] (Fig. 8–11). *The major source of blood to bone is through the nutrient artery.* A nutrient artery enters a bone through a nutrient foramen and

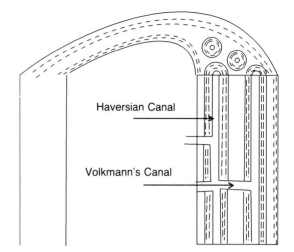

Figure 8–10. Illustration of cortical bone with haversian and Volkmann's canals.

bifurcates into ascending and descending branches. There are two parallel systems of blood flow from the nutrient artery, one supplying the marrow and the other supplying the cortex. Metaphyseal vessels are multiple and penetrate around joint capsule attachments. They anastomose in the medullary cavity with branches of the nutrient artery so that collateral circulation to all areas of the medullary cavity is achieved if any one of these blood supplies is obstructed.

Blood supply to cortical bone is centrifugal. There is a higher pressure within the medullary cavity that encourages blood to flow out. Cortical vessels from the nutrient or metaphyseal arteries enter the cortex and supply the cellular components of bone via the haversian system. Blood is then collected by venules within the periosteum. Venous return from the medullary vascular system is alternately achieved by a medullary venous sinus and nutrient vein exiting through the nutrient foramen.

The third source of blood to bone is periosteal vessels. In uninjured adult bone, this is the least important blood supply. Small arterioles enter the outer cortex. These vessels seldom penetrate beyond the outer third of the cortex, but they penetrate deeper in areas of tendinous or ligamentous attachments. They may be essentially nonexistent in areas far from muscular attachments to long bones.

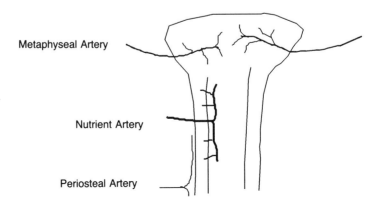

Figure 8–11. The three vascular supplies to bone.

Secondary Bone Healing

Secondary bone healing applies to healing of bone by the metamorphosis of granulation tissue into normal bone.[7] This occurs when there is motion at the fracture site and gaps between fragments. An unstable fracture is methodically transformed back into a stable, rigid bone. The effect of motion is more critical for bone healing than for the healing of many other tissues. Bone healing can be divided into the general overlapping phases of inflammation, repair, and remodeling.

INFLAMMATORY PHASE

The inflammatory phase of secondary bone healing starts at the time of injury. Tissue is damaged, and hemorrhage fills the disrupted area. Hemorrhage comes from surrounding tissue, endosteum, and periosteum. The normal blood supply to the affected bone fragments, specifically nutrient arteries and periosteum, is often lost or compromised. The blood will clot as a result of tissue thromboplastin and initiation of contact activation and the intrinsic coagulation system. The clot can prevent early revascularization of bone. It is removed during the repair of bone and does not serve as a scaffold. The blood clot, in conjunction with disruption of normal blood supply, leads to ischemic necrosis of bone adjacent to fracture sites. Dead bone is characterized by loss of osteocytes, although the structural integrity of the bone may still remain.

The permeability of adjacent vessels changes, and exudate is present in the internal wound. Inflammatory changes stimulate a vascular response that leads to initiation of an extraosseous blood supply soon after the initial insult.[10] The establishment of this additional blood supply is hastened by a lack of obstructing clot and intact soft-tissue attachments.

The newly established blood vessels allow cellular infiltration of neutrophils and macrophages, which serve to remove necrotic debris and the fracture clot. Fibroblasts follow the macrophages and, with neovascularization, form granulation tissue. Granulation tissue encircles the fracture fragment and initiates the process of fracture repair within 3 to 4 days.[11] Motion and surgical intervention will disrupt this process.

REPAIR PHASE

Even during formation of granulation tissue around a fracture, pluripotential mesenchymal cells are migrating to unite the fracture fragments. The origins of these cells are unknown. They are classically described as originating from the cambium layer of the periosteum, but they also may come from endosteum or bone.[7, 12–14] These cells differentiate into fibroblasts, chondroblasts, or osteoblasts and are the fracture callus. A fractured tubular bone will form an endosteal and periosteal callus. The pluripotential cells differentiate into the types and numbers of cells necessary to eliminate interfragmentary motion and reunite the bone fragments.

The main determining factor of cellular differentiation is the local environment, mainly oxygen tension.[7, 15] Osteocytes develop in environments of greatest oxygen tension, chondroblasts develop in areas of lower oxygen tension, and fibroblasts develop in areas of very low oxygen tension and motion. Oxygen tension is directly related to two factors: blood supply and motion. Adequate blood supply to the fracture depends on the surrounding soft-tissue attachments. Additionally, although the new extraosteal blood supply is important to fracture repair, medullary blood flow to the endosteal callus is also important. The occurrence of nonunions of distal radial fractures in small breed dogs is probably due to the lack of medullary blood flow and paucity of soft-tissue coverage. Motion between fragments will disrupt newly formed capillaries and cause inadequate oxygen delivery.

The size of a callus is directly related to interfragmentary motion. Increased motion produces a large callus as long as there is an adequate blood supply. The exact mechanism determining callus size is unknown, but the result serves an important mechanical purpose. Forces acting on a fracture must be opposed by pluripotential cells in the fracture callus. Since some motion is present and oxygen tension is low, osteoblasts are less likely to form and chondroblasts and fibroblasts proliferate. Production of many cells has two mechanical advantages. First, many cells produce a large amount of collagen to inhibit distractive forces at the fracture site. Second, as the diameter of the callus increases, the outer aspect of the callus has a mechanical advantage in opposing forces placed on the limb[16] (Figs. 8–12 and 8–13). This mechanical advantage on the outside of the callus leads to less micromotion and results in osteogenic cells forming on the outside of the callus. This produces the characteristic topography of a healing callus (Fig. 8–14).

Once the fracture is stable enough for osteogenic elements to differentiate, cartilage and necrotic bone are replaced by bone. Cartilage is replaced through endochondral ossification, a process similar to endochondral ossification of the physes of growing animals.[17] Osteoblasts advance through mineralized cartilage and deposit osteoid, which calcifies. The cartilage is thus replaced with woven bone.

Necrotic bone is replaced in a different manner. The necrotic bone, either cortical or cancellous, behaves much like autologous bone grafts. In cortical bone, the haversian system is used by advancing osteoclasts to replace the necrotic bone with new haversian systems. Large cortical fragments often maintain their mechanical integrity during this process. Old bone is resorbed, and new osteoid is deposited with osteocytes in their lacunae. Small fragments of cortical and cancellous bone can be incorporated into the fracture callus. As the callus ossifies, these bone elements are replaced by new bone in the same manner.

In areas of low oxygen tension and motion, only fibrous tissue is usually formed. This situation is unfavorable for bone union. Fibrous tissue does not allow vascular ingrowth and cannot maintain sufficient stability for chondrocytes or osteocytes to differentiate. Also, fibrous tissue is slow to differentiate into cartilage or bone. A fracture gap filled with fibrous tissue often leads to an atrophic nonunion.

REMODELING PHASE

Once the fracture gap is bridged with an ossified hard callus and is strong enough to provide support, the fracture has healed. It has not, however, reached maximum strength and size. The fracture gap has healed through formation of an endosteal and periosteal callus made of woven bone and a considerable extraosseous blood supply. Remodeling of the callus continues until the normal cortical architecture of bone is reestablished and normal (intraosseous) blood supply is regained.

The woven bone of the endosteal and periosteal callus is less rigid than cortical bone, but because of the diameter of the callus, the new bone is quite strong. Once forces are transmitted through the callus, the bone

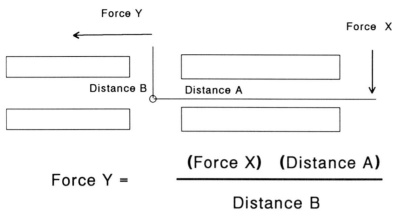

$$\text{Force Y} = \frac{(\text{Force X}) \ (\text{Distance A})}{\text{Distance B}}$$

Figure 8–12. An angular force to a limb (force *X*) will lead to forces that must be opposed at the fracture (force *Y*). The magnitude of the resulting force *Y* at the fracture is related to force *X*, the length of the lever arm to the fracture (distance *A*), and the length from the center of motion of the fracture to the outside of the fracture (distance *B*).

responds to these forces and the callus changes. The response of bone to loading forces is classically referred to as *Wolff's law*.[18] The exact mechanism of the bone response is unknown. It is assumed that the crystalline component of bone (hydroxyapatite) has piezoelectric properties.[8, 11] When this crystal is deformed by loading forces, charges are established across the crystals. These charges cause a remodeling response into more rigid cortical bone. In the same manner, bone that is not stressed tends to be resorbed.

As ossification of the callus progresses, greater stresses will occur close to the axis of the fracture and adjacent to cortices of the fracture ends. Bone at the outer aspect of the callus, owing to its mechanical advantage, will be

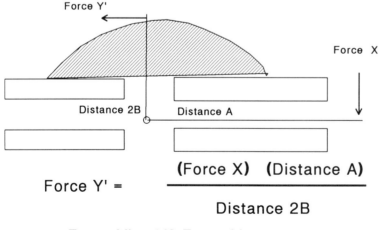

$$\text{Force Y}' = \frac{(\text{Force X}) \ (\text{Distance A})}{\text{Distance 2B}}$$

$$\text{Force Y}' = 1/2 \ \text{Force Y}$$

Figure 8–13. Callus formation results in greater distances from the center of motion to the outer aspect of the fracture site. In this example, the distance from the center of motion to the outside of the callus has doubled. This results in opposing forces (force *Y'*) only half as great as those on the outside of the fracture without a callus (force *Y* in Fig. 8–12).

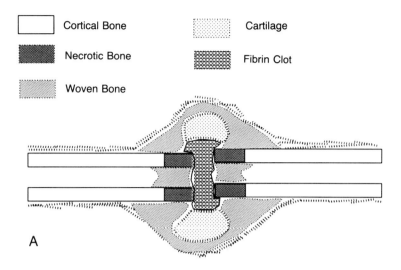

Cortical Bone

Necrotic Bone

Woven Bone

Cartilage

Fibrin Clot

A

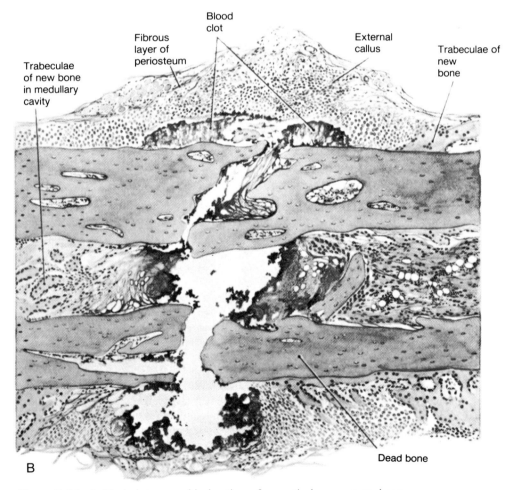

Blood clot

Fibrous layer of periosteum

External callus

Trabeculae of new bone

Trabeculae of new bone in medullary cavity

Dead bone

B

Figure 8–14. *A*, Typical topographic location of necrotic bone, woven bone, cartilage, and fibrin clot in a fracture stabilized by secondary bone healing. *B*, Diagrammatic representation of a longitudinal section of a 1-week-old rib fracture (rabbit). (From Ham AW, Harris WR: Repair and transplantation of bone. In Bourne GH (ed): The Biochemistry and Physiology of Bone, vol 3, 2d ed. New York: Academic Press, 1971, p 338.)

less stressed and will rarify. Bone is remodeled through osteoclastic activity, which replaces the porous woven bone with cortical bone.

The blood supply to the bone also returns to its prefracture state. The endosteal callus, which has been obstructing the medullary cavity, also resorbs. As the medullary cavity is reestablished, endosteal blood supply returns. Also, as woven bone is remodeled into cortical bone, haversian systems allow the return of centrifugal blood flow. The outer aspect of the fracture callus is resorbed and the temporary extraosseous blood supply to the fracture callus is lost.

CLINICAL IMPLICATIONS OF SECONDARY BONE HEALING

The mechanisms of secondary bone healing involve several clinical principles. *Blood supply and limited motion are necessary for fracture healing.* An extraosseous blood supply is essential to nourish a callus and promote formation of osseous (versus cartilaginous) tissues. Fractures that occur in bones not covered by soft tissue or where the blood supply to soft tissue is compromised are less likely to heal by secondary bone healing.

The extraosseous blood supply is established early in the healing process. Disruption of this blood supply by surgical intervention will postpone healing until the blood supply can be reestablished. If surgical intervention does not result in limitation of motion at the fracture site, it may even be detrimental to the healing process. The vital extraosseous blood supply is best and most quickly established in areas of soft-tissue attachment. Aggressively removing these soft-tissue attachments is detrimental to bone healing.

Motion is inherently related to blood supply because tenuous capillaries are easily damaged in the newly formed callus. Motion probably also has a direct effect on the differentiation of pluripotent mesenchymal cells. The size of a callus is directly proportional to the amount of motion at the fracture site. Slight strains are the mechanism for bone to remodel into strong cortical bone. Some motion may be beneficial to the formation of a unifying callus. Because motion has deleterious effects on bone healing, only slight, visually inappreciable motion should be allowed at the fracture site. Quantifying the amount of motion is impossible. Relatively large amounts of motion can be tolerated in fractures of young animals in areas of great soft-tissue coverage where a substantial callus will stabilize the fracture. On the other hand, in fractures with poor vascularity in adult animals, even slight motion may result in lack of bone union.

Primary Bone Union

Secondary bone union involves formation of a callus composed of cartilage and fibrous tissue that later ossify and are replaced by bone. *Under conditions of little or no fracture gap and high stability, bone can heal directly through formation of cortical bone without cartilage, fibrous tissue, or even woven bone.* This type of bone healing is called *primary bone healing.*[16, 19, 20]

Motion is the stimulus for callus formation and the lack of motion is essential for primary bone healing. Because conditions of absolute stability were rarely achieved with pin and cerclage fixation, it was not until the advent of internal fixation with bone plates and screws that primary bone healing became well described. The mechanism for primary bone healing is essentially the same as for bone remodeling and haversian system formation—it is characterized by the *resorption cavity.* The anatomy of a resorption cavity, or "cutter cone," is illustrated in Figure 8–15. Leading the cone are a group of multinucleated osteoclasts that resorb bone or calcified matrix as they advance. They are capable of advancing at rates of 70 to 100 μm per day.[16] Under most conditions, the osteoclasts advance in directions longitudinal to the long axis of the bone. The impetus for this osteoclastic activity is probably related to the electric charges established within bone during stresses, as well as to systemic hormones and local growth factors.[12, 21] Following the advancing osteoblasts, is a capillary loop that provides nutrition to the metabolically active osteoclasts and osteoblasts. Osteoblasts follow the resorbing osteoclasts and line the resulting tunnel. These cells deposit osteoid and establish the proper environment within the osteoid for hydroxyapatite crystals to form on collagen fibrils.[22] Osteoblasts become incorporated in the resorption cavity by successive layers of osteoid deposition. They form

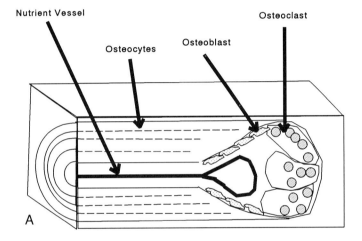

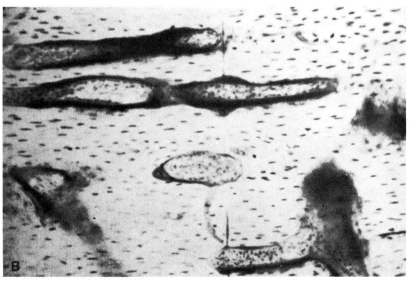

Figure 8–15. *A*, The components of a resorption canal ("cutter cone"). *B*, Histologic characteristics of primary bone healing 12 weeks after internal fixation with a compression plate. There is direct haversian system remodeling and no resorption of the compressed surfaces. (From Hayes WC: Biomechanics of fracture treatment. In Heppenstall RB (ed): Fracture Treatment and Healing. Philadelphia: WB Saunders, 1980, p 140.)

lacunae that communicate with the center of the resorption cavity by means of canaliculi. Thus, the characteristic haversian system is formed.

Conditions that do not allow callus formation result in the bone being healed by these resorption cavities uniting the fracture. This occurs in two situations: contact and gap healing.[16, 20] *Contact healing* occurs when direct contact of cortical bone is present or there is a gap of less than 0.01 to 0.02 mm. In this instance, resorption cavities form and cross the fracture. The resorption cavities align with the longitudinal axis of the bone. Increased osteoclastic activity continues until the fracture line and surrounding bone have been remodeled into new haversian systems.

Gap healing occurs when there is absolute stability, but the gap between the fracture fragments is greater then 0.02 mm but less than 0.08 mm. This width cannot be crossed directly by a resorption cavity but can be entered by one. In gap healing, osteoclasts and their accompanying capillary loops and osteoblasts enter and follow the gap, depositing lamellar bone much like an advancing haversian resorption cavity. The resorption unit may first subdivide the gaps into smaller units with woven bone into which the lamellar bone is then deposited. These resorption units first travel in the direction of the fracture line. Later, remodeling occurs, resulting in longitudinally oriented haversian systems much like primary contact healing.

In fractures that heal by primary bone union, contact and gap healing occur within different aspects of the same fracture. Because plastic deformation occurs when bone fails, fragments are distorted. Prefect alignment of distorted fragments is impossible. Also, the most meticulous surgeon cannot truly approximate fragments to gaps less than 0.01 mm.

Radiographically, primary bone union is characterized by a lack of callus formation. As the osteoclastic and remodeling activities increase, the fracture line becomes more lucent. Slowly the fracture line becomes unnoticeable, and the original continuity of the bone is reestablished.

Factors Affecting Bone Healing

In addition to the factors of motion and vascularity, many other factors can affect bone healing. Nutritional factors, specifically vitamins and minerals, can significantly affect bone healing.[7] High doses of vitamin A result in thinning of cortical bone and probably inhibit bone healing. Although deficiencies of vitamin A promote deposition of bone, they cannot be safely advocated to promote bone healing. Vitamin C is integral in the formation of collagen. Deficiencies in vitamin C, which are rare in small animals, can inhibit bone healing.

Vitamin D is specifically associated with bone and calcium metabolism. Deficiencies in vitamin D will lead to delayed bone healing. These deficiencies are also uncommon in small animals.

Prostaglandins, especially those of the E series, are known to have a vital role in promoting regional resorption and remodeling.[23] Antiprostaglandins such as aspirin are commonly used to control pain associated with orthopedic injuries, but could theoretically inhibit bone healing.

Electric charges occurring from the deformation of piezoelectric hydroxyapatite crystals promote bone formation. Results of numerous investigations involving the application of charges have suggested a positive influence on bone healing. Electric currents can be applied directly with current generators and electrodes or indirectly by inducing electric fields from time-varying magnetic fields.[24, 25] This area of research still needs development prior to clinical application, and is currently less important then surgical technique.

Implications of Bone Healing Biomechanics for Fracture Repair

Integral to bone healing are stability and vascularity. When choosing a fixation strategy, the surgeon should evaluate the fracture in a systematic and routine method, as described earlier. Once the forces acting on the fragments are assessed, appropriate instrumentation is based on fixation techniques that counteract these forces. The method of fixation should be based on the mechanical characteristics of the specific bone, as well as bone vascularity and healing potential. Although there may be more than one appropriate technique for repairing a fracture, there are many incorrect methods.

SPLINTS

Splints, such as a lateral splint, spica splint, Schoeder-Thomas splint, or metatarsal/carpal splint, are often misused in veterinary medicine. These external coapting devices support a limb but do not immobilize bones. Therefore, splints should be used for inherently stable fractures, such as "greenstick" fractures of the tibia or radius and fractures of some, but not all, metatarsal and carpal bones. Since splints do not immobilize bone, there will be considerable motion between fracture fragments. The bones will heal through secondary bone healing and considerable callus formation. The advantage of these devices is that they do not require surgical intervention.

CYLINDER CASTS

Properly applied casts will immobilize a limb. If the joints above and below the fracture can be immobilized by a cast, sufficient stability can be achieved to allow secondary bone healing. As with a splint, the size of the callus depends on interfragmentary motion. The amount of interfragmentary motion depends on fracture conformation and the ability of the cast to immobilize that limb. The advantage of a cast is that it does not require surgical intervention. Surgery disrupts the newly forming extraosseous blood supply and can slow the onset of bone healing. Casts can be an excellent form of fixation, especially in young animals where healing is rapid and bone is too soft for metallic implants. Disadvantages include a cast not being able to directly stabilize bone, and immobilization of a limb can have deleterious effects on muscle and joint functions.

INTRAMEDULLARY PINS

Intramedullary pins oppose angular forces. The fracture fragments will slide along the smooth pin surfaces; therefore, a pin cannot oppose compressive, distractive, and rotational forces. Pins best stabilize fractures if they align the bone and normal compressive forces along the pins in association with proper fracture geometry. This results in neutralization of rotational, shear, and distractive forces. Intramedullary pins can be placed without extensive soft tissue dissection. This is important for maintaining vascular supply to the fracture. The disadvantage of intramedullary pins is that they disrupt the normal intraosseous vascular supply in the medullary cavity of bone. In fact, a round pin that fills the medullary cavity will completely obstruct the blood supply to the inner cortex.[26] Pins with diameters one-half to two-thirds the diameter of the medullary cavity should be chosen, or smaller, multiple pins can be used to provide rotational stability and allow vessels to form in the spaces between pins. Very often, intramedullary pins are used in conjunction with other forms of fixation.

BONE PLATES

Bone plates allow the most rigid fixation of long bones. In many cases, bone plates permit sufficient stability and fragment alignment to cause primary bone union. However, even under ideal conditions, some fractures stabilized with a bone plate heal with a callus.[21] Often, primary and secondary bone healing occurs in different areas of the fracture simultaneously. Dynamic compression plates permit fragments to be compressed. Internal compression of fracture fragments decreases the fracture gap and increases stability. Increased stability occurs because the force needed to slide two fragments against each other is related to their coefficient of friction and the force pushing them together. Interfragmentary compression dynamically pushes fragments together. *Bone plates can oppose bending, compressive, distractive, shearing, and rotational forces*, and the screws do not interfere with the intramedullary blood supply to the bone.

The disadvantage of bone plating is removal of soft tissue from the bone surface and between fracture ends. Placement of a plate disrupts newly forming blood supply to the fracture.[26] If adequate stability cannot be achieved, plate fixation can be deleterious to fracture healing.

EXTERNAL FIXATOR

External fixation devices stabilize fracture fragments by means of percutaneous pins held rigidly by external connecting devices. Properly applied, external fixation devices can achieve good stability. *These devices can oppose distractive, compressive, bending, shearing, and rotational forces.* Pins do not disrupt intramedullary blood supply and can be placed without disruption of early extraosseous blood supply or soft-tissue attachments.[26] Under ideal situations, interfragmentary compression also can be achieved. Smaller fracture fragments cannot be stabilized. Since the rigidity is determined by external connecting devices, rigidity can be reduced externally as the fracture heals to stimulate osteogenesis (dynamization).

ANCILLARY DEVICES

Cerclage wires, hemicerclage wires, and lag screws can be used in many situations to fix and compress two bone fragments. Such devices act directly at fragment interfaces and do not support the entire bone. They must be used with other forms of fixation that support the bone over a greater length. Although wires have no deleterious effect on extraosseous vascular supply, soft-tissue dissection prior to placement of wires and screws should be limited and atraumatic.

SUMMARY

Advances and improvements in orthopedic surgery are occurring as the basic principles of bone repair are being elucidated. An orthopedic surgeon must understand fracture mechanics and bone healing before using a surgical technique. Each fracture is different, and repair requires numerous decisions unique to each case. Using techniques described by others without understanding the biomechanical principles will result in improper application and failure. Surgical decisions based on a thorough understanding of fracture mechanics and healing will most likely lead to satisfactory results.

REFERENCES

1. Natali AN, Meroi EA: A review of the biomechanical properties of bone as a material. J Biomed Eng 1989; 11:266–276
2. Carter DR, Spengler DM: Mechanical properties and composition of cortical bone. Clin Orthop 1978; 135:192–217
3. Carter DR, Spengler DM: Biomechanics of fracture. In Sumner-Smith G (ed): Bone in Clinical Orthopedics. Philadelphia: WB Saunders, 1982
4. Nordin M, Frankel VH: Biomechanics of whole bones and bone tissue. In Frankel VH, Nordin M (eds): Basic Biomechanics of the Skeletal System. Philadelphia: Lea & Febiger, 1980
5. Owen R, Goodfellow P, Bullough P: Scientific foundations of orthopedics and traumatology. Philadelphia: WB Saunders, 1980
6. Herron AJ: Review of bone structure, function, metabolism, and growth. In Bojrab MJ (ed): Pathophysiology in Small Animal Surgery. Philadelphia: Lea & Febiger, 1981
7. Peacock EE: Wound Repair, 3d ed. Philadelphia: WB Saunders, 1984
8. Tothill P, Hooper G, McCarthy ID, et al: The pattern of distribution of blood flow in dog limb bones measured using microspheres. Clin Phys Physiol Meas 1987; 8:239–247
9. Wilson JW: Vascular supply to normal bone and healing fractures. Semin Vet Med Surg (Small Anim) 1991; 6:26–38
10. Rhinelander RW: Blood supply of healing long bones. In Newton CD, Nunamaker DM (eds): Textbook of Small Animal Orthopedics. Philadelphia: Lippincott, 1985
11. Schenk RK: Histology of fracture repair and non-union. A-O Bull (Bern) 1978; p 14
12. Canalis E, McCarthy T, Centrella M: Growth factors and the regulation of bone remodeling. J Clin Invest 1988; 81:277–281
13. Aro HT, Kelly PJ, Lewallen DG, et al: The effects of physiologic dynamic compression on bone healing under external fixation. Clin Orthop 1990; 256:260–273
14. Shapiro F: Cortical bone repair. J Bone Joint Surg 1988; 70A:1067–1081
15. Brand RA, Rubin CT: Fracture healing. In Albright JA, Brand RA (eds): The Scientific Basis of Orthopaedics, 2d ed. Norwalk, Conn: Appleton and Lange, 1987, pp 325–345
16. Prieur WD, Sumner-Smith G: General considerations. In Brinker WO, Hohn RB, Prieur WD (eds): Manual of Internal Fixation in Small Animals. Berlin: Springer-Verlag, 1984
17. Ham AW, Cormack DH: Bone and bones. In Ham AW, Cormack DH (eds): Histology, 8th ed. Philadelphia: Lippincott, 1979
18. Sissons HA: Bones. In Symmers W (ed): Systemic Pathology, vol 5, 2d ed. New York: Churchill-Livingstone, 1979
19. Bagby GW, Janes JM: The effect of compression on the rate of fracture healing using a special plate. Am J Surg 1958; 95:761–767
20. Kaderly RE: Primary bone healing. Semin Vet Med Surg (Small Anim) 1991; 6:21–25
21. O'Sullivan ME, Chao EYS, Kelly PJ: The effect of fixation on fracture healing. J Bone Joint Surg 1989; 71A:306–310
22. Boskey AL: Current concepts of the physiology and biochemistry of calcification. Clin Orthop 1981; 167:225–273
23. Shih MS, Norrdin RW: Effect of prostaglandin E_1 on regional haversian remodeling in beagles with fractured ribs: A histomorphometric study. Bone 1987; 8:87–90
24. Lavine LS, Grodzinsky AJ: Electrical stimulation of bone. J Bone Joint Surg 1987; 69A:626–630
25. Clark DM: The use of electrical current in the treatment of nonunions. Vet Clin North Am (Small Anim Pract) 1987; 17:793–798
26. Smith SR, Bronk JT, Kelly PJ: Effect of fracture fixation on cortical bone blood flow. J Orthop Res 1990; 8:471–478

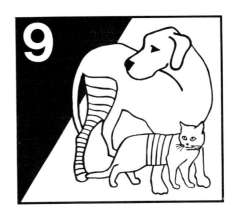

ROBERT M. RADASCH

OSTEOMYELITIS

Osteomyelitis is inflammation of bone involving the marrow cavity, cancellous trabeculae, cortex, or periosteum.[1-4] In veterinary medicine, osteomyelitis is caused most frequently by bacteria.[3,5] Therefore, the emphasis of this chapter will be bacterial-induced osteomyelitis. Systemic mycotic infections with bone manifestations are the second most common cause of osteomyelitis.[6,8] These diseases have specific geographic distributions and the route of entry for infection is the respiratory or gastrointestinal system. Viral and parasite-induced osteomyelitides have been reported, but are exceptionally rare.

Pathogenic bacteria are not the only prerequisite for the establishment of osteomyelitis.[1,9] Inoculation of bacteria intravenously or into the medullary cavity of bone has inconsistently produced osteomyelitis.[6,10,11] *Vascular obstruction concurrent with bacterial colonization of bone is necessary for osteomyelitis to develop.*[1,4,6] The disease can be experimentally produced by inoculation of bone with *Staphylococcus aureus* and damaging the local blood supply of bone.[11,12] Recently, prostaglandins and their precursor, arachidonic acid, have been implicated as potential agents contributing to the vascular obstruction necessary for the development of osteomyelitis.[11,13] Animals with experimentally induced osteomyelitis treated with an antiprostaglandin had less radiographic and pathologic bone changes as compared with animals not treated with the drug.[11,14] The exact role of prostaglandins in the formation of osteomyelitis is currently being investigated.[11]

The typical presentation of osteomyelitis in small animals is a chronic, protracted disease often as a result of a previous surgical procedure or traumatic incident.[1,3,15] An acute hematogenous infection is not commonly detected in small animals. Often, there is not a clear delineation in terms of pathogenesis between acute and chronic stages of the disease.

ROUTES OF BONE CONTAMINATION

Bacterial inoculation of bone can occur by a hematogenous route, extension from a soft-tissue infection, or secondary to trauma.[1,5,6] The hematogenous spread of bacteria from cystitis to the vertebral endplates and disk space, as seen in diskospondylitis, is an example of hematogenous osteomyelitis. Secondary extension of a preexisting soft-tissue infection to an adjacent bone is another potential route of contamination. However, the most common route of contamination resulting in osteomyelitis occurs when exogenous organisms gain access to bone following a traumatic or surgically created wound. This form of bone infection is termed *posttraumatic osteomyelitis*.[1–3, 5, 9, 15]

Hematogenous Osteomyelitis

Approximately 6% of reported small animal osteomyelitis cases are due to the hematogenous spread of bacteria.[16] Acute hematogenous osteomyelitis is more frequently reported in people, foals, and calves than in small animals.[15] A temporary bacteremia develops that allows organisms to "seed" the metaphyseal regions of long bones.[9] Omphalophlebitis, pneumonia, enteritis, or other systemic infections usually precede the bone lesions.[17, 18] Neonatal animals with hematogenous osteomyelitis are suspected to be immunoincompetent, possibly due to failure of passive transfer of maternal immunoglobulins.[1] Preferential seeding of the metaphyseal region of long bones is due to the unique vascular anatomy of the neonate.[1, 9, 17–19] Ascending metaphyseal arteries form a series of end-arterial loops just below the metaphyseal growth plate. The vessels take a hairpin turn, travel back toward the diaphysis, and enter a system of large, dilated venous sinusoids.[9, 17] Bacteria settle in the region where end-arterial loops anastomose with the venous sinusoids. Possible theories to explain preferential bacterial seeding in this area include (1) a paucity of phagocytic cells, (2) sluggish blood flow due to a large increase in the cross-sectional area and a decrease in local blood pressure, (3) increased turbulence of blood flow, and (4) stretching and bursting of metaphyseal loop vessels during bone growth that allows bacteria to escape and proliferate in the extravascular tissues.[1, 9, 17]

Neonatal humans and foals also have vessels that traverse the growth plate and enter the epiphysis.[1, 9, 20] It is possible for hematogenous osteomyelitis to develop in the epiphyseal bone with further spread to the joint resulting in septic arthritis in these species. Neonatal dogs and cats do not have these transphyseal vessels.[1] Therefore, hematogenous osteomyelitis is restricted to the metaphyseal side of the growth plate, and septic arthritis rarely occurs.

One of the most common examples of hematogenous osteomyelitis in the dog is diskospondylitis, an infection of the intervertebral disk and adjacent vertebral endplates.[1, 21, 22] This disease usually occurs in large, middle-aged, male dogs of the sporting breeds.[21] Orchitis, bacterial endocarditis, and lower urinary tract infections are the most commonly reported sources of the primary infection.[21, 22] Bacterial lodgment in the subchondral bone of the vertebral endplates follows the same pathophysiologic principles as hematogenous metaphyseal osteomyelitis of the neonate.[21, 22]

Osteomyelitis Due to Extension of a Soft-Tissue Infection

Contiguous spread of a soft-tissue infection to bone has been reported in approximately 26% of all cases of osteomyelitis in small animals.[16] The majority of these cases were infections involving the metacarpals, metatarsals, or phalanges. Severe periodontal disease with secondary infection of the surrounding mandibular or maxillary alveolar bone is also a common example of this form of osteomyelitis in small animals. End-stage otitis with the subsequent formation of bacterial osteomyelitis of the osseous tympanic bullae is another example of extension of a soft-tissue infection. Other soft-tissue infections potentially causing osteomyelitis are lick granulomas, chronic pododermatitis, bite wounds, abscesses, and decubital ulcers.

Posttraumatic Osteomyelitis

Posttraumatic osteomyelitis (contamination of bone as a consequence of an open fracture or open reduction of a closed fracture) is the most common form of osteomyelitis in animals.[1-3, 5, 9, 15] In one study, 10% of all cases of osteomyelitis were secondary to open fractures and 55% were associated with open reduction and internal fixation of closed fractures.[16]

Open fractures usually involve bones with limited soft-tissue coverage such as the radius/ulna, tibia/fibula, metacarpal, and metatarsal bones. All open fractures are classified as contaminated or dirty wounds depending on the amount of debris in the wound and the duration of injury.[23, 24] Open fractures are also four times more likely to harbor bacteria at the time of surgery than a closed fracture.[25] The development of postoperative osteomyelitis in an open fracture is directly related to the severity of the soft-tissue injury. Open fractures are classified as grade I, II, or III.[26, 27] In grade I open fractures, bone fragments penetrate the muscle and skin from within. In grade II open fractures, external trauma causes a penetrating wound of the soft tissues with exposure of the bone. The degree of soft-tissue damage is similar in grade I and II open fractures. Grade III open fractures are caused by the same forces as grade II injuries, but extensive loss and damage to the surrounding soft tissue is present. Grade I and II open fractures, if properly managed, are no more likely to develop postoperative osteomyelitis than a closed fracture.[27, 28] However, because of extensive vascular impairment and contamination, grade III open fractures have a higher risk for the development of osteomyelitis.[27] Therefore, these injuries require aggressive treatment and carry a more guarded prognosis than grade I and II open fractures.

Development of osteomyelitis after open reduction and internal fixation of a closed fracture continues to be one of the most serious postoperative complications of orthopedic surgery. A break in sterile surgical technique usually is the cause of this form of osteomyelitis.[1, 3, 6, 15] However, other factors can predispose an animal to develop osteomyelitis. These include excessive surgical trauma, retraction and dehydration of tissues.[29] In people, the rate of postoperative infection correlates positively with the duration of surgery.[23, 28, 30] Therefore, it cannot be overemphasized that expedient, sterile, atraumatic surgical technique by an experienced surgeon is necessary for successful fracture management. Host factors such as age, nutritional status, immunocompetence, and condition of the patient can also be potential factors affecting the development of osteomyelitis after surgical management of a closed fracture.[23]

Recently, a chronic focal form of posttraumatic osteomyelitis associated with bone plates and screws has been described.[31-33] Characteristically, there is chronic bacterial proliferation at the site of a healed fracture and no overt clinical signs of infection. The bacteria often remain dormant for years until an undetermined stimulus causes a reduced adherence of the organism to the implant and subsequent development of a delayed local infection. This type of osteomyelitis is termed a *cryptic infection*.[31, 32] It is believed the bacteria gain access to the implant during open reduction of the fracture. The causative bacteria produce a polysaccharide, mucoid, peribacterial film, called a *glycocalyx*, that covers the organisms, promoting bacterial growth and adherence to the implant.[31, 32, 34] Furthermore, the glycocalyx is impervious to the immune system, inhibits bacterial phagocytosis, and significantly reduces the effectiveness of most antimicrobial agents.[31] A cryptic infection can persist until the implant is removed. In a recent study, 38% of dogs with closed fractures repaired with bone plates had positive cultures at the time of plate removal.[32] Clinical complications, however, were not documented.

PATHOGENESIS OF OSTEOMYELITIS

The Inflammatory Reaction[23, 25, 36]

Regardless of the route of bacterial inoculation, the sequence of events that leads to osteomyelitis is identical at the cellular level. Initially, there is a local acute inflammatory response. Vessels temporarily vasoconstrict and then actively vasodilate. Vasodilation is initiated and maintained by the vasoactive substances histamine, serotonin, bradykinin, and kallidin. Concurrent with vasodilation is a separation of the vascular endothelial cells, thus increasing the permeability of the vessel. The functions of vasodilation and increased vascular permeability are to provide access for the components of circulation to the site of the injury and contamination in order to contain and eliminate the infection. Plasma proteins, immunoglobulins, complement, chemotactic substances, fibronectins, neutrophils, macrophages, and lymphocytes can be found in the extravascular space shortly after insult and contamination. Initiation of the clotting cascade occurs as a result of activation of the Hageman factor (clotting factor XII) by exposure of subendothelial collagen and tissue thromboplastin (clotting factor III) due to damaged cells. The resultant fibrin clot gives neutrophils a matrix against which bacteria are phagocytized. The fibrin also blocks surrounding lymphatics to locally contain the infection.

Humoral Immunity and the Complement Cascade[23, 36]

Immunoglobulins, primarily IgG and IgM, react with specific antigenic determinants on the bacterial cell wall. The interaction of the antibody and bacterial antigen results in a stearic configurational change of the antibody that allows a specific protein, C1, to bind to the antibody–antigen complex. Activation of C1 stimulates the enzymatic cascade of the complement system. The end products of the complement cascade are biologically active particles that (1) further increase vascular permeability, (2) lyse bacterial cell walls, (3) promote antibody–antigen recognition and adherence, and most important, (4) give directional motility and guidance to the cells (neutrophils and macrophages) of phagocytosis.

The Phagocytic System[23, 35]

Neutrophils are the primary cells in the early cellular response to bacterial contamination of bone. Initially, neutrophils bind with antibody-coated bacteria. The microorganisms are engulfed by neutrophils and lysosomal enzymes kill and subsequently digest the bacteria. The life span of a neutrophil is relatively short (several hours), and after it has phagocytized bacteria, it also dies. Autolysis of the dead neutrophils allows their contents to escape into the extracellular space. The accumulation of bacteria, neutrophils, and released lysosomal enzymes is collectively referred to as *pus* (purulence) or, more correctly, *exudate*. Later in the inflammatory response, macrophages are present in increasing numbers. Macrophages further phagocytize bacteria and remove dead neutrophils. Unlike the neutrophil, macrophages have a long half-life (days to months) and release only small quantities of lysosomal enzymes into the extracellular space. In addition, the macrophage is instrumental in providing bacterial antigens to lymphocytes for immunologic processing and antibody production. The combined efforts of phagocytic cells, the immune system, and the complement cascade are an attempt by the body to eradicate offending organisms prior to the development of extensive bone pathology.

The Response of Bone to Bacteria

Whether bone infection is contained and eradicated or allowed to progress depends on many factors. It is generally agreed that 10^5 to 10^6 organisms per gram of tissue are required for a contaminated wound to become infected.[15, 23, 27] However, contaminated bone can become infected with fewer bacteria if the host's inflammatory response is insufficient or overwhelmed. If the host's inflammatory response is successful in overcoming the infection, a sterile abscess surrounded by granulation tissue and compact cancellous bone will form. This sterile bone abscess is termed a *Brodie's abscess* and is usually 1 to 3 cm in diameter.[1, 2, 4, 6, 9] This lesion is more common in humans but has been reported in small animals.[1, 37]

As previously stated, vascular occlusion is mandatory, along with bacterial colonization, for osteomyelitis to develop.[1, 4, 6, 10–12] As the inflammatory reaction progresses, exudate accumulates within the medullary cavity of the bone. Septic thrombophlebitis of diaphyseal vessels causes venous stasis.[4, 6, 11, 16] Necrosis of the medullary trabecular bone results from the vascular compromise and the proteolytic enzymes released by neutrophils. With an increasing volume of exudate, pressure within the medullary cavity rises.[9] Eventually, the pressure is sufficient to force the exudate into and through the nonexpansible Volkmann and haversian canals of cortical bone[1–3, 9] (Fig. 9–1). Small vessels lying within these canals collapse or are destroyed, resulting in death of surrounding osteocytes. The exudate also passes through these canals to enter the adjacent subperiosteal or endosteal spaces, thus allowing further spread of the infection and vascular damage to healthy bone.[1–3, 5, 9] The overall result is the isolation of a segment of cortical bone from its blood supply. This avascular, infected segment of cortical bone is called a *sequestrum*.[1–3, 9] In an attempt to isolate the infection, a layer of granulation tissue surrounded by a layer of newly formed compact bone, collectively termed the *involucrum*, encases the sequestrum.[1, 2, 9] Unfortunately, the involucrum not only walls off the infected avascular bone from the body but also prevents blood vessels, antibodies, and antibiotics from reaching the nidus of infection.[1–3, 9]

On rare occasions, the sequestrum is reabsorbed by osteoclastic activity or incorporated back into the living bone by osteoconduction. It is also possible for infected avascular bone to be extruded from the body through a draining tract.[2, 39] However, the most likely occurrence is bacterial proliferation in the sequestrum and stimulation of an acute inflammatory response and formation of septic exudate.[1, 2, 9] As the exudate accumulates and pressure rises,

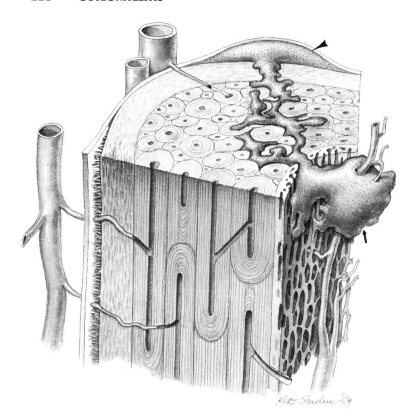

Figure 9–1. Diagram of the manner in which infection in the medullary canal (*arrow*) permeates the cortex and collects beneath the periosteal membrane (*arrowhead*). (Reprinted with permission from Resnick D, Niwayama G: Diagnosis of Bone and Joint Disorders. Philadelphia: WB Saunders, 1981.)

holes in the involucrum will form, and draining sinus tracts to the skin develop. The draining tracts are called *cloacae* and are a cardinal sign of chronic suppurative osteomyelitis[1, 2, 5, 9] (Fig. 9–2). Periods of quiescence, followed by exacerbation of acute osteomyelitis, will continue to occur until the sequestrum is either removed, reabsorbed, or incorporated back into bone.

DIAGNOSIS OF OSTEOMYELITIS

A tentative diagnosis of osteomyelitis is based on the history, clinical presentation, and radiographic signs. Identification of the causative micro-

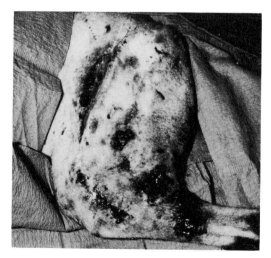

Figure 9–2. Multiple draining sinus tracts developed 16 months after bone plating of an open femur fracture. Draining tracts are considered a cardinal sign of chronic osteomyelitis. After plate removal and wound debridement, the osteomyelitis resolved. (Reprinted with permission from Daly WR: Orthopedics infections. In Slatter DH (ed): Textbook of Small Animal Surgery. Philadelphia: WB Saunders, 1985, p 2024.)

organisms is necessary, however, to confirm the diagnosis and initiate effective antimicrobial therapy.

Signalment, History, and Clinical Signs

Acute hematogenous osteomyelitis usually affects dogs less than 6 months of age.[9] Typically, an infection elsewhere in the body precedes the signs of osteomyelitis. The animal usually has a sudden onset of a non–weight-bearing lameness without a history of trauma. Deep palpation of the metaphyseal regions of the involved bones will cause moderate to severe pain. In addition, the involved bones and surrounding soft tissue may be warm and swollen. The animal is often depressed, anorectic, and febrile. Leukocytosis is not always present and, therefore may not be useful in establishing a diagnosis.

Diskospondylitis is a disease primarily of large, male sporting dogs.[21, 22] However, the disease has been reported in small chondrodystrophic breeds following prophylactic disk fenestration or laminectomy.[21, 22] Animals with diskospondylitis usually have acute back pain and reluctance to move. Palpation over the affected vertebral endplates and disk space will elicit a painful response. Typically, a protracted waxing and waning history of anorexia, weight loss, and fever is reported by the owner. If the condition is allowed to progress, severe paresis or paralysis due to spinal cord compression can occur. The disease may mimic the clinical signs of intervertebral disk herniation.

The clinical signs of posttraumatic osteomyelitis will depend on the stage of the disease. Repair of an open contaminated fracture or open reduction and internal fixation of a closed fracture is a usual precipitating cause.[1–3, 5–7, 9, 15, 16, 25] This is often associated with a technical error during surgery, such as a break in sterile technique or inadequate fracture stabilization.

The acute stages of osteomyelitis become clinically apparent approximately 5 days after bone contamination.[9] Localized pain, warmth, swelling, and lameness, followed by systemic signs of depression, anorexia, and fever, are the common clinical signs.[1–3, 9] However, the early signs of acute osteomyelitis can be confused with normal postoperative inflammation, making clinical differentiation between the two conditions difficult. Normal postoperative inflammation results in a low-grade fever lasting for several days with subsequent daily improvement.[1] In contrast, animals with acute suppurative osteomyelitis have a progressive rise in temperature. If a sufficient quantity of exudate accumulates around the bone, it may drain through a partially open skin incision.[3] Otherwise, the exudate remains as a localized abscess of the bone and surrounding soft tissue. The acute stages of posttraumatic osteomyelitis often are never recognized and the disease progresses to chronic osteomyelitis.

The classic clinical signs of chronic osteomyelitis are muscle atrophy, lameness, pain, and draining sinus tracts.[1, 2, 9, 16] With exudate accumulation, it is common to have multiple, temporary episodes of depression, anorexia, fever, and localized soft-tissue swelling.[7, 9] As the exudate finds new routes for drainage, signs compatible with acute infection subside and are replaced by a prolonged period of quiescence. Eventually, the draining tracts close, and exudate once again accumulates internally, thus causing recurring clinical signs similar to those of acute osteomyelitis. This process will be repeated until the cause of bone infection is removed. Except during periods of acute exacerbations, chronic osteomyelitis is rarely accompanied by leukocytosis.[7, 38] Therefore, hematologic evaluation often does not aid in the diagnosis of chronic osteomyelitis.

Radiology

Radiographic signs of acute hematogenous osteomyelitis usually include focal lysis of metaphyseal trabecular bone (Fig. 9–3) and adjacent soft-tissue swelling.[1, 17] If the disease progresses into septic arthritis, joint capsule distension and collapse of the subchondral bone, causing irregular joint surfaces, also may be visualized. Because the condition may involve several bones, radiography of all long bones is prudent in suspected cases of acute hematogenous osteomyelitis.

During the acute stages of posttraumatic osteomyelitis, the consistent radiographic signs are soft-tissue swelling and generalized loss of fascial planes.[1, 9] Radiographically detectable bone changes will not occur until 10 to 14 days after onset of infection.[9] At that time, local cortical bone lysis, sclerosis, or irregular periosteal bone formation may be detected[1–4, 9, 15, 16, 39] (Fig. 9–4). Pathologic fractures also may be seen in regions of cortical lysis due to a reduced load-carrying capacity.

The degree of new periosteal bone formation depends on timing of therapy, bacterial virulence, and the animal's age. Young animals with loosely attached periosteum tend to have more bone reaction than mature animals. As subperiosteal exudate accumulates and lifts the loosely attached periosteum off the cortex, the cambium layer reacts by forming new bone.[9] In a mature patient, the periosteum is more tightly adhered to the cortex, thus inhibiting accumulation of subperiosteal exudate. Instead, the medullary and cortical abscesses rupture directly through cloacae in the periosteum to create sinus tracts to the exterior of the body.[9] Since less trauma occurs to the cambium layer of the periosteum, a reduced amount of new periosteal bone formation occurs in the adult patient.

Sequestrum and involucrum formation are occasional radiographic signs seen in chronic osteomyelitis[1–4, 9] (Fig. 9–5). The sequestrum often appears more radiodense than surrounding bone. Because the sequestrum has no blood supply, it does not undergo demineralization, thus allowing it to maintain its original radiodensity.[3, 9] However, the adjacent vascular bone

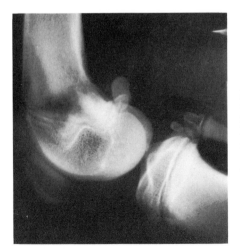

Figure 9–3. Lateral radiograph of the stifle joint of a 4-month-old male Labrador retriever with hindlimb lameness. Lysis of the metaphyseal bone is typical of acute hematogenous osteomyelitis. Bone biopsy and culture revealed a coagulase-negative *Staphylococcus* species. (Reprinted with permission from Gilson SD, Schwarz PD: Acute hematogenous osteomyelitis in a dog. J Am Anim Hosp Assoc 1989; 25: 685.)

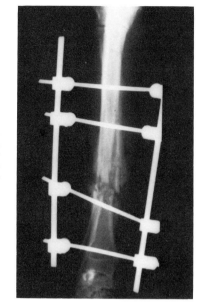

Figure 9–4. Craniocaudal radiograph of a grade III open comminuted radius and ulna fracture 4 weeks after stabilization with type II external fixation. Cortical bone lysis and irregular periosteal bone reaction are present along the radius just proximal to the fracture. Culture of the bone at the time of surgery revealed *E. coli*, *Klebsiella* species, and *Staphylococcus aureus*. Osteomyelitis resolved after 4 months of antimicrobial therapy.

can become somewhat radiolucent owing to demineralization caused by an increased blood supply, prostaglandins, and other inflammatory products.[11, 39, 40] Therefore, a radiographic demarcation between vascular bone and the sequestrum is apparent.

Another radiographic technique that may provide useful information in animals with chronic osteomyelitis and draining tracts is fistulography.[3, 9] A sterile Foley catheter (Akron Catheter, Inc., Akron, Ohio) is introduced into a fistula, and an appropriate amount of sterile, aqueous contrast material is injected through the catheter to fill the entire fistulous tract. A fistulogram aids in locating the origin of the infection, especially if a large metallic implant, such as a plate, obscures visualization of the underlying bone. If a sequestrum is identified under a bone plate, direct fragment excision without

Figure 9–5. *A*, Craniocaudal radiograph of an ulnar fracture associated with a gunshot injury. Wound debridement and antibiotic therapy were used for treatment of the injury. A bone sequestrum is present along the lateral aspect of the proximal ulna 2 months after treatment (*arrows*). *B*, The avascular bone is identified (*arrow*) prior to removal at surgery. After sequestrectomy and 6 weeks of antibiotic therapy, the fracture healed uneventfully.

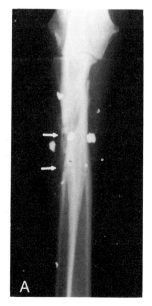

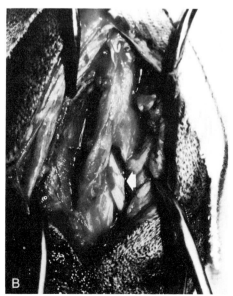

excessive soft-tissue dissection can be performed. A fistulogram also helps approximate the internal extent of sinus tract formation, which may not be readily apparent from the exterior drainage site(s). When treating chronic osteomyelitis, removal of the sinus tracts and nidus of infection is necessary to obtain healing. The actual extent of the sinus tracts, however, may be underestimated by evaluation of a fistulogram.[9]

Nuclear scintigraphy has been used in experimental animal models and human clinical cases to diagnose osteomyelitis earlier and with a higher degree of specificity than conventional radiography.[39, 40] Within a short time after establishment of osteomyelitis, an increase in blood flow, capillary permeability, and bone metabolism occurs. Bone scans are more sensitive because they detect changes in local blood flow of infected tissue. Radiographs detect bone-density changes due to demineralization or osteoid production. The radiographic changes lag several weeks behind the metabolic changes detected by a nuclear scan. Even though radionuclide imaging is extremely sensitive, radiographs are currently the most practical diagnostic procedure in veterinary medicine. The expense of the scanning equipment and necessary facilities may limit this diagnostic modality to large referral institutions.

Diagnosis of osteomyelitis based on radiographic signs should be made cautiously because numerous bone diseases have similar characteristics. Concomitant evaluation and interpretation of other parameters such as clinical signs, history, bone biopsy, and culture are necessary to avoid a misdiagnosis. Instability at the fracture site, neoplastic diseases, and normal bone reaction to trauma may appear radiographically similar to chronic osteomyelitis, thus making differentiation difficult.[3, 9] Bone lysis and new periosteal and endosteal bone formation due to fracture instability are usually limited to the region adjacent to the fracture. In contrast, osteomyelitis usually causes a more aggressive and diffuse pattern of bone lysis and new periosteal bone production. However, at times, the two conditions can appear identical, and a bone culture is required for diagnosis.

Primary bone tumors generally have a more "sunburst" radiographic appearance than osteomyelitis.[3, 41, 42] Metastatic bone tumors are primarily lytic, with minimal periosteal proliferation, compared to osteomyelitis.[42] In addition, the region of bone pathology is usually different with bone tumors and osteomyelitis. Bone tumors are located primarily in the metaphyseal regions of long bones.[41, 42] Most lesions of osteomyelitis are located near a fracture, which is often in the diaphysis of the bone. Because of the possible radiographic similarities between a tumor and osteomyelitis, a bone biopsy should always be performed in questionable cases to prevent a misdiagnosis.

Radiographically, diskospondylitis is initially characterized by focal bone lysis of vertebral endplates. As the infection progresses, sclerosis of endplates, collapse of the disk space, and bridging spondylosis occur[21, 22] (Fig. 9–6). Radiographic changes of the disease often lag behind the onset of infection by 4 to 6 weeks.[22] In the spine, vertebral spaces T5–T10, C6–C7, and L7–S1 are most commonly affected.[21, 22] A myelogram should be performed if neurologic signs indicate spinal cord compression. Cord compression can be due to disk-space collapse, secondary vertebral body subluxation, or excessive bone and fibrous tissue deposition within the neural canal.

Microbiology

The most common aerobic bacterial species isolated from osteomyelitides in small animals is *Staphylococcus aureus*. The occurrence of this organism

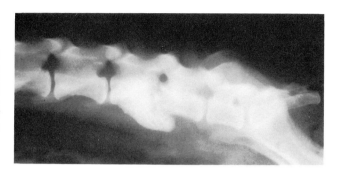

Figure 9–6. Diskospondylitis in a dog caused by *Staphylococcus aureus*. Radiographic changes include vertebral body and endplate lysis along with ventral bone bridging along vertebral spaces L5–L6. (Reprinted with permission from Rudd R: Diagnosis and treatment of osteomyelitis. Compend Contin Educ Vet Pract 1986; 8: 225.)

varies from 45% to 88%.[3, 9, 15, 16, 43–45] Other aerobic bacteria isolated are *Escherichia coli*, beta-hemolytic streptococcus, *Proteus* and *Pseudomonas* species.[1, 3, 4, 9, 15, 16, 42–46] Osteomyelitis is caused by a single bacterial species in approximately 50% of cases.[46, 47] Polymicrobial infections occur in the remaining cases, including isolation of up to six organisms.[46] A combination of gram-negative and gram-positive bacteria is usually present in polymicrobial infections, with *E. coli* the most common gram-negative isolate.[47] The number of different bacteria present in the wound has clinical relevance. In a recent study, animals with a polymicrobial infection suffered significantly more postoperative complications than those with one bacterial isolate.[24]

The importance of anaerobic bacteria in the pathogenesis of osteomyelitis has recently become evident. In one report, 74% of osteomyelitides contained an anaerobic organism.[48] In addition, 16% had only anaerobic bacteria, whereas 58% had both aerobic and anaerobic organisms. The most common anaerobic genus was *Bacteroides*, whereas the most frequently encountered organism was *Peptococcus anaerobius*. Isolation of anaerobes seems to be especially high in animals with osteomyelitis due to bite wounds.[43]

The clinical importance of anaerobic bacterial osteomyelitis has been demonstrated in people.[47] Patients with anaerobic infections had three times higher treatment failure rates than patients with aerobic bacterial osteomyelitis. The presence of anaerobic bacteria also may help explain previously reported high failure rates of osteomyelitis treatment, since anaerobic cultures were not routinely performed and antibiotic selection was based on incomplete antimicrobial sensitivity results.

Obtaining an appropriate sample for culture is imperative when dealing with an osteomyelitis case. The animal should not be given antimicrobial medication for several days prior to culture and sensitivity testing. The culturing of a sinus tract is highly discouraged because the predictive value of the culture is low.[1, 49] Culturing the soft tissues adjacent to the infected bone or the sequestrum at the time of surgery is the preferred technique. Fine-needle aspiration of exudate surrounding the bone also will provide reliable samples for culturing. All samples should be submitted for both aerobic and anaerobic culture and antimicrobial sensitivity. Anaerobic culturettes are available commercially and should be analyzed within 48 hours after obtaining the sample.[1]

Patients suspected of having hematogenous osteomyelitis should have blood cultures performed. Approximately 50% of humans with hematogenous osteomyelitis have positive blood cultures yielding the causative agent.[1, 9, 17, 50] The frequency of diagnostic blood cultures in small animals with hematogenous osteomyelitis is unknown. However, pathogenic bacteria cultured from multiple blood samples are assumed to be the causative organisms.

Diskospondylitis is usually caused by *Staphylococcus* species.[1, 21, 22] Proper identification of the causative organism can be done by culturing blood, urine, or affected bones. Blood cultures are positive in approximately 75% of dogs with diskospondylitis.[22] The causative organism also can be identified in the urine of 25% of the cases.[22] Routine serial blood and urine cultures are recommended, therefore, because they often yield the causative agent and are relatively noninvasive techniques. Bone cultures are obtained if a laminectomy is performed because of deteriorating neurologic signs.[22] Bone cultures are not routinely performed because they inconsistently yield the causative organism.[1] Cerebrospinal fluid culturing usually does not yield bacterial growth in affected animals and is also not recommended.[21] If an organism cannot be identified by one of the recommended culture (blood, urine) techniques, it could be assumed that a *Staphylococcus* species is involved and the appropriate antimicrobial drug selected.[22] Approximately 10% of diskospondylitis cases are due to *Brucella canis*.[22] Because of the possible public health significance, all intact animals with diskospondylitis should have a tube agglutination test performed for *B. canis*. A titer of 1:250 to 1:500 indicates an active bacteremia, and a titer between 1:50 and 1:100 suggests previous exposure.[22]

TREATMENT

Before initiating treatment of osteomyelitis, treatment protocols, potential short- and long-term costs of therapy, and complication rates should be discussed with the pet owner. Since considerable progress has been made in the management of osteomyelitis, results of proper treatment are generally favorable. However, since some conditions have a guarded prognosis, limb amputation may eventually be the only means for a cure.

In general, hematogenous osteomyelitis, diskospondylitis, and select cases of acute posttraumatic osteomyelitis can be treated medically; occasionally, some lesions require surgical drainage. The chronic stages of posttraumatic osteomyelitis, however, usually require a combination of surgical debridement, stabilization, and prolonged postoperative antimicrobial therapy.[1, 3, 4, 6, 9, 15] Unfortunately, chronic osteomyelitis is often treated solely with high doses of new and expensive antibiotics, resulting in poor long-term success. Antibiotics alone will suppress clinical signs of the disease but will not eradicate infection. In the management of acute and chronic posttraumatic osteomyelitis, absolute fracture stability is the cornerstone to a successful treatment protocol.[1-3, 6, 9] It is important to understand that a fracture will heal in the face of infection if adequate stability is provided (Fig. 9–7). Therefore, concurrent bone infection is not a contraindication for the use of internal fixation.[1, 6, 9, 15]

The treatment protocol used to manage osteomyelitis will depend on the form of the disease. Throughout the course of treatment, the veterinarian should radiograph the affected bone to evaluate the progression of the disease and effectiveness of therapy. If necessary, modifications and changes in the initial treatment plan are made. Occasionally, a new treatment modality or protocol may be required to obtain a successful outcome.

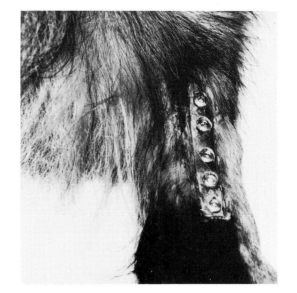

Figure 9–7. The medial aspect of a tibia with exposure of a bone plate 9 months after surgery. Although the skin over the plate sloughed several weeks after surgery, the owner did not seek veterinary attention until persistent drainage occurred. The fractured tibia had completely healed, and drainage subsided after plate removal, soft-tissue coverage of bone, and prolonged antibiotic therapy.

Treatment of Posttraumatic Osteomyelitis

ACUTE OSTEOMYELITIS

Appropriate antimicrobial therapy, begun within 72 hours after bone contamination, can prevent bone necrosis and subsequent development of chronic osteomyelitis.[1] Early diagnosis and initiation of treatment are necessary for medical therapy to be successful. Antibiotic selection should be based on bacterial culture and antimicrobial sensitivity results. While culture results are pending, a combination of a first-generation cephalosporin (cefazolin, cephalothin, cephaloridine) and an aminoglycoside (gentamicin, amikacin) can be used against a broad spectrum of organisms. The antibiotic(s) can then be changed, if necessary, once results of the antimicrobial sensitivity testing or the causative organism or organisms are known. During the first several days of therapy, the animal's cardiovascular status should be monitored for signs of septicemia. If clinical signs and laboratory parameters reveal septic shock, specific therapy should be initiated.[51]

In general, antibiotic treatment for acute osteomyelitis should cause an improvement in the animal's condition within 2 to 3 days of initiation of treatment. A failure in response to drug therapy characterized by a worsening of the animal's general condition or development of an abscess near the fracture(s) may necessitate surgery. The general principles used for the management of any wound infection apply to the treatment of acute suppurative posttraumatic osteomyelitis. The treatment goals are (1) stability of the fracture by internal or external fixation, (2) aggressive soft-tissue and bone debridement, (3) drainage of the infected tissue, and (4) appropriate antibiotic therapy based on bacterial culture and antimicrobial sensitivity testing.[3, 9]

Surgical intervention requires general anesthesia and wound exploration using aseptic surgical conditions. Samples from bone and soft tissues are submitted for aerobic and anaerobic cultures. All necrotic bone and soft tissues should be debrided, and unnecessary foreign material, such as suture material, should be removed from the wound. Debridement should spare vital neurovascular structures. Avascular fragments of bone must be removed or stabilized within the repair. If the bone fragment is small and will not provide structural support, it should be discarded. Large bone fragments that aid in fracture stability should be saved and reattached using full- or hemicerclage wire or, preferably, an interfragmentary lag screw.[3, 9] Fragments of bone with an intact periosteal blood supply should remain in place even if they cannot be incorporated into the repair. Such fragments still maintain an osteogenic capacity that is beneficial for callus formation and bone healing.

The initial fracture stabilization should be critically assessed; if the fracture is stable, then all implants should be left in place. Any motion, however, detected at the fracture site while rotating and bending the limb will be detrimental to bone healing and will contribute to the development of chronic osteomyelitis. Motion deleteriously affects newly forming vessels at the fracture that are necessary for supplying osteogenic cells, cellular and humoral components of the immune system, and antimicrobial agents to the wound.[2] Therefore, the primary goal in the management of an infected, unstable repair is to provide absolute fracture stability.[1–3, 5–7, 9, 15, 46, 47] This can be provided by internal fixation, such as a bone plate and interfragmentary screws, or external fixation. Intramedullary pinning should be used with caution because this technique can spread infection proximally and distally along the intramedullary cavity.[3, 7] Once bone union has occurred, internal implants usually have to be removed to obtain a cure of osteomyelitis.

All hematomas present in the wound must be surgically removed. One study suggests that 20% of fracture-associated hematomas are colonized by *Staphylococcus* organisms.[52] In addition, a hematoma can inhibit the local immune system and prevent an adequate concentration of antibiotics from reaching the infected bone. Meticulous hemostasis of bleeding vessels and closure of large pockets of dead space should be performed to prevent hematoma formation. A light, soft, padded bandage over the limb during the immediate 2 to 3 days after debridement is also effective in minimizing hematoma formation and obliterating dead space.

During surgery, the wound should be copiously lavaged with 2 to 5 L of a sterile solution. The specific lavage fluid used is not as important as the volume and pressure under which it is applied.[3, 53] The purpose of lavage is to mechanically remove necrotic tissue and dilute microorganisms left behind after debridement. To obtain high-pressure irrigation, a Water-Pik (Teledyne Aquatec, Fort Collins, Colo.) or a 19-gauge needle attached to a 35-ml syringe is an economical and useful lavage system.[9, 15, 23, 53] Lavage solutions that have been used include sterile normal saline, lactated Ringer's solutions, diluted sterile solutions of 1% povidone-iodine (Betadine solution, Purdue Frederich, Co., Norwalk, Conn.), 0.05% chlorhexidine diacetate (Nolvasan Solution, Fort Dodge Laboratories, Fort Dodge, Iowa), or lavage fluids containing antimicrobial agents.[3, 4, 6, 53, 54] The effectiveness of antiseptics and antibiotics in the lavage fluid is somewhat controversial. If an antiseptic or antibiotic is combined with lavage fluid, the surgeon should be aware that these agents can have deleterious effects on local tissues and wound healing.[9, 23, 53] These substances are also absorbed into the general circulation and have potential systemic side effects if used in excessive concentrations.[3, 6]

An intramedullary irrigation system is an effective technique to lavage the infected bone during surgery.[6] In addition, intramedullary lavage can be continued during the postoperative period. Two holes, one proximal and one distal, are made at each end of the affected bone. A flexible tube is inserted into the proximal hole, guided into the medullary cavity, and exits from the distal hole. The portion of tube within the medullary cavity is fenestrated to permit lavage fluid access into the intramedullary cavity. If this system is used during the postoperative period, the ends of the tube can be closed with sterile injection caps and incorporated into a sterile bandage to reduce the chance of a nosocomial infection. Drainage techniques, subsequently described, will be necessary during the postoperative period.

After wound debridement, lavage, and fracture stabilization, establishment of wound drainage is mandatory. If the wound is not adequately drained, proteolytic enzymes produced by dying neutrophils and bacteria will cause further bone lysis. In addition, these enzymes can damage the surrounding microvasculature and soft tissues, allowing progression of the disease. Numerous techniques are available for orthopedic wound drainage. The technique utilized will depend on the degree of wound contamination, postoperative monitoring facilities, and patient cooperation. Ingress–egress irrigation and suction drains can be used in selected patients. One of the most effective and practical techniques in the veterinary patient, however, is nonclosure of the wound. The specific techniques, advantages, and disadvantages of the various drainage systems are discussed under the treatment of chronic osteomyelitis.

During the postoperative period, the animal receives antibiotic treatment for 6 to 8 weeks based on culture and sensitivity testing.[1, 3, 6] The response to treatment can be evaluated by serial radiography. In select cases, short-term limb immobilization with a Robert-Jones bandage may help reduce soft-tissue swelling. If an irrigation–drainage system or an open drainage technique is used, a sterile bandage over the wound helps reduce colonization with organisms indigenous to the hospital environment. A light, soft, padded bandage is extremely useful for this purpose. Prolonged limb immobilization should be avoided. It can cause fracture disease and restrictive joint motion as a result of periarticular joint fibrosis.[6, 9] The technique used for fracture stabilization should be rigid enough to allow early limb function without the need for external coaptation.

CHRONIC OSTEOMYELITIS

Chronic osteomyelitis is a disease of bone ischemia, infection, and possible instability.[9] Even though some cases of acute osteomyelitis can be treated medically, most cases of chronic osteomyelitis require surgical treatment.[1–3, 5–7, 9, 15] The dead, infected sequestrum is isolated from the systemic circulation and therefore is a perpetual nidus of infection. Because of the chronic nature of the disease, the surrounding soft tissues are often infected, nonviable, and fibrotic, resulting in restricted joint mobility, muscle atrophy, restrictive fibrosis, and adhesions ("tie down"). The goals of treatment include (1) thorough soft-tissue and bone debridement, (2) sequestrectomy, (3) fracture stabilization, (4) obliteration of dead space, (5) wound drainage, (6) prolonged antimicrobial therapy, and (7) aggressive postoperative physical therapy to reverse the clinical signs of fracture disease.[9]

The surgical approach to the affected bone and sinus tracts is based on preoperative radiography, including fistulography. Alternative or multiple approaches to the bone may be required owing to extensive bone and soft-tissue pathology. Because of extensive fibrous tissues deposition, normal surgical planes of dissection and useful landmarks may be obscured and difficult to identify. A good understanding of regional topographic anatomy is mandatory to preserve vital neurovascular structures.

When performing wound debridement, all necrotic tissues should be removed. A thick, fibrous capsule usually surrounds the bone, with sinus tracts leading to the skin surface. If possible, *en bloc* resection of all abnormal tissues, including skin, fascia, muscle, scar tissue, and necrotic bone, should be performed. Projections of sinus tracts should be identified and carefully excised from normal, healthy tissues. Evaluation of the preoperative fistulogram will help in dissection of the sinus tracts. An additional technique that is valuable, especially if multiple tracts are present, is the injection of sterile dye into the fistula prior to surgery. This allows identification and meticulous removal of all diseased tissues, including sinus tracts and bone sequestrum. A 1% solution of sterile methylene blue is injected into the tracts 12 to 24 hours preoperatively. Healthy vascular tissues clear the dye and appear normal, whereas avascular tissue, including sinus tracts and the sequestrum, stain a deep blue.[1, 3, 9] An alternative procedure is injection of disulphine blue intravenously 1 hour before surgery. This dye stains vascular tissue blue, while avascular tissue appears white.[1, 3, 9]

Necrotic, infected bone is still mineralized and not easily resorbed by the body.[6, 9, 55] Therefore, after adequate soft-tissue debridement, sequestrectomy is necessary. If a dye is not used, the avascular sequestrum will be yellow and have irregular surfaces and edges[1, 15] (see Fig. 9–5B). Internal implants, such as bone plates, occasionally must be removed in order to visualize and remove the sequestrum (Fig. 9–8). The preoperative fistulogram will usually identify cases in which the sequestrum is hidden by the plate. Regardless of its size, the sequestrum must be removed to eradicate infection.[1–7, 9, 15, 46, 47] In addition, the involucrum should be curetted until healthy, bleeding bone is encountered ("paprika" sign).[3, 56] The medullary cavity will generally be exposed during debridement. Any avascular cancellous bone encountered within the cavity must be removed. The resulting bone and soft-tissue defect left after debridement resembles a saucer. Therefore, the entire procedure

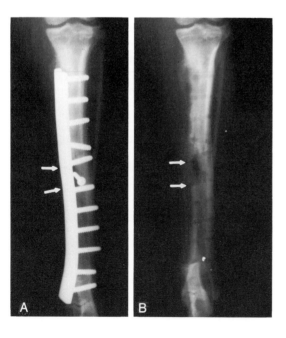

Figure 9–8. Craniocaudal radiographs of a tibia that developed draining tracts 9 months after surgery. *A,* A focal area of cortical lysis (*arrows*) could be seen on the medial aspect of the tibial cortex beneath the plate. Following plate removal, a sequestrum hidden by the plate was identified as the source of drainage. *B,* After sequestrectomy, a cortical deficit was apparent along the medial aspect of the tibia (*arrows*).

is often referred to as wound *saucerization*.[9] After debridement, the defect should be lavaged with a copious volume of irrigation solution, as described under the treatment for acute osteomyelitis.

After wound saucerization and lavage, fracture stability should be assessed. Implants that are providing rigid stability are left in place until the bone has healed. If the fracture has already healed, implants can be removed. If fracture instability is present, implants should be removed and an alternative stabilization technique utilized. Bone union is the initial treatment priority in septic delayed or nonunion cases.[1, 3, 9, 15] After fracture healing has occurred, the infection is finally eradicated by implant removal and antibiotic therapy. Absolute stability at the fracture site allowing early return to function of the limb is best achieved with bone plates. However, some cases also may respond favorably to treatment with external fixation.

If large segments of bone are removed during debridement, a cancellous bone graft should be used. Some osteogenic cells will survive the grafting procedure and produce osteoid.[5, 57, 58] The greatest benefits of a cancellous graft include osteoinduction and osteoconduction. The graft stimulates and guides formation of new trabecular bone from the surrounding soft tissues and viable bone. Timing of the grafting procedure depends on the condition of the wound. Grafting can be performed during the initial surgical procedure if minimal exudate is present. At worse, the cancellous graft will be extruded from the wound, resorbed by the body, or dissolved by proteolytic enzymes generated by bacteria and neutrophils. However, a cancellous graft will not become a sequestrum in the face of infection.[58] If a closed suction and drainage system is used or heavy exudation of the wound is expected, cancellous grafting should be delayed.[3] Delay of the grafting procedure until adequate granulation tissue has covered the wound will allow a higher chance of graft "take" and survival. Usually, the graft can be placed into the wound 7 to 14 days after initial debridement. When cancellous grafting is performed, special precautions should be taken in order to prevent contamination of the graft donor site with organisms from the infected bone. This is accomplished by (1) separate draping of the graft donor site and the infected bone, (2) use of separate instruments, gowns, and gloves for the two surgical procedures, and (3) harvesting the cancellous graft before surgical manipulation of infected tissue.

Wound drainage and obliteration of dead space are necessary in the management of chronic osteomyelitis. The most effective and practical method to accomplish this goal is nonclosure of the wound. The procedure is referred to as the *Papineau open cancellous technique* in human orthopedic surgery and, with several modifications, has been used successfully in veterinary patients.[1, 3, 9, 59] In one study, this technique resulted in successful treatment of chronic osteomyelitis in 92% of the small animal patients.[59] Initially, wound saucerization and debridement, along with rigid fracture fixation, are performed. The wound is left open, and sterile sponges soaked in saline, antibiotic, or antiseptic solutions are packed into the wound defect to obliterate dead space and facilitate exudate removal. A sterile, soft, padded bandage or a tie-over bandage (a wet-to-dry bandage held in place over a wound by umbilical tape secured to circumferential loose skin sutures) is then applied to hold the sponges in place and prevent further contamination of the wound. The bandage is changed twice a day, and the wound is flushed with a sterile solution. After exudate formation has diminished, bandage changes can be reduced to once a day. Wound lavage and bandage changes are continued until healthy, bleeding granulation tissue covers the bone and begins to fill the soft-tissue defect (7 to 14 days). At this stage, delayed cancellous bone grafting and secondary closure of the wound can be performed or the soft tissues allowed to close by second intention. The Papineau technique provides excellent wound drainage, requires minimal skill or specialized equipment, and is well tolerated by veterinary patients. The animal should be monitored daily, and an Elizabethan collar should be used to prevent inadvertent removal of the protective bandage.

Another technique to allow wound drainage and obliteration of dead space is closed suction drainage and irrigation of the wound[1, 3, 9, 60, 61] (Fig. 9–9). This system requires an ingress fenestrated delivery tube placed proximal to the wound along the bone and a second fenestrated egress tube placed parallel and superficial to the first tube exiting distal to the wound. The wound is closed in layers to eliminate dead space. The ingress tube is irrigated continuously with a sterile solution. Some surgeons advocate the addition of an antiseptic or antibiotic to the irrigation solution. The egress tube should be connected to a suction apparatus (Snyder Hemovac, Snyder Laboratories, Dover, Ohio) to evacuate the irrigation solution under gentle negative pressure. The ingress–egress tubes and the suction apparatus should be maintained as a closed system to minimize secondary wound contamination. Furthermore, components of the system should be incorporated into a bandage to prevent premature patient removal.

The principal function of closed suction drainage and irrigation is to obliterate dead space by suction while granulation tissue fills the cavity left by debridement.[61] The irrigation solution is used primarily to prevent clogging of the suction system.[3] Fluids used to irrigate the system are detrimental to cancellous bone. Therefore, cancellous bone grafting should always be delayed until the irrigation–drainage system has been removed.[3] The system is left in place until all dead space has been obliterated by granulation tissue. A radiograph of the region after injection of a sterile aqueous contrast agent into the irrigation tube will help determine if this has occurred. The closed suction drainage and irrigation system has been used in human patients with reported success rates ranging from 33% to

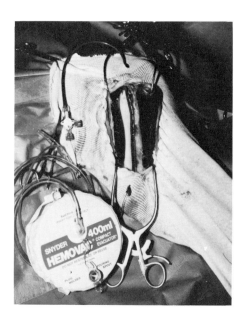

Figure 9–9. Closed suction drainage and irrigation provide wound drainage and obliteration of dead space. During the postoperative period, it is necessary to incorporate the ingress and egress tubes in a sterile bandage to prevent secondary ascending infections and patient removal of the system.

90%.[59] The success rate of the system has not been documented in veterinary medicine. Potential complications encountered with the system include (1) premature clogging of the irrigation–drainage tubes, (2) secondary ascending wound infections via the drains, and (3) removal of the system by an uncooperative patient.[3, 9, 60, 61] Constant 24-hour patient monitoring is necessary to prevent these potential complications. This system may offer no advantages over the Papineau open cancellous technique, and requires intensive patient and system monitoring.

Extensive soft-tissue loss over the infected bone can occur as a result of infection or wound debridement. The use of local muscle flaps in such circumstances can be beneficial to eliminate dead space, improve local bone blood supply, promote new bone formation, and improve delivery of antibiotics to the bone.[3, 62] In addition, more radical debridement of the tissues may be performed if local muscle flaps are incorporated to cover the resulting defect. The muscle, with an intact arterial and venous blood supply, is transplanted over the bone. A myocutaneous flap, incorporating muscle and overlying skin, also can be used. Local muscle or myocutaneous flaps used in small animal surgery have included cranial tibialis, caudal sartorius, and cranial sartorius muscle flaps, and cutaneous trunci and latissimus dorsi musculocutaneous flaps.[63–66] In human orthopedic surgery, free-muscle transfers with microvascular anastomoses have been used in regions where adequate tissue is not available to create a local muscle flap.[67] This technique also may be beneficial in veterinary patients, although it may be limited to large referral centers with trained surgeons and microvascular surgical equipment.

In addition to surgical debridement, sequestrectomy, and establishment of wound drainage, broad-spectrum bactericidal antibiotics should be used. Definitive antibiotic selection should be based on culture and sensitivity results of the soft tissue and sequestrum. The duration of antibiotic therapy required for a cure is not known, although a minimum of 8 weeks of therapy may be necessary. Antibiotics can be continued until radiographic examination reveals smooth lamellar bone in the region of the previous pathology. If internal implants were used, a cure cannot be expected until osseous union has occurred and implant removal performed.

Early return to limb usage is best accomplished by initiating aggressive, early physical therapy. Passive flexion and extension exercises of the limb should be performed to minimize muscle atrophy, fibrosis, and adhesions. Once the wound is closed, controlled leash walks and swimming should be encouraged. When performing fracture stabilization, the surgeon should therefore select a technique that is rigid enough to withstand physical therapy exercises.

Cryptic Infections

By definition, this type of osteomyelitis occurs at the site of a healed fracture, and no overt clinical signs of infection are present.[31, 32] The clinical significance of this infection in veterinary patients has yet to be determined. The causative organisms are surrounded by a biofilm that protects the bacteria from systemic antibiotics.[31, 32, 34] Therefore, antimicrobial therapy alone is an ineffective treatment. Surgical removal and culturing of the metal implant, followed by appropriate antibiotic therapy for 6 weeks, is necessary to eradicate a cryptic infection.[31] Because large metal implants may stimulate biofilm-mediated infections, the routine removal of large implants may be advisable. Generally, this form of osteomyelitis has an excellent prognosis once the implant is removed and antibiotic therapy initiated.

Neonatal Acute Hematogenous Osteomyelitis

Acute hematogenous osteomyelitis of the neonate can be managed successfully with medical therapy. After blood culture or needle aspiration of the bone lesion(s), the animal should receive a broad-spectrum antimicrobial agent until a definitive drug can be chosen based on culture and sensitivity results. If microorganisms cannot be cultured, an empirical combination of a first-generation cephalosporin and an aminoglycoside can be used. During the first several days of treatment, antibiotics are given parenterally (IV or IM), followed by an oral route of administration. Antimicrobial therapy is continued for 30 days after the clinical signs of lameness and focal swelling have subsided.[17] The bone should be radiographed weekly to monitor the effectiveness of treatment. Because this form of osteomyelitis can be associated with generalized septicemia, the patient should be monitored carefully.

If the condition is going to respond to antibiotic therapy, a general improvement in the animal's demeanor should be seen within 24 to 48 hours after initiation of treatment. Early diagnosis and aggressive treatment are vital for a successful outcome. Most cases that do not respond to medical therapy are due to a delay in the initiation of treatment or improper antibiotic selection.[1, 17] Indications for surgical intervention include failure to respond to medical therapy, formation of a soft-tissue abscess with swelling over the bone lesion, and radiographic enlargement of the bone abscess.[6]

Surgical decompression and drainage of the bone are necessary if medical management of the disease is unsuccessful. An incision is made over the point of maximum swelling and tenderness. After retraction of the adjacent soft tissues and exposure of the involved bone, the intramedullary abscess should be decompressed (Fig. 9–10). This involves drilling multiple small holes through the periosteum and cortex into the medullary abscess.[6, 9]

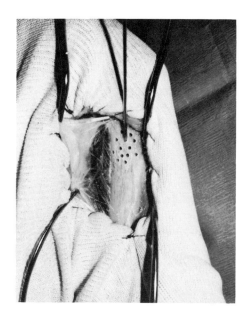

Figure 9–10. Decompression of a metaphyseal abscess can be accomplished by drilling multiple small holes through the cortex with a pin or small drill bit.

Culture of the bone and exudate should be performed. If a large abscess is encountered, the removal of a "window" of cortex may provide better drainage.[9] If necessary, the limb can be supported with external coaptation to prevent pathologic fracture at the site of bone decompression. A lavage and drainage system also may be utilized in order to reduce accumulation of exudate around the bone. The wound over the lesion should not be closed. The limb is wrapped in a sterile bandage and the wound allowed to close by second intention. Alternatively, delayed secondary closure of the wound, after granulation tissue has covered the bone, can be performed. Based on the culture and sensitivity results, the animal is given an appropriate antibiotic for at least 6 weeks.

Diskospondylitis

Diskospondylitis can be treated medically and have a favorable prognosis if minimal neurologic deficits are present. Based on blood or urine culture and sensitivity results, an appropriate antibiotic is selected. If an organism cannot be cultured, it is assumed that the infection is caused by *Staphylococcus aureus*, and antibiotics are chosen accordingly.[1, 21, 22] In one report, the first-generation cephalosporins cephradine and cephalexin were effective in treating 97% of the diskospondylitis cases due to *S. aureus*. Cloxacillin also was found to be highly effective.[22] The duration of therapy necessary to establish a cure has not been determined. However, a minimum of 8 weeks of antibiotic therapy should be used as a general guideline. Therapy can be used until there is radiographic evidence that lytic vertebral endplates have been remodeled and replaced with healthy, new lamellar bone.

Dogs with severe paresis or paralysis may require surgical decompression of the spinal cord in addition to prolonged antibiotic therapy.[22] A liberal hemilaminectomy is preferred over a dorsal laminectomy to save the dorsal spinous processes for spinal stabilization.[22] After adequate exposure of the spinal cord, offending bone and proliferative fibrous tissue are carefully removed from the spinal canal. The lytic portions of the involved vertebral endplates and disk spaces are curetted to remove any necrotic tissue. A portion of the necrotic bone should be submitted for histologic evaluation and bacterial culture. If large bone deficits are created by curettage, a cancellous bone graft may be beneficial in stimulating new bone formation. Spinal instability resulting from the disease process or curettage of necrotic bone should be treated with a dorsal spinous plate, a vertebral body plate, vertebral body cross pinning, or spinal segmented stapling.[21, 68] When internal implants are utilized for the management of diskospondylitis, the owner should be informed that implant removal will be necessary once permanent vertebral stability has been achieved and the lesion healed.

Diskospondylitis due to *Brucella canis* has been treated using oral tetracycline hydrochloride (20 mg/kg) for 3 weeks in combination with streptomycin (20 mg/kg) during the initial 5 days of treatment.[22] After completion of treatment, medications are stopped for 3 weeks, followed by a second therapy of tetracycline and streptomycin.[22] Intact animals should be neutered. Clinical signs of the disease can usually be prevented with periodic antibiotic treatment. However, *B. canis* is a difficult organism to eliminate. Repeated treatments are often required, with control rather than a cure of the disease being possible in some cases. In addition, owners of dogs infected with *Brucella* should be informed of the zoonotic potential of the infection.

Individuals with high exposure to the animal should seek medical advice from a physician.

General Guidelines for Antibiotic Therapy for Osteomyelitis

For successful treatment of bacterial osteomyelitis, therapeutic concentrations of the antimicrobial agent must be present in the bone–interstitial fluid space.[69–72] Current recommendations indicate that bacteriostatic antibiotics have no role in the treatment of osteomyelitis. Because many cases of osteomyelitis involve β-lactamase–producing bacteria, drugs such as penicillin, amoxicillin, and ampicillin are often ineffective. The choice of antibiotic should always be based on culture and sensitivity results. Responsible antibiotic selection is necessary to prevent the emergence of resistant organisms, and selection of narrow-spectrum agents is encouraged. If available, the minimal inhibitory concentration (MIC) is the best guide for antibiotic selection.[70] As a general rule, an antibiotic should be selected that will produce a continuous serum concentration at least four times the MIC required to prevent bacterial growth. Other variables such as antibiotic toxicity, frequency and route of administration, drug interactions, and cost of treatment also must be considered when selecting an appropriate antimicrobial agent. Generally, the least toxic, most readily available, and most cost-effective bactericidal antibiotic should be chosen. While waiting for culture results, a first-generation cephalosporin plus an aminoglycoside is an effective empirical combination.

Initially, an IV or IM route of administration is used. The IV route will provide the highest and most reliable tissue concentration of the drug.[70] However, IV therapy is usually the most expensive route of administration, which often limits its practicality for long-term use in the veterinary patient. An acceptable protocol is the use of an IV or IM route of administration for the first several days of therapy, followed by oral medications. Therefore, it is beneficial to select an agent that is available in both parenteral and oral forms. Table 9–1 is a list of common antimicrobial agents, including dosages and available routes of administration, that are currently used in the management of osteomyelitis in small animals.

A special note should be made regarding a new family of antimicrobial agents, the fluoroquinolones.[73–75] These agents are active against *Staphylococcus* species and many gram-negative agents, such as *Pseudomonas* species, that are often resistant to other commonly used antibiotics. Fluoroquinolones, however, are not effective against anaerobes. Ciprofloxacin is the principal fluoroquinolone that has been used clinically in human osteomyelitis cases. This drug reaches high therapeutic bone concentrations and is available in oral forms for prolonged treatments. Enrofloxacin (Baytril, Mobay Animal Health Co., Shawnee, Kans.) is the licensed fluoroquinolone in veterinary medicine. It has been shown to be extremely effective in soft-tissue infections; however, efficacy of its use for the treatment of osteomyelitis is currently unavailable. The author has used the drug successfully for the treatment of select chronic osteomyelitis cases in which other antimicrobial agents failed to give satisfactory results.

Experimental Protocols for the Treatment of Osteomyelitis

Polymethylmethacrylate bone cement impregnated with antibiotics has been used as a prophylactic technique to prevent osteomyelitis following

TABLE 9–1. Commonly Used Antimicrobial Agents for Small Animal Orthopedic Infections

AGENT	DOSE (mg/kg)	ROUTE	INTERVAL (hours)
Amikacin*†	10	IV, IM, SC	6
Amoxicillin†	22–30	IV, IM, SC, PO	6–8
Amoxicillin clavulanate	22	PO	6–8
Ampicillin	22	IV, IM, SC, PO	6–8
Cefadroxil	22	PO	8–12
Cefazolin	22	IV, IM, SC	6–8
Cefotaxime	20–40	IV, IM, SC	6–8
Cefoxitin	22	IV, IM	6–8
Ceftazidime‡	25	IV, IM	8–12
Cephalexin	22–30	PO	6–8
Cephalothin	22–30	IV, IM, SC	6–8
Cephapirin	22	IV, IM, SC	6–8
Cephradine	22	IV, IM, SC, PO	6–8
Ciprofloxacin	11	PO	12
Clindamycin§¶	11	IV, IM, PO	8–12
Cloxacillin	10–15	IV, IM, PO	6–8
Enrofloxacin	5–11	PO	12
Gentamicin*†	2	IV, IM, SC	8–12
Oxacillin	22	IV, IM, SC, PO	6–8
Penicillin G (aqueous)	20,000–40,000 IU	IV	6

*Nephrotoxic and ototoxic; renal function must be monitored throughout use.
†Limit use to 1 week.
‡Only effective against *Pseudomonas*.
§Painful on IM injection; can cause phlebitis if given IV.
¶Parenteral dose every 8 hours; oral dose every 12 hours.
Source: Reprinted with permission from Budsberg S: Antimicrobial distribution and therapeutics in bone. Compend Contin Educ Vet Pract 1990; 12:1759.

total hip replacement and long bone fractures.[3, 76–78] Gentamicin is the antibiotic usually incorporated into the cement. The cement–antibiotic composite is formed into small beads and placed around a stainless steel wire, similar to a necklace. The beads are implanted next to the bone following surgical debridement. The cement acts as a carrier vehicle for the antibiotic, which slowly leaches from the beads. After 2 weeks, the beads are removed from the wound and replaced with a new strand. A major technical difficulty is production of beads with a known and standard release of antibiotic. Conflicting results have been reported on the use of this technique in experimental models and clinical cases of osteomyelitis.[76] The technique has been used clinically in people. However, the effectiveness of this technique, based on major clinical trials, must be established before it can be recommended for the routine treatment of osteomyelitis in animals.

Plaster of Paris beads impregnated with antibiotic also have been used in a fashion similar to the bone cement beads.[79] Plaster beads fill dead space while slowly being absorbed and replaced by bone. The plaster does not cause adverse tissue reactions, does not hinder bone growth at the fracture site, and does not become a sequestrum. Similar to the polymethylmethacrylate beads, plaster beads bind antibiotics in such a way that the antibiotic is slowly released into the surrounding tissue. In contrast with the polymethylmethacrylate beads, plaster beads impregnated with antibiotics are relatively inexpensive to prepare and are spontaneously absorbed. This technique, therefore, may be more feasible in veterinary medicine.

Extremely high local levels of antibiotics have been achieved in infected bone by venous profusion of antibiotics under pressure.[80, 81] Pneumatic tourniquets are placed distally and proximally to the infected bone. The antibiotic is then infused at a pressure of 100 to 150 mmHg into a superficial vein distal to the site of osteomyelitis. Perfusion time is approximately 1 hour, twice daily, for 5 to 7 days. By intravenous infusion of antibiotics under pressure with concurrent venous obstruction proximal to the lesion, the venous flow rich in antibiotic is shunted into the deep venous plexus of the bone. This procedure has achieved local antibiotic concentrations 100 times those found in the systemic circulation.[1, 81, 82] Local wound debridement, sequestrectomy, and systemic antibiotic therapy should be used in combination with local venous perfusion of antibiotics. Results from human surgeries have been very encouraging. The technique may be beneficial in selected small animal osteomyelitis cases. However, because of equipment costs, time necessary for perfusion, and possible poor patient cooperation, the technique may not be practical.

Another technique to achieve high local concentrations of antibiotics is use of an implantible pump.[82] A two-chambered pump that can be filled percutaneously with antibiotics is placed subcutaneously near the site of infection. The pump automatically forces antibiotics through an outflow catheter that is placed at the site of infection. The technique is currently being used with success in human patients.

Silver ion iontophoresis, which is the electrical generation of silver cations from silver wire or mesh, has been used in human orthopedics to treat refractory cases of osteomyelitis.[83, 84] The exact effect of silver cations on bacteria is not known. It is speculated that they interfere with cell-membrane function, cellular DNA, or the respiratory chain of enzymes.[84] In addition, silver cations are toxic only to bacteria, not to mammalian tissue. Silver cations have a broad spectrum of activity against gram-positive, gram-negative, aerobic, and anaerobic organisms. Development of bacterial resistance to silver cations is extremely rare.[83] After thorough debridement of the infected bone and soft tissue, silver mesh is placed in contact with all infected tissue. The mesh is then electrically stimulated by an external battery source for 2 to 3 months. The silver mesh bandage is changed every other day until the wound has healed by second intention. The main disadvantage of the technique is the limited zone of penetration by silver cations, which is approximately 1 cm.[83, 84] Another potential problem in veterinary patients would be patient interference with the wires and external battery source.

In severe cases of human osteomyelitis with little hope of success by the use of standard surgical procedures, free microvascular osseous bone grafts have permitted aggressive resection and replacement of diseased bone.[67] Large segmental replacements of femoral and tibial defects have been performed. The procedure is technically demanding and requires special training and equipment to perform the microvascular anastomoses. Clinical trials of the procedure have not been reported in veterinary medicine. However, in a recent study, autogenous free ulnar bone grafting in the dog by microvascular anastomoses was found to be a feasible and successful technique.[85] Its use for the treatment of refractory osteomyelitis should warrant future consideration.

The use of hyperbaric oxygen as an adjunct treatment for osteomyelitis has been reported in people.[86, 87] No reports are available regarding its use in veterinary medicine. Unfortunately, the expense of the necessary equipment may limit its use in veterinary medicine.

PERIOPERATIVE PREVENTION OF OSTEOMYELITIS

Most cases of osteomyelitis occur as a direct result of a technical error made by the surgical team. Therefore, proper patient and surgeon preparation, strict adherence to accepted surgical techniques, and prophylactic antibiotic therapy are the foundations to prevent osteomyelitis.

Liberal hair clipping, well beyond the area of the intended incision, will help minimize inadvertent contamination while manipulating the limb during surgery. Wrapping the foot with an impervious material such as a surgical glove or waterproof tape also helps prevent contamination. If surgery is being performed on a long bone, suspending the wrapped foot from any overhead structure will allow surgical scrubbing and draping without contaminating the limb with body regions not surgically prepared. A minimum of five 3-minute scrubs of the entire area is necessary.[15] Numerous antiseptic scrubs are available. However, product selection is not as important as the contact time the antiseptic has with the skin. Following surgical scrubbing, the skin should be sprayed or painted with an antiseptic solution.

Two layers of sterile drapes should cover regions of the animal not surgically scrubbed. At least one layer of the drapes should be waterproof, to prevent lavage fluids and blood from soaking through to the animal or table. A drape that is soaked is no longer a sterile barrier between the animal and the surgical field. In addition, one drape should cover the table down to the surgeon's knees. As the animal's limb is manipulated during orthopedic surgery, short drapes tend to creep up and allow regions of the table or animal to contaminate the surgical team or field. Placing a sterile drape or towel circumfrentially around the wrapped foot further helps to prevent bacterial spread to the surgical field. Finally, a sterile stockinette or an impervious, self-adherent wrap (Via-Drape, Desert Medical Inc., Sandy, Utah) should be placed over the entire limb, secured to the drapes, and fenestrated over the proposed incision site. After incision of the skin and hemostasis of bleeding vessels, the edge of the stockinette is sutured to the subcutaneous region of the skin incision. This process reduces contact of the surgeon and wound with the skin, which can be a source of contamination. Some surgeons advocate changing gloves after subdraping the skin and using different scalpel blades for deeper dissection to prevent contamination with organisms endogenous to the skin.

Proper preparation of the surgeon and surgical instruments is mandatory when performing orthopedic surgery. Surgical caps and masks should be worn by the surgical team and any individual entering the operating room. All members of the surgical team should scrub from the elbows down to the fingertips for a minimum of 5 minutes prior to surgery. Sterile surgical gowns and gloves should be worn to prevent wound contamination during the procedure. The surgeons should periodically check their gloves for punctures. Studies have found that over 50% of visibly intact gloves were perforated by the end of an orthopedic procedure.[15] Some surgeons advocate double gloving when handling sharp objects such as pins, drill bits, and bone fragments. All instruments, implants, and suture materials should be sterilized. The use of cold sterilization solutions for instruments and covering of unsterile instruments, such as a power drill, with sterile wraps are not considered aseptic techniques and should be avoided. These practices generally result in wound contamination. If an instrument or implant cannot be steam sterilized, gas sterilization with ethylene oxide is necessary.

Surgical technique also can influence the development of osteomyelitis. Using accepted surgical approaches to the bone will prevent unnecessary tissue damage. Incisions should be made through intermuscular planes. If necessary, subperiosteal elevation of muscle is preferred to muscle transection. Gentle soft-tissue handling and frequent lavage to prevent desiccation are important. Fastidious hemostasis and elimination of dead space during wound closure will prevent hematoma formation during the postoperative period. The overall goal is to prevent vascular insult and damage to the soft tissues and bone. Vascular, healthy tissue should be able to tolerate and eliminate acceptable levels of bacterial that are present in all surgical wounds. However, avascular tissue or hematomas are ideal growth media for bacteria and can allow an acceptable level of bacterial contamination to develop into infection.

Prophylactic antibiotic therapy is useful in orthopedic surgery to prevent osteomyelitis, especially when implants are used or a prolonged surgical procedure is anticipated.[88] Unfortunately, prophylactic antibiotic therapy is seldom used correctly. Timing of therapy is crucial. An antibiotic must be present in therapeutic interstitial fluid concentrations at the time of bacterial contamination if it is to be considered a prophylactic measure in the prevention of osteomyelitis. Giving antibiotics after completion of surgery is not considered prophylactic therapy and will not reduce the incidence of osteomyelitis. It is generally accepted that the antibiotic should be given immediately prior to surgery and repeated every 2 to 3 hours during prolonged procedures. Ideally, the drug is given as an IV bolus. The antibiotic should not be continued during the postoperative period. The selection of an appropriate prophylactic antibiotic should be based on the known common hospital pathogens. If these agents are not known, an antibiotic should be selected that is effective against β-lactamase–producing bacteria. A first-generation cephalosporin alone or in combination with an animoglycoside is usually an excellent choice for prophylactic therapy.

The initial management of open fractures is important in the prevention of osteomyelitis. All open fractures are contaminated. Immediate surgical debridement of the soft tissues and bone is necessary, assuming the patient can be safely anesthetized. Delayed soft-tissue closure is necessary after wound debridement and fracture stabilization. A study involving human open wound management found that 73% of wounds that were debrided and closed on the day of the trauma became infected.[89] If wound closure was performed 2 to 3 days after debridement, 22% of the wounds became infected. However, only 3% of the wounds became infected that were managed by debridement, open drainage for at least 4 days under a sterile dressing, followed by delayed wound closure. Therefore, it is recommended that open fractures not be closed immediately after surgery. The wound is left open to drain and is protected by a sterile bandage. After 4 days, the wound can be closed if no exudate formation has occurred. The wound also can be left open and allowed to close by second intention.

REFERENCES

1. Rudd RG: A rational approach to the diagnosis and treatment of osteomyelitis. Compend Contin Educ Pract Vet 1986; 8:225–234
2. Aron DN: Pathogenesis, diagnosis, and management of osteomyelitis in small animals. Compend Contin Educ Pract Vet 1979; 1:824–830

3. Parker RB: Treatment of posttraumatic osteomyelitis. Vet Clin North Am 1987; 17:841–856
4. Harari J: Osteomyelitis. J Am Vet Med Assoc 1984; 184:101–102
5. Brinker WO, Piermattei DL, Flo GL: Treatment of acute and chronic bone infections. In Handbook of Small Animal Orthopedics and Fracture Treatment. Philadelphia: WB Saunders, 1990, pp 59–64
6. Sumner-Smith G: Osteomyelitis. In Whittick WG (ed): Canine Orthopedics. Philadelphia: Lea & Febiger, 1990, pp 571–581
7. Nunamaker DM: Osteomyelitis. In Newton CD, Nunamaker DM (eds): Textbook of Small Animal Orthopedics. Philadelphia: Lippincott, 1985, pp 499–510
8. Newton CD, Siemering G: Skeletal diseases. In Ettinger SJ (ed): Textbook of Veterinary Internal Medicine. Philadelphia: WB Saunders, 1983, pp 2236–2260
9. Daly WR: Orthopedic infections. In Slatter DH (ed): Textbook of Small Animal Surgery. Philadelphia: WB Saunders, 1985, pp 2020–2035
10. Norden CW: Experimental osteomyelitis: II. Therapeutic trials of antibiotic levels. J Infect Dis 1970; 122:410–418
11. Norden CW: Lessons learned from animal models of osteomyelitis. Rev Infect Dis 1988; 10:103–110
12. Deysine M, Rosario E, Isenberg H: Acute hematogenous osteomyelitis: An experimental model. Surgery 1976; 79:97–99
13. Rissing JP, Buxton TB, Fisker J, et al: Arachidonic acid facilitates experimental chronic osteomyelitis in rats. Infect Immun 1985; 49:141–144
14. Dekel S, Francis MJO: The treatment of osteomyelitis of the tibia with sodium salicylate: An experimental study in rabbits. J Bone Joint Surg 1981; 63B:178–184
15. Braden TD: Posttraumatic osteomyelitis. Vet Clin North Am 1991; 21:781–811
16. Caywood DD, Wallace LJ, Braden TD: Osteomyelitis in the dog: A review of 67 cases. J Am Vet Med Assoc 1978; 172:943–946
17. Gilson SD, Schwarz PD: Acute hematogenous osteomyelitis in the dog. J Am Anim Hosp Assoc 1989; 25:684–688
18. Turner S: Diseases of bones and related structures. In Stashak TS (ed): Adams' Lameness in Horses. Philadelphia: Lea & Febiger, 1987, pp 305–308
19. Ressnick D, Niwayama G: Diagnosis of Bone and Joint Disorders. Philadelphia: WB Saunders, 1981
20. Martens RJ: Pathogenesis, diagnosis and therapy of septic arthritis in foals. J Vet Orthop 1980; 2:49–58
21. Walker TL, Tomlinson J, Sorjonen DC, Kornegay JN: Diseases of the spinal column. In Slatter DH (ed): Textbook of Small Animal Surgery. Philadelphia: WB Saunders, 1985, pp 1367–1395
22. Kornegay JN: Diskospondylitis. In Kirk RW (ed): Current Veterinary Therapy, vol 9: Small Animal Practice. Philadelphia: WB Saunders, 1986, pp 810–814
23. Daly WR: Wound infections. In Slatter DH (ed): Textbook of Small Animal Surgery. Philadelphia: WB Saunders, 1985, pp 37–51
24. Wallace LJ: Classification and initial treatment of open fractures. 1987 Scientific Proceedings, 15th Annual Veterinary Surgical Forum, Chicago, Ill, 1987, p 50
25. Stevenson S, Olmstead ML, Kowalski J: Bacterial culturing for prediction of postoperative complications following open fracture repair in small animals. Vet Surg 1986; 15:99–102
26. Muller ME, Allgower M, Willenegger H: Manual of Internal Fixation. New York: Springer-Verlag, 1970
27. Richardson DC: Fracture first aid: The open (compound) fracture. In Slatter DH (ed): Textbook of Small Animal Surgery. Philadelphia: WB Saunders, 1985, pp 1945–1949
28. Brown PW: The fate of exposed bone. Am J Surg 1979; 137:464
29. Vasseur PB, Levy J, Dowd E, Eliot J: Surgical wound infection rates in dogs and cats: Data from a teaching hospital. Vet Surg 1988; 17:60–64
30. Cruse PJE, Foord R: The epidemiology of wound infections: A ten-year prospective study of 62,939 wounds. Surg Clin North Am 1980; 60:27–40
31. Gristina AG, Costerton JW: Bacterial adherence and the glycocalyx and their role in musculoskeletal infection. Orthop Clin North Am 1984; 15:517–535
32. Smith MM, Vasseur PB, Saunders HM: Bacterial growth associated with metallic implants in dogs. Am Vet Med Assoc 1989; 195:765–767
33. Petty W, Spanier S, Shuster JJ, Silverthorne C: The influence of skeletal implants on incidence of infection. J Bone Joint Surg 1985; 67A:1236–1244
34. Mayberry-Carson KJ, Taber-Meyer B, Smith JK, et al: Bacterial adherence and glycocalyx formation in osteomyelitis experimentally induced with *Staphylococcus aureus*. Infect Immun 1984; 43:825–833
35. Peacock EE: Wound Repair, 3d ed. Philadelphia: WB Saunders, 1984, pp 1–14, 414–418
36. Miller C, Trunkey DD: Immunobiology of sepsis. In Flint LM, Fry DE (eds): Surgical Infections. Garden City, NY: Medical Examination Publishing Co, 1982
37. Berzon JL: Brodie's abscess: A case report in a dog. J Am Anim Hosp Assoc 1979; 15:749–752

38. Smith CW, Schiller AG: Osteomyelitis in the dog. J Vet Orthop 1980; 2:11–18
39. Gibson KL, van Ee R, Watters J: Radiographic diagnosis. Vet Radiol 1987; 28:229–231
40. Hoskinson JJ, Daniel GB, Patton CS: Indium-111 chloride and three-phase bone scintigraphy: A comparison for imaging experimental osteomyelitis. J Nucl Med 1991; 32:67–75
41. Park RD: Radiographic diagnosis of long bone neoplasms in the dog. Compend Contin Educ Pract Vet 1981; 3:922–928
42. Probst CW, Ackerman N: Malignant neoplasia of the canine appendicular skeleton. Compend Contin Educ Pract Vet 1981; 4:260–271
43. Wong WT, Mason TA: Survey of 44 cases of canine osteomyelitis. Aust Vet Pract 1984; 14:149–151
44. Smith CW, Schiller AG, Smith AR, Dorner JL: Osteomyelitis in the dog: A retrospective study. J Am Anim Hosp Assoc 1978; 14:589–592
45. Hirsh DC, Smith TM: Osteomyelitis in the dog: Microorganisms isolated and susceptibility to antimicrobial agents. J Small Anim Pract 1978; 19:679–687
46. Stevenson S: Acute and chronic bacterial osteomyelitis. 1984 Scientific Proceedings, 12th Annual Veterinary Surgical Forum, Chicago, Ill, 1984, p 59
47. Fossum TW: Infections after internal fixation. 1988 Scientific Proceedings, 17th Annual Canine Basic ASIF Course, Columbus, OH, 1988
48. Walker RD, Richardson DC, Bryant MJ, Draper CS: Anaerobic bacteria associated with osteomyelitis in domestic animals. J Am Vet Med Assoc 1983; 182:814–816
49. Mackowiak PA, Jones SR, Smith JW: Diagnostic value of sinus-tract cultures in chronic osteomyelitis. JAMA 1978; 239:2772–2775
50. Septismus EJ, Musher DM: Osteomyelitis: Recent clinical and laboratory aspects. Orthop Clin North Am 1979; 10:347–359
51. Goodwin JK, Schaer M: Septic shock. Vet Clin North Am 1989; 19:1239–1258
52. Burri C: Posttraumatic Osteomyelitis. Bern: Hans Huber, 1975
53. Bright RM, Probst CW: Management of superficial skin wounds. In Slatter DH (ed): Textbook of Small Animal Surgery. Philadelphia: WB Saunders, 1985, pp 431–443
54. Swaim SF, Henderson RA: Wound lavage solutions. In Swaim SF (ed): Small Animal Wound Management. Philadelphia: Lea & Febiger, 1990, pp 44–47
55. Kahn DS, Pritzker KPH: The pathophysiology of bone infection. Clin Orthop 1973; 96:12
56. Cierney G, Mader JT: Adult chronic osteomyelitis. Orthopedics 1984; 7:1557–1564
57. Fox SM: Cancellous bone grafting in the dog: An overview. J Am Anim Hosp Assoc 1984; 20:840–848
58. Stevenson S: Bone grafting. In Slatter DH (ed): Textbook of Small Animal Surgery. Philadelphia: WB Saunders, 1985, pp 2035–2048
59. Bardet JF, Hohn RB, Basinger R: Open drainage and delayed autogenous cancellous bone grafting for treatment of chronic osteomyelitis in dogs and cats. J Am Vet Med Assoc 1983; 183:312–317
60. Kelly PJ, Martin WJ, Coventry MB: Chronic osteomyelitis: II. Treatment with closed irrigation and suction. JAMA 1970; 213:1843–1848
61. Clawson DK, Davis FJ, Hansen ST: Treatment of chronic osteomyelitis with emphasis on closed suction–irrigation technique. Clin Orthop 1973; 96:88–97
62. Fitzgerald RH, Ruttle RE, Arnold PG: Local muscle flaps in the treatment of chronic osteomyelitis. J Bone Joint Surg 1985; 67A:175–185
63. Basher AWP, Presnell KR: Muscle transposition as an aid in covering traumatic tissue defects over the canine tibia. J Am Anim Hosp Assoc 1987; 23:617–628
64. Weinstein MJ, Pavletic MM, Boudrieau RJ: Caudal sartorius muscle flaps in the dog. Vet Surg 1988; 17:203–210
65. Chambers JN, Purinton PT, Moore JL, Allen SW: Treatment of trochanteric ulcers with cranial sartorius and rectus femoris muscle flaps. Vet Surg 1990; 19:424–428
66. Pavletic MM, Kostolich M, Koblik P, Engler S: A comparison of the cutaneous trunci myocutaneous flap and latissimus dorsi myocutaneous flap in the dog. Vet Surg 1987; 16:283–293
67. Kelly PJ, Fitzgerald RH, Cabanela ME, et al: Results of treatment of tibial and femoral osteomyelitis in adults. Clin Orthop 1990; 259:295–303
68. Matthiesen DT: Thoracolumbar spinal fractures/luxations: Surgical management. Compend Contin Educ Pract Vet 1983; 5:867–878
69. Papich MG (ed): Clinical pharmacology. Vet Clin North Am 1988; 18:1141–1182, 1267–1285
70. Budsberg SC, Kemp DT: Antimicrobial distribution and therapeutics in bone. Compend Contin Educ Pract Vet 1990; 12:1758–1763
71. Penwick RC: Use of antimicrobial drugs in surgery. In Slatter DH (ed): Textbook of Small Animal Surgery. Philadelphia: WB Saunders, 1985, pp 52–70
72. Aronson AL, Kirk RW: Antimicrobial drugs. In Ettinger SJ (ed): Textbook of Veterinary Internal Medicine. Philadelphia: WB Saunders, 1983, pp 338–366
73. Neer TM: Clinical pharmacologic features of fluoroquinolone antimicrobial drugs. Am Vet Med Assoc 1988; 193:577–580

74. Aucoin D: The fluoroquinolone antibiotics: Use in companion animal medicine. In Scientific Proceedings, Texas Veterinary Medical Association Annual Meeting, Dallas, Texas, 1990
75. Bahri LE, Blouin A: Fluoroquinolones: A new family of antimicrobials. Compend Contin Educ Vet Pract 1991; 13:1429–1433
76. Hedstrom S: Antibiotic-containing bone cement beads in the treatment of deep muscle and skeletal infections. Acta Orthop Scand 1980; 51:863–869
77. Fitzgerald RH: Experimental osteomyelitis: Description of a canine model and the role of depot administration of antibiotics in the prevention and treatment of sepsis. J Bone Joint Surg 1983; 65A:371–380
78. Wahlig H, Dingledein E, Bergmann R, Reusi K: The release of gentamicin from poly-methylmethacrylate beads. J Bone Joint Surg 1978; 60B:270–275
79. Mackey D, Varlet A, Debeumont D: Antibiotic-loaded plaster of paris pellets: An in vitro study of a possible method of antibiotic therapy in bone infection. Clin Orthop 1988; 167:263–268
80. Finsterbusch A, Weinberg H: Venous perfusion of the limb with antibiotics for osteomyelitis and other chronic infections. J Bone Joint Surg 1972; 54A:1227–1234
81. Finsterbusch A, Argaman M, Sacks T: Bone and joint perfusion with antibiotics in the treatment of experimental staphylococcal infections in rabbits. J Bone Joint Surg 1970; 52A:1424–1432
82. Perry CR, Pearson RL: Local antibiotic delivery in the treatment of bone and joint infections. Clin Orthop 1991; 263:215–226
83. Webster DA, Spadaro JA, Becker RO, Kramer S: Silver anode treatment of chronic osteomyelitis. Clin Orthop 1981; 161:105–114
84. Becker RO, Spadora JA: Treatment of orthopedic infections with electrically generated silver ions. J Bone Joint Surg 1978; 60A:871–881
85. Levvitt L, Fowler JD, Longley M, et al: A developmental model for free vascularized bone transfers in the dog. Vet Surg 1988; 17:194–202
86. Schweitzer VG: Management of chronic staphylococcal osteomyelitis of the temporal bone: The use of hyperbaric oxygen. Henry Ford Hosp Med J 1990; 38:16–20
87. Horgood G, Elkins AD, Hill RK: Hyperbaric oxygen therapy: Mechanism and potential applications. Compend Contin Educ Vet Pract 1990; 12:1589–1597
88. Nichols RL, Condon RE: Prophylactic antibiotics in surgery. In Kagan BM (ed): Antimicrobial Therapy, 3d ed. Philadelphia: WB Saunders, 1980, pp 350–360
89. Edlich RF, Rogers W, Kasper G, et al: Studies in the management of the contaminated wound: I. Optimal time for closure of contaminated open wounds. II. Comparison of resistance to infection of open and closed wounds during healing. Am J Surg 1969; 117:323–329

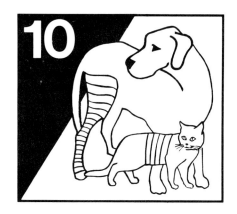

TRAUMATIC, SEPTIC, AND IMMUNE-MEDIATED JOINT DISEASES

SCOTT GUSTAFSON

The inflammatory response in a joint to traumatic, septic, or immune-mediated injury is nonspecific and directly proportional to the degree of insult. Following injury, pathways are activated that cause further synovitis or cartilage injury. Much information has been published on the relationship between inflammatory mediators in joints and the development of degenerative joint disease. From our understanding of the pathways contributing to degenerative joint disease, new treatments are being advocated. Accurate diagnosis and proper management of traumatic, septic, and immune-mediated joint diseases must be based on an understanding of articular pathophysiology.

There is a plethora of information on articular injury. Part of the difficulty in deciphering the information is the lack of a consistent definition of such terms as *osteoarthritis, osteoarthrosis, degenerative joint disease*, and *degenerative arthritis*. Furthermore, does the diagnosis of "degenerative joint disease" listed on the radiographic report mean the same to the attending clinician as it did to the consulting radiologist? The following definitions are interpretations of terms found in the literature.

ARTHRITIS AND ARTHROSIS

The prefix *arthr-* is derived from the Greek word *arthros* meaning "joint." The suffix *-osis* denotes an abnormal or disease condition, whereas *-itis* is an inflammatory disease condition. *Consequently, arthrosis is defined as an abnormal condition or disease of a joint. Arthritis is a disease with an inflammatory component.* A number of words or prefixes may be added to make the definition more specific.

One difficulty in defining *arthritis* arises in deciding which part of the joint is injured and the degree of severity of the injury. For example, does an inflamed synovium (synovitis) constitute a diagnosis of arthritis or must there be concurrent cartilage injury? If synovitis is the major component of the injury and articular cartilage injury is minor, *synovitis* is a more descriptive term. Cartilage injury is a prerequisite for a diagnosis of arthritis, and the damage must be macroscopic and have evidence of fibrillation. The most important prognostic indicator is determination of the reversible or irreversible nature of the lesion.

OSTEOARTHRITIS AND OSTEOARTHROSIS

The prefix *osteo-* ("bone") is frequently added to specify that change is occurring in subchondral or marginal bone concurrently with articular cartilage disease. Joint disease in animals is generally secondary to traumatic, infectious, neoplastic, developmental, metabolic, or immune-mediated disorders. Since there is usually an inflammatory component, the term *osteoarthritis* is frequently used. In much of the older human and veterinary literature, the term *osteoarthrosis* is used, thereby classifying the condition as a noninflammatory joint disease.[1] Older theories of osteoarthritis focused on mild inflammatory changes in the synovial membrane (synovium) and synovial fluid (synovia) and considered them secondary to the degeneration of articular cartilage. More recent theories on the pathophysiology of osteoarthritis include pathways whereby the mildly inflamed synovium augments further injury to articular cartilage.[2] These inflammatory pathways may be causing continuous cartilage degeneration despite nearly complete resolution of pain and inflammation. The term *osteoarthrosis* has also been used previously to describe mild clinical and histologic abnormalities in contrast to severe inflammatory conditions such as rheumatoid or septic arthritis.[3]

Cartilage injury is a major component of osteoarthritis. This inclusion of cartilage injury in the definition is rational because of the intimate physiologic relationship between subchondral bone and articular cartilage. Generalized subchondral bone changes characterized by irregular joint surfaces, sclerosis, and lysis correlate well with cartilage injury.[4, 5] Osteophytes or bone spurs, which occur at the articular margin, are evidence of current or previous inflammation or instability. The presence of marginal osteophytes does not necessarily signify cartilage injury nor does it indicate an active problem. Since the inciting cause may no longer be present and osteophytes may form with reversible cartilage injury, their presence is not sufficient to diagnose osteoarthritis.

DEGENERATIVE JOINT DISEASE

Degenerative joint disease combines the morphologic changes of osteoarthritis with the clinical manifestations of pain, decreased range of motion, and limb or joint dysfunction. The term *degenerative* suggests irreversible and progressive cartilage injury. Consequently, degenerative joint disease is treatable but not curable. In the biomedical literature, *osteoarthritis* and *osteoarthrosis* are listed as synonyms for *degenerative joint disease*.[1]

ARTICULAR STRUCTURE

Diarthrodial joints are composed of the subchondral bone covered by hyaline articular cartilage, a fibrous joint capsule lined with synovium, and a joint cavity filled with fluid. Most diarthrodial joints are supported by ligaments, some have articular synovial fossae, and two joints (femorotibial and temporomandibular) contain menisci.

Articular Cartilage

Hyaline articular cartilage is primarily (70%) composed of water. Of the dry matter, 60% is approximately collagen and 30% is proteoglycan, and the remainder is made up of chondrocytes and lipids. There are relatively few cells (chondrocytes) living in a highly hydrated proteoglycan matrix (Fig. 10–1A). These cells are supported by a collagen framework. The surface is not completely smooth and contains a number of 6-nm–diameter pores that allow water, electrolytes, and small solutes, such as glucose, to pass through. Most of the components of synovial fluid, except for sodium hyaluronate, can diffuse through these pores. Since mature articular cartilage in humans, dogs, cats, and horses does not contain blood vessels, all substances required for chondrocyte function and health must diffuse through the articular surface. Passive diffusion alone is not sufficient for nutrient transport. Joint motion and weight-bearing aid in squeezing some of the matrix fluid into the synovial fluid. Fluid is restored into the matrix by the osmotic pressure generated by the proteoglycan.

The proteoglycan molecule has a molecular weight of approximately 1×10^6 and is composed of numerous glycosaminoglycan chains covalently bound to a central core protein molecule (Fig. 10–2). The glycosaminoglycan chains (50,000 daltons) are composed of repeating subunits of closely related, highly sulfated, polyanionic disaccharides (either chondroitin-4 sulfate, chondroitin-6 sulfate, or keratan sulfate). Without being bound to the proteoglycan, the glycosaminoglycan would diffuse out of the articular cartilage matrix into the synovial fluid. The large number of negative charges on the glycosaminoglycan chains attract water molecules. Large numbers of proteoglycan

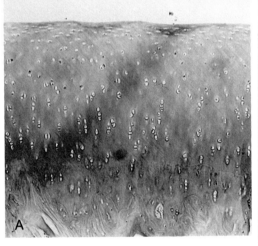
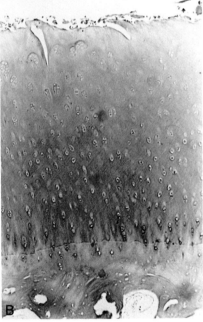

Figure 10–1. *A*, Photomicrograph of normal articular surface of the medial femoral condyle in the canine stifle joint. *B*, Photomicrograph of damaged articular surface of the medial femoral condyle in the canine stifle joint 4 months following repair of a torn cranial cruciate ligament. Disruption of the normal superficial cartilage architecture is evident (Safranin O stain; × 50, courtesy Dr. J. Dupuis).

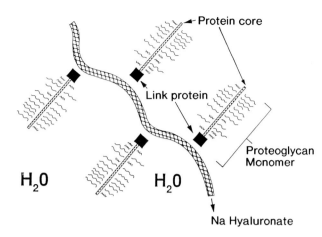

Figure 10–2. Proteoglycan aggregate composed of glycosaminoglycan chains bound to central core proteins that are loosely bound to sodium hyaluronate.

Legend

▨ Na Hyaluronate
▥ Protein Core
〜 Chondroitin Sulfate
∿ Keratan Sulfate
■ Link Protein

molecules are nonconvalently bound to sodium hyaluronate (hyaluronic acid) by hyaluronate binding sites, called *link proteins*, on the end of each central core protein. The resulting proteoglycan aggregate may have a large molecular weight, thus making it relatively immobile within the articular matrix and providing compressive stiffness to cartilage. Sodium hyaluronate is a nonsulfonated glycosaminoglycan with a molecular weight between 5×10^5 and 3×10^6.

Type II collagen provides tensile strength and a framework for the hydrated proteoglycan aggregate. Alpha chains of procollagen are wound into a triple helix, forming a collagen molecule (tropocollagen unit). These units are bundled and cross-linked into collagen fibrils. The orientation of these fibrils is essential for resistance to shear stresses and attachment of cartilage to bone. Type I collagen is the primary type in tendons, ligaments, joint capsules, and the fibrocartilaginous repair tissue for articular cartilage defects. Identification of type II collagen is used as an indicator of how similar the repair tissue is to hyaline (articular) cartilage or fibrocartilage.[6] Fibrocartilaginous repair tissue is less resilient to shear stresses than hyaline cartilage and is, therefore, less desirable.

Chondrocytes are fairly active metabolically despite lacking a direct vascular supply. Proteoglycan and procollagen are synthesized within the cell and exported to the matrix for proteoglycan aggregation and collagen cross-linkage. Chondrocytes synthesize a number of enzymes for intracellular and extracellular use. These endogenous enzymes are often contained in lysosomes and, if released, may attack proteoglycan or collagen molecules. Synovial fluid contains a number of natural enzyme inhibitors; however, their relatively large size often precludes their presence in the articular matrix. The lysosomal enzymes, cathepsin D and B_1, are acid and neutral proteases, respectively, capable of degrading proteoglycan. Acid and alkaline phosphatases, arylsulfatase, metalloproteinases, and lysozyme also may play important roles. Products from the release of lysosomes also contain super-oxide and hydroxyl radicals that are destructive to cell membranes and protein molecules. Collagenase has been isolated from diseased articular cartilage. Although hyaluronidase could be destructive to the proteoglycan aggregate, it has not yet been identified in articular cartilage.

Collagen and chondrocytes change in orientation at different levels within the articular cartilage and are categorized into four characteristic zones (see Fig. 10–1A). The most superficial zone, the *tangential zone*, contains oblong cells and a relatively high concentration of collagen fibrils parallel to the articular surface. Much of the tensile strength of the surface of the articular cartilage is provided by this parallel orientation of collagen and is lost when this layer is damaged. Deep to the tangential zone is the *transitional zone*, which contains a random orientation of cells and fibrils. Collagen orientation is in transition between the horizontally oriented tangential zone and the more vertically oriented collagen fibrils in the deeper *radial zone*. In the radial zone, the cells start to form vertical columns resembling those in the physeal plate of growing long bones. Deep to the radial zone is a *calcified zone* of articular cartilage that conforms with the irregular subchondral bone. This calcified layer is separated from the noncalcified radial zone by a tidemark (visible with most histologic stains) and acts as a buffer between the pliable articular cartilage and stiff subchondral bone. The vertically aligned collagen fibrils traverse from the radial zone through the calcified cartilage and attach firmly in the subchondral bone. The junction between the calcified articular cartilage and the subchondral bone is irregular and strongly resists shear forces.

Subchondral Bone Plate

Subchondral bone is responsible for joint congruity and is the greatest single contributor to shock absorption in the joint.[7] Remodeling of the subchondral bone occurs in response to articular cartilage damage and is characterized by increased bone production (sclerosis) or increased resorption (lysis). These changes may result in decreased shock absorption, decreased support of articular cartilage, or loss of joint congruency.

Synovium (Synovial Membrane)

Synoviocytes (synovial lining cells) have a mesenchymal origin and form a one- to four-cell-layer-thick intima without a detectable basement membrane. Synoviocytes are classified ultrastructurally into types A (macrophage-like) and B (fibroblast-like). The presence of intermediate cells suggests that cell type is a reflection of cell function: phagocytosis, regulation of synovial composition, or self-regeneration.

Synovia (Synovial Fluid)

Synovia is a dialysate of plasma to which hyaluronate produced by syno-viocytes is added. Sodium hyaluronate is a polymer of repeating subunits of nonsulfated glycosaminoglycan produced by either synoviocytes or subintimal fibroblasts. The principal function of hyaluronate is boundary lubrication of the convoluted synovium. It is important to realize that most of the resistance to flexion originates from synovium sliding past synovium and not from cartilage sliding past cartilage.

Fibrous Joint Capsule

The joint capsule attaches firmly to the periosteum and connects to bone via Sharpey's fibers (Fig. 10–3A). Unlike cartilage and synovium, the joint capsule contains nociceptors for detection of pain. The adjacent periosteum also contains nociceptors. Nerve fibers have rarely been identified in subchondral bone.

The joint capsule is not uniform in thickness or composition. Orientation and elasticity of collagen, degree of cellularity, and thickness vary with the biomechanical need for range of motion and support.

TRAUMATIC JOINT DISEASE

There are many forms of trauma. Fractures may directly disrupt the articular surface. Supporting structures can be disrupted partially or completely, producing some degree of luxation. Joints may be subjected to continuous trauma as a result of abnormal conformation or absence of stability. The progression of morphologic changes in response to instability has been described, but the pathways for the development of these changes are not fully understood.[2, 8]

The amount of preexisting articular injury may have a dramatic effect on the clinical signs that develop after a traumatic insult. Traumatized joints with concurrent primary or secondary osteoarthritis may be associated with

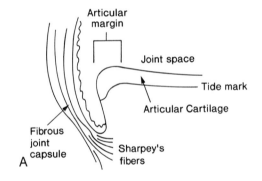

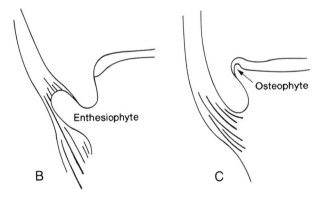

Figure 10–3. Diagrammatic representation of a sagittal section of normal and abnormal articular margin that includes joint capsule, subchondral bone, and articular cartilage. A, Normal articular margin. B, Enthesiophyte. C, Osteophyte.

more pain and prone to more severe injury requiring longer convalescence than normal joints that are traumatized.

Pathogenesis

Traumatic injury may arise from a single episode or repeated joint use with a predisposing biomechanical abnormality (conformational defect). A single traumatic injury may result in direct cartilaginous, bone, or ligamentous damage. Alternatively, "use trauma" may occur as a result of long-term stresses of excessive weight-bearing associated with obesity or strenuous exercise. A house pet often suffers use trauma during excessive participation in normal activities (frisbee chasing, jogging).

Many theories exist concerning the role of trauma in the etiopathogenesis of degenerative joint disease (Fig. 10–4). Some are oversimplifications and others are extrapolations from limited biomechanical or biochemical studies. A basic understanding of the pathways leading to degenerative joint disease will prove useful in choosing the most rational treatment(s) for a patient.

In understanding the pathogenesis of degenerative joint disease, it is convenient to classify the joint into three compartments: cartilage, synovium/joint capsule, and subchondral bone (including articular margin). Each area can be involved primarily or secondarily depending on the disease process.

CARTILAGE

Trauma to articular cartilage may result in chondrocyte damage, tearing of collagen fibrils, or disruption of the articular surface (see Fig. 10–1B). Damaged chondrocytes may have decreased proteoglycan synthesis, libera-

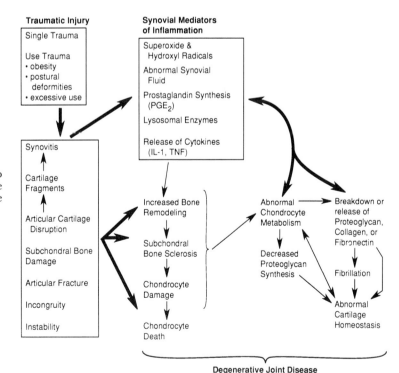

Figure 10–4. The relationship between traumatic injury and the development of degenerative joint disease.

tion of lysosomal enzymes and superoxide and hydroxyl radicals resulting in cellular or matrix damage, release of cytokines [interleukin 1 (Il-1) and tumor necrosis factor β (TNF-β)], or increased synthesis and release of prostaglandin E_2 (PGE$_2$). Interleukin 1 and PGE$_2$ have different chemical structures yet both act to modify chondrocyte activity to become degradative to the matrix. This occurs by release of enzymes which digest glycosaminoglycan, core protein, or collagen. Trauma also may result in intracellular release of lysosomal products directly causing cell death. With matrix degradation, the cartilage loses its ability to resist compressive forces and this results in damage to the supporting collagen network. With loss of collagen, cartilage loses its ability to resist tensile or shear forces and blisters develop. These can lead to superficial and deep fibrillation. With lack of support, further chondrocyte damage occurs and results in subsequent loss of matrix. Chondrocytes in damaged cartilage attempt to repair the tissue by increasing their metabolism, and they divide once or twice to form clumps of chondrocytes called *clones*; however, once significant disruption has occurred, repair is relatively ineffective.

Synovitis may develop secondary to this primary articular destruction. This is due to cartilage fragments or cellular enzymes released into the joint fluid and changes in subchondral bone, supporting ligaments, and joint capsule. Cartilage damage also may be an age-related phenomenon. In older animals, the congruity of the joint may become more exact. This increased congruity is due to subchondral bone remodeling during weight-bearing. However, this increased fit may result in increased contact at the joint margin during full range of motion. For example, a shallow ball-and-socket joint has too little congruity and allows trauma to occur through excessive motion. A normal ball-and-socket joint has adequate congruity for stability while preserving the full range of motion. An excessively deep ball-and-socket joint has more exact congruity than an ideal joint, but there is more potential for wear and trauma at the articular margin. The resulting trauma to the cartilage at the articular margin in deep joints may be one basis for osteoarthritis/osis.[9]

SYNOVIUM AND JOINT CAPSULE

Chronic traumatic synovitis and capsulitis result in the release of cellular intermediaries, enzymes, and metabolites from the synoviocytes and leukocytes. These compounds are deleterious to articular cartilage. Recently, much interest has been focused on cellular messengers called *cytokines*. Interleukin 1 and TNF-β released from synoviocytes and monocytes not only potentiate synovitis, but also act on chondrocytes to stimulate release of degradative enzymes and PGE$_2$. Prostaglandin E_2 is also released from synoviocytes and acts on chondrocytes to cause decreased matrix production and matrix degradation. Superoxide and hydroxyl radicals released by polymorphonuclear cells (PMNs) and synoviocytes have the capability to destroy cell membranes of chondrocytes or synoviocytes, depolymerize hyaluronate, cleave core protein, and damage collagen fibrils. Lysosomal enzymes released from synoviocytes also have the capacity to decrease the matrix content of proteoglycan. This secondary loss of cartilage matrix decreases its ability to withstand compressive and tensile forces and may result in a degenerative cascade leading to articular cartilage destruction.

Synovitis also results in the production of an increased volume of synovial fluid with poor quality. Blood flow may be increased to the synovium and capsule, resulting in higher hydrostatic pressure. Inflamed synovium is a poor selective filter of plasma that causes production of a synovial fluid with an increased total protein and fibrinogen content. This enables synovial fluid to clot. Hyaluronate content and the mean molecular weight of the hyaluronate are reduced, which results in less effective boundary lubrication of the synovium. This decreased lubrication may result in more synovitis. Reduced hyaluronate–synovium contact may further decrease the quantity and quality of hyaluronate produced by the synoviocytes. Likewise, the decreased synovium–hyaluronate molecular contact may alter synovial composition by loss of selectivity in filtration based on steric hindrance. Abnormal joint fluid may not entirely meet the metabolic demands of chondrocytes. Chronically inflamed synovium may become hypertrophied or fibrotic, resulting in further synovial fluid changes. Without the presence of normal synovial fluid and synovial membrane, the homeostasis of the chondrocyte ground substance and collagen is adversely affected.

Joint capsule inflammation and disruption also may occur secondary to trauma. Pain and lack of stability may result in cartilage injury through abnormal joint loading. In an attempt to heal capsular injury or restabilize the joint, the joint capsule may fibrose and result in a decreased range of motion. Trauma also may result in tearing at the bone–joint capsule–periosteal interface, resulting in bone proliferation or enthesiophyte formation (see Fig. 10–3B). This differs from formation of osteophytes, which develop at the articular margin within the joint.

SUBCHONDRAL BONE

Subchondral bone may play a role in the health of the overlying articular cartilage. Because of the shock-absorptive capabilities of subchondral bone, microfractures may occur which, when healed, result in increased stiffness. This increased stiffness may result in decreased shock absorption and increased stress on the articular cartilage. Eventually, large areas of focal or generalized subchondral sclerosis may lead to articular cartilage damage progressing to osteoarthritis.

Increased stress on the subchondral bone at the articular margin from instability or cartilage injury may result in osteophyte formation (see Fig. 10–3C). Cytokines, prostaglandins, and breakdown products of articular cartilage also may stimulate marginal endochondral ossification leading to the development of osteophytes. This new bone formation occurs below the tidemark at the articular margin and not between the cartilage surfaces.

Classification, Diagnosis, and Treatment

Regardless of the type of trauma, the goal of treatment is to return the joint, biomechanically and physiologically, to a near-normal state and prevent degenerative joint disease. The presence of preexisting degenerative joint disease will complicate recovery. In order for treatment to be effective, a diagnosis must be made. In general, the following diagnostic categories are useful.

POSTURAL OR CONFORMATIONAL DEFECTS

Many animals with abnormal weight-bearing or abnormal joint surface angulation have repeated trauma to a joint. Abnormally excessive weight-bearing may be due to an injury in the contralateral limb. When possible, surgical correction of the abnormal angulation or improved weight-bearing in the contralateral limb is indicated. Restricted activity and the judicious use of nonsteroidal anti-inflammatory agents may be beneficial.

Sprain Trauma

Simple sprains are the result of stretching of the joint capsule with varying degrees of capsular disruption and synovitis but without obvious instability. Clinical signs may include lameness, joint pain, warmth, and effusion. The exact degree of anatomic damage may be impossible to determine. Radiographs may contain evidence of joint effusion. There is often poor correlation between radiographic changes and clinical signs.[5] In people, magnetic resonance imaging (MRI) may be the best technique for identifying a soft-tissue injury.[10] Occasionally, intraarticular anesthesia or local infiltration may be necessary to localize the lameness. Mild sprains in which the lameness regresses within hours of injury probably do not result in significant anatomic damage and may only require 1 week of restricted activity.

In moderate sprains, the lameness may persist for a week. There is mild joint capsule tearing. Consequently, palpation for ligamentous laxity and radiographic examination are indicated. Radiographs may contain evidence of preexisting articular pathology. This could alter the prognosis and therapeutic recommendations. Nonsteroidal anti-inflammatory therapy for 3 to 5 days is indicated for the synovitis, along with restricted activity for 3 to 4 weeks.

With severe sprains, clinically significant joint capsule tearing occurs, resulting in a lameness that slowly improves over several weeks. Thorough palpation of the joint while the patient is anesthetized, along with a complete radiographic study, is indicated. Careful scrutiny of the radiographs for fissure fractures, avulsion of a flake of bone with a tendon or joint capsular insertion, or subluxation during stressed views should be performed. Initial treatments include alternating warm and cold packs, support bandages, and nonsteroidal anti-inflammatory drugs. Palpable instability may only become apparent after the resolution of local swelling. Strict rest for 2 to 3 weeks is required for early granulation tissue to form in the capsular defects. This rest is followed by 4 to 6 weeks of restricted exercise, during which maturation and alignment of collagen fibrils occur. Early, excessive activity may result in tearing of this immature collagen and result in increased fibrosis and scar tissue.

Chronic sprains of the same joint may result in decreased range of motion by fibrosis of the joint capsule and adhesions between the plications of the synovial membrane. With forced movements, tearing of these adhesions and fibrotic areas may cause recurring bouts of synovitis and capsulitis. As mentioned previously, cellular intermediaries may be released that have deleterious effects on articular cartilage.

Instability

Palpable instability usually warrants further diagnostics and surgical intervention to correct the anatomic abnormality and arrest progression of the disease. The clinical outcome of the repair is best assessed by palpation and correlates poorly with the later development of radiographic changes. The joint should be examined at the time of surgical stabilization for other problems, such as meniscal damage or tendon or cartilage fragments.

Damaged tissues should be debrided to decrease mechanical and enzymatic sources of further articular injury.

LUXATION OR SUBLUXATION

Diagnosis of a luxation is made by palpation and radiography. A joint may have characteristic directions for a luxation based on disruption of a particular anatomic structure. A specific review may be found in small animal surgery textbooks.[1, 11]

Acute subluxations (incomplete luxations) are treated as a severe sprain and may respond within a week to conservative therapy. The joint must be protected from excessive activity to minimize articular pathology.

Chronic subluxations (greater than 1 week duration) may require extracapsular stabilization or joint capsule imbrication. The temptation exists to wait for fibrous tissue to stabilize the joint; however, this decision depends on the size and expected activity of the patient.

Acute luxations are preferably reduced within the first 48 to 72 hours. In this time, luxations may be reduced with closed technique. After closed reduction, the joint must be palpated for range of motion and stability. It may be necessary to determine if a blood clot or torn joint capsule is preventing complete reduction. Radiographs are obtained (at least two views) to confirm reduction. The joint must then be supported in a non–weight-bearing position for 10 days to 2 weeks, followed by restricted activity for the next 6 to 8 weeks to allow for collagen maturation.

Luxations of greater than 3 days' duration, incompletely reduced luxations, and recurrent luxations must be reduced and stabilized by open repair. During surgery, integrity of the joint capsule, supporting ligaments, and articular cartilage should be evaluated. Appropriate surgical intervention may include debridement of damaged intraarticular ligaments, menisci, or cartilage; replacement or repair of a damaged ligament; imbrication or fortification of the joint capsule; or translocation of a tendon.

FRACTURE

Articular fractures are diagnosed by palpation and radiography. Nondisplaced fractures may not be apparent radiographically until 10 to 14 days after injury. Nondisplaced fractures are generally treated conservatively.

Displaced fractures should be reconstructed as soon as possible, preferably within the first 5 days. The basic principles to follow include (1) accurate anatomic reconstruction of the joint articular surface, (2) even compression of the fracture at the articular surface to provide stability, and (3) avoidance of metallic implant placement through the articular surface. The degree of weight-bearing allowed postoperatively depends on the fracture configuration and stability of repair. Chronic, irreparable articular fractures may require arthrodesis or limb amputation.

Treatments of Degenerative Joint Disease: Current Concepts

Many patients are predisposed to or already have some degree of degenerative joint disease. Much information on well-established and new, potentially useful treatments is being accumulated based on a greater understanding of joint pathobiology. The following sections will review current recommendations for these treatments.

SUPPORT, WEIGHT REDUCTION, HEAT, MASSAGE, AND PHYSICAL THERAPY

Supportive care (e.g., padded bandage, Robert Jones bandage, cast) and weight reduction, when appropriate, are important adjuncts to successful management of degenerative joint disease. Topical heat (warm towels) and local massage may decrease soft-tissue pain associated with degenerative joints (see Chap. 17). Deep-heating therapeutic ultrasound machines are utilized in human and equine patients with variable degrees of success. Range-of-motion exercises and continuous passive motion have been shown to improve the healing of articular cartilage defects.[12]

JOINT LAVAGE

Joint lavage, using warm lactated Ringer's solution or saline, may be used to temporarily remove degradative enzymes, cellular debris, and inflammatory mediators from the synovial cavity.[13] This removal will decrease the degree of synovitis and result in restoration of synovial fluid of more normal quality. Joint lavage is frequently performed during joint surgery (especially arthroscopy), and can also be used in severe cases of traumatic arthritis.

NONSTEROIDAL ANTI-INFLAMMATORY DRUGS

Nonsteroidal anti-inflamatory drugs (NSAIDs) have analgesic and anti-inflammatory properties. Indepth reviews of their pharmacologic and pharmacokinetic properties are available.[14] They are the most widely used class of drugs in the treatment of degenerative joint disease in companion animals. The basic mechanism of action is inhibition of prostaglandin synthetase enzyme within the cyclooxygenase pathway of prostaglandin and prostacyclin synthesis from arachidonic acid (Fig. 10–5). By decreasing production of prostaglandins, most notably PGE_2, NSAIDs may decrease the resultant negative effects that prostaglandins have on articular cartilage in the inflamed joint. In addition to modulating the inflammatory response, prostaglandins sensitize pain receptors to chemical and mechanical stimuli; therefore,

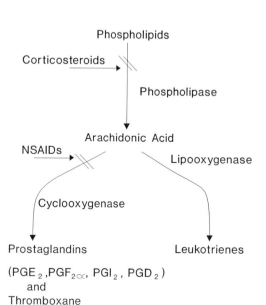

Figure 10–5. A schematic diagram of the metabolism of phospholipids to prostaglandins, thromboxane, and leukotrienes.

NSAIDs provide some analgesia.[15] NSAIDs are typically administered systemically but also have been used intraarticularly.

Possible complications from NSAIDs include gastrointestinal tract upset, ulceration, and hemorrhage; nephrotoxicity; and platelet dysfunction. Generally, these toxicities are dose-related and are exacerbated by dehydration or the concurrent use of steroids or other NSAIDs. Consequently, the dose of NSAIDs used should be the lowest effective dose. Feline patients are susceptible to toxicity (owing to their relative lack of glucuronidase), and the use of NSAIDs, other than aspirin, is not recommended.[14]

Aspirin. Aspirin (acetylsalicylic acid) is one of the most commonly used NSAIDs in companion animals. Aspirin is often effective in reducing the inflammatory response associated with traumatic arthritis and degenerative joint disease. Aspirin may have deleterious effects on the cartilage of osteoarthritic humans and animals. Proteoglycan synthesis is depressed by salicylates in osteoarthritic cartilage.[16] This depression of proteoglycan synthesis is probably unrelated to its ability to inhibit prostaglandin synthesis and more directly related to concentration of the drug in synovial fluid. However, the synthesis of prostaglandins in the F series, which may stimulate proteoglycan synthesis, are inhibited by NSAIDs. *Clinically, there is no evidence to indicate that the use of NSAIDs causes progressive articular cartilage destruction, and the benefits of decreased inflammation outweigh the possible risks of decreased proteoglycan synthesis.* In the future, however, other NSAIDs may be used that do not share these potentially deleterious effects on articular cartilage. Aspirin is frequently chosen as a first treatment in dogs because of its efficacy and low occurrence of toxic side effects. The recommended dosage range of aspirin for dogs is 10 mg/kg per 12 hours to 25 mg/kg per 8 hours. The maximum dose to be used in severe cases is 40 mg/kg per 18 hours.[17] The dose of aspirin in cats is 10 mg/kg per 52 hours up to a maximum of 40 mg/kg per 72 hours.[18]

Phenylbutazone. Phenylbutazone is preferred by some veterinarians who subjectively feel that patients have a more profound improvement in clinical signs than with aspirin. Some dogs that develop mild signs of aspirin toxicity are not affected by phenylbutazone. Phenylbutazone has a greater potential for bone marrow supression than other commonly used NSAIDs. The canine dose of phenylbutazone is 10 to 15 mg/kg per 8 hours PO up to a total daily dose of 800 mg.[17]

Ibuprofen or Flunixin Meglumine. Ibuprofen or flunixin meglumine (Banamine) may be used for injuries that are more severe or nonresponsive to aspirin or phenylbutazone. However, owing to their lower therapeutic index, they are not frequently utilized. Specific indications include *short-term use* for treatment of severe local trauma or to allow an animal to become ambulatory to facilitate a neurologic or postoperative musculoskeletal examination.[19] Neither drug is approved for use in the dog. Recommended canine doses of flunixin include: a single dose of 0.5 to 1.0 mg/kg IV or IM, 1.0 mg/kg per 24 hours IV or PO for not more than 3 days, or 0.25 mg/kg per 24 hours IV for not more than 5 days.[20] The suggested dose for ibuprofen is 2 to 3 mg/kg per 12 hours PO.[17]

CORTICOSTEROIDS

Corticosteroids are powerful anti-inflamatory agents. They block the cyclooxygenase and lipooxygenase pathways of arachidonic acid metabolism by inhibiting the phosphorylase enzyme, thereby blocking the conversion of phospholipids to arachidonic acid (see Fig. 10–5). Consequently, in addition to inhibiting prostaglandin and prostacyclin production as done by NSAIDs, corticosteroids inhibit leukotriene synthesis. Corticosteroids stabilize cell membranes and lysosomes, suppress leukocyte superoxide production, block leukocyte kinin production, retard leukocyte migration, and inhibit fibrin deposition and fibrous tissue formation. The pharmacology of corticosteroids is reviewed in more depth elsewhere.[21]

Corticosteroids have been utilized systemically or intraarticularly to treat the clinical signs associated with traumatic arthritis and degenerative joint disease. The systemic use of corticosteroids should be considered carefully because of the risk of gastrointestinal or renal toxicity, immunosuppression, and depression of endogenous glucocorticoid synthesis.[21] There is much debate over the use of intraarticular corticosteroids in the treatment of degenerative joint disease. Intraarticularly, corticosteroids are the most potent anti-inflamatory agents and may give dramatic relief of clinical signs. Multiple injections of intraarticular steroids in dogs, horses, and humans have been anecdotally associated with dramatic articular cartilage destruction and osteoproliferation or "steroid arthropathy." However, there is very little supporting evidence that the corticosteroids specifically induced the rampant destruction of cartilage seen in cases of steroid arthropathy. Intraarticular corticosteroids are used to alleviate the pain and dysfunction of degenerative joint disease in humans.[22] In canine patients, intraarticular medications are infrequently utilized.

Two commonly used glucocorticoids in the treatment of degenerative joint disease in dogs and cats are dexamethasone and prednisone. Recommended doses for prednisone are an initial dose of 1 to 2 mg/kg parenterally followed by 0.5 to 1.0 mg/kg per day PO. Recommended doses for dexamethasone are 0.2 to 0.3 mg/kg given parenterally initially, followed by 0.1 to 0.15 mg/kg per day PO. Both drugs should be reduced to every-other-day dosage regimens as soon as possible.[17]

POLYSULFATED GLYCOSAMINOGLYCAN

Polysulfated glycosaminoglycan (PSGAG) (Adequan) has been used intra-articularly for treatment of degenerative joint disease in people in Europe and equine patients in North America since the early 1980s. PSGAG inhibits the loss of glycosaminoglycan induced by enzymes, most notably metallopro-teinase,[23–25] scavenges free radicals,[26] blocks the inflammatory complement cascade,[27] and stimulates the metabolism of synoviocytes.[28] In addition, PSGAG blocks Il-1–mediated loss of glycosaminoglycan in cartilage tissue culture explants.[29] The *in vivo* use of PSGAG is chondroprotective in monoiodoacetate-mediated articular cartilage injury models of osteoarthritis in dogs and horses.[30, 31] Over the last several years, there has been consider-able interest in intramuscular delivery of PSGAG for treatment of synovitis and degenerative joint disease in dogs, and clinical studies are currently under way to help determine its efficacy and dosage. In experimental models, a dose rate of 4 mg/kg IM twice weekly has been shown to protect cartilage in dogs.[31a] Although PSGAG is currently available for use in the horse, no product is currently licensed in dogs.

SODIUM HYALURONATE

Although intraarticular sodium hyaluronate is beneficial in establishing a more healthy synovial membrane and reducing synovial inflammation and adhesions in horses, there has been little interest in its therapeutic use in dogs.[32] This may be due to its relatively high cost and need for intraarticular administration. Research is currently under way evaluating an intravenously administered hyaluronate product in horses.

SUPEROXIDE DISMUTASE

Superoxide dismutase (Paloscein, Orgotein) is a free-radical scavenger used systemically and intraarticularly to reduce synovial inflammation, cellular damage, and proteoglycan, hyaluronate, and collagen disruptions. These products are used in horses and utilized more frequently prior to the availability of PSGAG.

DIMETHYL SULFOXIDE

Dimethyl sulfoxide (DMSO) (Domoso) has been utilized topically and intraarticularly to decrease soft-tissue inflammation and scavenge free radicals. A 10% solution of DMSO in an articular lavage solution resulted in no pathologic response by articular cartilage in horses.[33] The use of a 10% solution of DMSO by the author to treat cases of traumatic arthritis and septic arthritis in horses produced variable results.

ARTICULAR GRAFTING

There is considerable interest in articular grafting techniques for the replacement of injured articular cartilage because of the limited capacity for repair or regeneration by osteoarthritic cartilage. Although currently there are no small animal clinically applicable techniques, it is a field of possible future promise.

SEPTIC JOINT DISEASE

Bacterial agent(s) associated with septic arthritis may originate from endogenous or exogenous sources. In neonates and juvenile animals, bacteremia may result in bacterial showering of the synovium, physis, or epiphysis. Bacterial colonization and extension into the joint cavity cause joint infection. In most skeletally mature animals, exogenous bacteria are directly deposited into a joint. This inoculation of bacteria may occur from an open joint injury, arthrocentesis, intraarticular injection, open joint surgery, or as a direct extension of local infection. In this section, the focus will be on open joint injuries and postoperative joint infection.

Open Joint Injuries

If open joint injuries can be diagnosed early and managed appropriately, septic arthritis may not develop. In 58 cases of open joint injury in horses diagnosed within 24 hours, 50% of the injuries became infected. In cases diagnosed after 24 hours, 92% became septic.[34]

DIAGNOSIS

Traumatic injuries resulting in wounds near joints must be investigated thoroughly for the possibility of joint involvement. Early after injury, these wounds have varying degrees of foreign material (including bacterial) contamination and tissue trauma. Consequently, clinical signs of pain and inflammation are variable. If infection has not developed and the degree of tissue trauma is not severe, the animal may exhibit minimal or no lameness.

Before focusing on the wound, the entire animal must be examined for the presence of other injuries. Radiographs of the joint may show articular involvement characterized by gas in the joint cavity.[34] The presence of articular fracture, effusion, or foreign bodies also may be determined radiographically. Eighty per cent of equine open joint injuries could be detected on radiographic examination.[34] Examination of the wound begins with clipping the hair over the joint and carefully examining for puncture wounds. Placing a sterile, water-soluble gel over the wound prior to clipping may help decrease the amount of hair deposited in the tissues from clipping. The hair is rinsed from the wound with the gel. The wound is cleansed, lavaged, and debrided. With sterile gloves and a blunt probe, the wound should be examined. Occasionally, radiographic examination with sterile, water-soluble contrast medium injected into a puncture wound may help determine joint involvement.

Arthrocentesis of the joint, from a site distant to the wound, may provide valuable information. First, synovial fluid is collected for cytologic analysis and bacterial culture. Sterile saline may be injected into the joint if sufficient joint fluid cannot be aspirated for laboratory analysis. Further injection of saline will distend the joint capsule if it is intact or leak out of the wound if the joint capsule is damaged. If the joint capsule is torn and saline leaks from the joint, more saline can be injected as a through-and-through lavage agent. Some clinicians add povidone-iodine or chlorhexidine to the lavage solution. Concentrations of chlorhexidine that exceed 0.5% are deleterious to articular cartilage.[35] Since most recent studies support the use of intraarticular antibiotics as adjunctive therapy in bacterial arthritis, and because there are minimal potential side effects, in equine patients, saline infusion is followed by an injection with an antibiotic, generally an aminoglycoside, in an amount not to exceed one systemic dose. The high concentrations achieved with intraarticular aminoglycoside antibiotics will initially far exceed the minimum inhibitory concentration (MIC) for virtually all potential pathogens. Minimum inhibitory concentrations of gentamicin for *Staphylococcus aureus* were exceeded for 36 hours in the equine antebrachiocarpal joint.[36] Despite its acidic pH, intraarticularly administered gentamicin does not result in significant synovitis.[37]

MANAGEMENT

Once synovial samples have been collected for cytologic analyses, bacterial culture, and antimicrobial susceptibility testing, and the joint has been irrigated with saline, systemic antibiotics are used. The antibacterials should be broad-spectrum and started prior to receiving bacterial culture results.

In most cases, the wound should be left open until there is no evidence of sepsis. If the wound is less than 4 hours old, with minimal tissue trauma, the wound margins can be debrided aggressively, and primary closure performed. Primary closure of a contaminated joint may potentiate the development of infection by preventing drainage. Puncture or bite wounds, degloving injuries, and abrading pavement injuries should not be closed early in the treatment process.

The wound should be covered with a sterile absorbent bandage that is changed once to twice daily to decrease the likelihood of retrograde infection.

Immobilization or stabilization with a bandage and splint, or even an external fixator in cases of articular fracture or ligamentous disruption, may enhance granulation of the wound and closure of the joint capsule.

Most open joints, if not infected, will close spontaneously within 5 to 7 days after injury. Prior to closure, granulation tissue will appear pink and healthy, and the volume of fluid in the bandage will decrease. Secondary closure may be appropriate in some joints that do not close by this time. Prior to closure, repeated synovial fluid samples (aspirated from the wound) should appear grossly normal, and clinical signs should be resolving. Joint infection has occurred if synovial fluid becomes copious, purulent, or fibrinous; granulation tissue becomes purple and unhealthy; and the joint becomes swollen and painful. Joint fluid should be analyzed and cultured again, and more aggressive treatment should be instituted.

Septic Arthritis

It is much more desirable to prevent septic arthritis than to treat an infected joint. Most open joint injuries can be managed effectively without the development of bacterial infection. Once the joint becomes infected, it is managed similarly regardless of the cause of injury. The incidence of postoperative septic arthritis following joint surgery in small animal patients is unknown. Since most surgeons monitor their own patients, there is a tendency to hope that excessive inflammation is not due to infection.

Two basic principles exist in treating septic arthritis: sterilize the joint and prevent bacterial and enzymatic joint destruction. If sepsis is identified early and treatment instituted, bacterial numbers decrease and joint damage is minimized.

DIAGNOSIS

Definitive diagnosis of septic arthritis is made by bacterial isolation from joint fluid or synovial membrane. Unfortunately, culture results often lag by 12 hours to 3 days from the time of sample collection. Bacteria are recovered from 50% to 70% of synovial fluid samples in humans, dogs, and horses.[38, 39] Studies have differed on the impact of prior antibiotic administration on recovery of the etiologic agent. Since it is imperative to institute early treatment, and because negative culture results are not reliable indicators of noninfection, the diagnosis of septic arthritis is generally based on clinical signs and laboratory data. It may be difficult to distinguish inflammation due to infection from postoperative inflammation.

Clinical signs of an infected joint secondary to bacterial deposition during surgery may be fulminant and develop acutely as early as 12 hours after surgery. Less commonly, signs may be related to a low-grade infection for 1 to 2 weeks before producing dramatic clinical signs.

Infected joints are warm, swollen, and painful. In light-skinned animals, they may appear reddened secondary to increased local blood flow. The joint swelling is often periarticular and intracapsular. Initially, the swelling consists of edema and engorged blood vessels. Effusion causes the intracapsular swelling. Fluid in effusive large joints may be pushed from one side to the other. In deep joints, such as the coxofemoral joint, effusion may be impossible to detect owing to the relatively large amount of tissue overlying the joint. Lameness is often a predominant clinical sign in animals with an infected joint. An initially favorable postoperative progression and weight-bearing followed by a warm, swollen joint with increased lameness and persistent 1 to 2 degree elevation in rectal temperature are signs of infection, and further diagnostics are warranted.

In cases of postoperative infection, early radiographic changes may include periarticular swelling and increased joint space width (effusion). Radiographic changes of osteolysis may occur 1 to 2 weeks after infection. In cases of chronic infection with a sudden onset of severe clinical signs, radiographic changes are likely to be seen. The presence of preexisting radiographic changes, as seen in degenerative joint disease, or rheumatoid arthritis may complicate the interpretation of radiographic changes. In chronic septic arthritis, osteolysis and bony proliferation occur at the articular margin. Joint space width begins to narrow radiographically during weight-bearing as articular cartilage loses compressive stiffness and becomes eroded. Supporting ligaments or their osseous attachments may fail, resulting in radiographic evidence of subluxation.

Synovial fluid analysis is often the most valuable parameter used to establish the diagnosis of septic arthritis. Refractometric estimate of total protein or total solids, total nucleated cell count, and cytologic examination are three parameters of synovial fluid analysis that frequently give strong indications of sepsis.

Refractometric estimates of total protein are imprecise but useful owing to their simplicity. Estimates of total protein may reliably reflect infection. A total protein greater than 3 gm/dl but less than 4 gm/dl may indicate a joint condition with an inflammatory component severe enough that sepsis may be present. In horses, a synovial fluid total protein greater than 4 gm/dl is most consistent with the degree of inflammation associated with an infected joint.[40] There are no published reports of confirmed septic arthritis with total protein estimates of less than 2.5 gm/dl.

Synovial total nucleated cell counts are usually markedly elevated in septic arthritis, with values often exceeding 50,000 to 100,000/μl.[41] However, cell counts as low as 2000 to 3000 may occasionally be observed, especially in neonates, joints injected with medications, or patients with compromised immunity. Consequently, low cellularity of synovial fluid does not rule out septic arthritis unless the total protein is less than 3 gm/dl.

Cytologic examination of synovial fluid samples from septic joints reveals greater than 90% polymorphonuclear cells (neutrophils). These cells are frequently nondegenerate with minimal toxic changes, which is uncharacteristic of neutrophils in septic body cavities. Analysis of sediment from a cytospin of septic joint fluid is rarely necessary because of the cellularity of the fluid. However, a cytospin may increase the chance of finding bacteria. The observation of bacteria confirms the diagnosis of an infected joint. The absence of identifiable bacteria on cytologic examination is common in subsequently confirmed cases of septic arthritis. Evaluation of these slides as "nonseptic" purulent inflammation does not permit confirmation of sepsis, thus leaving the interpretation of sepsis up to the clinician. Rheumatoid arthritis is more common in human beings and may appear similar cytologically. Therefore, human diagnostic laboratories are uncomfortable reporting these cytologies as "consistent with sepsis."

Isolation of a bacterial agent is an important step in the confirmation of sepsis and selection of appropriate antimicrobials. Bacterial isolation may be performed using synovial fluid or synovial membrane samples. These samples may be collected via aspiration (arthrocentesis) or during exploratory surgery (arthrotomy or arthroscopy). There are two basic methods for recovering bacterial isolates: inoculation of blood agar plates and inoculation into brain–heart infusion broth blood culture bottles. Direct inoculation of synovial fluid onto blood agar plates may result in earlier growth and lead to higher rates of isolation than sending transport swabs long distances to a microbiology laboratory. If sufficient fluid is present, it is prudent to use both plates and blood culture bottles.

Brain–heart infusion broth blood culture bottles contain *para*-aminobenzoic acid (PABA), 0.1% agar, vitamin K, hemin, CO_2, and sodium polyanetholesulfonate (SPS, Fisher Diagnostics, Orangeburg, N.Y.). In addition to providing an excellent medium for bacterial growth, relatively large samples of synovia with proportionately greater numbers of bacteria are inoculated into blood culture bottles compared with agar plates, thus increasing the chance for bacterial isolation.[42] Synovial fluid containing endogenous (complement, enzymes, antibodies) and exogenous (antibiotics) factors that inhibit bacterial growth is also diluted by blood culture bottles. Consequently, preexisting synovial fluid concentrations of antibacterial substances may be diluted in the broth to levels below their effective concentrations. Contaminants may grow in blood culture bottles to mask a pathogenic isolate, so proper technique is essential. Using proper techniques, 50% to 80% of bacterial isolates may be recovered,[35, 38, 43] but up to 15% of cultures from normal sterile joints may result in the growth of contaminants.[44] Significant isolates are typically *Staphylococcus aureus*, *Streptococcus* spp., *Pseudomonas* spp., and various coliforms. *Salmonella, Chlamydia, Mycoplasma,* and anaerobes also have been reported. A recent study in dogs suggests that blood culture bottles inoculated with synovia are more reliable than direct culture of synovial membrane biopsies.[45]

MANAGEMENT

If joint infection is suspected, the following steps should be followed:

1. *Aggressively pursue a diagnosis.* Clinical signs of excessive warmth, pain, and swelling warrant aspiration of joint fluid for analysis and culture. Samples should be collected for culture prior to instituting or changing antibiotic therapy. Septic postoperative joints warrant vigorous treatment and drainage, and are not likely to respond only to a change in antibiotics. Consequently, it is desirable to pursue diagnostics actively, before destruction of articular cartilage occurs while trying one more change in systemic antibiotics. Aspiration may be beneficial in the treatment of infected joints by removing infected joint fluid and enzymes potentially deleterious to articular cartilage.[46] Simple aspiration, combined with systemic antibiotics, was effective in the treatment of 39 of 71 joints of children with septic arthritis.[43] Fibrin accumulations and redundant, swollen, and inflamed synovium may make arthrocentesis extremely difficult and traumatic. In postoperative joints or joints such as the hip which are relatively inaccessible to arthrocentesis, it may be necessary to obtain samples surgically for analysis and culture. Blood culture bottles should be used to maximize the chance for recovery of an etiologic agent. Intraarticular and systemic antibiotics following aspiration of the synovial sample should be considered.

2. *Administer broad-spectrum antibiotics.* In general, systemically administered antibiotics will attain similar levels in synovial fluid to those achieved in plasma. Cephadrine and flucloxacillin administered systemically, however, do

not achieve adequate synovial levels in infected human joints.[47] Sodium ampicillin levels are relatively higher in the synovial fluid of inflamed equine joints than in normal joints.[48] Penicillin and aminoglycoside combinations or certain cephalosporins are appropriate choices for systemic administration. Because of the effect of enrofloxacin on cartilage development, it is only appropriate for use in skeletally mature animals.

Intrasynovially administered antibiotics achieve concentrations in milligrams per milliliter (compared with micrograms per milliliter with systemic administration). In an experimental model of equine septic arthritis using *E. coli*, peak synovial fluid concentrations (4.7 mg/ml) were approximately 1000 times greater than those found in serum (5.1 µg/ml). Twenty-four hours after injection, bacteria could not be isolated in any of the five horses receiving intraarticular unbuffered gentamicin, compared with heavy growth in four of five horses receiving intravenous gentamicin.[49] Consequently, intraarticular antibiotics should be considered in select cases of septic arthritis as an adjunct to systemically administered antibiotics, drainage, lavage, and nonsteroidal anti-inflammatory drugs. Forced regional limb and carpal joint perfusion has recently been described in equines for local antibiotic delivery to infected tissues.[49a, b] After intravenous or intramedullary injection and tight limb bandaging, high antibiotic concentrations were present in infected joints and bones. This treatment protocol may be useful in patients with joint or bone lesions that have poor vascularity.

3. *Nonsteroidal anti-inflammatory drugs are important to reduce pain and inflammation associated with septic arthritis.* The production of some of the mediators of the severe inflammatory response associated with septic arthritis, namely, PGE$_2$, may be blocked by NSAIDs. Consequently, prudent NSAID use may help prevent secondary cartilage damage.

4. *Institute an appropriate drainage technique.* Lavage is frequently used to increase the effectiveness of a drainage technique. Drainage and lavage techniques may be intermittent or continuous. Closed drainage includes needle aspiration, saline distension and aspiration, and through-and-through lavage using needles, catheters, arthroscopic portals, or drainage tubes. Closed drainage techniques are not nearly as effective in preventing fibrin accumulation within the joint.[50] After a few hours, the lavage solution in most closed drainage techniques probably follows the same pathway within the joint and does not effectively irrigate the entire joint. In one series of clinical cases of equine tarsocrural septic arthritis, continuous egress with a soft Silastic catheter was a highly effective treatment. However, most authors and clinical investigators in human and veterinary medicine recommend open drainage via arthrotomy in cases of septic arthritis that do not respond rapidly (within the first 12 to 24 hours) to needle aspiration and antibiotics alone. Open drainage techniques utilize arthrotomy to provide continuous drainage with or without fluid ingress.

Drainage is often the key to successful resolution of any body-cavity infection. Infected joints are no exception. Drainage reduces the pain that accompanies distension of an inflamed joint capsule. Deleterious enzymes, products of the inflammatory response, and fibrin should not be allowed to accumulate within the joint capsule. The potential risk of introduction of bacteria into the joint is of concern with any drainage technique, but it should not intimidate the clinician from providing necessary treatment.

The particular lavage solution utilized is much less important than the volume used. The key is to use a solution that will cause little damage, such as lactated Ringer's solution. DMSO has been utilized as a 5% to 20% solution, in lavage solutions for septic joints, for its antibacterial and anti-inflammatory effects. Experimentally, DMSO has no deleterious effect on articular cartilage. However, when DMSO is mixed with antibiotics (aminoglycosides), an exothermic reaction occurs and this may inactivate the antibiotic. The importance of this potential inactivation is unknown in light of DMSO's antibacterial effects.

5. *Surgically explore and debride infected, devitalized, or necrotic tissue.* A surgical approach to an infected joint may be necessary for collection of fluid or tissue samples, instillation of ingress or egress fluid drainage systems, assessment of articular damage, or debridement of infected and necrotic cartilage, tendon, synovium, or subchondral bone. Areas of osteomyelitis, based on radiographic evidence of subchondral radiolucency, should be curetted to bleeding subchondral bone. Frayed and necrotic ends of tendons or joint capsule margins should be identified and debrided. Accumulations of fibrin may be peeled or scraped away from the synovial membrane. If needed, an attempt can be made to debride as much pyogranulomatous, necrotic, infected synovial membrane as can be visualized. Undermined cartilage flaps should be removed. When debridement has been completed, the joint cavity should be thoroughly irrigated. Based on surgical findings, the joint should be left open (arthrotomy), or opened more widely (after arthroscopy), to ensure adequate drainage. The surgical drainage site should be protected from exogenous contamination with a sterile absorbent wrap and changed often to prevent exudate from soaking through.

6. *Reevaluate the patient's progress.* Septic joints should be monitored frequently for signs of increased or decreased severity. Repeat radiographic examinations may provide useful information. Changes in the character of the joint fluid may warrant repeat synovial fluid analysis with culture and antimicrobial susceptibility. In a resolving infected joint, the granulation tissue surrounding the wound will become pink and healthy, fluid volume will decrease, the joint capsule will spontaneously seal, and the fluid will have serial decreases in total protein and total nucleated cell count. Synovial fluid may clot and trap large quantities of neutrophils, resulting in a dramatic decrease in the apparent total nucleated cell count. This falsely low total nucleated cell count should not be misinterpreted as an indication of improvement of the joint's condition. Antibiotic administration should continue for 3 weeks beyond the successful resolution of clinical signs.

PROGNOSIS

The prognosis for resolution of the infection and painless joint movement depends on the length of time from onset to treatment, duration of treatment, severity of the lesion, and virulence of the bacteria.[51] Often, the most significant prognostic indicator for infected joints and open joint injuries is the length of time before treatment is instituted.[34]

The potential exists for long-term disablement and severe degenerative joint disease. Many intraarticular medications used to treat degenerative joint disease, especially polysulfated glycosaminoglycan, may potentiate infection and should not be used to prevent secondary degenerative cartilage injury when the potential for sepsis exists.[52]

IMMUNE-MEDIATED JOINT DISEASES

Immune-mediated, noninfectious causes of inflammatory joint disease can be classified as erosive and nonerosive. Rheumatoid arthritis is the most common cause of *erosive*, noninfectious arthritis in dogs and humans.[3, 53] Lyme disease also may cause an intraarticular immune reaction resulting in erosive cartilage and degenerate ligamentous and meniscal lesions.[54, 55] Systemic lupus erythematosus (SLE), arthritis associated with chronic infectious diseases, and SLE-like joint disease without serologic evidence of SLE are the most common noninfectious, *nonerosive* inflammatory arthritides.[56] Immune-mediated joint diseases are being recognized frequently in veterinary practice. All these diseases result in synovial fluid parameters similar to those of infectious arthritis, including extremely high numbers of nondegenerate neutrophils and increased total protein concentration.

Rheumatoid Arthritis

The exact cause of rheumatoid arthritis in humans and dogs is unknown. The pathogenesis of rheumatoid arthritis involves formation and deposition of immune complexes in the joint. Rheumatoid factors IgG and IgM, antibodies that have reacted with altered endogenous IgG protein, activate the complement cascade. Large numbers of leukocytes, attracted by products of the complement cascade, enter the joint and phagocytose immune complexes. Lysosomal enzymes and superoxide radicals released by the leukocytes (neutrophils) cause further synovitis and articular cartilage destruction. The inflammatory pathways activated by rheumatoid arthritis are the same pathways involved in osteoarthritis (see Fig. 10–4). The synovial membrane has hypertrophic, inflamed villi. The histologic appearance of the synovial membrane consists of hyperplasia of the intima and subintimal infiltration with lymphocytes and plasma cells.

There are two causes for the articular erosions characteristic of rheumatoid arthritis. First, subchondral deposition of immune complexes and the resultant local inflammatory cascade result in erosion through the articular cartilage. Second, proliferative granulation tissue (pannus) migrating from the synovial membrane at the articular margin invades the subchondral bone and directly resorbs the articular cartilage surface that it covers.

Dogs affected with rheumatoid arthritis have progressive polyarthritis that typically involves small joints of the appendicular skeleton. The clinical signs may include fever, anorexia, depression, and variable degrees of lameness and joint swelling. These signs may wax and wane with the progression of the disease.

The diagnosis of rheumatoid arthritis is not easy to confirm. The American Rheumatism Association recommends that a minimum of 7 of 11 criteria must be recognized for the diagnosis in people[57] (Table 10–1).

Rheumatoid factor can be demonstrated in the serum of 60% to 80% of people with rheumatoid arthritis. This differs from the disease in dogs, where rheumatoid factor may be identified in as few as 30% of suspected cases.[58] Many clinical laboratories use human IgG in the latex particle rheumatoid factor test. This gives poorer results in the dog than tests using canine IgG.[58]

Periarticular subcutaneous nodules are a manifestation of rheumatoid arthritis in 20% of people. In dogs, subcutaneous nodules have not been reported.

TABLE 10–1. Criteria for the Diagnosis of Rheumatoid Arthritis in People

1. Morning stiffness
2. Pain or tenderness on joint motion
3. Soft-tissue or fluid swelling in one or more joints
4. Swelling of another joint
5. Symmetrical onset of joint swelling and symptoms
6. Subcutaneous nodules (periarticular)
7. Radiographic changes typical of rheumatoid arthritis
8. Positive rheumatoid factor test
9. Poor mucin precipitate of synovial fluid
10. Characteristic histologic changes of synovial membrane
11. Characteristic histologic changes in nodules

Source: From Primer of Rheumatic Diseases, 7th ed. New York: American Rheumatism Association, The Arthritis Foundation, 1973.

Radiographic changes consistent with rheumatoid arthritis include periarticular swelling, subchondral bone lysis, marginal articular erosions, and decreased joint space width. Osteoporosis and osteophytes are seen later in the course of the disease.[59]

Treatment of early rheumatoid arthritis is aimed at reducing the inflammatory response. NSAIDs, particularly aspirin, are used. Although salicylates may control the clinical signs of dysfunction, they do not prevent development of secondary degenerative joint disease. Systemic corticosteroids gave temporary improvement in clinical signs in eight dogs but did not arrest progression of the arthritis.[53] Gold salts may be useful in some cases, but there is little available published information. Cytotoxic drugs such as cyclophosphamide and azathioprine may decrease inflammation by limiting the immune response.[60]

Lyme Disease

Musculoskeletal and joint pain are characteristics of Lyme disease in dogs. Lyme disease is caused by the spirochete *Borrelia burgdorferi,* which is primarily transmitted by the tick *Ixodes dammini.* The spirochete causes an immune-mediated response; therefore, clinical signs may involve many systems. Diagnosis is made by analysis of history, clinical signs, and positive antibody titers using ELISA or IFA tests. Treatment is with systemic antibiotics. Tetracyclines, including doxycycline and minocycline, are all effective against *B. burgdorferi* and are the treatment of choice. The most effective beta-lactam antibiotics include ampicillin, amoxicillin, ceftriaxone sodium, and cefotaxime.[61] A prolonged treatment period of 4 weeks should be used to avoid persistent infection. Improvement on antibiotic therapy should be evident within 1 week to 10 days. This fact is helpful in diagnosing Lyme disease (while waiting for the titer results) and may be difficult to interpret if anti-inflammatory drugs are used concurrently.

Systemic Lupus Erythematosus (SLE)

Systemic lupus erythematosus is a type III immune response in which excessive antibodies are deposited in tissues. When deposited in the synovial membrane, these antigen–antibody complexes cause inflammation, activation of the complement cascade, and stimulation of the release of leukotactic factors. The resultant synovitis is responsible for the clinical signs of joint swelling and pain. In contrast to the erosive arthritides, primary radiographic changes are limited to soft tissue. Important laboratory tests include serologic examination for anti-DNA antibodies (ANA titers), lupus erythematosus (LE) cell factor, and direct Coombs' antibody test. Not all dogs with SLE will have positive results with these tests. False-positive results may be obtained in dogs with chronic infectious diseases.

The treatments for SLE are similar to those used for rheumatoid arthritis. Systemic corticosteroids seem to be more efficacious in the treatment of SLE than rheumatoid arthritis.[53, 56]

Arthritis Associated with Chronic Infectious Diseases

Because of chronic antigenic stimulation, excessive antibodies are produced in this condition. These antigen–antibody complexes are deposited in tissues and result in similar pathophysiology and clinical signs as SLE. These cases may have false-positive results to ANA titers, the LE test, and the direct Coombs' antibody test. Consequently, chronic infectious disease must always be ruled out before diagnosing SLE and initiating immunosuppressive therapy. Treatment of the primary condition results in remission of the synovitis.

REFERENCES

1. Brinker WO, Piermattei DM, Flo GL: Handbook of Small Animal Orthopedics and Fracture Management. Philadelphia: WB Saunders, 1990, pp 285–304, 312–340
2. Lipowitz AJ, Wong PL, Stevens JB: Synovial membrane changes after experimental transection of the cranial cruciate ligament in dogs. Am J Vet Res 1985; 46:1166–1170
3. Hollander JL: Introduction into arthritis and the rheumatic diseases. In Hollander JL and McCarty DJ (eds): Arthritis and Allied Conditions. Philadelphia: Lea & Febiger, 1972, pp 3–14
4. Altman RD, Bloch DA, Bole GG, et al: Development of clinical criteria for osteoarthritis. J Rheum 14:3–6, 1987
5. Spector TD, Hart DJ, Huskisson EC: The use of radiographs in assessing the severity of knee osteoarthritis. J Rheumatol 1991; 18:38–39
6. Vachon AM, McIlwraith CW, Keeley FW: Biochemical study of repair of induced osteochondral defects of the distal portion of the radiocarpal bone in horses by use of periosteal autografts. Am J Vet Res 1991; 52:328–332
7. Radin EL, Rose RM: Role of subchondral bone in the initiation and progression of cartilage damage. Clin Orthop 1986; 213:34–40
8. McDevitt C, Gilbertson E, Muir H: An experimental model of osteoarthritis: Early morphological and biochemical changes. J Bone Joint Surg 1977; 59B:24–35
9. Bullough PG: The geometry of diarthrodial joints, its physiologic maintenance and the possible significance of age-related changes in geometry to load distribution and the development of osteoarthritis. Clin Orthop 1981; 156:61–66
10. Martel W, Adler RS, Chan K, et al: Overview: New methods in imaging osteoarthritis. J Rheumatol 1991; 18:32–37
11. Arnoczky SP: Musculoskeletal system. In Slatter DH (ed): Textbook of Small Animal Surgery. Philadelphia: WB Saunders, 1985, pp 1925–2330
12. Salter RB, Bell RS, Keeley FW: The protective effect of continuous passive motion on living articular cartilage in acute septic arthritis. Clin Orthop 1981; 159:223–247
13. McIlwraith CW: Diseases of joints, tendons, ligaments, and related structures. In Stashak TS (ed): Adams' Lameness in Horses, 4th ed. Philadelphia: Lea & Febiger, 1987, pp 339–485
14. Rubin SI, Papich MG: Nonsteroidal anti-inflammatory drugs. In Kirk RW (ed): Current Veterinary Therapy, vol 10. Philadelphia: WB Saunders, 1989, pp 47–54
15. Short CR, Beadle RE: Pharmacology of antiarthritic drugs. Vet Clin North Am (Small Anim Pract) 1978; 8:401–417
16. Palmoski MJ, Colyer RA, Brandt KD: Marked suppression by salicylate of the augmented proteoglycan synthesis in osteoarthritic cartilage. Arthritis Rheum 1980; 23:83–91

17. Moore GA: Degenerative joint disease: Pharmacology and therapeutics of treatment. Vet Med Rep 1990; 2:89–96
18. Table of common drugs: Approximate dosages. In Kirk RW (ed): Current Veterinary Therapy, vol 10. Philadelphia: WB Saunders, 1989, pp 1370–1380
19. Klause SM: Personal communication, 1992
20. Conlon PD: Nonsteroidal drugs used in the treatment of inflammation. Vet Clin North Am (Small Anim Pract) 1988; 6:1115–1131
21. Papich MG, Davis LE: Glucocorticoid therapy. In Kirk RW (ed): Current Veterinary Therapy, vol 10. Philadelphia: WB Saunders, 1989, pp 54–62
22. Gray RB, Gottlieb NM: Intraarticular corticosteroids: An updated assessment. Clin Orthop 1983; 177:235
23. Howell DS, Muniz OE, Carreno MR: Effect of a glycosaminoglycan polysulfonate ester on proteoglycan-degrading enzyme activity in an animal model of osteoarthritis. In Otterness I, Lewis A, Capetola R (eds): Advances in Inflammation Research, vol 2. New York: Raven Press, 1986, pp 197–206
24. Verbruggen G, Veys EM, Luyten FP, et al: Some "antiarthritic" properties of an oversulfated glycosaminoglycan in degenerative joint disease. In Willoughby DA, Giroud JP (eds): Inflammation: Mechanisms and Treatment. Baltimore: University Park Press, 1980, pp 183–191
25. Verbruggen G, Veys EM: Influence of sulfated glycosaminoglycan upon proteoglycan metabolism of the synovial lining cells. Acta Rheumatol 1977; 1:75–92
26. Tsuboi I, Matsura T, Shichioo O, Yokoyama M: Effects of glycosaminoglycan on human neutrophil function. Jpn J Inflamm 1988; 3(2):131–135
27. Rashmir-Ravin AM, Coyne CP, Fenwick BW, et al: Inhibition of equine complement activity by polysulfated glycosaminoglycans. Am J Vet Res 1992; 53(1):87–90
28. Glade MJ: Polysulfated glycosaminoglycan accelerates net synthesis of collagen and glycosaminoglycans by arthritic equine cartilage tissues and chondrocytes. Am J Vet Res 1990; 51:779–785
29. Bouakka M, Loyau G, Bocquet J: Effect of a glycosaminoglycan peptide complex (GP-C) on the biosynthesis of proteoglycans in articular chondrocytes treated with interleukin-1. Curr Ther Res 1988; 43:588–599
30. Hannan N, Ghosh P, Bellenger C, Taylor T: Systemic administration of glycosaminoglycan polysulfate (arteparon) provides partial protection of articular cartilage from damage produced by meniscectomy in the canine. J Orthop Res 1987; 5:47–59
31. Yovich JV, Trotter GW, McIlwraith CW, Norrdin RW: Effects of polysulfated glycosaminoglycan on chemical and physical defects in equine articular cartilage. Am J Vet Res 1987; 48(9):1407–1414
31a. McKellar QA, May SA, Lees P: Pharmacology and therapeutics of non-steroidal anti-inflammatory drugs in the dog and cat. J Small Anim Pract 1991; 32:225–235
32. Rose RJ: The intraarticular use of sodium hyaluronate for the treatment of osteoarthrosis in the horse. NZ Vet J 1979; 27:5–8
33. Adair HS, Goble DO, Vanhooser SL, et al: Intraarticular lavage using dimethyl sulfoxide in the clinically normal equine (abstract). Vet Surg 1989; 18:72
34. Gibson KT, McIlwraith CW, Turner AS, et al: Open joint injuries in horses: 58 cases. J Am Vet Med Assoc 1989; 194:396–404
35. Bertone AL, McIlwraith CW, Jones RL, et al: Povidone-iodine lavage treatment of experimentally induced equine infectious arthritis. Am J Vet Res 1987; 48:712–715
36. Lloyd KC, Stover SM, Pascoe JR, et al: Plasma and synovial fluid concentrations of gentamicin in horses after intraarticular administration of buffered and unbuffered gentamicin. Am J Vet Res 1988; 49:644–649
37. Lloyd KC, Stover SM, Pascoe JR, et al: Effect of gentamicin sulfate and bicarbonate on the synovium of clinically normal equine antebrachiocarpal joints. Am J Vet Res 1988; 49:650–657
38. Koch DB: Management of infectious arthritis in the horse. Comp Contin Educ Pract Vet 1979; 1:S45–S50
39. Brown SG: Infectious arthritis and wounds of joints. Vet Clin North Am 1978; 8:501–510
40. Gustafson SB, McIlwraith CW, Jones RL, Dixon-White HE: Further investigations into the potentiation of infection by intraarticular injection of polysulfated glycosaminoglycan and the effect of filtration and intraarticular injection of amikacin. Am J Vet Res 1989; 50:2018–2022
41. Werner LL: Arthrocentesis and joint fluid analysis: Diagnostic applications in joint diseases of small animals. Comp Contin Educ Pract Vet 1979; 1:855–862
42. Von Essen R, Holtta A: Improved method of isolating bacteria from joint fluids by the use of blood culture bottles. Ann Rheum Dis 1986; 45:454–457
43. Morrey BF, Bianco AJ, Rhodes KH: Septic arthritis in children. Orthop Clin North Am 1975; 6:923–934
44. Gustafson SB: Unpublished data 1988
45. Montgomery RD, Long IR, Milton JL, et al: Comparison of aerobic culturette, synovial

membrane biopsy, and blood culture medium in detection of canine bacterial arthritis. Vet Surg 1989; 18:300–303

46. Rahkoff ES, Burkhalter WE, Mann RJ: Septic arthritis of the wrist. J Bone Joint Surg 1983; 65A:824–828

47. Schurman DJ, Hirshman HP, Nagel DA: Antibiotic penetration of synovial fluid in infected and normal knee joints. Clin Orthop 1978; 136:304–310

48. Firth EC, Klein WR, Nouws JFM, Wensing TH: Effect of induced synovial inflammation on pharmacokinetics of sodium ampicillin and kanamycin sulfate after systemic administration in ponies. J Vet Pharmacol Ther 1988; 11:56–62

49. Lloyd KC, Stover SM, Pascoe JR, Adams P: Synovial fluid pH, cytologic characteristics, and gentamicin concentration after intraarticular administration of the drug in an experimental model of infectious arthritis in horses. Am J Vet Res 1990; 51(9):1363–1369

49a. Whitehair KJ, Blevins WE, Fessler JF, et al: Regional perfusion of the equine carpus for antibiotic delivery. Vet Surg 1992; 21:279–285

49b. Whitehair KJ, Adams SB, Parker JE, et al: Regional limb perfusion with antibiotics in three horses. Vet Surg 1992; 21:286–292

50. Bertone AL, McIlwraith CW, Jones RL, et al: Comparison of various treatments for experimentally induced equine infectious arthritis. Am J Vet Res 1987; 48:519–529

51. Gustafson SB, McIlwraith CW: Intraarticular infection following intraarticular injection of medication: Diagnosis, possible etiologic factors and prevention. In Proceedings of the Annual Meeting of the American Association of Equine Practitioners, 1988, pp 283–289

52. Gustafson SB, McIlwraith CW, Jones RL: Comparison of the effect of polysulfated glycosaminoglycan, corticosteroids, and sodium hyaluronate in the potentiation of a subinfective dose of *Staphylococcus aureus* in the midcarpal joint of horses. Am J Vet Res 1989; 50:2014–2017

53. Pedersen NC, Pool RC, Castles JJ, Weisner K: Noninfectious canine arthritis: Rheumatoid arthritis. J Am Vet Med Assoc 1976; 169:295–303

54. Steere AC: Lyme disease. N Engl J Med 1989; 321:586–596

55. Kornblatt AN, Urband PH, Steere AC: Arthritis caused by *Borrelia burgdorferi* in dogs. J Am Vet Med Assoc 1985; 186:960–964

56. Pedersen NC, Weisner K, Castles JJ, et al: Noninfectious canine arthritis: The inflammatory, nonerosive arthritides. J Am Vet Med Assoc 1976; 169:304–310

57. Primer of the Rheumatic Diseases, 7th ed. New York: American Rheumatism Association, The Arthritis Foundation, 1973

58. Lipowitz AJ, Newton CD: Laboratory parameters of rheumatoid arthritis in the dog: A review. J Am Anim Hosp Assoc 1975; 11:600–606

59. Biery DN, Newton CD: Radiographic appearance of rheumatoid arthritis in the dog. J Am Anim Hosp Assoc 1975; 11:607–612

60. Gilman AG, Rall TW, Nies AS, Taylor P (eds): Goodman and Gilman's The Pharmacological Basis of Therapeutics, 8th ed. New York: Pergamon Press, 1990, pp 1264–1272

61. Luft BJ, Gorevic PD, Halperin JJ, et al: A perspective on the treatment of Lyme borreliosis. Rev Infect Dis 1989; 2(suppl 6):S1518–S1525

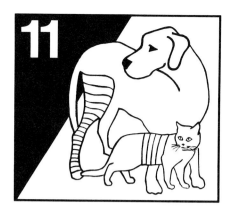

NOSOCOMIAL INFECTIONS

JAMES K. ROUSH

Nosocomial infections are infections not present or incubating at the time of admission to a hospital but develop during hospitalization. These infections may become clinically apparent during hospitalization or shortly after discharge from the hospital. Nosocomial infections include all primary surgical wound infections and secondary remote infections caused by the same organism. Culture of different organisms from a previous site of nosocomial infection should be considered a separate episode of nosocomial infection.[1]

Nosocomial infections are commonly perceived by veterinarians as epidemics caused by organisms from the hospital environment, but they are more frequently caused by endogenous microorganisms that normally comprise the patient's flora. Thirty-five per cent of nosocomial infections are polymicrobial. Single pathogens have been identified less frequently in respiratory tract infections (44%) and surgical wound infections (47%).[2] Urinary tract infections, respiratory infections, surgical wound infections, and bacteremia associated with intravenous (IV) catheters are common veterinary nosocomial infections. While many surgeons refer to postoperative infection as a "complication," each surgical wound infection should be considered an episode of nosocomial infection regardless of the number or type of pathogen. Nosocomial epidemics in veterinary medicine most often involve outbreaks of bacterial diarrheas such as *Salmonella* spp. or *Clostridium perfringens*,[3-5] infectious viral agents such as canine parvovirus or canine distemper,[6] or opportunistic bacteria such as *Klebsiella* spp., *Pseudomonas* spp., *Enterobacter* spp., *Escherichia coli,* or *Serratia* spp.[7]

Nosocomial infections are responsible for increased morbidity, mortality, and cost in human hospitals.[2] Surgical wound infections prolong hospitalization of human patients by an average of 7 days and add thousands of dollars to an average hospital bill.[8] The rate of nosocomial infection in veterinary hospitals has not been well documented but may be similar to human hospitals, in which approximately 5% of hospitalized patients are affected.[2, 9, 10] Three studies in the veterinary literature attempted to document the incidence of nosocomial infection. In one instance, 3 nosocomial infections were found in 183 dogs (1.5%) undergoing surgery in a teaching hospital in 1976–1977.[1] In another, 24 of 677 horses admitted to a university equine clinic developed nosocomial infections with non-*Salmonella* spp. gram-negative bacteria (3.5%).[11] Nosocomial infection in this report was underestimated because infections that developed after release were not included. In another study of surgical wound infection rates in a veterinary teaching hospital, a clean wound infection rate of 2.5% was found in 1100 cats and dogs.[12] Two additional reports describe the occurrence rate of epidemic nosocomial infection outbreaks due to individual organisms. Twenty-three dogs and one cat were identified with nosocomial *Klebsiella* spp. infection in a university veterinary hospital over a 16-month period (0.85% infection among hospitalized dogs for the period).[13] *Salmonella travis* infection occurred in 2% of 833 hospitalized dogs over a 5-month period at another university hospital.[3]

EPIDEMIOLOGY

Development of nosocomial infection requires that a potential pathogen must be transmitted to a susceptible host site. Nosocomial pathogens are commonly endogenous patient microflora that cause disease by entering sterile tissues through anatomic, physiologic, or biochemical defects in the host defenses, or exogenous organisms that colonize body surfaces and cause infection similar to endogenous flora.[2] Rarely, exogenous hospital microflora may directly contaminate body tissues and cause infection. Shortly after admission to a hospital, most animals, especially immunocompromised or terminal animals, become colonized with organisms from the hospital reservoir. The animal then provides the major reservoir of pathogenic nosocomial organisms. Common reservoir sites are the lower intestinal tract, lower urinary tract, and nasopharyngeal area. Colonization of the gastrointestinal tract by antimicrobial-resistant, nosocomial *Klebsiella* spp. organisms is a significant intermediate step in the development of *Klebsiella* spp. nosocomial infection.[14] Coagulase-positive staphylococci have been reported to colonize nasal passages in 19.8% of hospitalized animals.[15] The primary reservoir sites for bacterial organisms found during microbial survey of a small animal surgery room were the upper respiratory tract, digestive tract, and integument.[1] The site of colonization also varies with the organism. Outbreaks caused by *Klebsiella pneumoniae* often are carried in the gastrointestinal tract, whereas *Serratia marcescens* and *Pseudomonas rettgeri* are carried in genitourinary tracts.[16] The hospital, including animals, personnel, and environment, thus provides an excellent ecologic reservoir for a multitude of potential pathogenic organisms.[2] Hospitalized patients are the primary reservoir for multiple resistant pathogens in urinary tract infection outbreaks in humans.[16]

Most recent outbreaks of nosocomial infection are caused by opportunistic bacteria that infrequently cause infections in healthy, nonhospitalized animals. Significant nosocomial pathogens are usually first recognized by veterinarians when they occur as epidemics. These disease outbreaks are usually caused by the same exogenous organism that often has a unique pattern of resistance to antimicrobials. When the incidence of nosocomial infection is low, infections tend to occur sporadically and are caused by a variety of opportunistic or endogenous organisms.[10]

Ninety per cent of nosocomial infections in humans involve four sites: urinary tract, surgical wound, respiratory tract, and circulatory system.[17] The actual prevalence of each site of infection varies and depends on the environment and hospital division under study. In one study that tabulated nosocomial infections by site for patients on surgical services, urinary tract infections accounted for 39%, surgical wound and skin infections 32%, respiratory tract infections 16%, and bacteremia 4% of nosocomial infections.[8] The distribution of nosocomial infection on medicine services in this study was similar, except total surgical infections accounted for only 3% of infections. In a similar study, the most common sites of infection were urinary tract (61%) and respiratory tract (14%), followed by surgical infections and septicemia.[18] In a study of patients in a surgical intensive care unit, urinary tract infections were most common (15%), followed by wound infections (10%), respiratory infections (8%), and bacteremia (8%).[9] During a *Klebsiella* spp. outbreak in a university veterinary hospital, surgical wounds were the most common site of infection (15 of 24 animals), followed by urinary tract infection (6 animals) and septicemia (3 animals).[13]

Transmission

Transmission of nosocomial pathogens occurs through contact between animals, or between hospital staff and animals. Transmission also may occur through contaminated vehicles. Airborne spread of nosocomial pathogens has been reported in human outbreaks of *Legionella* spp. respiratory infections,[19] but airborne spread is unlikely with the nosocomial pathogens common in veterinary medicine.[6] Classic contagious diseases of animals are usually well controlled in veterinary hospitals by immunization, isolation, or clinic hygiene. Colonized and infected animals are the most common sources of nosocomial infections, and, thus, handwashing of hospital personnel between animals and isolation of animals who are reservoirs of nosocomial agents (wound infections, respiratory infections, and so on) is the most important means of transmission control. Transmission of the organisms in seven human nosocomial urinary tract infection epidemics was from patient to patient by the hands of personnel in all outbreaks.[16] Cultures from hands of personnel yielded the epidemic strain in three of the five outbreaks in which such cultures were taken.[16] Clustering of patients in specific rooms was noted in all outbreaks.

Contaminated vehicles are unlikely sources of nosocomial pathogen transmission unless there is a breakdown in aseptic technique, disinfection, or sterilization procedures. Rectal thermometers and stethoscopes have been contaminated with nosocomial strains of *Klebsiella* spp. and should be disinfected between animals.[6] Fluorescein solutions used for diagnosis of corneal abrasions in dogs were sources of *Pseudomonas* spp. which caused penetration of ulcers.[1] *Pseudomonas aeruginosa* has been associated with nosocomial folliculitis outbreaks from physiotherapy pools.[20]

In a large veterinary hospital, 62% of aqueous benzalkonium chloride (0.025%) sponge pots were noted to be a reservoir for *Serratia marcescens,* resulting in contamination of 50% of intravenous catheters over a 1-year period.[21] Chlorhexidine solutions also become contaminated with gram-negative organisms and have been responsible for nosocomial infections.[22] One outbreak of nosocomial *Pseudomonas cepacia* in humans was associated with contamination of rubber tubing in the pharmacy through which deionized water passed during the dilution of chlorhexidine gluconate.[23]

Nosocomial infection epidemics have been associated with intravenous therapy.[17, 24, 25] Contamination of a vacuum system in an IV-additive preparation room was implicated in an outbreak of fungemia where 21% of patients receiving intravenous fluids became infected.[24] In this hospital, medications were added to IV fluids in the pharmacy using sterile techniques under a laminar flow hood.

The general environment of a hospitalized animal is probably the least likely cause of nosocomial infection if a reasonably clean environment is maintained. A study of bacterial flora in a small animal surgery area indicated that routine cleaning of operating room surfaces reduces overall bacterial contamination by 60%, although disinfection "loopholes" such as foot pedals and cabinet tops were found.[1] An 8-day closure of the room subsequently reduces bacterial count by 95%, but this closure is not necessary or useful from a practical standpoint.[1] In animals, transmission of many gram-negative nosocomial organisms is by oral ingestion of feces of infected animals.[4] The primary requirement for prevention of this mode of transmission is removal of organic material in cages and runs through normal cleaning routines.

Risk Factors

Multiple factors may contribute to the risk of nosocomial infection in hospitalized animals (Table 11–1). Risk factors for nosocomial infections can be divided into hospital and individual risk factors, although a few risk factors, such as antimicrobial use, are affected by hospital policy and the needs of the individual patient. When an animal is exposed to more than one risk factor, each additional procedure or exposure appears to increase the risk of nosocomial infection.[16]

Hospital Factors. Factors related to the hospital are the type of hospital, number of personnel in contact with the patient,[6] number of days of hospitalization per patient, and number of days of intensive care support. Nosocomial surgical infections are more likely in municipal (7%) and university hospitals (5.7%) compared with community hospitals (4.3%).[8] The highest rate of nosocomial infections is seen in large referral or teaching institutions.[6] The incidence of nosocomial infections increases with increased length of hospitalization.[6, 8] It is important to release animals as soon as they can be

TABLE 11–1. Risk Factors Associated with Nosocomial Infection

Hospital Factors

Type of hospital
Number of personnel in contact with animal
Average days of hospitalization per animal
Average days of intensive care support per animal
Policies on antibiotics
Policies on use of invasive devices

Individual Factors

Susceptibility to infection

    Age (neonate or aged animal)
    Surgical procedures
    Severe illness (malignant or chronic disease)

Immunosuppressive therapy (chemotherapy or glucocorticoids)
Prolonged hospitalization
Remote infections
Surgical or urinary drains
Use of antimicrobials or invasive devices

given adequate care at home, particularly animals with impaired resistance, those already weakened by a medical condition, or animals recovering from a surgical procedure.[1] The incidence of nosocomial infections increases with increased number of days of preoperative hospitalization and with each additional day of intensive care support. In small animals, the incidence of nocosomial urinary tract infections increased with increased hospitalization in an intensive care unit.[26] Only 1 of 23 dogs with nosocomial *Klebsiella* spp. infection had not been in an intensive care unit (ICU) and catheterized.[13]

Individual Factors. Individual factors that contribute to nosocomial infection include susceptibility to infection, therapy with immunosuppressive agents, prolonged periods of hospitalization (especially preoperative hospitalization), increased severity of illness, preexisting or remote infections, surgical or body cavity drains, and virulence of the nosocomial agent. Individual susceptibility to infection is affected by age (both younger and older animals are more susceptible); malignant, chronic, or debilitating disease; nature of exposure to the agent; and surgical procedures. Host defenses are impaired by steroid or immunosuppressive therapy and by altering normal anatomic barriers with invasive instruments such as catheters and endoscopes.

In a recent report in humans, patients with increased risk of nosocomial infection included older patients and patients with extended preoperative hospitalization, increased duration of surgery, prolonged urinary catheterization, use of steroid or immunosuppressive therapy, and continuous ventilatory support.[2] Patients with extremity injuries are also likely to develop nosocomial infection.[18] While urinary infection rates are 1% to 2% in normal, healthy adults, urinary infection rates may be as high as 10% to 20% in elderly patients, diabetic patients, and patients with significant residual urine in the bladder.[27]

Use of Invasive Devices. Almost half of nosocomial infections in humans are related to invasive procedures or therapies.[9] Invasive devices may increase susceptibility to infection by transgressing natural host defenses. Invasive devices also may be associated with increased risk of nosocomial infections because they act as "markers" or indicators of more serious illness. In a study of the effects of invasive devices in humans, variables associated with increased risk of nosocomial infection included increased duration of urinary catheter placement (>10 days versus 3–10 days), increased number of days in an intensive care unit (3–10 days versus <3 days), "shock" on admission, duration of indwelling arterial lines, and presence of intracranial pressure monitors.[9] When the effects of invasive devices were excluded from the study, the number of days in an ICU, "shock" on admission, administration of corticosteroids or chemotherapy, and creatinine levels greater than 130 μmol/L indicated significant increased risk of nosocomial infection. Arterial pressure transducers have been implicated in human medicine as the site of contamination of *Enterobacter cloacae*, *Pseudomonas aeruginosa*, and *Candida* spp. infections.[8, 28] Intravenous catheter–related infection may be widespread in small animals.[29] Duration of IV catheterization was not a significant factor determining a positive catheter-tip culture in animals, whereas duration of urinary catheterization in the animals developing urinary tract infections (5.78 ± 3.53 days) was significantly longer compared with the noninfected group (2.52 ± 1.12 days).[26] In a large veterinary teaching hospital, 17 of 65 jugular catheters (26%) were positive for infection after an average of 2.70 days in place.[26]

Nosocomial catheter-associated urinary tract infections are frequent in veterinary medicine.[30] In animals, nosocomial urinary tract infections have been related to the use and duration of indwelling urinary catheters.[26] In one report, 11 of 21 animals (52%) developed positive urine bacterial cultures after a mean of 4 days of indwelling catheterization and closed drainage system.[31] The incidence of nosocomial urinary tract infection increased with the duration of catheterization. In another report of 28 animals with indwelling urethral catheters, 9 (32%) developed a nosocomial urinary tract infection.[26] In an experimental study in cats, indwelling urinary catheters were associated with a 60% rate of infection after 5 days of catheterization and may have caused urethral blockage.[32] Combination of perineal urethrostomy with indwelling urinary catheters in this group of cats also increased the incidence of infection and resulted in more mixed infections (39%) than catheterization alone. Nosocomial urinary tract infections of *Klebsiella* spp. in five of six dogs were associated with prior urinary catheterization.[13] Urinary tract infections are more frequent after catheterization in female than in male dogs.[33] Confirmed nosocomial urinary tract infections over a 5-year period at a large veterinary teaching hospital occurred in approximately 1 case per 700 hospital admissions.[34] Total number of nosocomial urinary tract infections was unchanged over the 5-year period, but the number of infections caused by *Klebsiella pneumoniae* declined significantly. In one prospective study, the type of bacteria changed during the urinary catheterization period in six animals, all of which were given antimicrobials.[31] In this study, the bacteria isolated from animals given antimicrobials seemed to become increasingly antimicrobial-resistant.

Inappropriate Antimicrobial Use. Antimicrobial use is a two-edged sword: it prolongs the survival of critically ill animals, yet may result in extended hospitalization and increased risk of nosocomial infection. Antimicrobial treatment is the most important predisposing factor allowing colonization with unusual organisms. In the normal animal, resistance to colonization by potentially pathogenic bacteria occurs through the synergistic action of the host immune defenses and the ubiquitous anaerobic bacterial flora of the digestive tract. Antimicrobials suppress normal enteric flora and increase the risk of colonization of the animal with antimicrobial-resistant opportunistic pathogens.[35] Suppression of normal flora is most damaging when the antimicrobial selectively affects the anaerobic bacterial population, thus providing a new ecologic niche for establishment and proliferation of gram-negative enteric organisms. Antimicrobials can be classified as to their effect on commensal anaerobic flora[7, 14] (Table 11–2).

Inappropriate antimicrobial therapy can lead to antimicrobial resistance of indigenous nosocomial pathogens. In 24 small animals with a nosocomial *Klebsiella* spp. infection in a university veterinary hospital, prophylactic use of antimicrobials increased the risk of infection and antimicrobial resistance of the organism.[13] All the *Klebsiella* isolates were resistant to the antimicrobials used before culture.[13] In a university equine hospital, *Escherichia coli* and *Klebsiella* spp. isolated on day 7 from hospitalized horses were resistant to a significantly higher number of antimicrobials compared with day 1 isolates.[11] In horses not treated with antimicrobials, no significant difference in antimicrobial resistance was found in these organisms. Although spread of antimicrobial resistance through a single strain of nosocomial pathogen can occur, different bacteria with the same resistance pattern are frequently seen in outbreaks of nosocomial infections. Separate outbreaks of nosocomial

TABLE 11–2. Antimicrobial Effects on Host Resistance to Microbial Colonization

Suppress Colonization Resistance

Ampicillin
Cloxacillin
Metronidazole
Furazolidone

Moderately Suppress Colonization Resistance

Amoxicillin
Tetracycline
Chloramphenicol

No Effect on Colonization Resistance

Cephalosporins
Aminoglycosides
Penicillin (parenteral)
Trimethoprim
Sulfonamides
Doxycycline
Erythromycin

Enhance Colonization Resistance

Trimethoprim–sulfamethoxazole
Nalidixic acid
Neomycin (oral)
Polymyxin B (oral)

Source: Data from Jones RJ: Control of nosocomial infections. In Kirk RW (ed): Current Veterinary Therapy IX. Philadelphia: WB Saunders, 1986, pp. 19–24 and Kaufman J: Nosocomial infections: *Klebsiella.* Compend Contin Educ Pract Vet 1984; 6:303–310.

infections caused by *Pseudomonas aeruginosa* and *Serratia marcescens* over a 5-year period in humans were related by transmission of a common plasmid-mediated gentamicin resistance.[36] As previously noted, use of antimicrobials to treat urinary tract infections in animals with indwelling urinary catheters can result in colonization of the urinary tract by opportunistic bacteria.[31]

Surgical Procedures. The surgeon has the primary opportunity and responsibility for control of surgical nosocomial infections by limiting the spread of pathogenic nosocomial organisms and controlling the sources of exposure to the patient. A 10-year prospective study of 62,939 human surgical wounds identified factors that influence wound infection rate (nosocomial infection rate).[10] Overall, 4.7% of these patients became infected, with 1.5% of clean wounds becoming infected. Review of the factors indicated that shaving the operative site, improper skin preparation, increased length of preoperative hospitalization, and increased duration of the operation also increased the rate of nosocomial infections in animals.[10] The type and site of surgery and the presence of surgical implants also increase the risk of nosocomial infection.[2] In animals, bacterial wound contamination is often associated with open fractures and, specifically, radial or tibial fractures.[37] Adequate procedures for surgical preparation and aseptic surgical technique are outlined in many sources.[6, 38]

AGENTS

Any microbial organism is a potential agent for nosocomial infection. These microbes include viruses, *Chlamydia* spp., *mycoplasma* spp., fungi, and protozoa, although bacteria remain the most common nosocomial pathogens. Bacteria most frequently isolated in human nosocomial infections include *Escherichia coli* (21%), *Staphylococcus aureus* (11.5%), group D streptococci (10.1%), *Pseudomonas aeruginosa* (8.8%), *Klebsiella* spp. (8.5%), *Proteus* spp. (8%), *Enterobacter* spp., *Staphylococcus epidermidis,* and *Candida* spp.[2] Nosocomial urinary tract pathogens in a veterinary study included *Mycoplasma canis, Serratia liquefaciens, Enterobacter cloacae, Corynebacterium* spp., *Escherichia coli, Pseudomonas aeruginosa, Proteus mirabilis, Klebsiella pneumoniae, Pasteurella multocida,* and *Streptococcus* spp.[26] Nosocomial epidemic outbreaks in animals are usually associated with a single pathogen. *Serratia marcescens* was isolated from 50% of all contaminated IV catheters from dogs and cats in a large veterinary hospital in one outbreak.[21] Nosocomial diarrhea has been associated with multiple serotypes of enterotoxigenic *Clostridium perfringens* in dogs in a teaching hospital.[5] *Salmonella* spp. and *Klebsiella* spp. have been isolated in several veterinary nosocomial epidemics.[3, 4, 13]

Bacteria involved in nosocomial infections tend to display increasing environmental and antimicrobial resistance.[6, 35] Before antimicrobials were introduced, penicillin-susceptible gram-positive cocci of *Streptococcus* spp. and *Staphylococcus aureus* were the most common infectious agents. The rate of *S. aureus* and *Streptococcus* spp. infections has decreased substantially over time in human and veterinary medicine, infections with *Klebsiella* spp. have slightly declined, and *Serratia marcescens* infections have increased over the past few decades.[8, 14]

The actual prevalence of isolated bacteria depends on the area of infection, coexisting risk factors such as invasive devices, antimicrobial therapy, and aseptic technique. In human urinary tract infections, bacteria isolated were *Klebsiella* spp., *Escherichia coli, Candida* spp. and *Pseudomonas* spp., while in human wound infections, *Candida* spp. were less prevalent and *Klebsiella* spp., *Pseudomonas* spp., and *Serratia* spp. were most prevalent.[9] Seven outbreaks of nosocomial urinary tract infection in humans were associated with three different organisms: *Klebsiella pneumoniae, Serratia marcescens,* and *Proteus rettgeri.*[16]

SURVEILLANCE

Surveillance of hospitalized animals for nosocomial outbreaks should be established to recognize infection, and identify the agent and infection reservoir (Table 11–3). A complete surveillance program should provide for the following:

1. Recognition of an atypical infectious disease problem. Epidemics and clusters of infections must be identified quickly.
2. Timely identification of the agent.
3. Prompt reporting of nosocomial infections.
4. Determination of the endemic level in hospitalized animals.

In most large veterinary institutions, clinical microbiology personnel are often first to recognize an unusual cluster of isolates of a single pathogen. Repeated isolation of bacterial species with a similar antimicrobial resistance pattern may lead to recognition of a nosocomial epidemic or endemic situation.[7] Periodic microbiologic sampling of the hospital environment to monitor the level of contamination is neither cost-effective nor recom-

TABLE 11–3. Nosocomial Surveillance and Control Measures

1. Appoint an infection control officer or committee.
2. Develop written standards for medical asepsis and hospital sanitation.
3. Develop a practical system of surveillance, identification, and accurate reporting of infections.
4. Establish an adequate microbiology service.
5. Educate hospital personnel in hospital asepsis standards.
6. Isolate infected or immunocompromised animals.
7. Eliminate identifiable sources of nosocomial infection.
8. Decrease contact spread of nosocomial organisms:
   a. Proper handwashing techniques.
   b. Monitor sterilization, disinfection of equipment.
   c. Aseptic technique where indicated.
   d. Sterile wound bandaging for open wounds.
   e. Complete, frequent cleaning of environment.
9. Eliminate risk factors:
   a. Periodic review of antimicrobial use.
   b. Change catheters every 48 hours.
   c. Aseptic catheter placement and maintenance.
   d. Closed urinary and surgical wound drainage.
   e. Decrease preoperative hospitalization.

mended,[39, 40] although it has been used to evaluate the effects of cleaning and disinfection in small animal hospitals.[1] Random microbial sampling should be limited to investigation of epidemics caused by a single organism originating from a contaminated object. For effective microbiologic sampling, precise identification of the agent is required and may include biotyping, phage typing, serotyping, and plasmid fingerprinting. Bacteria should be identified to the species level at a minimum. Identification of common resistance patterns may help connect the nosocomial organism to the environmental reservoir.

Hospital equipment is divided into critical, semicritical, and noncritical categories (Table 11–4) for determination of necessary disinfection levels.[6] Microbial sampling of sterilized critical equipment is not necessary if sterilization procedures are adequately monitored by biologic testing. Disinfection of semicritical equipment should kill all live organisms. Semicritical equip-

TABLE 11–4. Categorization of Hospital Equipment for Disinfection

Critical items (devices directly introduced into the body)

Surgical instruments
Intravenous and other internal catheters
Surgical implants
Surgical drains
Intravenous solutions
IV, IM, SC pharmaceuticals

Semicritical items (devices that come in contact with mucous membranes)

Thermometers
Oral and vaginal speculums
Endotracheal tubes
Stethoscopes
Physiotherapy equipment

Noncritical items (environmental surfaces)

Floors, walls
Tables
Cages
Clippers

ment is often inadequately disinfected in veterinary hospitals, and surveillance techniques should be directed to this equipment early in outbreaks of nosocomial infections. Visual inspections are usually an adequate means of evaluation of cleaning and disinfection of noncritical items, and these items do not require additional microbial surveillance. Surveillance for infections in small animals has been reported rarely.[26] Although floor cultures are an excellent method to determine the prevailing bacteria and potential degree of infectivity of the environment, they have limited use in control of nosocomial outbreaks.[41]

CONTROL

Control of nosocomial epidemics and sporadic infections depends on establishment of standard surveillance and reporting procedures and strict adherence to hospital sanitation and protocol (see Table 11–3). Identification of nosocomial infections should not be based on the ability of an individual to perceive a cluster of nosocomial infections, nor should control of the outbreak be dependent on temporary actions by an *ad hoc* group.

Control of nosocomial infections generally consists of eliminating the source of infection, interrupting contact spread of the organisms, and modifying risk factors. Clinic personnel should be educated about hospital protocol or "universal precautions," and this knowledge should be reinforced periodically. One-time educational efforts have little or no effect on modifying behavior leading to universal precaution violations.[42] In some instances, surveillance data may provide a means of control because clean-wound postoperative infection rates often drop when surgeons are informed of their infection rates and the comparative averages of their peers.[10]

The most important aspect of nosocomial infection control is to develop and follow standards of care that prevent introduction of microorganisms into normally sterile body sites and spread of microorganisms between animals. Unfortunately, the demands of daily practice often lead to repeated noncompliance with standard hospital protocols. Infractions of standard universal blood and body fluid precautions occurred in 57% of 549 observed procedures in one human hospital despite the threat of transmission of hepatitis B or human immunodeficiency virus (HIV) to enhance compliance.[42]

Eliminating Infection Sources

The most important factor in eliminating a source of nosocomial pathogens is identification of the outbreak and organism through surveillance mechanisms previously discussed. Identified sources of infection should be discarded, and new procedures for disinfection or sterilization should be instituted for contaminated equipment.[21]

Animals with nosocomial infections or animals that are reservoirs of potential nosocomial organisms should be isolated, and special vigilance should be taken to prevent transmission of nosocomial infection. In addition, immunocompromised animals at risk for development of nosocomial infection should be isolated.[7] Animals with existing nosocomial infections require isolation by mode of transmission rather than individual isolation (isolating the disease, not necessarily the animal). Isolation efforts should be aimed at eliminating routes of microbial exit and entry and fomite transmission of the organisms. Environmental survival of the organism should be considered. Transmission of nosocomial organisms via oral ingestion of feces is easily prevented by diligent cleaning of clinical veterinary facilities. To facilitate cleaning, hospital wards and cages should be constructed from nonporous materials.

Decreasing Contact Spread

Proper handwashing before and after contact with each animal is considered the most important measure to prevent nosocomial infections because many of these infections are caused by organisms transmitted on the hands of personnel.[6, 16, 17, 21, 22] In a survey of hospital protocol infractions, 9% were from absence of handwashing between patients.[42] Handwashing with soap, water, and mechanical friction are sufficient to remove most transiently acquired organisms.[22] Any form of soap is effective, although contaminated liquid soap dispensers have been associated with nosocomial outbreaks.[22] Abrasive scrubbing and irritating antiseptics should be avoided because they dry skin excessively, lead to dermatitis, and thus lessen the desire of hospital personnel to wash their hands frequently.[7] Antiseptic solutions for handwashing should be used before surgery, high-risk invasive procedures, and the care of newborns.[22]

Where disinfectants are needed for semicritical equipment, glutaraldehyde, povidone-iodine, and chlorhexidine are acceptable if fresh solutions are used for disinfection and immediately discarded. Povidone-iodine and chlorhexidine are also acceptable antiseptics for surgical preparation. Hexachlorophene and benzalkonium chloride are unacceptable antiseptics for nosocomial control.[21, 22] Hexachlorophene preparations have minimal activity against gram-negative bacteria and fungi and may even enhance growth of these organisms. *Pseudomonas aeruginosa*, *Serratia marcescens*, and *Alcaligenes faecalis* have been found to grow in these preparations. Benzalkonium chloride products are relatively ineffective antiseptics and are rapidly inactivated by contact with protein, cellulose fibers, and other organic materials.[15, 22] *Pseudomonas* spp. and *Enterobacter* spp. have frequently been isolated from benzalkonium chloride solutions.

Critical, semicritical, and noncritical equipment should be monitored periodically for proper cleansing and disinfection. Critical equipment should be sterilized in an acceptable manner. Sterilization methods (autoclaves and gas sterilizers) should be monitored for proper sterilization with a biologic monitoring device. Semicritical equipment should be disinfected with proper concentrations and contact times with appropriate antiseptics or disinfectants. Closed system drainage should be used for surgical drains and urinary catheters to prevent luminal contamination by environmental organisms.[43] Noncritical equipment requires only routine cleaning and disinfection, concentrating on removal of organic debris. The only special care required during cleaning and disinfection of noncritical areas is cleansing of hidden surfaces.[1]

Controlling Risk Factors

To control nosocomial infections, identified risk factors should be monitored and corrected if possible. Important risk factors associated with surgery

TABLE 11–5. Preventing Nosocomial Surgical Infections

Limit preoperative hospitalization.
Shave animal immediately prior to surgery.
Limit tissue devitalization during surgery.
Reduce intraoperative time.
Make incisions on clean, dry, body surfaces.
Avoid foreign bodies or surgical implants if possible.
Postpone surgery in animals with remote infections.
Provide information about clean-wound infection rates to individual surgeons.

can be controlled easily with attention to surgical preparation and aseptic technique (Table 11–5). Immunocompromised animals should be isolated and treated by separate medical teams to prevent disease transmission to them. Invasive devices, such as intravenous or urinary catheters and surgical drains, should be placed aseptically. Intravenous and urinary catheters should be removed or replaced every 48 hours. Intravenous catheters should not be used to draw blood or administer treatment.[14] Intravenous fluids should be prepared only under the strictest guidelines, and partial bottles of intravenous fluids should be discarded.

Prophylactic antimicrobial use should be monitored and controlled carefully. Prophylactic antimicrobials should be administered prior to likely contamination with the organism and should not be continued beyond the period of contamination. Antimicrobials chosen for prophylactic use against the expected pathogen should be of narrow spectrum, effective against the expected organism, and not affect the normal flora of the patient.[35] Prophylactic antimicrobial use is justified only in animals with a high risk of developing a postoperative infection.[44] Antimicrobials chosen for prophylactic use should be the least expensive, least toxic, and most convenient to administer among the available choices. Oral antimicrobial administration should be avoided for prophylactic antimicrobial use and for administration in intensive care units.

Particular attention to correct dosage and duration of antimicrobial therapy is imperative. Therapeutic antimicrobials should be given beyond clinical recovery to eliminate recurrent infections and development of antimicrobial resistance. Programs to provide education in antimicrobial use by veterinarians should be developed and instituted. These programs should cover antimicrobial pharmacokinetics, pharmacodynamics, selection, indications, and therapy duration.[6] Highly potent bactericidal antimicrobials such as the third-generation cephalosporins should be restricted from general use unless reviewed by the infection control officer.

The high incidence of nosocomial urinary tract infections in small animals mandates special actions for control. Urine specimens for diagnostic purposes should be collected routinely by cystocentesis rather than urinary catheterization. If a urinary catheter is used, aseptic technique is necessary to prevent contamination of the catheter. Indwelling urinary catheters should be connected to a closed drainage system and secured to prevent movement or dislodgment.[14] Prophylactic antimicrobials should not be used because they promote selection of antimicrobial-resistant organisms and development of antimicrobial resistance in existing organisms of the urinary tract.[26, 30, 45]

REFERENCES

1. Bech-Nielsen S: Nosocomial (hospital-acquired) infection in veterinary practice. J Am Vet Med Assoc 1979; 175:1304–1306

2. Jay SJ: Nosocomial infections. Med Clin North Am 1983; 67:1251–1277
3. Ketaren K, Brown J, Shotts EB, et al: Canine salmonellosis in a small animal hospital. J Am Vet Med Assoc 1981; 179:1017–1018
4. Calvert CA: *Salmonella* infections in hospitalized dogs: Epizootiology, diagnosis, and prognosis. J Am Anim Hosp Assoc 1985; 21:499–503
5. Kruth SA, Prescott JF, Welch MK, Brodsky MH: Nosocomial diarrhea associated with enterotoxigenic *Clostridium perfringens* infection in dogs. J Am Vet Med Assoc 1989; 195:331–334
6. McCurnin DM, Jones RL: Principles of surgical asepsis. In Slatter DH (ed): Textbook of Small Animal Surgery. Philadelphia: WB Saunders, 1985, pp 250–261
7. Jones RJ: Control of nosocomial infections. In Kirk RW (ed): Current Veterinary Therapy, vol 9. Philadelphia: WB Saunders, 1986, pp. 19–24
8. Brachman PS, Dan BB, Haley RW, et al: Nosocomial surgical infections: Incidence and cost. Surg Clin North Am 1980; 60:15–25
9. Craven DE, Kunches LM, Lichtenberg DA, et al: Nosocomial infection and fatality in medical and surgical intensive care unit patients. Arch Intern Med 1988; 148:1161–1168
10. Cruse PJE, Foord R: The epidemiology of wound infection. Surg Clin North Am 1980; 60:27–40
11. Koterba A, Torchia J, Silverthorne C, et al: Nosocomial infections and bacterial antibiotic resistance in a university equine hospital. J Am Vet Med Assoc 1986; 189:185–191
12. Vasseur PB, Levy J, Dowd E, Eliot J: Surgical wound infection rates in dogs and cats. Vet Surg 1988; 17:60–64
13. Glickman LT: Veterinary nosocomial (hospital-acquired Klebsiella infections.) J Am Vet Med Assoc 1981; 179:1389–1392
14. Kaufman J: Nosocomial infections: *Klebsiella*. Compend Contin Educ Pract Vet 1984; 6:303–310
15. Silberg SL, Blenden DC, Novick A: Risk of staphylococcic infection among human beings and animals in a veterinary hospital environment. Am J Vet Res 1967; 28:267–273
16. Schaberg DR, Weinstein RA, Stamm WE: Epidemics of nosocomial urinary tract infection caused by multiply resistant gram-negative bacilli: Epidemiology and control. J Infect Dis 1976; 133:363–366
17. Harris AA, Levin S, Trenholme G: Selected aspects of nosocomial infections in the 1980s. Am J Med 1984; 77:3–8
18. Pories SE, Gamelli RL, Mead PB, et al: The epidemiologic features of nosocomial infections in patients with trauma. Arch Surg 1991; 126:97–99
19. Eickhoff TC: Nosocomial infections—A 1980 view: Progress, priorities, and prognosis. Am J Med 1981; 70:381–387
20. Schlech WF, Simonsen N, Sumarah R, Martin RS: Nosocomial outbreak of *Pseudomonas aeruginosa* folliculitis associated with a physiotherapy pool. Can Med Assoc J 1986; 134:909–913
21. Fox JG, Beaucage CM, Folta CA, Thornton GW: Nosocomial transmission of *Serratia marcescens* in a veterinary hospital due to contamination by benzalkonium chloride. J Clin Microbiol 1981; 14:157–160
22. Steere AC, Mallison GF: Handwashing practices for the prevention of nosocomial infections. Ann Intern Med 1975; 83:683–690
23. Sobel JD, Hashman N, Reinherz G, Merzbach D: Nosocomial *Pseudomonas cepacia* infection associated with chlorhexidine contamination. Am J Med 1982; 73:183–186
24. Plouffe JF, Brown DG, Silva J, et al: Nosocomial outbreak of *Candida parapsilosis* fungemia related to intravenous infusions. Arch Intern Med 1977; 137:1686–1689
25. Duma RJ, Warner JF, Dalton HP: Septicemia from intravenous infusions. N Engl J Med 1971; 284:257–260
26. Lippert AC, Fulton RB, Parr AM: Nosocomial infection surveillance in a small animal intensive care unit. J Am Anim Hosp Assoc 1988;24:627–636
27. Kunin CM: Urinary tract infections. Surg Clin North Am 1980; 60:223–231
28. Weinstein RA, Stamm WE, Kramer L, Corey L: Pressure monitoring devices: Overlooked source of nosocomial infection. JAMA 1976; 236:936–938
29. Burrows CF: Inadequate skin preparation as a cause of intravenous catheter-related infection in the dog. J Am Vet Med Assoc 1982; 180:747–749
30. Lees GE, Osborne CA: Urinary tract infections associated with the use and misuse of urinary catheters. Vet Clin North Am 1979; 9:713–727
31. Barsanti JA, Blue J, Edmunds J: Urinary tract infection due to indwelling bladder catheters in dogs and cats. J Am Vet Med Assoc 1985; 187:383–388
32. Smith CW, Schiller AG, Smith AR, et al: Effects of indwelling urinary catheters in male cats. J Am Anim Hosp Assoc 1981; 17:427–433
33. Biertuempfel PH, Ling GV, Ling GA: Urinary tract infection resulting from catheterization in healthy adult dogs. J Am Vet Med Assoc 1981; 178:989–991
34. Wise LA, Jones RL, Reif JS: Nosocomial canine urinary tract infections in a veterinary teaching hospital (1983–1988). J Am Anim Hosp Assoc 1990; 26:148–152

35. Weinstein RA, Kabins SA: Strategies for prevention and control of multiple drug-resistant nosocomial infection. Am J Med 1981; 70:449–454
36. Rubens CE, Farrar WE, McGee ZA, Schäffner W: Evolution of a plasmid-mediating resistance to multiple antimicrobial agents during a prolonged epidemic of nosocomial infections. J Infect Dis 1981; 143:170–180
37. Stevenson S, Olmstead ML, Kowalski J. Bacterial culturing for prediction of postoperative complications following open fracture repair in small animals. Vet Surg 1986; 15:99–102
38. Altemeier WA, Burke JF, Pruitt BA, Sandusky WR (eds): Manual on Control of Infection in Surgical Patients. Philadelphia: Lippincott, 1984
39. Eickhoff TC: Perspectives in hospital infection. In Cundy KR, Ball W (eds): Infection Control in Health Care Facilities: Microbiological Surveillance. Baltimore: University Park Press, 1977, pp 1–9
40. Mallison GF: Monitoring of sterility and environmental sampling in programs for control of nosocomial infections. In Cundy KR, Ball W (eds): Infection Control in Health Care Facilities: Microbiological Surveillance. Baltimore: University Park Press, 1977, pp. 23–31
41. Smith CW, Schiller AG, Smith AR: Monitoring the cleanliness of your surgery room floor. J Am Anim Hosp Assoc 1980; 16:531–532
42. Courington KR, Patterson SL, Howard RJ: Universal precautions are not universally followed. Arch Surg 1991; 126:93–96
43. Alexander JW, Korelitz J, Alexander NS. Prevention of wound infections. Am J Surg 1976; 132:59–63
44. van den Bogaard AEJM: Antimicrobial prophylaxis in veterinary surgery. J Am Vet Med Assoc 1985; 9:990–992
45. Osuna DJ: Postoperative management of urinary tract surgical patients. Compend Contin Educ Pract Vet 1987; 9:873–881

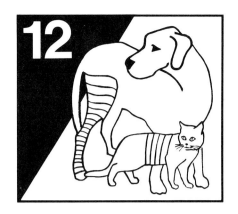

I will prescribe regimen for the good of my patients according to my ability and my judgement and never do harm to anyone.

HIPPOCRATIC OATH

PERIOPERATIVE ANTIBIOTIC THERAPY

JOSEPH HARARI

Perioperative antibiotics are given prior to, during, and after surgery against known or expected pathogens. Antibiotic usage is classified as prophylactic or therapeutic based on timing and goal of the treatment. *Prophylactic antibiotics are administered before the onset of infection, whereas therapeutic antibiotics are used against established infection.*

The basic principles of infection control were proposed by Lister, Pasteur, and Semmelweis in the late 1800s. Recognition of these principles and development of antimicrobial agents in the 1900s have changed surgery from a dreaded event, with infection and death expected, to one that now provides meaningful alleviation of suffering and prolongation of life.[1] Although preoperative prophylactic antibiotics have reduced wound infection rates in some clean and clean-contaminated operations, antibiotic therapy has, in general, often failed to reduce infection rates in people[1, 2] (Table 12–1) for the following reasons:

1. Complex and long procedures are being performed.
2. An increased number of geriatric patients with chronic diseases are being presented for surgery.
3. New procedures involving implants of foreign material have been developed.
4. Concurrent chemotherapy and irradiation may cause suppression of normal host resistance.
5. Drug-resistant, nosocomial pathogens have emerged.
6. Laxity and disregard for surgical principles and aseptic technique still exist.
7. There may be unwarranted reliance on prophylactic antibiotic treatments.

In veterinary medicine, wound infection rates at referral centers have been documented[3, 4] (Table 12–2). Control and reduction of surgical infections at

TABLE 12–1. Wound Infection Rates in People

TYPE OF WOUND	DEFINITION	RATE OF INFECTION
Clean	Atraumatic; no break in asepsis; respiratory, alimentary, or genitourinary tract not entered	<3%
Clean-contaminated	Minor break in asepsis; gastrointestinal or respiratory tract entered without spillage; oropharynx, vagina, or noninfected genitourinary or biliary tract entered	4%
Contaminated	Traumatic wound; major break in asepsis; spillage from gastrointestinal tract; entrance into infected genitourinary or biliary tract	9%

Source: Wenzel RP: Preoperative antibiotic prophylaxis. N Engl J Med 1992; 326:337–339.

teaching hospitals may be difficult due to variability in the quality and quantity of surgeons (students, house officers, and senior clinicians). In private surgical practices, however, infections can be controlled effectively by a combination of proper antibiotic use, recognition of infection sources, and strict adherence to principles and guidelines of proper surgical technique.

This chapter reviews the basis for antibiotic treatments of surgical wound infections. Because of the constant emergence of new drug treatments, however, the reader should review package inserts, product information, and pharmacology texts for current, detailed information regarding specific antimicrobial therapy.

SURGICAL WOUND SEPSIS

Causes of Wound Infection

Occurrence of surgical wound infections depends on a complex interaction between bacteria and host.[5] Most surgical wounds are contaminated with bacteria although progressive growth of pathogens leading to infection is inconsistent.[1] In animals, the origins of bacterial contamination include endogenous skin flora (*Staphylococcus* spp.); environmental sources (soil, hospital equipment); or respiratory, alimentary, and genitourinary tracts.[3]

TABLE 12–2. Wound Infection Rates in Animals

REFERENCE	TYPE OF WOUND	INFECTION RATE
Daly[3] (private referral center)	Clean*	5.7%
	Clean-contaminated	2.5%
	Contaminated	21%
	Dirty	25%
Vasseur et al.[4] (university referral center)	Clean*	2.5%
	Clean-contaminated	4.5%
	Contaminated	5.8%
	Dirty	18.1%

*The majority (>50%) of cases were clean wounds and included neurologic, orthopedic, and soft-tissue surgeries. *Clean* = uninfected, atraumatic wounds, no break in asepsis; *clean-contaminated* = visceral structures and tracts entered with minimal spillage, minor break in asepsis; *contaminated* = traumatic wounds, inflamed visceral structures or tracts entered, major break in asepsis; *dirty* = traumatic wounds more than 4 hours old, perforated viscera, abscessation, and fecal contamination encountered.
Note: Data for the number of animals in each wound category receiving antibiotics are not available.

Proliferation of bacteria and subsequent infection from these sources depend on microbial, local tissue, and systemic patient factors.[1, 3, 5]

Bacterial factors that affect wound sepsis include the number of organisms, virulence, and growth requirements. A dose greater than 10^5 organisms per gram of tissue is usually necessary to initiate infection.[1, 3] Wounds less than 4 to 6 hours old ("golden period") often have bacterial counts smaller than this number and can undergo primary closure.[3] Virulence factors include cell capsule and envelope, toxins, and degradative enzymes (streptokinase, hyaluronidase) that promote dissemination of infection. In addition, recent studies of human orthopedic infections involving *Staphylococcus* spp. and *Escherichia coli* have identified bacterial production of a protective polysaccharide biofilm ("glycocalyx") that protects bacteria from phagocytic cells and antibiotics.[6] This "layer of slime" potentiates deep-seated, chronic infections associated with internal fixation devices, sutures, catheters, and vascular grafts. Bacterial growth requirements are based on tissue oxygenation, available nutrients, and tissue redox potential (oxidation–reduction or the chemical transfer of electrons).[7] Some enteric organisms are facultative and can grow in aerobic or anaerobic conditions. In addition, polymicrobial infections containing aerobic and anaerobic bacteria also can occur.

Local tissue factors may be the most important aspect in the development of wound infection.[1] Reduced tissue viability and vascularity, lack of accurate tissue approximation, hematoma formation, and the presence of a foreign body (metal implants, prostheses, sutures) can deleteriously affect healing and promote bacterial infection.

Systemic patient factors in people that contribute to infection include old age, uremia, vascular collapse, excessive glucocorticosteroid administration, severe trauma, and cancer.[1] These conditions directly affect migration and intracellular killing of bacteria by neutrophils and monocytes. In addition, low serum opsonins, such as complement and antibodies in immunodeficient or chronically malnourished patients, cause an anergic state associated with an increased occurrence of complications and infections.[8]

Prevention of Wound Infections

Prevention of infectious complications is more practical and less expensive than treatment of established infections.[5, 9] Proper antibiotic usage, wound and patient preparation, surgical protocols, and postoperative care can reduce infection and patient morbidity.

Preoperative reduction of bacterial contamination and patient preparation involve avoidance of prolonged hospitalization prior to surgery, hair removal by gentle shaving immediately prior to the operative procedure, and adequate skin preparation with povidone-iodine (0.75% available iodine) or 0.5% chlorhexidine solutions.[1, 10] Contaminated wounds are treated with copious (500–1000 ml) lavage under pressure (35-ml syringe and 19-gauge needle) of a 0.05% chlorhexidine diacetate solution.[10] Aseptic debridement of necrotic tissue and removal of accessible foreign debris also should be performed.

Preoperative surgeon preparations include a 5-minute hand scrub with chlorhexidine or povidone-iodine antiseptic; use of a clean scrub suit, cap, and mask; careful gowning, gloving, and draping procedures; immediate replacement of torn surgical gloves; and limitation of traffic, activity, and talking in the operating room.[1, 10] Instrument preparation requires proper steam or ethylene oxide sterilization. The surgery suite should provide an environment as free of bacterial contamination as possible.[1, 11]

Surgical technique has a profound effect on patient morbidity and mortality in clean and contaminated wounds. The hallmarks of proper surgical technique are based on Halsted's principles and include gentle tissue handling, preservation of vascularity, removal of necrotic tissue, accurate hemostasis (precise and limited use of ligatures or electrocautery), anatomic approximation of tissues without tension, obliteration of dead space (including hematoma and seroma), and strict aseptic technique.[1, 3] In addition, proper technique for treatment of contaminated wounds includes delayed primary closure, use of monofilament nonabsorbable sutures (nylon, polypropylene), and proper tissue drainage.[1]

Postoperative reduction of infection rates is based on many factors. These include ward and patient surveillance for wound infection, adequate patient nutrition, a clean hospital environment, use of sterile dressings and drains, frequent bandage changes, limited use of indwelling urinary and intravascular catheters, and use of antibiotics based on bacterial culture and antimicrobial sensitivity results.[1] Additionally, physical therapy for nonambulatory patients, medicated baths to reduce patient urinary and fecal soiling, and avoidance of prolonged hospitalization are necessary.[1] Careful postoperative patient assessments by physical examination, hematologic (i.e., complete blood counts, serum biochemistry profiles, blood cultures) and radiographic evaluations, and aspiration cytology of suspected infected foci aid in the detection, treatment and, hopefully, reduction of surgical infections.

PROPHYLACTIC ANTIBIOTICS

Orthopedic Surgery

The principles of effective antibiotic prophylaxis are listed in Table 12–3. *In orthopedic patients, this is accomplished by administration of a narrow-spectrum bactericidal drug given intravenously and intramuscularly during induction prior to a prolonged (expected to last more than 3 hours) clean or clean-contaminated surgery.*[12–15] In contaminated and dirty surgeries, infection has already become established as a result of high bacterial concentrations ($>10^5$ bacteria per gram of tissue) or duration of injury (>4 hours), and antibiotic treatment is therefore considered therapeutic. The benefit of antibiotic prophylaxis is lost

TABLE 12–3. Principles of Effective Prophylaxis

1. Antibiotics should be used in procedures with high rates of postoperative sepsis or when the consequences of infection are serious.
2. The antimicrobial agent should be effective against major anticipated contaminating bacterial species.
3. The antibiotic should be nontoxic and inexpensive.
4. The drug should be given immediately prior to surgery to permit absorption and tissue distribution.
5. During surgery, serum and tissue levels of the agent should be maintained above the minimum inhibitory concentration of the contaminating species.
6. Prolonged (postoperative) administration of antibiotics is rarely indicated in clean or clean-contaminated surgery.
7. Postoperative sepsis may be caused by an organism resistant to the prophylactic antibiotic.

Source: Flynn NM: Antimicrobial prophylaxis. Med Clin North Am 1979; 63:1225–1243.

in operations lasting over 3 hours because of increased bacterial growth and drug pharmacokinetic properties (i.e., absorption, distribution, biotransformation, and excretion).[16]

Uncomplicated fracture repair utilizing internal fixation and not expected to last 3 hours would not require prophylactic antibiotic medication unless deleterious local (e.g., severe necrosis or hematoma formation) or systemic (e.g., diabetes mellitus, obesity, immunosuppression, multisystemic organ failure) host factors are present.[17] In a review of infection rates in veterinary orthopedic surgeries lasting less than 90 minutes, no beneficial effect of administering prophylactic antibiotics was noted.[4] In animals undergoing total hip replacement, prophylactic antibiotic coverage is provided regardless of operative time because of the catastrophic consequences of infection.[1, 13, 14, 18, 19]

Administration of antimicrobials intravenously produces rapid inhibitory concentrations of the drug in serum, interstitial fluid, and bone and also leads to rapid excretion. Intramuscular injection provides a sustained serum concentration and high levels in wound fluid because a concentration gradient forces entrance of the antibiotic into the injured area.[20] *Not all authors, however, recommend intramuscular administration of prophylactic antibiotics.*[6, 21, 22] *For prophylaxis to be effective, the antimicrobial must be in the tissues at the time of bacterial contamination (surgery), and dosing should be repeated during prolonged procedures.*[18] Repeat dosing with antibiotics during prolonged orthopedic procedures is based on pharmacokinetic properties of the drug. Recommendations, therefore, involve variable (1–3-hour) drug-related dosage intervals and use of an intravenous bolus.[13, 19, 21–24] Postoperative administration of antibiotics is not beneficial, promotes development of resistant organisms, or causes, rarely, untoward toxicities.[17, 18, 24–26]

Specific prophylactic recommendations for veterinary orthopedic patients have included:[14]

1. Cefazolin, 22 mg/kg, given IV and IM at induction and repeated IV every 3 hours, *or*

2. Oxacillin, 22 mg/kg, given IV and IM at induction and repeated IV every 2 hours.

Cefazolin is a first-generation, semisynthetic cephalosporin with bactericidal activity against gram-positive and gram-negative organisms. Cephalosporins are the most frequently used antibiotics in human surgical procedures.[1] Cefazolin is especially effective against β-lactamase–producing strains of *Staphylococcus aureus* in people and *S. intermedius* in animals. It is also effective against anaerobes except *Bacteroides fragilis*, in which case cefoxitin, a second-generation cephalosporin, can be used.[27] Cefazolin achieves higher concentrations and persists longer in serum and bone than other first-generation cephalosporins.[28, 29] Cephalosporin antibiotics have excellent penetration into bones and joints and are excreted by the kidneys.[17, 28, 29] In dogs undergoing total hip replacement, the mean inhibitory concentration (MIC) of cefazolin against *Staphylococcus* spp. was greatly exceeded by concentrations of the drug in serum, joint capsule, acetabulum, and femur.[19] The mechanism of action of cephalosporins is inhibition of bacterial cell wall synthesis. Side effects in animals are rare and involve gastrointestinal disturbances following oral administration.[28] Another first-generation cephalosporin used in people to control postoperative infections in clean orthopedic procedures is cephalothin.[25]

Oxacillin is a semisynthetic isoxazolyl penicillin with specific bactericidal activity against gram-positive bacteria such as β-lactamase–producing strains of *Staphylococcus aureus* and *intermedius*. As with other penicillins, the mechanism of action is inhibition of bacterial cell wall synthesis. Following intramuscular injection, peak serum concentrations appear in 30 to 60 minutes.[26] Isoxazolyl penicillins are rapidly excreted by the kidney. In people, oxacillin is sometimes used to treat musculoskeletal sepsis caused specifically by β-lactamase–producing strains of *Staphylococcus* and *Streptococcus* spp.[17]

Topical antibiotic agents used during intraoperative irrigation may be effective in preventing orthopedic infection although results of clinical trials are not conclusive.[6, 30] A recommendation, however, has been made for pulsatile lavage with a triple antibiotic solution containing neomycin, polymyxin, and bacitracin, and allowing it to remain in the wound for at least 1 minute.[30] Adverse effects were not reported.

Soft-Tissue Surgery

Cephalothin or cefazolin is given intravenously to people prior to cardiovascular or noncardiac thoracic surgery in an effort to reduce wound infections. This protocol is used in high-risk patients, if infection rates are high, and with cardiac valve or prosthetic material implantation.[25, 32] A similar regimen should probably be followed in veterinary patients.

For clean or clean-contaminated gastrointestinal surgeries, antibiotic prophylaxis involves enteral (intestinal antisepsis) and/or parenteral dosing.[9, 24, 25, 31, 32] Great variation exists in recommended protocols for abdominal operations. Antibiotic drug combinations are sometimes used rather than single-drug therapy because of the heterogeneous nature (e.g., aerobes, anaerobes, gram-positive cocci, gram-negative bacilli) of the intestinal microflora. Conversely, single-dose parenteral regimens using cephalosporins have been considered effective by some surgeons in preventing wound infections in upper bowel and urogenital operations.[9, 24, 32] For colorectal procedures in people, the benefit of adding oral antimicrobials to multiple-drug parenteral prophylactic regimens is unclear.[24, 33] Until definitive studies in veterinary patients are performed, the suggestion to utilize enteral and parenteral regimens for gastrointestinal surgery in animals may be difficult to refute.[31]

Enteral prophylaxis is designed to decrease the number of intestinal microflora during surgery and, therefore, to reduce the chances for contamination of the abdominal cavity or surgical wound.[31] Recommendations in veterinary medicine have included neomycin (25 mg/kg) and erythromycin (2 mg/kg) given orally every 8 hours on the day prior to surgery or metronidazole (30 mg/kg) given orally once a day for 1 to 5 days prior to surgery.[31]

Parenteral prophylaxis is used to produce high blood and tissue antibiotic concentrations to prevent infectious complications. Recommended protocols include:[1, 21, 31]

1. Cefazolin, 22 mg/kg, given IV and IM at induction, *or*
2. Trimethoprim–sulfadiazine, 30 mg/kg, given SC 2 hours prior to surgery, *or*
3. Gentamicin, 4.5 mg/kg, and clindamycin, 10 to 40 mg/kg, given IV at induction.

Neomycin is a bacteriostatic aminoglycoside with a broad spectrum of activity against gram-negative (*Enterobacter* spp., *E. coli, Klebsiella* spp.) and gram-positive (*Staphylococcus* spp. and *Streptococcus* spp.) organisms.[26] Its mechanism of action is inhibition of protein synthesis. The drug is poorly absorbed from the gastrointestinal tract and excretion is by the kidneys. Untoward effects include possible bowel overgrowth with yeasts.

Erythromycin is a macrolide antibiotic that is bacteriostatic or bactericidal depending on the microorganism and concentration of the drug.[26] It inhibits protein synthesis by binding to the 50 S ribosomal subunit of susceptible bacteria. Erythromycin is absorbed from the small intestine and excreted in bile. The drug is active against gram-positive cocci and bacilli, but not against most enteric aerobic gram-negative bacilli and anaerobes.[26] Its usefulness for surgical prophylaxis is limited to gastrointestinal bowel preparation for surgery when used in combination with neomycin. Concurrent administration of neomycin and erythromycin was found to reduce the occurrence of postoperative wound infection in people undergoing bowel surgery.[34]

Metronidazole is a bactericidal imidazole that is active against anaerobic bacteria and protozoa.[35] It has rapid and consistent bactericidal activity against *Bacteroides fragilis*. It inhibits bacterial DNA and nucleic acid synthesis. It diffuses passively into all tissues and body fluids, including bile, bone, abscesses, prostate gland, and vagina. The drug is metabolized by the liver and excreted by the kidneys.

In addition to its use in antibiotic prophylaxis for orthopedic infections, cefazolin is used in abdominal surgeries to prevent infections caused by gram-positive cocci, gram-negative Enterobacteriaceae (*Enterobacter* spp., *E. coli, Klebsiella* spp.) and some anaerobes.[9] Cefoxitin, a second-generation cephalosporin, is considered the most effective cephalosporin against enteric anaerobes, especially *B. fragilis*.[27]

Trimethoprim–sulfadiazine is a bactericidal drug combination used against aerobic gram-positive and gram-negative bacteria. Trimethoprim and sulfonamides have limited activity against anaerobic bacteria.[27] This combination of antimicrobials effectively inhibits bacterial nucleic acid synthesis. Although one veterinary report lists trimethoprim–sulfadiazine for chemoprophylaxis following subcutaneous injection, no clinical references were cited.[31] In people, trimethoprim–sulfamethoxazole has been given intravenously before surgery to prevent wound infections associated with colorectal and biliary operations.[24, 25] The equine veterinary formulation of trimethoprim–sulfadiazine is intended for intravenous administration and is twice the concentration of the canine formulation designed for subcutaneous use. Following parenteral dosing, there is rapid tissue distribution (including cerebral spinal and prostatic fluids), followed by urinary excretion. Trimethoprim achieves higher levels in tissues than in blood. Infrequent adverse effects include aplastic anemia and allergic immune-complex reactions.[36] This drug combination is contraindicated for use in animals with hepatic parenchymal damage.

Gentamicin is a bactericidal aminoglycoside that inhibits bacterial protein synthesis. It is an important agent for treatment of serious gram-negative bacillary infections.[26] Following intravenous injection, there is rapid and wide tissue distribution, followed by renal excretion. Untoward effects include oto- and nephrotoxicity. Extensive use of gentamicin in human hospitals has led to the emergence of antibiotic-resistant bacteria (e.g., *Klebsiella, Proteus, Pseudomonas* spp.).[26] Acquired resistance is most frequently due to drug inactivation by microbial enzymes and should be a concern in veterinary hospitals. Amikacin could be an effective alternative drug because of its resistance to the aminoglycoside-inactivating bacterial enzymes.

Clindamycin is a semisynthetic lincosamide used to treat infections caused by anaerobic bacteria or gram-positive cocci resistant to penicillins and cephalosporins. It has bacteriostatic (inhibition of protein synthesis) effects and can penetrate leukocytes to kill intracellular bacteria. It is degraded by the liver and excreted in bile and urine. Erythromycin and chloramphenicol competitively inhibit the action of clindamycin.[35] The human preparation (Cleocin, Upjohn) is used for parenteral administration.

Topical application of antibiotics during abdominal lavage has been recommended,[1, 31] although conclusive clinical results are lacking. One gram of kanamycin per liter of saline solution is considered an effective adjunct to parenteral antibiotic therapy and proper surgical technique.[1] Although this aminoglycoside may be less toxic than neomycin, its spectrum of activity is more limited than other members of this antibiotic class.[26] Irrigation of the peritoneal cavity with large volumes of aminoglycoside-containing solution can cause substantial systemic absorption and potentiation of previously administered neuromuscular blocking drugs or anesthetic agents in people.[26] This adverse reaction has not been reported in small animal patients, possibly due to the reduced volume and concentration of drugs used in lavage. Topical application of cefazolin (0.2 ml/kg of a 100 gm/L solution) was recently used in a canine soft-tissue wound model (muscle) to provide rapid and high concentrations in wound fluid and serum.[37] It may become useful in clinical cases.

Neurosurgery

Prophylactic antibiotics are indicated for complex and prolonged procedures involving bone plates, screws, pins, cortical bone grafts, or polymethylmethacrylate. Surgeries such as disk fenestration, spinal cord decompression, and fracture/luxation stabilization (simple pin or wiring techniques) would not require prophylactic antibiotic coverage unless severe tissue trauma and hematoma formation occur or the operation lasts more than 3 hours. In a recent retrospective review of wound complications following thoracolumbar laminectomies, prolonged procedures were associated with a higher incidence of complications compared with shorter operations.[38] Not all the complications (skin swelling, dehiscence) involved sepsis, however, and a specific wound infection rate was not reported.

In neurosurgical patients, potential bacterial pathogens arise from the skin and include *S. intermedius*, *Pseudomonas* spp., and *Proteus* spp.[39] For surgical procedures in animals and people, recommended prophylactic antimicrobials given at induction include chloramphenicol (50 mg/kg IV), trimethoprim–sulfamethoxazole (30 mg/kg IV), clindamycin (10–40 mg/kg IV), cefazolin (22 mg/kg IV), and oxacillin (22 mg/kg IV).[18, 25, 39–41] Based on results of clinical trials in people, drug availability, cost, and lack of untoward effects (see chloramphenicol later), cefazolin or, alternatively, oxacillin would be the drug of choice for antibiotic prophylaxis in veterinary neurosurgical procedures.

Chloramphenicol is a broad-spectrum bacteriostatic antibiotic that inhibits bacterial protein synthesis.[36] It is metabolized by the liver and excreted by the kidneys. It is highly lipid soluble and diffuses readily into most tissues, especially cerebrospinal fluid. Because of its bacteriostatic nature, potential for microsomal inhibition, and subsequent prolonged patient recovery from barbiturate anesthesia, the use of chloramphenicol for neurochemoprophylaxis is debatable.

TREATMENT OF ESTABLISHED INFECTION

Therapeutic antibiotics are used for the treatment of established infection and may be considered *empiric* if results of bacterial culture and antimicrobial sensitivity testing are pending or *definitive* if identification of the pathogen(s) and antimicrobial sensitivity have occurred.[21] The goal of therapy is to achieve antibiotic concentrations in plasma (or serum) and at the infection site that exceed by four- to sixfold the minimal inhibitory concentration (MIC) of the drug.[13, 42] This "excess" should provide effective bactericidal activity of the antibiotic.[29]

Prior to initiating therapy, the following questions need to be answered:[43] Is antibiotic treatment necessary? Which antibiotic(s) should be used? How should the drug be given? How often and how long should treatment be performed?

Antimicrobial therapy should be based on clinical assessment (e.g., vital signs, attitude, appetite, defecation/urination, voluntary movements) and laboratory evaluations (e.g., blood cultures, complete blood counts, aspiration cytology and Gram staining, and aerobic/anaerobic bacterial culture and antimicrobial sensitivity assay). Confirmation of disseminated infections (bacteremia) usually requires isolation of a known pathogen (not skin contaminant) from at least two blood samples obtained within a 1- to 2-hour time interval.[36, 44] Gram staining of material from a suspected focus of infection (not superficial drainage) aids in identifying presumptive pathogens and directs antibiotic therapy[23, 27, 28, 31, 35, 36, 46–50] (Tables 12–4 and 12–5). Specimens

TABLE 12–4. Bacteria Involved in Wound Sepsis and Commonly Used Antibiotics[23, 27, 28, 31, 36, 45–48, 50]

BACTERIA	WOUND SITE	ANTIBIOTICS
Aerobes		
Brucella	Vertebral, genital	Tetracycline or doxycycline and streptomycin or gentamicin
E. coli	Bacteremia, enteric, hepatobiliary, orthopedic, peritoneal, urogenital	Neomycin, cefazolin, trimethoprim–sulfonamides
Klebsiella	Bacteremia, enteric, nosocomial	Amoxicillin–clavulanate, cefazolin
Pasteurella	Percutaneous abscess, respiratory	Ampicillin, penicillin
Proteus	Bacteremia, urogenital	Amoxicillin–clavulanate, cefazolin
Pseudomonas	Bacteremia, burns, urinary	Amikacin, ciprofloxacin, enrofloxacin
Salmonella	Bacteremia, nosocomial	Chloramphenicol, trimethoprim–sulfonamides
Staphylococcus	Bacteremia, orthopedic, joints, skin and subcutaneous, urogenital, vertebrae	Amoxicillin–clavulanate, clindamycin, cefazolin, oxacillin
Streptococcus	Bacteremia, joints, urogenital	Penicillin G, ampicillin
Anaerobes		
Actinomyces	Abscesses, pyothorax	Penicillin G, clindamycin
Bacteroides	Abscesses, orthopedic, pyothorax	Clindamycin, metronidazole
Clostridium	Abscesses, bacteremia, orthopedic	Penicillin G, chloramphenicol, metronidazole
Nocardia	Abscesses, pyothorax	Amikacin, sulfonamides

obtained for bacterial isolation should be handled with care according to guidelines from the diagnostic laboratory especially in cases of mixed infections containing anaerobic pathogens. Anaerobic organisms should be suspected in chronic wound infections with a putrid odor, polymicrobial Gram staining characteristics, and poor response to therapy with antibiotics active against aerobic bacteria.[27] Following identification, bacterial sensitivity to antibiotics can be measured by standardized disk diffusion or, preferably, agar or both dilution techniques that yield quantitative data related to MIC. Commercially prepared microtiter plates are also being used in some laboratories.

Although "mild" surgical infections can be treated with oral antibiotics on an outpatient basis, "severe" cases require initial intravenous medication.[1] This is based on an unpredictable gastrointestinal absorption in systemically ill patients and discomfort associated with repeated intramuscular or subcutaneous injections. The duration of therapy is variable and depends on the type of infection (superficial or deep) and the host response.[1, 13] In general, most veterinary surgical infections are treated for 10 to 14 days, although duration of treatment should be based on clinical and laboratory parameters. These include normal temperature for 72 hours, normal white blood cell count, absence of drainage from infected sites, improved mental status, and return of normal bowel and bladder functions.[1]

Failure of antimicrobial therapy is characterized by persistence of abnormal clinical signs and laboratory data, and progressive deterioration of the patient. Causes include superinfection due to emergence of antibiotic-resistant bacteria, inappropriate antibiotic selection, inadequate drug delivery and concentration at the infection site(s), impaired host defense mechanisms, and requirement for adjunctive surgical or medical therapy (e.g., blood transfusion, fluid replacement, debridement, drainage).[1, 13, 45]

TABLE 12–5. Therapeutic Drugs and Dosages in Small Animals for Treatment of Surgical Infections[23, 28, 35, 36, 45, 48–50]

DRUG	DOSAGE (mg/kg) AND ROUTE	DOSAGE INTERVAL (h)
Amikacin	5–11; IM, SC, or IV	8
Amoxicillin	11–22; PO	8–12
	5.5–11; IM, SC, or IV	
Amoxicillin–clavulanate	12.5 (dog); PO	12
	62.5 (total per cat); PO	
Ampicillin	10–50 (dog); PO, IM, SC, or IV	6–8
	10–20 (cat); PO, IM, SC, or IV	
Cefazolin	15–25; IM, SC, or IV	4–8
Chloramphenicol	40–50; PO, IM, or IV	6–8 (dog)
		8–12 (cat)
Clindamycin	11–22; PO, IM, or IV	12
Doxycycline	2.5–5; PO	12–24
Enrofloxacin	2.5; PO, IM, or IV	12
Gentamicin	2–4; IM, SC, or IV	8
Metronidazole	7.5–15; PO or IV	8
Oxacillin	20–40; PO	8
	5–11; IM or IV	
Penicillin	20,000–40,000 U/kg; IM, SC, or IV	6
Oxytetracycline	25; PO	6–8
	7; IM or IV	12
Trimethoprim–sulfadiazine	30; PO or SC	12–24

Therapeutic Antibiotics

Many of the antibiotics (cephalosporins, aminoglycosides, clindamycin, metronidazole, trimethoprim–sulfadiazine) previously described for surgical prophylaxis are also useful in treating established infections. Other commonly used drugs are described next.

Ampicillin and amoxicillin are synthetic aminopenicillins with bactericidal activity against gram-positive, some gram-negative, and some anaerobic bacteria. Addition of a hydroxyl group to the amino benzyl group of ampicillin forms amoxicillin and improves penetration into gram-negative bacteria. The penicillins inhibit bacterial cell wall synthesis. Gastrointestinal absorption of ampicillin is less than that of amoxicillin. Both drugs lack resistance to β-lactamase production by *Staphylococcus* spp. These drugs have wide distribution into interstitial fluids, excluding prostatic fluid and brain tissue, and are excreted by the kidneys.[26] Amoxicillin combined with clavulanic acid (Clavamox, Smith, Kline, and Beecham) has broadened bactericidal activity due to lactamase binding by the acid and is useful against *Enterobacter, Pasteurella,* and *Proteus* spp. A similar combination of ampicillin and sulbactam (Unasyn, Roerig) is used to extend the antibiotic spectrum of the aminopenicillin. Another combination is a semisynthetic penicillin (ticarcillin) and clavulanic acid (Timentin, Smith, Kline, and Beecham). These combinations effectively provide broad-spectrum and β-lactamase inhibition. Penicillins or first-generation cephalosporins are often used in combination with aminoglycosides for synergistic activity against gram-negative enteric organisms.[28, 49] Penicillins are active against most anaerobic bacteria except penicillinase-producing *Bacteroides* spp.

Enrofloxacin and the human equivalent ciprofloxacin are fluoroquinolone antibiotics active against aerobic gram-negative and gram-positive bacteria.[35, 49] They have poor activity against anaerobic bacteria. Quinolones are bactericidal and inhibit bacterial DNA replication. They have rapid and good (including cerebrospinal fluid) tissue distribution and penetrate white blood cells. Quinolones are metabolized by the liver and excreted by the kidneys. Adverse reactions include gastrointestinal disturbances, neurotoxicity, and cartilage erosion in young dogs, although these effects were seen following excessive therapeutic dosing.

Tetracyclines, including doxycycline and minocycline, are bacteriostatic antibiotics that inhibit protein synthesis by binding to the 30 S unit of ribosomes.[26, 49] Historically, tetracyclines were used for treatment against many gram-negative and gram-positive organisms, including anaerobes. Recent emergence, however, of antibiotic-resistant strains and new antimicrobials has limited the current usefulness of tetracyclines for treatment of surgical infections.[1, 26] Dog with diskospondylitis caused by *Brucella canis* are often treated with tetracycline–aminoglycoside combination therapy.[36] Tetracyclines are concentrated in the liver and reabsorbed via enterohepatic recirculation. Most tetracyclines are excreted by the kidneys, except doxycycline, which is excreted in feces. Penetration of the drugs into body fluids and tissues is excellent. The lipid solubility of minocycline and doxycycline enhances their distribution and reduces chelation by dairy and antacid products.[26, 28] Untoward effects of tetracycline treatment include disturbances in neuromuscular transmission and myocardial contraction, as well as gastrointestinal disorders, including superinfections. Tetracyclines bind to calcium in bone and teeth and may alter normal structural development in young animals.

SUMMARY

Perioperative antibiotic therapy should be used to restore patient function and reduce patient morbidity. Judicious antibiotic usage is an adjunct (not a replacement) to proper surgical technique and excellent patient care in reducing surgery-associated morbidity. As stated by Wangensteen, "Antibiotics may turn a third-class surgeon into a second-class surgeon, but will never turn a second-class surgeon into a first-class surgeon."[51]

REFERENCES

1. Alexander JW, Dellinger ED: Surgical infections and choice of antibiotics, in Sabiston DC (ed): Textbook of Surgery. Philadelphia: WB Saunders, 1991, pp 221–236
2. Classen DC, Evans RS, Pestotnik SL: The timing of prophylactic administration of antibiotics and the risk of surgical-wound infection. N Engl J Med 1992; 326:281–286
3. Daly WR: Wound infections, in Slatter DH (ed): Textbook of Small Animal Surgery. Philadelphia: WB Saunders, 1985, pp 37–51
4. Vasseur PB, Levy J, Dowd E: Surgical wound infection rates in dogs and cats. Vet Surg 1988; 17:60–64
5. Davis JM, Shires GT: Principles and Management of Surgical Infections. Philadelphia: WB Saunders, 1991
6. Gustilo RB, Gruninger RP, Tsukayama DT: Orthopedic Infection: Diagnosis and Treatment. Philadelphia: WB Saunders, 1989
7. Dow SG, Jones RL: Anaerobic infections: I. Pathogenesis and clinical significance. Compend Contin Educ Pract Vet 1987; 9:711–719
8. Nichols RL: Surgical infections and choice of antibiotics, in Sabiston DC (ed): Sabiston's Essentials of Surgery. Philadelphia: WB Saunders, 1987, pp 141–168
9. Rotman N, Hay JM, Lacaine F: Prophylactic antibiotherapy in abdominal surgery. Arch Surg 1989; 124:323–327
10. Romatowski J: Prevention and control of surgical wound infection. J Am Vet Med Assoc 1989; 194:107–114
11. Hobson HP: Surgical facilities and equipment, in Slatter DH (ed): Textbook of Small Animal Surgery. Philadelphia: WB Saunders, 1985, pp 285–291
12. Flynn NM, Lawrence RM: Antimicrobial prophylaxis. Med Clin North Am 1979; 63:1225–1243
13. Penwick RC: Use of antimicrobial drugs in surgery, in Slatter DH (ed): Textbook of Small Animal Surgery. Philadelphia: WB Saunders, 1985, pp 52–70
14. Penwick RC: Preoperative patient preparation, in Newton CD, Nunamaker DM (eds): Textbook of Small Animal Orthopaedics. Philadelphia: Lippincott, 1985, pp 167–176
15. Wilcke JR: Use of antimicrobial drugs to prevent infections in veterinary patients. Prob Vet Med 1990; 2:298–312
16. Nichols RL: Postoperative wound infection. N Engl J Med 1982; 307:701–703
17. Fitzgerald RH, Thompson RL: Cephalosporin antibiotics in the prevention and treatment of musculoskeletal sepsis. J Bone Joint Surg 1983; 65A:1201–1205
18. Kaiser AB: Antimicrobial prophylaxis in surgery. N Engl J Med 1986; 315:1129–1137
19. Richardson DC, Aucoin DP, DeYoung DJ, et al: Pharmacokinetic disposition of cefazolin in serum and tissue during canine total hip replacement. Vet Surg 1992; 21:1–4
20. Alexander JW, Alexander NS: The influence of route of administration on wound fluid concentration of prophylactic antibiotics. J Trauma 1976; 16:488–495
21. Conte JL, Barriere SL: Manual of Antibiotics and Infectious Diseases. Philadelphia: Lea & Febiger, 1988
22. Papich MG: Tissue concentrations of antimicrobials. Prob Vet Med 1990; 2:312–329
23. Ferguson DC, Lappin MR: Antimicrobial therapy, in Lorenz MD, Cornelius LM, Ferguson DC (eds): Small Animal Medical Therapeutics. Philadelphia: Lippincott, 1992, pp 457–478
24. DiPiro JT, Cheung FPF, Bowden TA: Single dose systemic antibiotic prophylaxis of surgical wound infections. Am J Surg 1986; 152:552–559
25. Guglielmo BJ, Hohn DC, Koo PJ, et al: Antibiotic prophylaxis in surgical procedures. Arch Surg 1983; 118:943–955

26. Gilman AG, Goodman LS: The Pharmacological Basis of Therapeutics. New York: Macmillan, 1985
27. Dow SW: Management of anaerobic infections. Vet Clin North Am Small Anim Pract 1988; 18:1167–1182
28. Papich MG: Therapy of gram-positive infections. Vet Clin North Am Small Anim Pract 1988; 8:1267–1285
29. Budsberg SC, Kemp DT: Antimicrobial distribution and therapeutics in bone. Compend Contin Educ Pract Vet 1990; 1758–1762
30. Dirschl DR, Wilson FC: Topical antibiotic irrigation in the prophylaxis of operative wound infections in orthopedic surgery. Orthop Clin North Am 1991; 22:419–426
31. Penwick RC: Perioperative antimicrobial chemoprophylaxis in gastrointestinal surgery. J Am Anim Hosp Assoc 1988; 24:133–145
32. Van Scoy RE, Wilkowske CJ: Prophylactic use of antimicrobial agents in adult patients. Mayo Clin Proc 1987; 62:1137–1141
33. Kling PA, Dahlgren S: Oral prophylaxis with neomycin and erythromycin in colorectal surgery. Arch Surg 1989; 124:705–708
34. Clarke JS, Condon RE, Bartlett JG: Preoperative oral antibiotics reduce septic complications of colon operations. Ann Surg 1977; 186:251–259
35. Dow SW, Papich MG: An update on antimicrobials. Vet Med 1991; 86:707–715
36. Greene CG: Infectious Diseases of the Dog and Cat. Philadelphia: WB Saunders, 1990
37. Matushek KJ, Rosin EH: Pharmacokinetics of cefazolin applied topically to the surgical wound. Arch Surg 1991; 126:890–893
38. Hosgood G: Wound complications following thoracolumbar laminectomy in the dog: A retrospective study of 264 procedures. J Am Anim Hosp Assoc 1992; 28:47–52
39. Indieri RJ, Simpson SJ: Intracranial surgery, in Slatter DH (ed): Textbook of Small Animal Surgery. Philadelphia: WB Saunders, 1985, pp 1415–1429
40. Djindjian M, Lepresle E, Homs JB: Antibiotic prophylaxis during prolonged clean neurosurgery. J Neurosurg 1990; 73:383–386
41. Dempsey R, Rapp RP, Young B: Prophylactic parenteral antibiotics in clean neurosurgical procedures: A review. J Neurosurg 1988; 69:52–57
42. Eliopoulos GM, Moellering RC: Principles of antibiotic therapy. Med Clin North Am 1982; 66:3–16
43. Wilcke JR: Therapeutic decisions. Prob Vet Med 1990; 2:279–289
44. Dow SW, Jones RL: Bacteremia: Pathogenesis and diagnosis. Compend Contin Educ Pract Vet 1989; 11:432–443
45. Orsini JA: Wound infections and antimicrobial therapy, in Gourley IM, Vasseur PB (eds): General Small Animal Surgery. Philadelphia: Lippincott, 1985, pp 121–144
46. Wiseman DM, Rovee DT, Alvarez OM: Wound dressings: Design and use, in Cohen IK, Diegelmann RF, Lindblad WJ (eds): Wound Healing. Philadelphia: WB Saunders, 1992, pp 562–580
47. Hardie EM: Surgical infection, in Betts CW, Crane JW (eds): Manual of Small Animal Surgical Therapeutics. New York: Churchill Livingstone, 1986, pp 369–390
48. Davis LE: Antimicrobial therapy, in Kirk RW (ed): Current Veterinary Therapy VII. Philadelphia: WB Saunders, 1980, pp 2–16
49. Brown SA: Treatment of gram-negative infections. Vet Clin North Am Small Anim Pract 1988; 18:1141–1165
50. Plumb DC: Veterinary Drug Handbook. White Bear Lake, Minn: Pharma Vet Publishing, 1991
51. Van Den Bogaard AEJM, Weidema WF: Antimicrobial prophylaxis in canine surgery. J Small Anim Pract 1985; 26:257–266

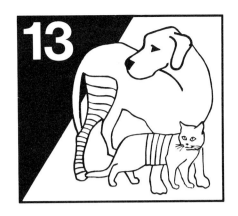

DETECTION OF SEPSIS IN THE POSTOPERATIVE PATIENT

DON R. WALDRON

The occurrence of sepsis in the postoperative patient depends on many factors. In simple terms, the risk of wound infection following surgery is related to the formula[1-3]

$$\frac{\text{Dose of bacterial contamination} \times \text{bacterial virulence}}{\text{Resistance of the host}}$$

Much of modern surgical practice concerning prevention of sepsis is aimed at modifying this formula. Despite intensive efforts to minimize complications, postoperative infections in humans continue to cause significant morbidity and mortality. Economic costs, morbidity and mortality data in veterinary surgery are not apparent; however, recent information from 2063 surgical procedures in a veterinary teaching hospital included the following infection rates: clean (2.5%), clean-contaminated (4.5%), contaminated (5.8%), and dirty (18.1%).[4]

The goals of infection treatment in the surgical patient are well known. Identification of an underlying cause (e.g., leaking intestinal anastomosis or specific microorganism), debridement, and proper drainage of infected wounds are fundamental concepts for successful treatment of sepsis in the surgical patient. Recognition of factors that predispose the patient to infection also assists the surgeon in prevention and treatment of sepsis.

The detection of infection is a prerequisite to appropriate therapy and, in most nonsurgical patients, is relatively simple. Fever, leukocytosis, anorexia, and depression are sufficient findings for a tentative diagnosis. Many of these abnormalities (e.g. pyrexia and elevated white blood cell count), however, are part of the normal response to stress and surgical procedures. Thus differentiation of sepsis from the normal physiologic response in a postoperative patient can be difficult. This chapter reviews the early detection of sepsis in the postoperative patient. In addition, local and systemic responses to infection, causes of fever, and laboratory diagnosis of sepsis are presented.

307

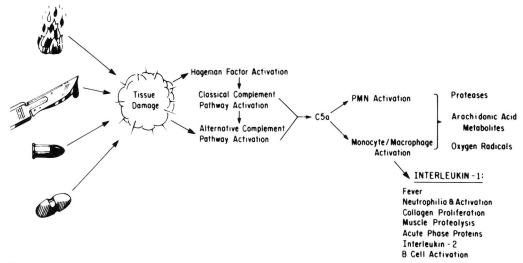

Figure 13–1. A framework whereby a "nonspecific" stimulus such as trauma could produce immunologic, inflammatory, and metabolic changes. (From Burke JF, Gelfand JA: Events in early "inflammation." In Howard RJ, Simmons RL (eds): Surgical Infectious Diseases. Norwalk, Conn: Appleton & Lange, 1988, p 204, with permission.)

LOCAL RESPONSE TO INFECTION

Surgical wounding results in activation of the complement, bradykinin, plasminogen, and clotting cascades.[5] Activation of the complement system causes production of C5a, which acts as a chemoattractant for neutrophils and macrophages (Fig. 13–1). Thrombin is produced as a result of clotting activation, and it activates platelets. Bradykinin causes local vasodilation, whereas plasminogen activation produces plasmin, which is responsible for fibrin degradation within the wound (Fig. 13–2). These processes begin soon after wounding and are beneficial and necessary for normal tissue healing.

The critical cell following wounding is the neutrophil. Normal function of the

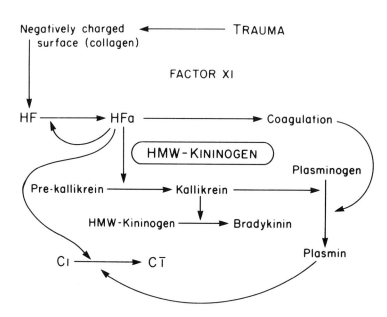

Figure 13–2. The interrelationships of the coagulation–kinin, fibrinolytic, and complement systems and their hypothetical activation by trauma. (From Burke JF, Gelfand JA: Events in early inflammation. In Howard RJ, Simmons RL (eds): Surgical Infectious Diseases. Norwalk, Conn: Appleton & Lange, 1988, p 203, with permission.)

host defense to local infection depends on timely delivery of neutrophils to the wound space, adequate function of the cell in the hypoxic and acidotic wound environment, and the capacity of the neutrophil to respond to bacterial challenge.

Clinically, the initial reaction to surgical wounding is inflammation. In most instances, heat, redness, swelling, pain, and loss of function are all present in varying degrees in the postoperative patient. The extent and duration of the inflammatory response depend on tissue damage, ability of the body to respond to injury, and presence of foreign bodies or bacteria. In animals, 10^5 or more bacteria per gram of tissue cause infection. The presence of a foreign body (e.g., suture, prosthetic devices, orthopedic implants, pacemakers, or drains) lowers the number of bacteria necessary for wound infection. In uncomplicated wound healing, there is elimination of the offending stimulus and normal tissue repair ensues. Inflammation of the noncontaminated wound peaks 72 to 96 hours postoperatively and then decreases.[6]

The clinical signs of inflammation and infection are similar, but in infected wounds the signs are exaggerated. Serum accumulation within the wound (seroma) appears as soft, fluctuant collection of fluid and indicates excessive dead space and tissue trauma. Seroma formation may lead to wound infection by preventing delivery of phagocytes to bacterial foci and interfering with opsonization of contaminating bacteria.[5, 7] Cellulitis is an excessive inflammatory response and an indication of wound infection. *Streptococcus* spp. frequently are associated with cellulitis. Abscess formation and wound exudate also are indications of infection; "sterile" abscesses are uncommon in veterinary patients. Anaerobic infections are characterized by a putrid exudate.

Appropriate samples should be collected from a suspected infected wound for Gram staining and culture (see Laboratory Diagnosis of Infection). In general, samples for culture are taken by aseptic needle aspiration or culturette contact of *deep* wound recesses. Culture of wound exudate from the skin surface or draining tracts may result in contamination and misleading information regarding the bacteria associated with infection.

Close monitoring and physical examination should be performed early in the postoperative period. Physical signs of wound infection are fever, erythema and edema of wound edges, changes in wound contour, and serosanguineous wound discharge. Treatment of infected wounds involves debridement, drainage, lavage, and appropriate systemic antibiotic therapy. If a surgical wound becomes infected and there is abscess formation, skin sutures should be removed and the wound left open for drainage. The wound is then healed by delayed closure or second-intention healing.

FEVER

Fever is an early and easily recognized sign of inflammation and infection. Normal body temperatures in dogs range from 100.2 to 102.8°F (37.9–39.3°C) and in cats from 100.5 to 102.5°F (38.0–39.2°C).[8] Fever is caused by exogenous pyrogens such as bacteria, viruses, fungi, and endotoxins. In addition, noninfective sources such as neoplasia and immune disease may cause fever. In the surgical patient, tissue trauma may activate the febrile response (Fig. 13–1). An exogenous pyrogen causes fever by stimulating release of endogenous pyrogen, also known as interleukin 1 (Il-1), from macrophages and monocytes. Lymphocytes and granulocytes produce little endogenous pyrogen, whereas some neoplastic cells can produce endogenous pyrogen.[9] Endogenous pyrogen (Il-1) causes an increase in the thermoregulatory set point of the hypothalamus, which causes an increase in heat generation and conservation by the body. The most likely mediators of fever at the central level are prostaglandins (PGE_1) or prostaglandin precursors.

Fever is commonly present in postoperative patients when there is no infection. *Inflammatory* fever is seen most commonly in orthopedic patients or patients with extensive soft-tissue trauma. Elevation in body temperature is usually mild (103–104°F), early (first 24 hours) in the postoperative period, and of short duration. No other clinical signs of infection are seen. Fever secondary to trauma or surgery has been ascribed to acute inflammation of tissues and subsequent release of endogenous pyrogen (Il-1); however, no component of the inflammatory response (except activated complement) has been shown to cause release of endogenous pyrogen.[9] The cause of inflammatory fever remains unclear, and the challenge for the surgeon lies in differentiating it from fever associated with infection.

Fever is the most *frequent* indicator of infection in the postoperative period, although its presence does not confirm infection. In one study, there was significant postoperative fever in 15% of postceliotomy patients.[10] Infection was confirmed by culture in one-fourth (27%) of the patients with fever, thus showing the low specificity of temperature elevation as an indicator of infection. The average time for the fever to peak was 2.6 days after surgery, and the duration of fever averaged 4.6 days in patients with infection compared with 2.9 days in febrile patients with no infection ($p > 0.05$). There was no attempt in this study to classify abdominal operations in terms of clean, clean-contaminated, or dirty procedures. Other studies were cited that showed that fevers associated with infection were higher and of longer duration than from other causes. In a series of septic canine surgical patients, only 59% of dogs had fever.[11] The lack of detected fever in infected dogs may be due to inadequate monitoring, low numbers of macrophages, or hypovolemic shock. Detection of normal temperatures in patients with sepsis who were later treated with surgery was a poor prognostic sign.[11]

Our knowledge of fever and available human surgical data confirm its role as an indicator of infection. A thorough physical examination is required in patients with postoperative fever to identify possible sources of infection (Table 13–1). Appropriate laboratory tests are useful in animals with clinical signs of illness and at risk for developing infection.

SYSTEMIC RESPONSE TO INFECTION

The invasion of the body by microorganisms in the face of inadequate host defenses will result in local and systemic responses to infection that are clinically important. The systemic responses are complex and affect patient morbidity and mortality. This section will briefly describe the circulatory and metabolic response to gram-negative infection and systemic sepsis. Physical signs also are described.

The dog has been used frequently in the laboratory as a model for endotoxic shock. When endotoxin is infused to cause peracute gram-negative

TABLE 13–1. Potential Causes of Fever in the Postoperative Patient

I. Acute inflammation and tissue trauma
II. Local infection
   A. Surgical incision or wounding
   B. Osteomyelitis
   C. Body cavity
      1. Abdomen
         a. Pyelonephritis
         b. Prostatitis/abscess
         c. Pyometra
         d. Liver
         e. Pancreas
      2. Thorax
         a. Pneumonia/atelectasis
   D. Intravenous catheter sepsis (phlebitis)
III. Systemic infection
   A. Bacterial endocarditis
   B. Systemic mycoses
      1. Histoplasmosis
      2. Blastomycosis
      3. Cryptococcosis
      4. Coccidioidomycosis
   C. Rickettsial disease
      1. *Ehrlichia*
      2. Rocky Mountain spotted fever
   D. Viral
      1. Distemper
      2. FeLV
      3. FIP
   E. Toxoplasmosis
IV. Other
   A. Neoplasia
      1. Necrosis
      2. Pyrogenic factors
   B. Immune mediated
      1. Rheumatoid arthritis
      2. Polyarthritis
   C. Pulmonary emboli
   D. Drug mediated

sepsis, there is a decrease in blood pressure and cardiac output and variable changes in pulmonary artery pressure, heart rate, and peripheral vascular resistance.[5, 11] There is also a decrease in blood pH, tachycardia, and pale mucous membranes. In the clinical patient, if there is long-standing systemic infection (wound infection or abscessation with gram-positive bacteria), hyperdynamic sepsis occurs. In this instance, cardiac output is increased, peripheral resistance decreases, and blood pressure is normal or low. Tachycardia and red mucous membranes are seen. Sepsis also induces progressive abnormalities in metabolism. Analysis of blood gas values often reveals metabolic acidosis. This acidosis will cause an increased respiratory rate in experimental models. This finding was not found in a clinical study and may be related to the dog's resistance to septic respiratory failure.[11, 12] Interestingly, blood glucose values in infected animals are variable and depend on the duration of infection. Initially, hyperglycemia occurs as a result of increased gluconeogenesis within the liver. Later, hypoglycemia occurs because of hepatic failure and increased peripheral uptake of glucose.[5, 11]

Clinical indications of systemic infection include pyrexia, tachycardia, weakness, severe depression, vomiting, or diarrhea. If infection is severe, circulatory collapse and shock occur. As described earlier, the presence of fever is variable and often unpredictable. Tachycardia usually occurs in the septic patient as a result of pain, elevated catecholamine levels, and increased metabolic needs. Other clinical signs are relatively nonspecific, and early recognition of sepsis depends on thorough physical examination in high-risk animals and correlation of clinical signs with appropriate laboratory tests.

Those animals at high risk for postoperative infection include patients undergoing surgeries classified as clean-contaminated, contaminated, or dirty. Most surgeons would agree that patients having intestinal surgery are at high risk for developing infection. The most common source of organisms in infection is the gastrointestinal tract.[11] Neurosurgical patients are also at risk for sepsis according to one study.[11] Generalized predisposing patient factors for development of infection are increased age, immunosuppression, and concurrent disease, such as diabetes mellitus. Some risk factors such as increased age and diabetes have been extrapolated from the human literature and have not been proven to predispose animals to postoperative infection.

LABORATORY DIAGNOSIS OF INFECTION

Hematologic values frequently may be abnormal in the presence of infection. Recognition of a normal versus abnormal response in the postoperative patient is important to prevent misinterpretation of the complete blood count (CBC). The normal canine or feline patient that undergoes surgery will often have a "stress" leukogram in the immediate postoperative period. A "stress" leukogram, or physiologic leukocytosis, is characterized by a mature neutrophilic leukocytosis.

Classic findings of purulent inflammation include neutrophilia with a left shift. Increased numbers of band neutrophils were found in 70% of dogs with postoperative sepsis.[11] Neutrophil counts may be low in the acute phase of gram-negative sepsis as a result of sequestration in the lung, liver, or spleen.[13] Neutropenia also may occur when there is massive utilization of neutrophils (abscess). Toxic changes within neutrophils consisting of prominent cytoplasmic granules or diffuse basophilia and cytoplasmic vacuolization may indicate severe toxemia. Platelet counts have not been evaluated in clinically septic canine patients, but thrombocytopenia is commonly recognized in experimental gram-negative sepsis in dogs.[12]

Serum biochemistry values may be abnormal during infection. Blood glucose values vary with time during the course of infection. Glucose values in dogs developing sepsis postoperatively are usually decreased; however, transient hyperglycemia may be seen in acute septic shock or in chronic sepsis. Proper handling of blood samples will preclude hypoglycemia due to erythrocyte glycogenolysis and a "false" low glucose value analysis. Other changes in serum biochemistries associated with infection include hypoalbuminemia and increased alkaline phosphatase values. Abnormalities of albumin and alkaline phosphatase may signal changes in liver function due to sepsis. Increased alkaline phosphatase and hypoalbuminemia were noted in 75% and 94% of septic dogs, respectively, in one study.[11] An increased alkaline phosphatase level may be the result of biliary stasis or elevated corticosteroid levels. Hypoalbuminemia reflects both a decrease in liver function and the effects of malnutrition.

A number of investigators in human surgery have sought blood tests that would reliably predict postoperative infection.[14, 15] The secretion of Il-1 (endogenous pyrogen) from macrophages stimulates the release of acute-phase proteins by the liver. One of these products, C-reactive protein, was shown to be consistently elevated in humans with postoperative sepsis.[14] In another test termed the *thrombotic index,* the recalcification time of blood incubated with saline was compared with the time of the same blood incubated with endotoxin. The test value was decreased in patients who were septic.[15] The value of such tests in veterinary surgical patients awaits further investigation.

Blood cultures are frequently performed in people and animals with suspected bacteremias. The lack of positive results with blood cultures, however, and the time and cost have limited their routine use in veterinary medicine. Nevertheless, periodic blood cultures are indicated in patients with fever of unknown origin and signs of systemic illness. In humans, the presence of *multiple-organism bacteremia,* defined as the growth of two or more organisms in the same blood culture, was an excellent indicator of intraabdominal sepsis in the absence of other polymicrobial sources such as burns.[16] In animals, mortality rates were not significantly different with monomicrobial versus polymicrobial bacteremia.[17] Gram-negative bacilli (*Escherichia coli*) and gram-positive cocci (*Staphylococcus* spp.) are most frequently cultured from canine blood.[18] Bacteremia occurring in the postoperative patient is often intermittent. Three separate blood cultures collected at hourly intervals and using a minimum of 5 to 10 ml of blood for each sample has been recommended for veterinary patients.[18]

Wound cultures may correlate with infection and identification of the offending organism. Cultures should be obtained by deep, aseptic aspiration. Positive bacterial identification may be adversely affected if samples are obtained from patients receiving antibiotics. Quantitative wound cultures ($>10^5$ organisms per gram of tissue) may prove valuable in determining if wound infection is present.[18a] Aerobic and anaerobic bacterial and fungal cultures are appropriate, and results often depend on the source of the wounding. Gram staining of wound contents provides early valuable information related to bacterial population and choice of antimicrobial drugs.

BODY CAVITY SEPSIS

Detection of sepsis in the thoracic or abdominal cavity may only require needle aspiration of purulent effusion from the body cavity. Frequently, however, the signs of postoperative infection and results of diagnostic techniques are inconclusive. Consideration of patients at risk for developing infection and a thorough search for the infection site are prerequisites to successful treatment. Animals at high risk for postoperative body sepsis include those with surgery of contaminated wounds. Penetrating abdominal wounds, pulmonary abscesses, and colonic resections and anastomoses are also associated with an increased incidence of postoperative sepsis. In a series of 50 canine patients with generalized peritonitis, the most common cause of infection was surgical wound dehiscence of the gastrointestinal tract.[19]

The problem of early detection of postoperative abdominal sepsis is a dilemma for the veterinary surgeon. Clinical signs such as anorexia, vomiting, fever, painful abdomen, and peritoneal effusion may be associated with enterotomy or anastomotic leakage, or postoperative abscess formation. The presence of a single clinical sign, such as fever early in the postoperative period, is a cause for concern. Multiple clinical signs, such as vomiting, fever, neutrophilia with a severe left shift, and toxic neutrophils, are usually diagnostic for sepsis. If there are no signs of incisional infection, abdominal sepsis is suspected and a diagnostic peritoneal lavage should be performed following abdominal radiography. Lavage is performed by infusion of 20 ml/kg of normal saline into the abdomen. A sample is collected and examined microscopically. Experimentally, dogs with intestinal resection and anastomosis have nondegenerate neutrophils and no bacteria within abdominal fluid.[20] Dogs with peritonitis have degenerate or toxic neutrophils and bacteria within abdominal fluid. A recent study of small intestinal dehiscence following enterotomy or anastomosis in dogs revealed a 15.7% dehiscence rate.[20a] Dehiscence was more frequent following trauma or foreign body ingestion compared with enterotomy. The band neutrophil counts in animals with dehiscence were similar to normally recovering animals during postoperative days 1 to 3, but significantly increased during days 4 to 6 after surgery.

Radiographic imaging techniques such as ultrasound and CT scanning have improved the diagnosis of postoperative abdominal abscess in humans. In animals, the problem of postoperative subphrenic abscessation is not often recognized, although retroperitonitis due to ligatures placed during ovariohysterectomy has been reported.[20b] Radiography of the animal with peritonitis may reveal peritoneal effusion and a "ground glass" appearance of the abdomen. The presence of free air within the abdomen has clinical significance if surgery or abdominocentesis was not previously performed. Free air may indicate a perforated viscus, leaking intestinal anastomosis, or abdominal abscess. The presence of free air is seen radiographically as an increased visibility of serosal surfaces of abdominal viscera. A horizontal-beam abdominal radiograph with the animal in lateral recumbency may demonstrate free air.[21] Because free air following abdominal surgery may persist for days to weeks, the presence of free air alone is not a reliable radiographic sign of complications following abdominal surgery.[22]

Computed tomography, ultrasound, and radionuclide scans are used in humans to diagnose abdominal abscesses.[23] Ultrasonography is widely available in veterinary medicine and may be useful in detection of a localized abdominal abscess in an animal.

ORTHOPEDIC INFECTION

Infection rates for animals undergoing clean orthopedic surgery are approximately the same as for other clean surgical procedures. Again, the surgeon should maintain an index of suspicion for those animals at risk for infection. Concerns related to infection increase if there is an open fracture, increased operative exposure time (>90 minutes), excessive soft-tissue damage, and use of orthopedic implants.

Osteomyelitis is classified as acute or chronic in nature. The most common cause of osteomyelitis in dogs is open surgical repair of a fracture. Bacteria that cause infection are usually introduced into the wound at the time of surgery by skin or airborne inoculation. Surgical procedures lasting longer than 90 minutes have an increased occurrence of infection. Increased exposure to airborne pathogens and drying of tissues exposed to surgical lights combine to decrease host resistance with a resulting increase in infection rates. Open fractures also have an increased incidence of infection.[24]

In a series of operated fractures (110) in animals, the duration of the surgical procedure, wound lavage, and method of fixation did not have a significant effect on bacterial contamination. Factors significantly affecting the incidence of wound contamination were the type of bone fractured, open or closed nature of the fracture, performing an initial surgery or reoperation, and extent of soft-tissue damage.[24] In this study, 72% of open fractures and 39% of closed fractures had bacterial contamination at the time of fracture repair. In addition, bacterial culturing at surgery was valuable in predicting postoperative complications. Animals with a contaminated wound (by culture) and postoperative fever greater than 103°F (39.4°C) 24 hours postoperatively were more likely to develop wound complications or osteomyelitis.[24] In animals with normal temperatures and negative cultures, postoperative complications or osteomyelitis did not occur.

The value of bacterial culture alone should not be overemphasized. Twelve of 13 dogs in one study had positive cultures obtained by deep aspiration and had normal bone healing without signs of infection and no treatment with antibiotics.[25] It is probable that rigid internal fixation was responsible for uncomplicated healing in these cases, since the presence of bacteria on plates and implants is not unusual.[26, 27] Bacteria present at the site of healed fractures without signs of osteomyelitis produce "cryptic" infections.[27] These infections are caused by bacterial production of a polysaccharide peribacterial film that promotes adherence to foreign material (i.e., metal). Because of latent infection, large surgical implants should be removed once bone healing has occurred.

Classic signs of acute postoperative osteomyelitis include soft-tissue swelling, drainage, fever, and depression. Soft-tissue (incisional) infection may not be evident. Fever caused by osteomyelitis is persistent or progressive as compared with inflammatory postoperative fever. Radiographic signs of acute bone infection include irregular productive periosteal reaction and, occasionally, gas in soft tissues. Development of fistulas or draining tracts and radiographic signs of sequestration of bone fragments indicate a chronic infection.

Culture and sensitivity testing should be performed to isolate the causative organism in animals with osteomyelitis. Caution should be used in interpreting culture of sinus tracts. If *Staphylococcus intermedius* is cultured, it is a probable causative organism; however, if gram-negative bacteria are cultured, they may not be the causative organism.[26] More reliable bacterial culture results are obtained by deep wound or sequestrum sampling and should include anaerobic as well as aerobic culturing. In one study involving animals, 74% of patients with osteomyelitis had positive anaerobic cultures.[28] The hallmarks of therapy for osteomyelitis are rigid internal fixation, proper drainage, sequestrectomy, and appropriate antibiotic therapy. Cancellous bone grafting is often used to aid fracture healing.

Another cause of infection in the orthopedic patient is related to prosthetic implants. Total hip replacement is a common surgery in animals, and implant-associated infection may be catastrophic, necessitating removal of the prosthesis and polymethylmethacrylate (PMM) bone cement. Exogenous contamination causes most of the infections in total hip procedures in dogs, although endogenous contamination may occur. The presence of PMM inhibits phagocytic cell and complement function within the wound. Polymethylmethacrylate acts as a foreign body and decreases the number of bacteria required to cause osteomyelitis.[27]

Clinically, animals may be systemically ill or have intermittent pain and lameness. Persistence of lameness following total hip replacement in the absence of technical error is suggestive of infection.[29] Evaluation of serial radiographs may reveal bone lysis and implant loosening characterized by lucency at the bone–cement interface. Aseptic aspiration of the surgical site is performed to recover samples for aerobic and anaerobic culture and Gram staining. Infected implants require complete removal of the prosthetic devices and bone cement.

SUMMARY

Detection of infection in the postoperative patient is sometimes difficult because clinical signs may be similar to those in the noninfected, normally recovering animal. Clinical signs such as fever and inflammation are often unreliable indicators of infection, and laboratory tests also may only be suggestive of infection. A combination of abnormal clinical signs and laboratory findings more clearly aids in the diagnosis of infection. The conscientious surgeon critically examines each patient with postoperative infection and assesses which causative factors should be modified to decrease patient morbidity and mortality.

REFERENCES

 1. Orsini J: Wound infections and antimicrobial therapy. In Gourley IM, Vasseur PB (eds): General Small Animal Surgery. Philadelphia: Lippincott, 1985, p 121
 2. Swaim SF: Surgery of traumatized skin. In Management and Reconstruction in the Dog and Cat. Philadelphia: WB Saunders, 1980, pp 120, 161
 3. Johnston DE: Wound healing. Vet Surg 1974; 3:30
 4. Vasseur PB, Levy J, Dowd E, Eliot J: Surgical wound infection rates in dogs and cats, data from a teaching hospital. Vet Surg 1988; 17:60–63
 5. Knighton DR, Hunt TK: The defenses of the wound. In Howard RJ, Simmons RL (eds): Surgical Infectious Diseases, 2d ed. Norwalk, Conn: Appleton & Lange, 1988, pp 201–208
 6. Peacock EE: Wound Repair. Philadelphia: WB Saunders, 1984, p 7
 7. Alexander JW: Surgical infections and choice of antibiotics. In Sabiston D (ed): Textbook of Surgery. Philadelphia: WB Saunders, 1986, pp 259–283
 8. Lusk RH: Thermoregulation. In Ettinger SJ (ed): Textbook of Veterinary Internal Medicine, 3d ed. Philadelphia: WB Saunders, 1989, pp 23–26
 9. McMillan FD: Fever: Pathophysiology and rational therapy. Compend Contin Educ Pract Vet 1985; 7:845–855
10. Freischlag J, Busuttil R: The value of postoperative fever evaluation. Surgery 1983; 94:358–363
11. Hardie EM, Rawlings C, Calvert C: Severe sepsis in selected small animal surgical patients. J Am Anim Hosp Assoc 1986; 22:33–41
12. Hardie EM: Early recognition of sepsis. Proc Vet Surg Forum 1990; 24–26
13. Duncan JR, Prasse KW: Leukocytes. In Veterinary Laboratory Medicine, 2d ed. Ames, Iowa: Iowa State University Press, 1986
14. Mustard RA, Bowen JM, Haseb S: C-Reactive protein levels predict postoperative septic complications. Arch Surg 1987; 122:69–73
15. Machiedo GW, Suval WD: Detection of sepsis in the postoperative patient. Surg Clin North Am 1988; 68:215–226
16. Ing AE, McLean PH, Meakins JI: Multiple-organism bacteremia in the surgical intensive care unit: A sign of intraperitoneal sepsis. Surgery 1981; 90:779–786
17. Dow SW, Curtis CR, Jones RL, Wingfield WE: Bacterial culture of blood from critically ill dogs and cats: 100 cases (1985–1987). J Am Vet Med Assoc 1989; 195:113–117
18. Dow SW, Jones RL: Bacteremia: Pathogenesis and diagnosis. Compend Contin Educ Pract Vet 1989; 11:432–443
18a. Daly WR: Wound infections. In Slatter DH (ed): Textbook of Small Animal Surgery, 1st ed. Philadelphia: WB Saunders, 1985, p 39

19. Hosgood G, Salisbury SK: Generalized peritonitis in dogs: 50 cases (1975–1986). J Am Vet Med Assoc 1988; 193:1448–1450
20. Botte RJ, Rosin E: Cytology of peritoneal effusion following intestinal anastomosis and experimental peritonitis. Vet Surg 1983; 12:20–23
20a. Allen DA, Smeak DD, Schertel ER: Prevalence of small intestinal dehiscence and associated clinical factors: a retrospective study of 121 dogs. J Am Anim Hosp Assoc 1992; 28:70–76
20b. Roush JK, Bjorling DE, Lord P: Diseases of the retroperitoneal space in the dog and cat. J Am Anim Hosp Assoc 1990; 26:47–54
21. Ticer JW: Radiographic Technique in Veterinary Practice. Philadelphia: WB Saunders, 1984, p 322
22. Probst CW, Stickle RL, Bartlett BC: Duration of pneumoperitoneum in the dog. Am J Vet Res 1986; 47:176–178
23. Gerzof SG, Oates ME: Imaging techniques for infections in the surgical patient. Surg Clin North Am 1988; 68:147–164
24. Stevenson S, Olmsteed M, Kolwalski J: Bacterial culturing for prediction of postoperative complications following open fracture repair in small animals. Vet Surg 1986; 15:99–102
25. Holmberg D: The use of prophylactic penicillin in orthopedic surgery: A clinical trial. Vet Surg 1985; 14:160–165
26. Rudd RG: A rational approach to the diagnosis and treatment of osteomyelitis. Compend Contin Educ Pract Vet 1986; 8:225–232
27. Smith MM, Vasseur PB, Saunders HM: Bacterial growth associated with metallic implants in dogs. J Am Vet Med Assoc 1989; 195:765–767
28. Walker RD, Richardson DC, Bryant MJ, Draper CS: Anaerobic bacteria associated with osteomyelitis in domestic animals. J Am Vet Med Assoc 1983; 182:814–816
29. Smith MM: Orthopedic infections. In Slatter DH (ed): Textbook of Small Animal Surgery, 2d ed. Philadelphia: WB Saunders (in press)

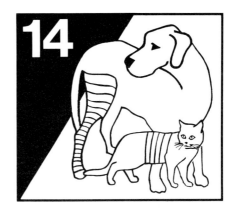

NANCY HAMPEL

SURGICAL DRAINS

At one time, over 5 million surgical drains were used yearly in U.S. hospitals. Their effectiveness, therapeutic indications, applications, and maintenance requirements, however, are still the subject of debate.[1] Controversy exists because the value of drains depends on method of application and case selection. Therefore, what is appropriate for one wound may not be useful for another. Many factors play a role in the success (improved wound healing) or failure (delayed wound healing) of a drainage system. These include the need for drainage, location and type of wound (clean versus infected), postoperative drain care, patient cooperation, and hospital environment. Hence, rather than absolute rules for drainage, general guidelines are more appropriate. It is important to evaluate each case and make decisions based on the advantages and disadvantages of drain use for each particular patient.

The objective of this chapter is to review the types of drains, indications for use, and complications. Guidelines are offered to aid in the practical application of surgical drains.

HISTORY OF DRAINS

The earliest recorded notes on surgical drains are attributed to Hippocrates (460–377 B.C.), who used "hollow pencils" to treat empyema. In the 3rd century B.C., Erasistratus of Alexandria also used drainage for empyema and introduced catheters for urinary drainage. During the 1st century A.D., Aurelus Celsus used conical metal tubes for drainage of ascitic fluid. Claudius Galen (A.D. 130–201), whose ideas were believed infallible over the next 15 centuries, also supported the use of lead tubes for drainage of abdominal fluid.[2]

The next recorded use of surgical drains was in 1363 by Guy de Chauliac in *Chirurgica Magna*. This is the earliest surgical treatise of modern times and contains translations of Greek and Arabic physicians. Wound drainage was accomplished with a "charpie" or "tente," which are pieces of linen.

Ambrose Paré (1510–1590) is credited with advancing surgery to the limits imposed by lack of anesthesia and antisepsis. Paré's indications for drainage included wounds that required debridement, purulent or contaminated

319

wounds, bites, ulcerated wounds, and orthopedic procedures. He used hollow tentes of lead. He also described the use of a large thread attached to the drain to prevent its loss.[3] Scultetus inserted a central wick into drainage tubes to improve their efficiency. This was the basis for capillary drainage, a principle that dominated surgical theory for 250 years. Benjamin Bell, who published the first textbook of surgery in America in 1791, advocated leaving the lower portion of the wound open and securing drains with many strands of silk. He cautioned against the use of tentes that do not absorb and serve to block discharge.[4]

Use of the first rubber drain was described in 1859 by Chassaignac of France. Application and knowledge of this type of drain remained limited until Lister began using them (1871). Lister believed that all wounds should be drained and used cloth drains.[5]

Charles Bingham Penrose was among the first to describe complications of drains. He used glass tubes and rubber sheets with gauze rolled inside. This drain was painful to remove. In 1890, Dr. Penrose developed a new drain made by cutting the end of a condom and placing gauze inside. The modern-day Penrose drain is a descendant of this drain and bears his name.[6]

With increasing use of drains during the next 30 years, reports of complications multiplied and debates on drainage became heated. Kelley believed that to use a drain implied imperfect surgery. Halsted agreed and stated that "no drainage at all is better than ignorant employment of it." His objections to prophylactic drainage were that "a drain invariably produces some necrosis of the tissue with which it comes in contact and enfeebles the power of resistance of the tissue toward organisms. But, given necrotic tissue plus infection, drains become almost indispensable."[1]

Suction applied to drains (active drainage) was initially tried before the close of the 19th century. Heaton described the use of a crude syphon (multilumen) drain.[7] In 1905, Yates, in a classic paper, described drainage as either secondary (curative) or primary (prophylactic). Further, he described drainage of the normal peritoneal cavity of dogs as a physiologic and physical impossibility.[8]

The use of drains in abdominal surgery greatly declined during World War I as mortality associated with abdominal injuries was reduced by 50%.[9] In the late 1920s, the final demise of gauze capillary drains for abscesses occurred. Chaffin likened placing gauze drains in purulence to placing the same wick in a jar of mayonnaise.[10] He introduced the first commercially available sump drain in 1932.[11] Intermittent closed suction drainage was first reported in 1947 by Murphy after a radical mastectomy.[12] Continuous closed suction drainage was used 3 years later. In 1954, the first radiopaque Penrose drains were made by addition of a mixture of barium by the Firestone Rubber Company.[13]

Yates' writing in 1905 remains true today that "a study of the history of surgical drainage has, aside from its intrinsic interest, some importance in showing the development of modern theory of practice."[8] Surgical drains maintain a place in modern surgery based on realization of strengths, weaknesses, and subsequent refinements in the product and application. As with other aspects of surgery, the patient will best be served by well-reasoned use of drains, thoughtful planning, careful placement, and conscientious postoperative care.

GENERAL INDICATIONS

"In all walks of life, drains are used to lead away unwanted material."[14] To a surgeon, unwanted material may be blood, purulence, bile, urine, serum, pancreatic exocrine products, foreign material, necrotic tissue, or air. A drain is used to decrease the accumulation of these materials and, subsequently, to decrease infection rate and shorten healing time. The three classic indications for drainage are:[1]

1. To eliminate unavoidable, incorrectable dead space.
2. To eliminate established and ongoing fluid collection (one that will recur after simple evacuation).
3. To provide a prophylactic measure against anticipated fluid or air collection within a wound.

Of these, the first two have sound scientific merit.

Dead Space

Dead space is defined as an abnormal space containing air within a wound. Elimination of dead space (one of Halsted's principles) promotes early union of divided tissues.[15] Dead space can be eliminated by surgical means, pressure wraps, or drainage. Surgical elimination of dead space can be achieved by placing internal sutures such as subcutaneous sutures or through-and-through skin-tacking sutures. Drainage can be used in combination with the first two methods of dead space elimination. If dead space can be completely eliminated through the use of suturing or pressure bandages, drains should be avoided.

The disadvantage of surgical methods of dead space elimination is placement of tacking sutures without visualization after skin edges are apposed. Sutures are placed from the skin surface into underlying muscle or subcutaneous tissue, thereby risking damage to underlying structures. Additionally, the more suture material present in a wound, the more likely infection is to occur as a result of increased foreign matter in the wound and decreased blood supply to ligated tissue. The disadvantages of pressure dressings are that pressure may be sustained only a few hours and it may not be feasible or advisable to compress the head, neck, or chest.[15, 16] The disadvantages of drains are discussed below, and all these factors must be evaluated critically in order to choose the ideal method of eliminating dead space.

Fluid

Early removal of wound fluid is recommended to prevent infection in contaminated wounds.[17, 18] It has been shown that wound fluid decreases host resistance to infection in three ways:[18]

1. The fluid progressively loses opsonins (proteins).
2. Fluid interferes with access of phagocytes to wound bacteria.
3. Fluid provides a substrate for bacterial growth.

Additionally, wound fluid may compromise blood supply to remaining tissues (e.g., skin flaps/grafts).[15, 19] Drainage is recommended if established fluid is likely to decrease after simple evacuation and strict adherence to Halsted's principles. Examples include infected fluid/tissue that cannot be surgically removed (e.g., abscess, bulla, osteotomy), wounds containing necrotic or foreign tissue that cannot be completely debrided (e.g., dog bite wounds), and noninfected wounds where fluid will be produced after surgery (e.g., elbow hygroma, salivary mucocoele, skin graft/flap).

The third indication for drainage, prophylaxis against fluid and air accumulation, is highly controversial.[1, 14, 20–25] Such use is rationalized as being an early warning system of fluid and air accumulation in a wound that has a low likelihood of complications (e.g., chest drain usage for 24 hours after patent ductus arteriosus repair). Prophylactic drainage, like antibiotics, should never be used in place of surgical techniques that follow Halsted's principles, including gentle tissue handling, accurate hemostasis, minimal tension on the wound edges, careful apposition of tissue, obliteration of dead space, strict asepsis, and preservation of blood supply. Because of the complications of drain usage and the availability of more satisfactory and less invasive alternatives (ultrasonography, radiography) to detect fluid and air accumulations, prophylactic drainage may be unjustified.[26, 27]

TYPES OF DRAINS

In selecting a drain, one must consider viscosity and volume of expected drainage, wound location, and patient factors such as nutrition and immunocompetency. Additionally, the type and technique of drainage are important in preventing postoperative sepsis. To select the most appropriate drain system for the patient, a thorough understanding of the drain's mode of action, efficiency, cost, and suitability to suction is necessary.

Active and Passive Drainage

Drains can be categorized by *active* or *passive drainage*. Passive drains function by overflow, are assisted by gravity, and are influenced by pressure differentials. They provide a path of least resistance to the exterior. Some capillary action may contribute to the function of passive drains if an absorbent dressing is applied. Passive drains placed nondependently (uphill) lose efficiency and depend on increased wound/cavity pressure to function. Active drainage occurs when an external source of vacuum is connected to a drainage tube. Active drainage that uses a continuous source of suction and is open to the atmosphere is a sump. Active drainage that uses a closed system is typified by the Hemovac apparatus.

The following drains are used frequently in veterinary medicine:

1. *The Penrose drain* (Fig. 14–1a) is a flattened cylindrical soft latex rubber tube that is a simple conduit drain (one lumen). Sizes range from ¼ to 2 inches in width by 12 to 36 inches in length.

The mode of action is gravity flow and capillary action (passive drainage).[14, 28, 29] The flow is intra- and extraluminal and directly related to surface area. Fenestrations decrease surface area and flow and are not advised when only using a Penrose drain. If the drains are not placed dependently, flow is reliant on increased pressure within the wound.[28, 29] This can be enhanced by a pressure dressing. An absorbent dressing also enhances the capillary action of Penrose drains.

When Penrose drains are used intraperitoneally and not placed depen-

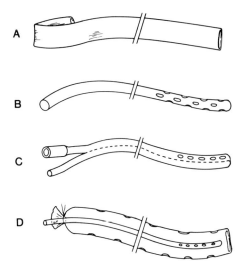

Figure 14–1. Four types of surgical drains. *a,* Penrose drain. *b,* Single-lumen tube drain. *c,* Sump drain. *d,* Sump–Penrose drain.

dently, flow can actually be toward the peritoneal cavity on expiration because of negative intraperitoneal pressure.[30] Positioning is of paramount importance, and care should be taken to place the drain dependently. In the normal canine peritoneal cavity, they drain 40% of the contained fluid.[31] A common mistake in Penrose drain placement is making the skin exit wound too small or tunneling the drain too far subcutaneously before entering the pocket or peritoneum, thus causing inadequate opening for fluid passage. Penrose drains are unsuitable for use with suction or placement in the thoracic cavity.

Latex and other types of rubber incite more tissue response than Silastic and polypropylene and therefore cause earlier formation of a fibrous tract.[32] This makes the Penrose drain more suitable for abscess drainage than Silastic drains because sinus tract extending from the abscess cavity to the skin is desirable.

2. *Simple tube drains* (one-lumen Sovereign feeding tubes) are made of moderately firm polyethylene or rubber and are fenestrated (Fig. 14–1*b*). If additional fenestrations are needed, oval holes can be cut with the hole diameter being less than one-third of the tube diameter. This reduces the chance of tube kinking. The cost of tube drains is similar to that for Penrose drains, and sizes range from 3½ to 30 French in diameter. They may function by gravity (passive) or closed suction (active) depending on the patient's needs and availability of a vacuum source. There is a small amount of capillary action, but flow is mostly intraluminal.[29] Tube drains are approximately 39% efficient in draining peritoneal fluid.[31] Disadvantages include obstruction by debris necessitating frequent flushing, and collapse when suction is applied.[33] Additionally, red rubber incites more inflammatory response than any other drain material, and an impurity in certain polyethylene tubes has been demonstrated to support bacterial growth.[32] Despite these disadvantages, tube drains are the only ones used in the pleural space and are useful in conjunction with closed suction of soft-tissue wounds.

3. *Sump drains have two or more lumens,* one primary lumen for the removal of materials and a second, smaller lumen as an air vent[14, 34] (Fig. 14–1*c*). In general, the more lumens in a drain, the greater the efficiency of drainage. The cost for commercially made sump drains (Shirley wound drains) is moderate, and such drains may include a bacterial filter for the air intake.

A sump drain can be made from a Foley catheter by removing the syringe adapter and bulb and adding more fenestrations (Fig. 14–2*a–d*). The air vent serves to keep the main tube from collapsing and helps move fluid up the drain. The drain can function by continuous vented suction. The efficiency in removing peritoneal fluid is approximately 60%.[31]

4. *The sump–Penrose drain* is the newest type of drain. It was first described in 1970[31] and has been improved through variations[28, 34] (Fig. 14–1*d*). The fenestrated Penrose covering increases the drainage efficiency in the peritoneal cavity to approximately 72%.[31] The gauze padding (described by Ranson[34]), encased by the Penrose drain, decreases tissue damage caused by the stiff sump drain without decreasing efficiency. It has been used experimentally in the peritoneal cavity for 3 weeks with no adverse results.[28, 34] Like the sump drain, its mode of action is continuous suction. It is useful in deep wounds and in the peritoneal cavity.

Suction Drainage (Active Drainage)

Closed suction is created when a vacuum is connected to a single-lumen tube with no external air vent. A vacuum is thereby created within the wound. The vacuum may be applied intermittently (chest drainage) or continuously (skin flaps). When used in wounds, suction is adequate to create an atmospheric bandage (obliterating spaces without excessive pressure), which is approximately 80 mmHg of pressure.[20] Many portable closed suction systems are available commercially. An example is a compressible plastic canister typified by the Snyder Hemovac (Fig. 14–3). The contents of the evacuator can reflux into the wound if the patient inadvertently lies on it.[35, 36] This problem is eliminated by the addition of a one-way valve device. The Hemovac device can be taped to the patient to provide a portable, continuous, even-pressure, and aseptic closed-suction device. The Snyder Hemovac reservoir container comes in three different sizes (200, 400, and 800 ml) with varied tubing sizes and lengths.

Vented suction is created when a vacuum source is applied to a multiple-

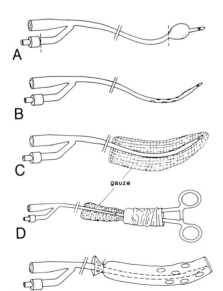

Figure 14–2. Foley catheter conversion to a padded Sump–Penrose drain. *a,* Removal of the syringe adaptor and bulb. *b,* Fenestration of the larger tube lumen. *c,* Placement of gauze padding around drain. *d,* Threading the padded drain through Penrose drain. *e,* Securing the Penrose drain and gauze to the Foley catheter; fenestrations are made in the Penrose drain.

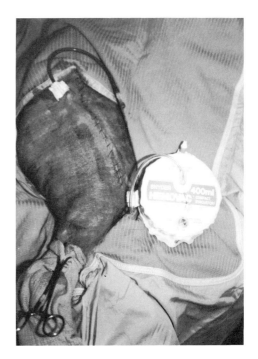

Figure 14–3. Photograph of inflow/outflow tube drains and a Hemovac portable continuous evacuation device. This is a 400-ml evacuator.

lumen drain.[37] Air is drawn from the room into the wound and back through the drain (Fig. 14–4). Bacterial filters may be fitted to the air intake and are helpful in decreasing contamination.[24, 37] Suction may be applied continuously or intermittently. High-volume suction (20 L/min) increases contamination compared to low-volume suction (4 L/min) because it draws a greater volume of room air through the wound.[38] It is also more traumatic to tissues than low-volume suction.

Properly applied suction drainage increases drain efficiency and reduces drain-related infection. Suction effectively decreases the "two-way street effect" of bacteria ascending into the wound while debris moves out of the wound. The suction thereby decreases stasis of effluence in the drain.[32] The contamination rate of the proximal end of Penrose drains in one study was 34% at the end of 24 hours,[25] whereas the contamination rate for drains with closed suction was 0%.[30] Closed, vented, and nonvented drainage should be further utilized in veterinary surgical patients.

Figure 14–4. Two variations of commonly used vented suction drains. The arrows trace the flow of air and wound fluid.

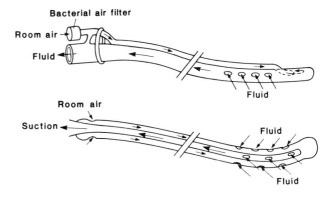

GENERAL COMPLICATIONS OF DRAIN USAGE

The complications of drain use can be more serious than the problem for which the drain is used.[19] An increased incidence of wound infection is a legitimate concern, but the problem can be tempered.[24, 25, 27, 32, 39, 40] This increased incidence of infection is related to two major factors: local tissue resistance and bacterial load.[41]

Tissue resistance to bacterial colonization is decreased by all types of drains. Even when the drain is buried, the infection rate is increased.[24] Cruse's study of 18,045 clean wounds supports the concept that drains increase infection rate and suction drainage reduces drain-induced morbidity[41] (Table 14–1). The mechanism for decreased local tissue resistance is not known, but may be related to tissue damage from foreign-body reaction, pressure ischemia, and adhesion breakdown at the time of drain removal.[42, 43] To combat the problem of decreased patient resistance, the fewest and smallest drains are used for drainage. The local bacterial population also affects wound infection rate. It is critical for drains to be placed and managed aseptically. Drains should be dressed and aseptically rebandaged as frequently as needed to maintain a dry bandage. Additionally, the fewest number of drain exit holes should be used for drainage. A generous area of skin around the drain should be clipped to ensure that the drain end is not contaminated by hair. It is possible for a drain to erode through the wall of a hollow viscus.[44] If a drain is placed near an anastomosis or large vessel, damage can occur at the time of drain removal if adhesions exist.[22, 34] Drains must be placed judiciously, and motion of the drain must be kept to a minimum.

An increased incidence of incisional dehiscence and hernia occurs when drains exit through the primary incision.[24, 40] Placing the drain through a separate stab incision diminishes this problem.[45]

Premature loss and retention of drains are common problems.[14] If a drain is not properly secured, it can easily fall or be pulled from the wound (Fig. 14–5). If strong adhesions have formed or a large suture penetrates the drain, the drain could break during removal and a portion retract into the wound. To minimize the chance of misplaced drains, the number, size, and date of removal should be recorded. Radiopaque-marked drains also should be used.[14] Appropriate restraining devices on the patient (Elizabethan collar, bandage) should be utilized. Skin sutures that incorporate the drain or tape on the drain should always be used.

Malfunction of drains from obstruction can be caused by tissue fragments or, in the peritoneal cavity, by omentum surrounding the drain. This occurs in a healthy abdomen within 24 hours after drain placement.[14, 26, 42] Periodic flushing with 30 to 40 ml of saline effectively removes the obstruction but also introduces contamination.[26] One may justifiably choose to flush a drain

TABLE 14–1. Influence of Drains on Wound Infection

CLEAN WOUNDS	INFECTION RATE
Undrained	1.5%
Closed suction	1.8%
Penrose through a separate stab	2.4%
Penrose through same incision	4.0%

Source: Cruse PJE, Arch Surg 1973; 107:206–210.

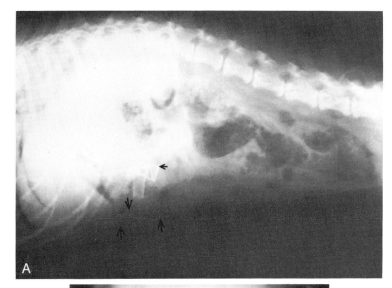

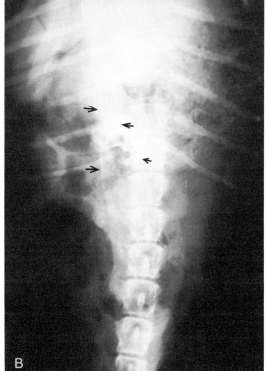

Figure 14–5. Lateral and ventro-dorsal view radiographs of a dog with a subcutaneous Penrose drain left in place *(larger arrows)* and a portion in the stomach *(smaller arrow)*. The patient chewed and ingested part of this subcutaneous drain. The ingested portion should pass without causing problems; however, the retained subcutaneous portion must be removed.

in a highly contaminated wound where drainage is essential (e.g., abscess, severe generalized/localized peritonitis). On the other hand, removal of an obstructed drain would be advisable in a clean wound if drainage is no longer critical (skin flap).

Pain associated with drains may be an overlooked problem in veterinary medicine. Drains have been shown to cause abdominal splinting and an elevated postoperative temperature in humans.[27, 40] This is termed *drain fever*. Upper abdominal drains can lead to decreased voluntary and involuntary respirations, predisposing the patient to atelectasis and pneumonia.[27, 46]

Discomfort may cause the veterinary patient to mutilate the drains. Appropriate restraint (Elizabethan collar) and analgesia are advisable.

Drain-tract cellulitis is another common, yet minor, problem.[26] It usually resolves without complication after drain removal.

A final drain-related problem is the surgeon's reliance on the drain to compensate for improper intraoperative and postoperative management. Drains cannot substitute for proper hemostasis, gentle tissue handling, and postoperative patient evaluation.[14, 23]

DURATION OF DRAINAGE

Between 3 and 5 days are required for a drain to establish a tract at sites of infection (abscess), and between 9 and 11 days are required in the biliary or urinary system.[25] As much as 50 ml daily of serosanguineous fluid can be induced by a drain in the thorax, abdomen, or a large subcutaneous wound.[23] This must be included in evaluation of the drain prior to removal. It is most often recommended that the entire drain be removed, although in patients with a large established abscess cavity, it may be best to withdraw only one-fourth of the drain daily and allow the cavity to close behind the drain.[14, 40]

SPECIFIC APPLICATIONS

Subcutaneous Drainage (Traumatic Wounds, Abscesses, and Incisions)

The most common method of draining a subcutaneous space (exclusive of skin flaps or grafts) is passive drainage by Penrose drains. Situations in which drains are commonly used include dog bite wounds with separation of the dermis from lower tissue levels, lacerations with loose skin, mastectomy incisions, some mammary lumpectomies or other large excision wounds, seromas, elbow and ischial hygromas, and cat bite abscesses.

The subcutaneous area to be drained should be evaluated, and the Penrose drain should be attached to the dorsal area by direct visualization (if a primary incision exists) or by blind placement (if no primary incision exists) through a stab wound. If there is a primary incision, a separate ventral stab incision is made away from the primary incision as a drain exit hole. For blind placement, a hemostatic forceps holding the drain is advanced through a ventrally placed stab wound. The hemostat and drain are tunneled as far dorsally as the wound pocket allows. A suture needle is passed through the skin and drain and out through the skin. This suture is tied loosely, and the hemostat is withdrawn. A gentle tug on the drain confirms that it is attached to the tissues. Ideally, contact of the drain under the main incision is kept to a minimum. A small length of drain should protrude through the stab wound (a 2–4-cm incision is adequate) with another tacking suture at the skin edge of the stab wound. There should be no tension on the drain. This is a single-exit drain (Figs. 14–6 and 14–7). If irrigation of the wound is desired, a double-exit drain may be more efficient. Placement in this instance involves two stab wounds and the drain is brought out both ends of the wound. Irrigation solution can then be instilled in the most dorsal or proximal opening and allowed to exit ventrally (Fig. 14–8).

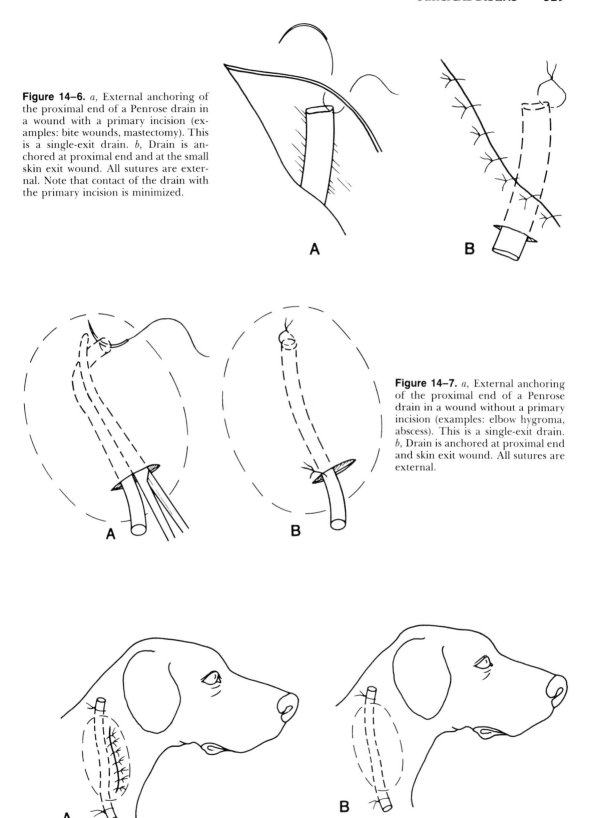

Figure 14–6. *a,* External anchoring of the proximal end of a Penrose drain in a wound with a primary incision (examples: bite wounds, mastectomy). This is a single-exit drain. *b,* Drain is anchored at proximal end and at the small skin exit wound. All sutures are external. Note that contact of the drain with the primary incision is minimized.

Figure 14–7. *a,* External anchoring of the proximal end of a Penrose drain in a wound without a primary incision (examples: elbow hygroma, abscess). This is a single-exit drain. *b,* Drain is anchored at proximal end and skin exit wound. All sutures are external.

Figure 14–8. Double exit drains can be flushed. *a,* With a primary skin incision, the drain should never exit through the primary incision. *b,* No primary incision.

The following specific guidelines should be used for the placement of Penrose drains:

1. The drain should be placed vertically to obtain maximum flow by gravity.
2. The exit wound should be adequate (1.5–2 times the width of drain) to permit flow of drainage fluid.
3. The drain's contact with the primary incision should be minimized, and drains should never exit through the primary incision.
4. Adequate wound preparation is essential (i.e., drain ends should not contact the haircoat).
5. A light, sterile bandage should be applied and changed to maintain asepsis.
6. Extruding drain and exit wound should be cleaned twice daily to avoid obstruction of the outflow tract and to minimize infection. The primary wound should be kept dry.
7. The patient should be kept inactive and in a clean, dry environment.
8. Duration of drainage may be from 2 to 14 days. The drain should be removed when drainage decreases. The following are general guidelines:

Hygroma or large seroma	10–14 days
Severe bite wound	4–6 days
Mastectomy	4 days

9. The drain should be protected from removal by using an Elizabethan collar or bandage. Drains should be examined daily and counted.
10. Penrose drains are not appropriate for intraoral or intrathoracic use (e.g., retrobulbar abscess or pleural effusion).
11. To remove the drain, cut all skin–drain tacking sutures and examine the drain to confirm it has been completely removed.

Deep-Pocket Drainage

Deep-pocket drainage can be achieved via passive Penrose drains or tubes and closed suction drainage. Deep-pocket drainage can be accomplished by use of Penrose drains if a sufficient pathway can be created from the pocket to the skin surface. Principles of subcutaneous drainage apply, with emphasis on an adequate, dependent pathway (primarily with Penrose use) and cleaning and bandaging the drain to decrease ascending bacterial infection (Penrose and closed suction drains). Examples of deep pockets where drains are commonly used include septic arthritis, osteomyelitis, and bulla osteitis.

Placement of the deep Penrose drain differs from subcutaneous placement by absence of external skin–drain tacking sutures. Generally, the pocket to be drained is deep enough to hold the Penrose drain in place simply by apposition of the overlying soft tissue. Additionally, more drain is left internally. An open approach is usually indicated to allow irrigation with or without debridement, culture, and biopsy of deep tissue (e.g., synovium, tympanic bulla, necrotic bone, implant removal associated with osteomyelitis). If the drain has a tendency to slip out, small (6-0) chromic catgut sutures can be placed loosely around the drain tip and secured to deep tissues although some surgeons prefer not to place internal sutures to avoid tearing the drain during removal.

Another appropriate method of draining deep pockets is closed suction drainage (intermittent or continuous). Red rubber tubes (Sovereign feeding

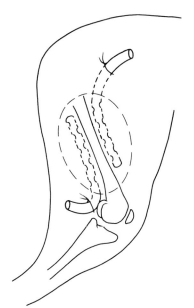

Figure 14–9. Illustration of an inflow and outflow tube drain system placed in a deep pocket adjacent to the femur. The tubes can be attached to continuous or intermittent closed suction.

tubes and urethral catheters) or polyvinyl chloride tubes (trocar catheters) are used singly or in pairs as an inflow/outflow system (Fig. 14–9). Injection plugs can be used to seal the system and can be removed to infuse irrigation solution or attach a suction device. The number of fenestrations in the distal end of the tube can be increased, if necessary, but in most instances this is not necessary. The drains are placed as described for Penrose drains, with attention to placing all the fenestrations within the cavity to be drained. If one fenestration is placed subcutaneously, fluid pockets will be created during infusion. If fenestrations are external to the wound, closed suction is not possible. When placing the drain, acute angles must be avoided to prevent tube kinking. Tube drains should never exit through the primary incision. Skin exit holes may be small because drainage should occur primarily through the lumen, not around the drain. Drains may be secured externally to the skin with butterfly tape and four-point fixation (Fig. 14–10) or the Chinese finger trap suture (Fig. 14–11).

The amount and frequency of irrigation depend on the degree of contamination. The amount of effluent is measured and should be equal to or greater than the amount of irrigation. Intermittent closed suction can be accomplished with a syringe or low-pressure suction machine. Aspiration should be performed at least every 6 hours. Continuous closed suction can be established with use of a Snyder Hemovac or other source of continuous suction (see Fig. 14–3).

The most common complication of this drainage is failure of the system

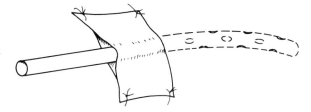

Figure 14–10. Butterfly tape applied to a tube drain with four-point suture fixation.

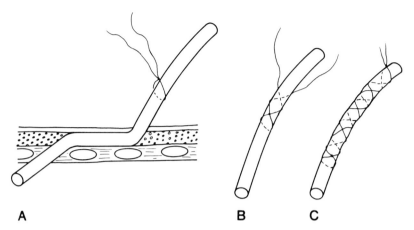

Figure 14–11. Chinese finger trap suture. *a,* A large bite of skin is taken 1 to 2 cm from the tube exit wound and the ends tied with two square knots. The ends are left long and in equal lengths. The ends are wrapped 180° around the tube and tied with a surgeon's knot. *b,* The suture ends are crisscrossed underneath the tube and tied with a constricting surgeon's knot on the near side. *c,* This process is repeated at least four times to complete the pattern.

due to obstruction (tissue particles or tube kinking). If flushing with sterile saline does not release the obstruction or the effluent removed is less than the irrigation inflow, the system must be removed or replaced.

Duration of deep pocket drainage varies with each case. Three to 5 days would be considered average drainage time although duration depends on the amount and character of the effluent. When the amount of effluent is diminishing and fluid is clearing (grossly and microscopically), the drain may be removed.

Care of deep-pocket drains includes:

1. Protection from patient removal with an Elizabethan collar placed on the animal.
2. Coverage with a sterile wrap when possible.
3. Complete drain removal.

Skin Flap and Graft Drainage

Hematoma or seroma formation under a full-thickness skin graft is the most common cause of graft failure. Drainage of fluid under full-thickness skin grafts is vitally important to maintain contact of the graft with the host bed. The following techniques are used and are listed in order of increasing efficiency of fluid removal: "pie crust" incisions, nonexpanded and expanded meshing, and continuous low-level suction.[47]

Two continuous low-level suction devices have been described by Swaim and Lee.[48] These consist of a butterfly catheter with or without an adapter, and a 5-ml red-top evacuated container or syringe (Figs. 14–12 and 14–13). They are easy to use, inexpensive, and effective.

The syringe adapter of the butterfly catheter is cut from the tubing, and fenestrations are cut into the tubing. The fenestrated portion of the tube is placed in the site to be drained and exited through a small, snug skin opening. The needle on the free end of the tubing is inserted into a 5- or 10-ml evacuated container (red-top tube) after the incision is closed. An

Figure 14–12. Placement of a closed suction drain under a skin flap. The device is made from a butterfly catheter by removing the syringe adapter and fenestrating this portion of the tube. The needle is inserted into a redtop tube after the skin has been sutured in place.

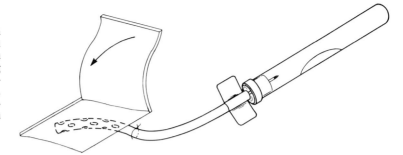

alternative device can be created by removing the needle portion of the butterfly catheter, fenestrating this end, and leaving the syringe adapter connected to a syringe. The syringe plunger is drawn back and held in position by a pin or needle to create negative pressure. The tubing can be attached with an encircling suture to the skin, and the entire apparatus lightly bandaged. It is important that movement of the tube under the skin flap or graft be eliminated. Movement of the drain will damage graft tissue vascularization. Correct placement of the drainage tubing under a skin flap through an exit skin wound that preserves the blood supply to the flap should be selected. The exit route should not involve the primary incision or damage the base of the pedicle.

When the drainage tubes are used to remove a hematoma due to capillary oozing, 24 hours is generally adequate for drainage.[48] A drain used to remove inflammatory fluids will generally be needed for 2 to 3 days if the wound is not infected. In an infected area, drains should be removed when infection is controlled. The character of the fluid changes from purulent to serosanguinous and fluid volume decreases.

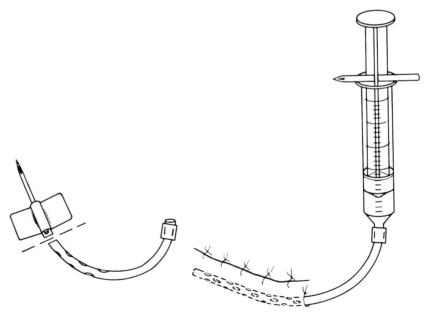

Figure 14–13. Placement of a closed suction device under a skin wound. The device is made from a butterfly catheter by removing the needle, fenestrating the tube, and connecting a syringe to the adapter. The plunger on the syringe creates negative pressure by being held in place by a needle put through the plunger.

Drain care involves the following procedures:

1. Protection from patient removal/mutilation.
2. Coverage with sterile wrap to reduce movement of the drain.
3. Complete removal of the drain.
4. If obstruction occurs, drains should be removed and not flushed.
5. Syringe or vacuum tube should be changed as needed to maintain suction.

Thoracic Drains

Only closed suction tube drains are used for draining the pleural space. Red rubber tubes (Sovereign feeding tubes) and clear polyethylene or polyvinylchloride tubes (trocar catheters) have been used. They can be placed by a closed (without thoracotomy) or open (during thoracotomy) technique. Thoracic drains are used to treat the following conditions:

1. Pyothorax
2. Air, blood, or fluid evacuation after thoracotomy
3. Chronic pleural effusion (e.g., chylothorax, hydrothorax)
4. Pneumothorax or hemothorax associated with trauma

Generalized Pyothorax. Open or closed placement technique is appropriate. Although there are no studies on mortality rates without thoracic drainage, pyothorax is generally considered fatal without such treatment. Survival rates increase to an estimated 40% to 60% with continuous closed suction thoracic drainage without thoracotomy.[49] Pyothorax also may be treated by thoracotomy involving debridement and lavage with postoperative drainage. There is no evidence to show that thoracotomy improves mortality. Intermittent evacuation (syringe) and lavage for the treatment of pyothorax is also appropriate. Evacuation should be done at least every 6 hours. Warm sterile saline (20 ml/kg) can be infused after each evacuation, removed immediately, and the procedure repeated. After several flush cycles, when the character of the fluid is less flocculent or if the tube is plugged, the thoracic wrap is replaced and the patient allowed to rest until the next scheduled treatment. The character and volume of evacuated fluid and air are monitored.

After Thoracotomy. After thoracotomy, a drain can be used for short- (minutes) or long-term (hours to days) duration depending on the need for continued drainage. Open placement is appropriate. For example, a patient undergoing a thoracotomy for repair of an uncomplicated patent ductus arteriosus (PDA), persistent right aortic arch (PRAA), or diaphragmatic hernia should not require drainage beyond initial evacuation of the pleural space. This can be completed within a few minutes. There should be no continued air or fluid leakage. One procedure is to place the drain intra-operatively and remove it shortly after the patient is extubated when negative pressure has been reestablished and the patient's respiratory excursions are normal. A patient undergoing removal of part of the respiratory tract (e.g., pneumonectomy, lung lobectomy) should have a chest drain for several hours postoperatively. This is especially necessary if the airway closure is tenuous or hemorrhage occurs. If a thoracotomy is performed, thoracic drains are best placed before the thoracotomy incision is closed (see Open Placement, below). The pleural space should be evaluated at least every 6 hours. Volumes of air and fluid should be monitored.

Chronic Pleural Effusion. Other indications for thoracic drainage include chronic hydrothorax and chylothorax. Open or closed chest tube placement is appropriate depending on the need for thoracotomy. Initially, conservative medical management is recommended for treatment of chylothorax and includes tube thoracostomy and dietary management.[50] Thoracic drains are not definitive treatment for the effusion. The thoracic drain's purpose is to evacuate fluid to relieve respiratory distress and seal the thoracic duct. Medical management also should include a diet high in protein and carbohydrates and low in fat with medium-chain triglycerides. This decreases the volume and flow of chyle from the thoracic duct. If the effusion persists longer than 2 to 3 weeks, an active or passive shunt, thoracic duct obliteration, pleuroperitoneal shunting, diaphragmatic meshing, or pleurodesis should be considered. Evacuation of the pleural space should be done at least every 6 hours initially and then as needed.

Trauma. Usually, closed placement is appropriate. Thoracic drains are uncommonly needed to treat thoracic trauma. Pneumothorax often can be treated and controlled by simple needle aspiration. If negative pressure in the pleural space cannot be established with needle aspiration, or if multiple aspirates per hour are required to maintain negative pressure, then a chest drain is indicated with continuous suction, a Heimlich one-way valve, or intermittent suction. Closed placement is generally used with severe pneumothorax because exploratory thoracotomy with open placement often yields multiple leaks that cannot be corrected surgically or the patient is an anesthetic risk. Likewise, hemorrhage into the pleural space does not often require chest drain placement. The respiratory distress seen with moderate amounts of hemorrhage into the pleural space is often due to pulmonary hemorrhage and edema, pain, and shock. In these cases, closed thoracic drainage may actually worsen the patient's condition as a result of anesthesia and postoperative discomfort. If hemorrhage occurs causing severe pulmonary compromise, drainage is necessary. Needle aspirate drainage should be attempted initially. If hemorrhage and respiratory compromise continue, then a thoracic drain should be placed in an open or closed manner. Closed placement should be considered if blood loss is not severe. Persistent anemia due to hemorrhage and respiratory embarrassment are indications for transfusion and open chest drain placement (thoracic exploratory).

Another cause for hemothorax is coagulopathies. Animals with warfarin toxicity can present only with hemothorax. Treating the primary problem with vitamin K, fresh whole blood transfusion, and supportive care often eliminates the need for placement of a thoracic drain. Needle evacuation of the pleural space can be done if respiratory compromise is severe.

CLOSED PLACEMENT

Closed placement of a thoracic drain refers to placement without a thoracotomy incision. This technique is commonly used with pyothorax, trauma, and chronic effusions. The catheter sizes are usually 10 to 12 French for adult cats and 18 to 26 French for large dogs. In patients with minimal subcutaneous fat and muscle (cats and small dogs), it is important not to overestimate the required tube size. A 14 to 16 French catheter in such patients can lead to subcutaneous leakage of pleural fluid and subcutaneous emphysema as a result of room air drawn into the wound. The hole in the thoracic wall and skin wound must not leak. The tube can be placed on the left or right side based on evaluation of chest radiographs. Radiographs are taken after careful fluid evacuation to check tube placement, function, and the presence of other lesions. Bilateral tubes may be required if the patient has bilateral fluid accumulation and an intact mediastinum or very viscous fluid.

Thoracic tube placement is painful and requires general anesthesia in all but moribund patients. With dyspneic patients, it is vitally important to relieve compromised respiratory function prior to anesthesia (e.g., via needle aspiration) or use an injectable anesthetic agent and gain control of the respiration via intubation and positive-pressure ventilation. The dose of induction agents for ill patients is often less than for healthy animals. If the patient has very mild tachypnea, pink mucous membranes, and is comfortable, gas induction may be used. Intubation and intermittent positive-pressure ventilation should be used soon after induction.

The entire lateral thoracic wall of the patient is clipped and prepared for aseptic surgery prior to induction with anesthesia. There should be minimal time delay from induction to surgery in patients with compromised respiration. A small vertical skin incision is placed at the level of the 10th rib midway between the dorsal and ventral midlines. A small, pointed hemostatic forceps (Kelly or mosquito) is used to hold the tube. The tip of the hemostat should extend 2 to 3 mm beyond the tip of the tube. The tube is tunneled cranially and subcutaneously past two ribs. The hemostat holding the tube is positioned perpendicularly to the body wall and pressure applied until the hemostat "pops" through the intercostal musculature (Fig. 14–14). The pressure required to achieve this is more than expected in many cases, thus making a controlled entry difficult. It is possible to penetrate the underlying lung and heart if care is not taken to control the depth of hemostat entry. The tips of the hemostat are opened to release the tube and part the soft tissues, and the tube advanced. The tube should be closed by a clamp or catheter plug to avoid pneumothorax.

The tube should be positioned along the sternum, with all fenestrations placed within the pleural space. A purse-string suture is used to close the skin opening around the entry wound to prevent subcutaneous emphysema. In patients with drains removed immediately after surgery (e.g., uncomplicated PDA, PRAA correction, or diaphragmatic herniorrhaphy), the purse-string suture is tied upon removal of the thoracic drain. A butterfly tape and four-point suture fixation or Chinese finger trap suture can be used to fix the tube to the patient[51] (see Figs. 14–10 and 14–11). A soft, padded sterile

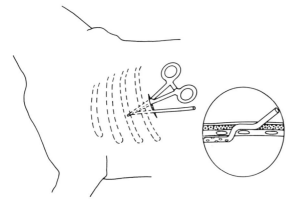

Figure 14–14. Using a hemostat to place a thoracostomy tube. The tube is tunneled subcutaneously two spaces rostral to the skin wound and forcibly passed into the thoracic cavity.

dressing is applied loosely over the drain entry wound and affixes the drain to the patient. The drain tip should be easily accessible without removing the entire wrap.

An intravenous male adaptor injection plug can be used in the end of the tube drain by cutting the drain back to a narrow diameter. The plug fits snugly and forms a watertight, airtight seal that prevents accidental pneumothorax. Also, fluid can be removed via the needle and syringe, or the plug can be removed at each treatment and the syringe attached directly to the tube. The Abbott male adapter plug will fit sizes 5 to 18 French feeding tubes. For larger feeding tubes, a Luer-Lok adaptor plug is necessary to fit the male adaptor plug into the end. A Heimlich, one-way valve also can be placed in the drain end if pneumothorax is the primary problem. It allows unidirectional airflow from the pleural space. It is bulkier and more cumbersome than an injection cap and should be reserved for patients with tension pneumothorax. With continuous closed suction, the tube drain is securely connected to the suction tubing via adapters. Patient monitoring must be intensive and continuous because accidental disconnection of the tubes may cause a pneumothorax. Two systems previously described for continuous closed suction thoracic drainage are the Thora-Klex Unit and Sentinel Seal Compact Drainage Unit.[49, 51] The pressure should be maintained between -15 and -25 cm H_2O.

OPEN PLACEMENT

Open placement of a thoracic drain refers to placement during a thoracotomy. It is commonly used for treatment of pyothorax, chronic effusions, or trauma (flail chest). This placement is technically easier and has less risk of damage to underlying organs than the closed technique. Thoracic drain placement alone, however, is not an indication for thoracotomy.

The small vertical skin incision for the drain is placed several inches caudal to the thoracotomy incision. For example, with a standard left 4th intercostal thoracotomy, the tube drain incision is placed at the 10th to 12th rib level, midway between the vertebrae and sternebrae. Use of a hemostat and subcutaneous tunneling is similar to closed placement. Upon entering the pleural space two to four ribs away from the primary incision, the surgeon's hand is placed inside the chest cavity to protect the heart and lungs. The remainder of tube placement is the same as described for closed thoracic drain placement.

Complications of thoracic drains are important and include:

1. Accidental, life-threatening pneumothorax. This can occur if the tube is left open to room air by failure or disconnection of the injection plug. Pneumothorax also can occur by leakage around the tube or partial removal of the tube and exposure of fenestrations to room air. Most situations causing accidental pneumothorax can be avoided by careful staff training, proper placement and fixation of the tube, proper restraint of the patient via bandages and Elizabethan collars, and constant observation.

2. Obstruction of the drain can be caused by particulate matter (tissue debris) and kinking of the drain. Kinking usually occurs at a fenestration if the fenestration is too large, wide, or irregular. It also can be caused by inserting excessive lengths of tubing into the pleural space. The drain then can curl, kink, or even form a knot. A clogged drain can be opened by flushing or readjusting the drain position (extract a small length), or the

drain should be removed. If the drain is still required, placement at a different site is recommended.

3. A functional obstruction occurs when the drain is not plugged by tissue or kinked but fails to drain fluid. This may occur because of fluid pocketing. This is common with pyothorax in cats. Warm sterile saline (50 ml) may be infused at one time, and only a portion of the fluid removed as effluent. The patient should be turned and held in different positions for removal of all pleural fluid. Gentle compression of the thoracic cavity also may improve the retrieval of fluid.

4. Drain tract cellulitis and subcutaneous emphysema can occasionally occur. Patients at risk for leakage are thin and have minimal musculature. Additionally, debility and pathogenic bacteria associated with pyothorax may predispose animals to subcutaneous abscessation at the drain site.

Duration of drainage will vary according to the problem and how long the tube remains functional. The drain should remain until the primary problem is sufficiently resolved so the patient no longer requires the regular evacuation of air or fluid. As a guideline, pyothorax drainage ranges 3 to 10 days in cats. In one study of pyothorax in dogs, the average duration of drainage was 5 to 6 days.[49] The character of fluid should be a modified transudate with diminishing volume. Idiopathic chronic effusion may require drainage for 1 to 2 weeks to determine if diminution of effluent volume will occur spontaneously.[50]

Removal of a thoracic drain is achieved by cutting the external suture attachments and quickly removing the entire length of tubing. A sterile, nonadherent pad with a small amount of bactericidal ointment is placed over the drain exit hole to provide an airtight seal and prevent pneumothorax. A light wrap holds the pad in position for 48 hours.

Thoracic drains, and tube drains in general, require more care than Penrose drains. Most critical is the need to prevent accidental pneumothorax by appropriate bandaging, suturing, use of an Elizabethan collar, and constant observation. "Stripping" the drain or backflushing sterile saline to ensure patency is done every 6 hours. Cleaning of the exit site is not recommended if the wound is dry because a reasonable seal exists around the tube. If the wound is scrubbed regularly, this seal will not readily form. Maintaining a sterile wrap is adequate to minimize local bacterial contamination.

Abdominal Drains

The two drains conventionally used in the abdominal cavity are the latex Penrose drain and the sump–Penrose drain.

The indications for their use are localized or generalized (diffuse) peritonitis with fluid accumulation. The reader is referred to Chapter 2 in this text and elsewhere for details of generalized and localized peritonitis.[17, 29]

LOCALIZED PERITONITIS

Localized peritonitis can be caused by rupture of the intestinal tract, body wall, reproductive organs, or urinary tract. In addition, pancreatitis and leakage of a hepatobiliary, lymph node, or prostatic abscess can cause localized peritonitis. One of the most common causes of localized peritonitis that requires drainage is prostatic abscessation. Use of a drain is indicated if septic fluid or necrotic debris accumulates and cannot be completely excised or marsupialized. Complete prostatectomy is an alternative to drainage, but requires greater surgical skill, demands longer operative times, and has major postoperative problems. Urinary incontinence is one of the foremost problems, and it occurs in 85% to 100% of surgical patients.[52, 53] Marsupialization is often not possible due to the position and friability of the prostate gland.

A new technique for surgical management of prostatic abscesses, called *prostatic parenchymal omentalization,* was recently reported.[54] The surgery was 100% successful for resolution of prostatic abscesses, although it only included a small number of cases and follow-up was only 6 months.

Since the majority of deaths in patients with prostatic abscessation occur from septic shock and because postoperative complications of prostate drainage are manageable, the simplest and quickest surgical procedure (i.e., drainage) seems advisable. In a study of 92 cases of prostatic abscess drained by Penrose drain, 82% of the surviving patients had fair to excellent postoperative results.[52] The method of Penrose drain placement within and around the prostate is described below.

Prostatic Abscess Drain Placement: Intraprostatic. Penrose drain placement for prostatic abscess was initially described by Zolton and Greiner.[55] After induction of the animal with general anesthesia, a urinary catheter is placed. The entire ventral abdomen is prepared for aseptic surgery. A parapreputial skin incision is made from the cranial border of the pubis to a point cranial to the prepuce. A midline entry is made into the abdominal cavity through the linea alba. The ventrolateral aspect of the prostate can be visualized from this approach in most cases. If the abscess has ruptured, gentle blunt dissection with scissors and fingers can be used to create a pathway for the drain. A sample should be taken for histologic evaluation, aerobic and anaerobic bacterial cultures; and antimicrobial sensitivity testing. If the prostate remains intact, two cube-shaped sections of the ventrolateral aspect of the prostate are removed on the left and right sides to gain access to the abscess cavity. The urethra, with the catheter in place, is easily identified by palpation. The abscess capsule may be thick and fibrous, and removing the initial sections may require scalpel dissection. Once the abscess cavity is open, suction and irrigation are instituted until the fluid appears clear and the lining is free of necrotic tissue. Two ventrolateral openings should be made as large as possible without damaging the urethra, dorsal vasculature, or nerves. The original technique described by Zolton and Greiner involves placing two to four ½-in Penrose drains via the ventral prostatic incision through the abscess cavity and exiting the prostate dorsolaterally (Fig. 14–15). These drain ends are then brought together through the paramedian aspect of the body wall. This is done on the left and right lobes if the abscess is generalized. The drains that are placed in the right lobe of the prostate exit to the right paramedian area and the left drains to the left paramedian area. Four to six additional Penrose drains are then placed externally around the gland and exit through a different paramedian incision. These drains are to be removed independently of the intraprostatic drains.

Another variation of this technique also avoids incising the dorsal portion of the prostate and damage to the neurovascular supply. The approach is similar to the preceding procedure but differs in drain placement. One to four wide (1–2-in) Penrose drains are placed through one ventrolateral

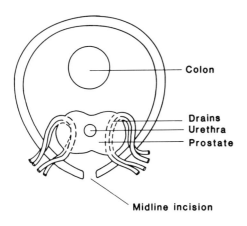

Figure 14–15. Cross-sectional view of prostate gland showing the path of the Penrose drains for the technique described by Zolton and Greiner. The drains exit through the left and right paramedian aspects of the ventral abdomen.

prostate opening, passed dorsally to the urethra, and exit through the opposite ventrolateral prostate opening (Fig. 14–16). The drain now has two ends, one exiting each side of the prostate. The ends are brought through two stab wounds in the body wall and skin at least 2 inches from the midline. Abdominal drains should never exit the primary wound because of the increased incident of dehiscence.[24, 40, 45] It is important that these openings in the body wall and skin are large enough to avoid pinching, allow extraluminal drainage, and still prevent herniation of abdominal contents. The drains should take a direct, short route to the body wall. The openings in the body wall and skin also should be fairly well aligned so that "scissoring" or subcutaneous tunneling of the drain does not occur. There should be no tension on the drains, which would cause discomfort for the patient. If one drain is used, the drain end will be visible externally on the left and right side. If two drains are used, two ends will be visible externally. The drains are tacked to the skin with one nonabsorbable suture. No internal drain suturing is necessary. No suturing of the prostate is necessary. If the prostatic abscess is severe and necrosis of the prostate capsule has occurred, placement of the Penrose drain is the same (i.e., encircling the urethra), but technically it may be periprostatic (see Fig. 14–16).

There are many postoperative problems associated with prostatic abscessation, but two reported problems directly related to the presence of the drain are premature removal of the drain and urine leakage from the Penrose drains. Other problems (e.g., urinary incontinence and recurrence of the abscess) occur with other methods of prostatic abscess treatment (total

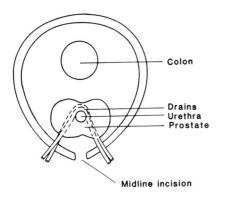

Figure 14–16. Cross-sectional view of the caudal aspect of the abdomen in a male dog. Two Penrose drains are placed through the ventrolateral aspect of the prostate, dorsally to the urethra, and exiting the opposite ventrolateral region of the gland. The drains exit the left and right paramedian aspects of the body wall.

SURGICAL DRAINS · 341

prostatectomy) and drainage.[52] Premature removal of the drains by the patient can be avoided by constant observation, Elizabethan collars, and bandaging. Urine leakage can be managed by placement of an indwelling urinary catheter for 5 to 7 days.

Penrose drains should be left in place at least 10 days and as long as 3 weeks depending on the amount and character of the effluent, results of patient's physical examination (prostate size, tenderness, texture), and laboratory data (complete blood count and urine sediment). When the drains are removed, the skin suture is cut, one end of the drain is cut short, and the area is cleaned. Tension applied to the longer uncut ends should aid in removal of the entire drain.

Other Abdominal Abscess Drainage. Placement of Penrose drains for other causes of localized peritonitis should follow the same principles: exposure, debridement, and irrigation of the septic area. Penrose drains should be positioned at the center of infection. They should exit by a direct ventral and paraincisional route. Internal suturing should only be used if there is concern for drain stability.

Penrose drains placed intraabdominally require the same attention as drains in subcutaneous pockets. The skin around the drain and the extruding drain should be cleaned with chlorhexidine or povidone-iodine solutions twice daily. The drains should be covered by a sterile, absorbent bandage. Retrograde flushing through the drain or around the drain is not recommended if the drain is functioning well. To prevent or identify internal retention of drains, the drains should be counted and numbers verified twice daily. The skin sutures through the drains also should be examined twice daily to identify tearing of the drain or suture failure. If the drain suture is disturbed, physical restraint of the patient should be increased. Elizabethan collars and side braces, as well as the absorbent bandage, will discourage patient destruction of the drainage system. Tube drains do not require frequent external cleaning but should be covered by a sterile wrap at the exit wound. Tube drains used for inflow of irrigation solution can be capped or left open if they provide drainage. As with Penrose drains, tube drain ends should be covered by an absorbent sterile bandage if left open. Sump drains also should be covered and may require periodic backflushing or "stripping" to clean debris or adhesions. This should be done only if the sump drain is obstructed. The suction line attached to the sump–Penrose drain requires frequent monitoring to ensure patency. Emptying the suction reservoir is done to prevent overflow.

GENERALIZED PERITONITIS

Until 1984, generalized peritonitis was usually treated by the use of drains. Penrose drains were used in a four-quadrant, multiple-drain pattern with or without an inflow tube for lavage.[29] However, conventional Penrose drains (latex) reportedly drain only 40% of a healthy peritoneal cavity and become obstructed or walled off within hours of placement.[31] This 40% efficacy may increase if the drains are used in a peritoneal cavity with severe generalized peritonitis. During inflammation, the omentum has decreasing ability to wall off foreign structures and create adhesions. The mortality rate of generalized peritonitis treated by this technique has not been reported.

In another study, silicone tube-type drains used in contaminated peritoneal cavities of dogs remained patent for at least 7 days after surgery.[56] Silicone incited a decreased tissue response compared to latex. When one or two of these drains were used with an inflow tube and lavage in animals with experimentally induced generalized peritonitis, the mortality rate was 25%.[57] There is no report of the efficacy of silicone drains used in clinical patients with generalized peritonitis.

Because of the low reported efficacy of latex Penrose (40%) and red rubber tube drains (39%) in the healthy canine peritoneum, alternative methods of peritoneal drainage were developed. The sump–Penrose drain increased efficiency to 72%; however, it was rigid and could readily damage adjacent organs. It also required labor-intensive continuous suction.[31] This system also may encourage patient destruction of drains as a result of discomfort. In one report when tubes and sump–Penrose drains were used for generalized peritonitis, mortality for both was 36%.[58]

The role of lavage in treating generalized peritonitis remains debated. The concern of spreading contamination through lavage is unfounded considering that the peritoneum's natural circulation will distribute contaminants within hours of introduction.[59] Warm sterile lavage fluid will dilute toxins and mobilize necrotic debris. Many reports in human as well as veterinary patients have shown lavage to be beneficial in decreasing mortality with generalized peritonitis.[29, 56, 57, 60–62] If the fluid is not entirely removed, however, it can increase mortality rates by diluting opsonins (proteins), decreasing surface area for white blood cells, and potentially supporting bacterial growth.[17] If lavage is employed, it is essential to remove all the fluid.

In 1984, open peritoneal drainage was introduced in veterinary surgery for treatment of generalized peritonitis.[62a] Open peritoneal drainage is accomplished by leaving a long laparotomy incision open (2–4 cm wide). The fluid drains into a large sterile bandage and no drain tube is employed. Treatment of generalized peritonitis with open peritoneal drainage has an overall mortality rate of 33% to 48%.[63, 64] A major disadvantage is the risk of evisceration and ascending infection. It appears that the mortality rates with generalized peritonitis in dogs treated by drain placement and by open peritoneal drainage are approximately equal. The best method depends on the ability to provide the required intense postoperative care. In a recent study, the clinicopathologic effects of open peritoneal drainage versus sump–Penrose drainage were compared in normal dogs.[64a] Neither technique caused detrimental effects, and drainage efficiencies were extremely variable.

As a generalization, if diffuse peritonitis is mild to moderate and the primary problem has been completely corrected, drainage may not be necessary. In this situation, postoperative observation and monitoring for peritonitis are critical. Human patients who develop peritonitis postoperatively have a high mortality due, in part, to delay of diagnosis and treatment.[65] If the peritonitis is severe or the primary problem cannot be corrected at the time of surgery, drainage is indicated. The methods described below include Penrose and sump–Penrose drains with an inflow lavage tube and open peritoneal drainage.

Placement of Drains. Closed placement of drains is rarely indicated. In general, if a patient has septic and intraabdominal fluid that requires drainage, then exploratory surgery, debridement, and lavage are needed. An exception may be a moribund patient with known septic peritoneal fluid and multiple-organ failure. Closed placement is utilized until the patient can survive anesthesia and surgical exploration. This requires aseptic preparation of the ventral aspect of the abdomen, using local anesthesia, making a 2-cm paramedian skin incision, and bluntly dissecting through the abdominal wall. Penrose drains are fed through the wound into the peritoneal cavity.

Open placement of Penrose drains for generalized peritonitis is done just before closure of the laparotomy incision. Four exit wounds are created in the skin, one in each quadrant of the abdomen (left, right, cranial, and caudal) (Fig. 14–17). Fenestrations in abdominal Penrose drains are not necessary or recommended. The skin wound should be approximately the same size as the Penrose drains being used (1–2 inches). A medium-sized curved hemostatic forceps (Pean) is used to separate the skin edges and penetrate the subcutaneous tissue and muscle. These tissue openings are stretched to allow comfortable passage of four Penrose drains. If the incisions are made lateral to the rectus abdominis muscle, the cranial and caudal epigastric vessels will be avoided. Minimal subcutaneous tunneling is advisable with the use of Penrose drains to avoid the "scissoring" effect of multiple tissue layers and obstruction of the periluminal flow. With the Pean forceps tip now inside the abdominal cavity, the four Penrose drain ends are grasped and pulled through the tissue layers. The length of drain protruding from the body should be 4 cm. Internal length of drain tubing should be adequate to fan out over much of the ventral abdomen. Drains should not be placed near an intestinal anastomosis. The drains are attached to the skin edge with a single nonabsorbable suture. This process is repeated in the remaining three quadrants using a total of 16 Penrose drains. Finally, an inflow tube of red rubber or silicone is placed paramedially in a caudal quadrant and by the same process. The tube is positioned obliquely across the ventral abdomen and secured to the skin with a butterfly device or Chinese finger trap suture. No internal suturing of drains is necessary. No drains exit through the laparotomy wound. Abdominal closure is routine and a sterile padded bandage is placed over all drains.

Lavage with warm sterile saline can be continuous or intermittent (two to

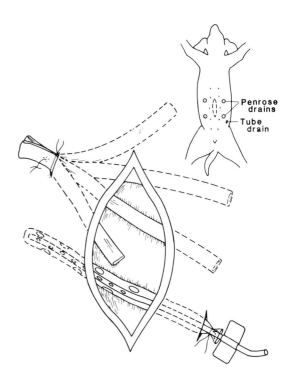

Figure 14–17. Four-quadrant technique of multiple Penrose drain and inflow tube placement. A total of 16 Penrose drains are placed within the abdominal cavity. The drain exit sites are marked on the ventral aspect of the abdominal wall. The tube drain can function as a vented suction device and for infusion of lavage fluid.

three times per day) with volume based on the size of the patient, efficacy of drains, and character of the effluent. Patients under 15 kg receive 500 ml of lavage, and those over 15 kg receive 1000 ml of lavage. There is considerable debate on the advantage of antibiotics or antiseptics mixed with the lavage fluid. Currently, saline lavage alone is considered as effective as saline plus antibiotics or povidone-iodine. Additionally, intraperitoneal use of many antibiotics and povidone-iodine can have deleterious effects.[66–68]

Placement of a sump–Penrose drain is similar to placement of a tube drain. The Penrose drain is fenestrated when used in this manner. The sump–Penrose drain is placed paramedially and parallel to the laparotomy incision. It may be placed in the cranial or caudal abdominal quadrant. The sump–Penrose drain must have all the fenestrations inside the abdominal cavity. Commercially made sump drains have a label marked "skin line" on the drain to indicate how far to insert them. The inflow tube may be placed in the opposite (left or right) quadrant. The sump–Penrose drain is attached to continuous suction after closure of the laparotomy wound. Sterile bandaging is recommended.

Open peritoneal drainage was first described in the veterinary literature by Orsher and Rosin and is accomplished by making a laparotomy incision from the xiphoid to the pubis.[62a] Exploration of the entire abdominal cavity, intraoperative lavage, and repair of the primary problem are completed. Upon closing the laparotomy wound, a simple continuous pattern using large nonabsorbable suture material is placed in the linea alba and skin. The wound edges are left 2 to 4 cm apart to allow ventral drainage and prevent evisceration. A large sterile bandage (including sterile hand towels) is placed over the wound prior to recovery from anesthesia. The wrap is changed aseptically once or twice daily as needed to maintain a dry external wrap. If the patient is uncooperative, brief anesthesia or sedation may be necessary. No drain tubes are employed, and final abdominal closure is performed 2 to 10 days after the initial surgery as the volume and character of the effluence improve.

Complications. Complications associated with Penrose drains include premature removal of drains and drain destruction with portions retained internally. Elizabethan collars, bandages, and close observation remedy this. Ascending infections, adhesions, and anastomotic breakdowns have not been reported in clinical veterinary cases. Malfunction of the drains is always a concern. Increasing peritoneal fluid can be difficult to detect in obese or painful patients. Additionally, if lavage is employed, the amount of effluent is difficult to measure because it is absorbed into bandage material. The amount of inflow is known, but the amount of outflow is only an estimate. If the drains are thought to be nonfunctional based on physical findings (increasing abdominal effusion), radiographic or ultrasound study, or paracentesis, the drains should be flushed with sterile saline. If they remain nonfunctional, they must be removed and another form of drainage instituted.

Complications associated with sump–Penrose drains are similar to those listed above, as well as problems related to maintaining continuous suction. Maintaining a patent suction line requires 24-hour care but is not technically difficult. Additionally, the amount of effluent can be measured and compared with the amount infused.

Complications specifically related to the technique of open peritoneal drainage could be increased risk of evisceration and ascending infection, although neither was reported to affect the outcome in two clinical studies.[63, 64] If bandage changes are performed with great care and the patient is properly restrained and observed, evisceration and ascending infection should be minimized. Patients did require monitoring and treatment for protein and fluid losses, however.

Duration of Drainage. For treatment of generalized peritonitis drainage will range from 2 to 10 days. For the average patient, lavage is needed for 2 to 3 days, with an additional day of drainage alone. The decision to discontinue lavage and drainage should be based on examination of the patient, laboratory results, ultrasonic evaluation for free fluid, and the amount and character of the effluent.

As with Penrose and sump–Penrose drainage of the peritoneal cavity, open peritoneal drainage may be necessary from 2 to 10 days. Most cases require 3 to 5 days. The decision to discontinue drainage is based on visualizing the exposed abdominal contents during wrap changes, the amount and character of the effluent, physical findings, and laboratory data. When open peritoneal drainage is no longer needed, the patient is anesthetized, intraoperative lavage and suction are repeated, and then routine closure of the laparotomy wound is accomplished.

PRODUCT LIST

Snyder Hemovac and one-way valve device, Zimmer, Inc., 727 North Detroit, Warshaw, IN 46580

Penrose drain, Davol, Inc., 100 Sockanossett Crossroad, Cranston, RI 02920

Sovereign feeding tube and Shirley wound drain, Monoject and Argyle, Division of Sherwood Medical, Inc., St. Louis, MO 63103

Foley catheter, CABARD, Inc., Murray Hill, NJ 07974

Male adapter plug, Abbott Hospitals, Inc., North Chicago, IL 60064

Butterfly catheter, Abbott Hospitals, Inc., North Chicago, IL 60064

Sovereign Luer-Lok adaptor plug, Argyle, Division of Sherwood Medical, Inc., St. Louis, MO 63103

Heimlich valve, Bard Parker/Becton Dickenson and Co., Lincoln Park, NJ 07035

Thora-Klex chest drainage unit, Davol, Inc., 100 Sockanossett Crossroad, Cranston, RI 02920

Sentinel seal compact chest drainage unit, Argyle, Division of Sherwood Medical, Inc., St. Louis, MO 63103

Nolvasan scrub, Fort Dodge Laboratories, Ft. Dodge, IO 50501

Povidone-iodine scrub, Camall, Washington, MI 48094

REFERENCES

1. Moss JP: Historical and current perspectives on surgical drainage. Surg Gynecol Obstet 1981; 152:173–527

2. Ludwig CH: The American Armamentarium. New York: George Tiemann, 1889
3. Castle FA: The antiquity of drainage tubes. Boston Med Surg J 1881; 104:356
4. Mumford JG: Surgical Memoirs. New York: Morrat and Yard, 1908
5. Dukes C: Lord Lister. London: Leonard Parsons, 1924
6. Penrose CB: Drainage in abdominal surgery. JAMA 1890; 14:264
7. Heaton G: Notes on the drainage of large cavities after surgical exploration. Br Med J 1898; 1:207
8. Yates JL: An experimental study of the local effects of peritoneal drainage. Surg Gynecol Obstet 1905; 1:473
9. Gray HMW: Some problems of drainage. Surg Gynecol Obstet 1924; 39:221–228
10. Chaffen RC: Drainage. Am J Surg 1934; 24:100
11. Ashhurst APC: Surgical drainage. Surg Clin North Am 1932; 13:372
12. Murphey DR: Use of atmospheric pressure in obliterating axillary dead space following radical mastectomy. South Surg 1947; 13:372
13. Flax LH: A new surgical drain. JAMA 1961; 177:150
14. Duthis HL: Drainage of the abdomen. N Engl J Med 1972; 287:1081–1083
15. Fox JW, Golden GT: The use of drains in subcutaneous surgical procedures. Am J Surg 1976; 132:673–674
16. McFarlane RM: The use of continuous suction under skin flaps. Br J Plast Surg 1959; 11:77–87
17. Crowe DT, Bjorling DE: Peritoneum and peritoneal cavity. In Slatter DH (ed): Textbook of Small Animal Surgery. Philadelphia: WB Saunders, 1985, pp 579–588
18. Alexander JW, Koewlitz J, Alexander NS: Prevention of wound infections: A case for closed suction drainage to remove wound fluids deficient in opsonic proteins. Am J Surg 1976; 132:59–63
19. Gupta S, Rauscher G, Stillman R, et al: The rational use of drains after cholecystectomy. Surg Gynecol Obstet 1978; 146:191–192
20. Garcia-Rinaldi R, Defore WW, Green ZD, et al: Improving the efficiency of wound drainage catheters. Am J Surg 1975; 130:372–373
21. Abel DL, Johnson JJ: Closed-wound irrigation of compound and contaminated fractures as a preventative and treatment for osteomyelitis. Vet Med/Sm Anim Clin 1975; 70:1425–1432
22. Abramson DJ: Charles Bingham Penrose and the Penrose drain. Surg Gynecol Obstet 1976; 143:285–286
23. Golovsky D, Conolly WB: Observations on wound drainage with a review of the literature. Med J Aust 1976; 1:289–291
24. Magee C, Rodeheaver GT, Golden GT, et al: Potential of wound infection by surgical drains. Am Surg 1976; 131:547–549
25. Nora PF, Vanecko RM, Bransfield JJ: Prophylactic abdominal drains. Arch Surg 1972; 105:183–176
26. Agrama HM, Blackwood JM, Brown CS, et al: Functional longevity of intraperitoneal drains. Am J Surg 1976; 132:418–421
27. Kassum DA, Gagic NM, Menon GT: Cholecystectomy with and without drainage. Can J Surg 1979; 22:358–360
28. Formeister JF, Elias EG: Safe intraabdominal and efficient wound drainage. Surg Gynecol Obstet 1976; 142:415–416
29. Withrow SJ, Black AP: Generalized peritonitis in small animals. Vet Clin North Am 1979; 9:363–379
30. Nora PF: Unpublished data, 1973, as stated in Cruse PJE: Arch Surg 1973; 107:206–210
31. Hanna EA: The efficiency of peritoneal drainage. Surg Gynecol Obstet 1970; 131:983–985
32. Casey B: Bacterial spread in polyethylene tubing: A possible source of surgical wound contamination. Med J Aust 1971; 2:718–719
33. Ross FP, Quinlan RM: Eight hundred cholecystectomies. Surgery 1975; 110:721–724
34. Ranson JHC: Safer intraperitoneal sump drainage. Surg Gynecol Obstet 1973; 137:841–842
35. Abramson DJ: A combined soft tissue and suction drain. Surg Gynecol Obstet 1967; 125:365–366
36. Wyatt AP: Hazards of Vacu-drain system. Lancet 1969; 2:1132
37. Worth MH, Anderson HW: The effectiveness of bacterial filtration in vented wound drains. J Surg Res 1979; 27:405–407
38. Baker MS, Borchardt KA, Baker BH, et al: Sump tube drainage as a source of bacterial contamination. Am J Surg 1977; 133:617–618
39. Higson RH, Kettelwell MGW: Parietal wound drainage of abdominal surgery. Br J Surg 1978; 65:326–329
40. O'Connor TW, Hugh TB: Abdominal drainage: A clinical view. Aust NZ J Surg 1979; 49:253–260
41. Cruse PJE: A five-year prospective study of 23,649 surgical wounds. Arch Surg 1973; 107:206–210

42. Berliner SD, Burson LC, Lear PE: Use and abuse of intraperitoneal drains in colon surgery. Arch Surg 1964; 89:686–690
43. Lessrer AJ: The place of wound drainage in surgery with description of a new drain. Arch Surg 1960; 81:870–876
44. Hubbard JG, Amin M, Polk HC: Bladder perforations secondary to surgical drains. J Urol 1979; 121:521–522
45. Todd GJ, Reemtsma K: Cholecystectomy with drainage. J Surg 1978; 135:622–623
46. Kambouris AA, Carpenter WS, and Allaben RO: Cholecystotomy without drainage. Surg Gynecol Obstet 1973; 137:613–617
47. Pope ER, Swaim S: Wound drainage from under full-thickness skin grafts in dogs: I. Quantitative evaluation of four techniques. Vet Surg 1986; 15(1):65–71
48. Lee AH, Swaim SF: Surgical drainage. Compend Contin Educ Pract Vet 1986; 8:94–103
49. Turner WD, Breznock EM: Continuous suction drainage of management of canine pyothorax: A retrospective study. J Am Anim Hosp Assoc 1988; 24:485–494
50. Birch SJ, Fossum TW: Chylothorax in the dog and cat. Vet Clin North Am 1987; 17:271–283
51. Smeak DD: Chinese finger trap suture technique for fastening tubes and catheters. J Am Anim Hosp Assoc 1990; 26:215–218
51. Wingfield WE, Bliven MT, Quirk PE: Use of continuous chest drainage in dogs and cats. J Am Anim Hosp Assoc 1985; 21:29–32
52. Mullen HS, Matthiesen DT, Scavelli TD: Results of surgery and postoperative complications in 92 dogs treated for prostatic abscessation by a multiple Penrose drain technique. J Am Anim Hosp Assoc 1990; 26:369–379
53. Hardi EM, Barsanti JA, Rawling CA: Complications of prostatic surgery; J Am Anim Hosp Assoc 1984; 20:50–56
54. White RAS, Williams JM: Prostatic parenchymal omentalization: A new technique for management of abscesses and retention cysts. (abstract) Vet Surg 1991; 20:351
55. Zolton GM, Greiner TP: Prostatic abscesses: A surgical approach. J Am Anim Hosp Assoc 1978; 14:698–702
56. Santos OA, Hastings FW, Mohamad KM: Effectiveness of silicone as an abdominal drain. Arch Surg 1962; 84:643–645
57. Hoffer RE, Prange JR, O'Neil GO, et al: Treatment of acute peritonitis in dogs by intermittent peritoneal lavage. J Am Anim Hosp Assoc 1970; 6:182–193
58. Parks J, Gahring D, Greene RW: Peritoneal lavage for peritonitis and pancreatitis in twenty-two dogs. J Am Anim Hosp Assoc 1973; 9:442–446
59. Rosato EF, Oram-Smith JC, Mullis WF, et al: Peritoneal lavage treatment in experimental peritonitis. Ann Surg 1972; 175:385
60. Hoffer RE: Peritonitis. Vet Clin North Am 1972; 2:189–194
61. McKenna JP, MacDonald JA, Mahoney LJ, Lonskail JC: The use of continuous postoperative peritoneal lavage in the management of diffuse peritonitis. Surg Gynecol Obstet 1970; 130:254–258
62. Hornanian AP, Saddawi N: An experimental study of the consequences of intraperitoneal irrigation. Surg Gynecol Obstet 1972; 134:575–578
62a. Orsher RJ, Rosin E: Open peritoneal drainage in experimental peritonitis in dogs. Vet Surg 1984; 13:222–226
63. Woolfson JM, Dulisch ML: Open abdominal drainage in the treatment of generalized peritonitis in 25 dogs and cats. Vet Surg 1986; 15:27–32
64. Greenfield C, Walshaw R: Open peritoneal drainage for treatment of contaminated peritoneal cavity and septic peritonitis in dogs and cats: 24 cases. J Am Vet Med Assoc 1987; 191:100–105
64a. Hosgood G, Salisbury SK, DeNicola DB: Open peritoneal drainage versus sump–Penrose drainage: Clinicopathologic effects in normal dogs. J Am Anim Hosp Assoc 1991; 27:115–121
65. Giacobine JW, Siler VE: Evaluation of diagnostic abdominal paracentesis with experimental and clinical studies. Surg Gynecol Obstet 1960; 110:676–686
66. Bolton JS, Bornside GH, Cohn I: Intraperitoneal povidine-iodine in experimental canine and murine peritonitis. Am J Surg 1979; 137:780–785
67. Lores ME, Ortiz JR, Rossello PJ: Peritoneal lavage with povidone-iodine solution in experimentally induced peritonitis. Surg Gynecol Obstet 1981; 153:33–38
68. Lagarde MC, Bolton JS, Cohn I: Intraperitoneal povidone-iodine in experimental peritonitis. Ann Surg 1978; 187:613–619

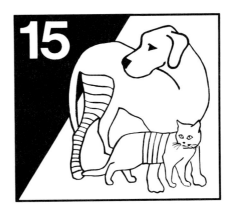

SURGICAL DEVICES AND WOUND HEALING

WILLIAM DERNELL
JOSEPH HARARI

LASER THERAPY

Laser is an acronym for *l*ight *a*mplification by *s*timulated *e*mission of *r*adiation. A laser emits a focused beam of radiation with identical and synchronized wavelengths in the infrared, visible, or near ultraviolet spectra. The theoretical basis of the laser stems from Einstein's work in quantum mechanics in the early 1900s. The first functional laser, using a ruby crystal, was developed in 1960 by Maiman. The argon and carbon dioxide lasers were developed during the 1960s and used for ophthalmic and general medical and surgical procedures in the late 1960s and early 1970s.[1] Over the past 20 years, extensive investigation into laser development and application has lead to development of a neodymium:yttrium–aluminum–garnet (Nd:YAG) laser with photodisruptive applications. During the 1980s and into the 1990s, considerable enthusiasm has arisen over the development of photodynamic therapy.[1] The latter modality involves selective laser destruction of photosensitized cells.

A review of the literature reveals that most of the basic biomedical research with lasers was performed in animals.[2] As clinical applications increase and the technology of lasers improves in human medicine, lasers will become more readily available to the veterinary profession. An understanding of the principles and tissue effects of lasers, therefore, becomes increasingly important.

The Basis of Laser Energy

Laser energy is emitted (stimulated) energy originating from the interaction of photons and excited atoms.[3] As these stimulated emissions interact further with excited atoms, a chain reaction occurs. The atoms are excited, or raised to a higher energy level, by electrical or photic stimulation. Once the number of atoms at a high energy level exceeds the rate of return to the original energy level, a state of population inversion exists and photons of energy are released, thus beginning the process of energy displacement. This reaction takes place in a chamber with mirrors at each end that reflect the energy to magnify the interactions and create a coherent photon beam. Once the beam is sufficiently strong, some of the photons are allowed to escape through a partially reflective mirror (Fig. 15–1). The wavelength of light energy produced by lasers depends on the medium within the excitement chamber and consists, most frequently, of either a gas or a crystalline solid.[1] Because the energy released is an identical (monochromatic) and synchronized (coherent) wavelength, it can be finely focused.

Laser effects depend on power per unit area (power density) and time of exposure. Thus power (measured in watts), focal spot diameter, and time of tissue contact are all important biologic considerations.[1] An equivalent amount of tissue will be destroyed by a given amount of radiant energy regardless of the rate of delivery. The rate, however, will affect the degree of tissue affected outside the destructive zone. A slow speed, for example, will cause increased peripheral damage.

Laser energy may be delivered by pulse or continuous wave. Long pulses (milliseconds to microseconds) are more common in medical uses because short, high-power pulses (nanoseconds) can spatter tissue and cause spread of microorganisms or tumor cells. These short-pulse lasers generate their power by a shutter within the pumping chamber optical path that creates a state of maximal inversion. Pulse lasers can obtain power levels 1000 times greater than their continuous-mode counterparts.[3] The operator controls the laser through use of a hand-held optical fiber, control of a mirrored micromanipulator, or computer programs.[1]

Interaction of light with tissue is characterized by absorption, reflection, scatter, or transmission and can result in various tissue reactions.[1] These depend on the wavelength of irradiation and properties of the tissue. *Photochemical reactions* induce or destroy chemical bonds and are typical of ultraviolet and visible light lasers. *Thermal reactions* are used for coagulation or vaporization and are caused by infrared and visible lasers. Photocoagulation is the result of raising tissue temperature to the point of protein denaturation and cell coagulation. Vaporization is caused by heating intra-

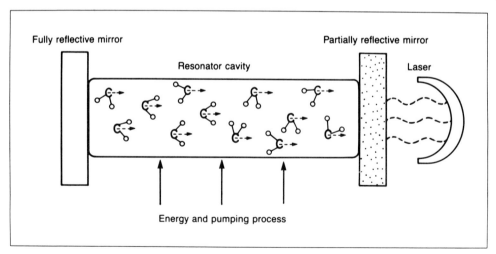

Figure 15–1. Diagram of a carbon dioxide laser apparatus. (From Klause SE, Roberts SM: Lasers and veterinary surgery. Compend Contin Educ Pract Vet 1990; 12(11):1569, with permission.)

cellular water to steam, which causes the cell to explode. *Photodisruption* is the result of concentrated photons stripping electrons from atoms and molecules to create free electrons and ions leading to a shock wave that blasts tissue apart. This occurrence is termed *optical breakdown* and does not rely on vaporization.

Types of Lasers

Lasers are divided into two categories: hot or high-energy lasers and cool or low-energy lasers. The CO_2, Nd:YAG, argon, and krypton lasers are the most commonly used hot lasers.[2]

CO₂ LASER

The CO_2 laser operates in the far-infrared region, and its effects are primarily thermal. The beam is invisible, so it is accompanied by a helium–neon pilot light to assist visualization during application. The CO_2 laser results in a three-dimensional zone of tissue injury characterized by a central void caused by vaporization, an inner zone of cauterized collagen, and an outer zone of edematous tissue[1] (Fig. 15–2).

Cutaneous wound healing patterns following CO_2 laser irradiation have been described.[4] Histologically, the initial wounds were characterized by a V-shaped zone of cauterized collagen with a depth dependent on the amount of energy applied. Transepidermal cauterization and basal cell vacuolization were noted at the periphery of the primary radiation site. As the wound healed, the cauterized collagen was slowly extruded and the crevice approximated (Fig. 15–3). Minimal granulation tissue was evident, and sutured wounds had prolonged retention of destroyed collagen. Wound contraction characterized laser wound healing because of the need for cauterized collagen

Figure 15–2. Concentric zones of laser–tissue impact (*A* = central crater; *B* = inner zone; *C* = desiccated zone; *D* = outer zone). (From Klause SE, Roberts SM: Lasers and veterinary surgery. Compend Contin Educ Pract Vet 1990; 12(11):1570, with permission.)

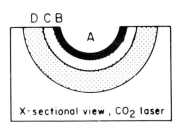

X-sectional view, CO_2 laser

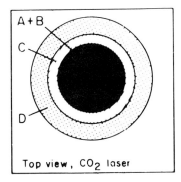

Top view, CO_2 laser

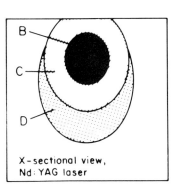

X-sectional view,
Nd:YAG laser

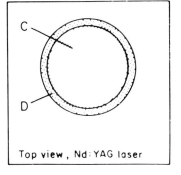

Top view, Nd:YAG laser

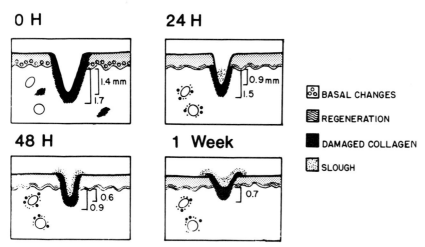

Figure 15–3. Diagram of cellular changes following cutaneous irradiation with a focused carbon dioxide laser. (From Kamat BR, Carney JM, Arndt KA, et al: Cutaneous tissue repair following CO_2 laser irradiation. J Invest Dermatol 1986; 87(1):271, with permission.)

extrusion. The inertness of collagen caused a decreased inflammatory response and white blood cell debridement. Granulation tissue formation was decreased due to denaturing of the collagen and absence of coagulation products (fibroblastic growth factors) within the wound. The lack of inflammatory mediators may be the basis for the painless nature of laser applications.

Biologic amplification must be controlled during laser therapy to minimize the extent of tissue damage.[5] This amplification is caused by substances released from cells as they are destroyed. Even in small amounts, histamine, chemotactic factors, and cellular toxins can cause inflammation, immunogenicity, and even muto- or carcinogenesis in tissues surrounding the target area. Amplification can be minimized by judicious removal of destroyed tissue during laser treatment. With CO_2 lasers, 90% of the laser energy is absorbed within 0.01 mm of impact, which yields protection for tissue a few cells away. Despite this precision, vital underlying structures such as vessels and nerves must be carefully avoided. In addition, the energy of the CO_2 laser is ineffective in fluid-filled cavities or areas of hemorrhage due to inactivation of thermal effects by fluid.

The CO_2 laser is used as a surgical scalpel, although its hemostatic effects are limited to vessels smaller than 0.6 mm in diameter. The CO_2 laser can lyse collagen bonds, which can re-form on cooling, resulting in tissue welding. This makes the CO_2 laser suitable for anastomosing nerves, tendons, and skin. Strength of skin anastomosed with a CO_2 laser is significantly greater than that of sutured wounds at 6 weeks, and healing progresses slightly faster owing to a shortening of the debridement phase.[1] A slight delay in epithelialization occurs as a result of thermal necrosis at the wound edge. Although seldom reported as a clinical problem, in one experimental study, a lower resistance to infection in wounds was created by a CO_2 laser compared with those made by scalpel.[6] This caused a delay in wound healing, although long-term outcome was not examined. This decreased resistance may be due to the lack of inflammation that occurs in response to the laser. When colonic anastomoses in rats were examined, no significant differences in wound strength were found between laser, scalpel, or diathermy at 7 days.[7] Lumen diameters in wounds created by laser and scalpel were similar. When examining split-thickness porcine skin grafts, no significant difference in healing occurred between grafts excised by laser or scalpel.

The advantages of the CO_2 laser include precision in confined areas; a clear, dry, blood-free field; decreased postoperative edema, reduced scarring, pain, and healing time; minimal, controlled tissue damage; and induced tissue sterility due to destruction of bacterial cells. The main disadvantages of the CO_2 laser are decreased hemostasis compared with photodisruptive lasers, and an inability to be used through flexible fiberscopes.[1]

Nd:YAG Laser

The Nd:YAG laser is produced by a solid-state crystal and can generate up to 100 W of power in the infrared region. The energy of the Nd:YAG is preferentially absorbed by pigmented tissue, can penetrate transparent tissue or fluid-filled cavities, and can be passed through fiberscopes. When the Nd:YAG laser is used in a continuous mode, the tissue effects are primarily thermal, with an unpredictable depth of penetration, although deeper than that of the CO_2 laser.[1, 3] This lack of depth control makes the Nd:YAG less precise than the CO_2 laser, but its high power and short exposure time result in minimal tissue effects outside the target area (see Fig. 15–2). Other advantages include the ability to penetrate transparent tissue, which makes it applicable to surgical ophthalmology, and coagulation effects due to heme pigment absorption, which makes it applicable to tumor debridement.[1] The Nd:YAG laser has the ability to deliver intense beams at ultrashort time intervals, thus making it an effective photodisruptor.

Argon and Krypton Lasers

Argon and krypton lasers are similar. They create a beam in the visible region, are able to penetrate transparent tissues, and can be preferentially absorbed by pigmented tissues. Their effects are thermal and have a limited depth of penetration when compared with CO_2 or Nd:YAG lasers. They are primarily used in ophthalmic procedures.[1]

Low-Energy Lasers

The second category of lasers consists of low-energy lasers (approximately 1 W). Dye-tuned lasers, which can be adjusted to deliver varying wavelengths of light, are becoming popular because of the continued development of photodynamic therapy.[2] Photodynamic therapy involves systemic injection of a photoreactive dye that is preferentially absorbed into a target tissue such as a neoplastic lesion. Absorption of a specific wavelength of laser energy allows identification or selective destruction of the affected tissue. Other applications of low-energy lasers are induction of wound healing, various diagnostic procedures, and treatment of musculoskeletal diseases through acupuncture.

Complications of Laser Therapy

There are two dangers for the patient undergoing laser therapy. The first is the risk of fire caused by combustible materials ignited by the laser. Alcohol solutions should be avoided, and antiseptics should be dried prior to laser contact with the surgical site. The surgical areas should be isolated with moistened towels, since dry paper drapes and sponges are flammable. Rubber and plastic materials can be ignited with a laser. The hazards of endotracheal tube combustion can be reduced by using a noncombustible tube, coating the tube with metallic tape or wet muslin, avoiding oil-based lubricant ointments, or using injectable anesthetics.[1] The potential for ignition of the anesthetic gases passing through the tube should be considered.[8] In cases of airway fire, the patient should be treated immediately for shock and pulmonary edema.[9]

The second risk to the patient is inadvertent damage to nontargeted tissues. This can occur through scatter of the laser beam by reflection and is avoided by cautious use of metallic instruments in the surgical field. The primary organ at risk from scatter is the eye, and it should be protected or fixed closed. Because of the intense power of the laser, undesired tissue damage can occur within a fraction of a second. Preplanning of surgical procedures, preoperative adjustment of the laser beam, cautious use of the laser by the operator, and maintenance of a clear field are essential in avoiding complications.[1]

Risks also can exist for operating room personnel during laser surgery. Because a laser beam can be reflected without any loss to its properties, beam scatter can produce harmful effects. Cautious use of the laser and other surgical instruments is essential, as well as protective eye wear for all operating personnel.

Clinical Applications of Laser Therapy

Lasers are used extensively in human medicine and surgery.[10] Lasers have been used in many surgical procedures in which a scalpel was used previously. Lasers are used for procedures where surgical exposure is minimal or unfeasible, such as the globe and through a fiberoptic endoscope. They are particularly useful in procedures complicated by hemorrhage or where total tissue destruction is essential, such as in the treatment of neoplasia.[11] Emphasis is being placed on research and clinical use of low-power lasers in photodynamic therapy and nonsurgical (laser) treatment of wounds, arthritis, and other medical disorders. Reports of surgical complications beyond inadvertent tissue contact are few and primarily involve scar-tissue formation in dermatologic use.[10, 12] In ophthalmic cases, postoperative complications have included hemorrhage, adhesions, and posterior uveitis.[3]

Laser use in large animal surgery has involved oral, pharyngeal, and laryngeal surgeries because of endoscopic accessibility and minimal granulation tissue response. Complications (recurrence of tumor or cyst and aryepiglottic adhesion) were infrequently encountered.[9] A laser has been used to treat limbic squamous cell carcinoma.[13]

In small animal surgery, lasers have been applied in experimental situations during development of techniques for human use and, more recently, in clinical practice as the instrumentation becomes available. Most veterinary clinical use is based on human applications, inaccessibility for conventional therapy, or when complete tissue destruction is desired.[1] Ophthalmic use began with applications of the argon laser in the repair of retinal attachment and has expanded to removal of lesions within the uveal tract, trabeculoplasty for glaucoma, and treatment of adnexal neoplasms.[3] The Nd:YAG laser is now the preferred instrument for posterior capsulotomy in the treatment of cataracts. Complications are similar to those associated with human laser ophthalmology and are less frequent than complications following conventional surgical methods.[3] Laser treatment for pharyngeal and laryngeal conditions is gaining popularity because of laser precision and accessibility with endoscopy.[1] In a recent study of 13 cases of intraoral ventriculocordectomy with a CO_2 laser, only one dog had a complication (small inflammatory granuloma).[8] Successful long-term results of CO_2 laser ventriculocordectomy were reported in 9 dogs.[14] Lasers are useful in the treatment of lesions where hemostasis is important, such as removal of neoplasms, treatment of gastrointestinal ulcers, and excisions or biopsies of splenic and hepatic tissues.[1] In conditions (neurologic neoplasms) where consistent and predictable tissue destruction is desirable, lasers have shown immense potential.[1] In a recent study of subtotal prostatectomy, the Nd:YAG laser was a useful adjunct to prostatic tissue debridement.[15] The only reported complication was mucosal perforation in cases where the beam was passed too closely to the urethra.

Summary

There are many advantages of laser surgery, although safety requirements and technical expertise may limit widespread use by the veterinary profession. Use of lasers in human medicine and surgery has become more commonplace, and their utilization in animals should steadily increase due to animal model development and an increase in the availability of equipment. Lasers are presently becoming a useful therapeutic tool in veterinary medicine and, when used properly, result in few complications.

ELECTROSURGERY

Historical Perspective

Cautery dates back to the use of a fire rod by Egyptians to control hemorrhage and is first described in the medical literature by Hippocrates for the treatment of hemorrhoids.[16] Refinement of hemostasis was described by Celcus, who outlined the use of styptics, astringents, ligatures, and cautery.

Electrosurgical instruments were first described by d'Arsonoval and Oudin, who devised an electrical apparatus with a 5- to 14-mm spark gap that caused local analgesia.[16] This device was later revised by Nagelschmidt in 1897, who placed patients within an electrical circuit to create heating of tissues (diathermy) for treatment of arthritis. At the turn of the century, Riviere described the use of the spark generated by d'Arsonoval's apparatus to treat indolent ulcers, and tumorous and tubercular lesions (fulguration). Doyen added a second wire to d'Arsonoval's apparatus and placed it under the patient. He described the different uses for contact of the tissue with the electrode (coagulation) and utilization of a spark on the tissue (carbonization).

Beer, in 1908, used fulguration through a cystoscope to treat bladder tumors.[16] In 1923, Wyeth developed a practical machine capable of creating both cutting (desiccation) and coagulation currents. A more economical unit was developed by Cushing and Bovie in 1926. This apparatus remained unchanged until 1970, when solid-state equipment replaced vacuum tubes.

Recently, two new electrosurgical instruments have been devised. The first is similar to a conventional scalpel except the blade is heated with electric current, resulting in coagulation of the edges of incised tissue.[17] The second is a plasma scalpel that involves passage of electric current through argon or helium gas at the surgical tip, thus creating thermal energy at the instrument–tissue interface.[18] Since both these instruments rely on heat for their tissue effects, they will be included in the following discussion of electrosurgery.

Principles of Electrosurgery

Electrocautery and electroincision are the direct result of heat created by tissue resistance to the passage of electric current.[16] This current is generated by the electrosurgical unit, passes to the patient by the surgical handpiece, travels through the patient, passes into a ground plate placed under the patient, and then travels back to the electrosurgical unit to complete the circuit. The current is concentrated at the tip of the electrosurgical handpiece, and as the current is dispersed throughout the body, current density and resistance are greatly diluted, thus eliminating heating of peripheral tissues. Concentration of the current density can be refined by monopolar cautery as the current is passed between the tips of electroforceps, thereby eliminating the passage of current through the patient.[12]

The greater the tissue resistance to the current, the greater is the heat production at the handpiece–tissue interface. Factors that affect local resistance include age, disease, current frequency, and patient environment. Electrosurgical units utilize currents greater than 10,000 Hz because lower (less than 3000 Hz) currents will result in muscle contraction and pain or heat damage to tissues (currents between 3000 and 5000 Hz).[16] Modern electrosurgical units use currents in the range of 250,000 to 2 million Hz.[12]

The waveform of the electric current determines the electrosurgical effect (cutting or coagulation).[16] Continuous sine or square waves result in a cutting current. Interrupted waves produce a coagulation current. A blend of continuous and interrupted waves results in a combination of cutting and coagulation capabilities. *Fulguration is the result of a spark gap of greater than 1 mm between the handpiece and the tissue*[19] (Fig. 15–4). *Cutting is the result of a spark gap produced at a tissue–handpiece interface of less than 1 mm* (Fig. 15–5). *Coagulation is the result of electric current passing directly through tissue* (Fig. 15–6).

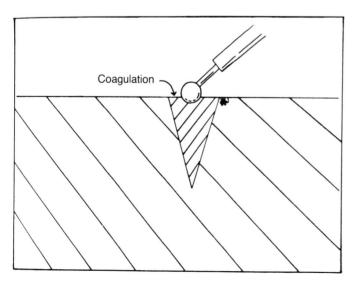

Coagulation

Figure 15–4. Diagram of electrosurgical fulguration, a technique used for superficial dehydration or coagulation of tissue. (From Greene JA, Knecht CD: Electrosurgery: A review. Vet Surg 1980; 9(1):29, with permission.)

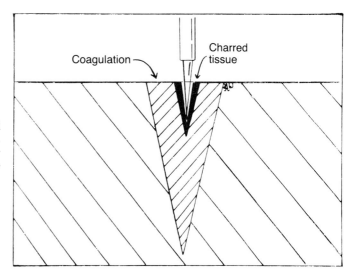

Figure 15–5. Diagram of electrosurgical desiccation used for incision or excision. (From Greene JA, Knecht CD: Electrosurgery: A review. Vet Surg 1980; 9(1):29, with permission.)

Effects of Electrosurgery

Use of the cutting current through tissue produces a zone of carbonized tissue at the edges of the incision approximately one cell wide.[16] This is the result of vaporization and pyrolysis of the cells. This area is surrounded by a zone of desiccated and coagulated cells associated with cellular death without protein or molecular breakdown. Cells immediately adjacent to this latter zone elongate and have mild thermal injury. Blood vessels at the edge of the wound are thrombosed.

Wound healing following electroincision follows the same chronologic inflammatory patterns as scalpel-associated inicisional healing except the inflammatory stage occurs away from the immediate wound edge. This is due to the layer of carbonized debris that must be cleared by phagocytosis prior to epithelial migration. This results in a slight delay in wound healing.[12, 16–18] Electrosurgical wounds have decreased tensile strength 50 days after wounding compared with scalpel incisions.[12, 16, 17, 20] Susceptibility to infection is increased, and the diameter of the anastomotic lumen in bowel

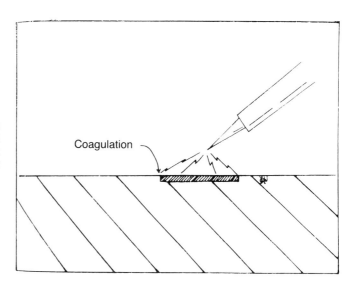

Figure 15–6. Diagram of electrosurgical coagulation resulting in the sealing of small blood vessels. (From Greene JA, Knecht CD: Electrosurgery: A review. Vet Surg 1980; 9(1):29, with permission.)

surgery is decreased when electrosurgery is compared with sharp incision.[6, 7, 12, 16–18] These results may be due to an increase in the inflammatory response and tissue debris at the surgical wound. These factors (decreased wound strength and increased susceptibility to infection) may contribute to increase in wound dehiscence following electroscalpel incision of abdominal cavities.[21] The potential for greater delay in wound healing, decrease in wound strength, and increase in susceptibility to infection exists when current is increased.[16]

As coagulation currents are applied to tissues, initial desiccation occurs as a result of intracellular water evaporation. Depending on the application of the instrument, desiccation is followed by obliterative or coaptive coagulation. *Obliterative coagulation* is a result of current passing through a vessel and causing shrinkage and contraction of the vessel with subsequent thrombosis. Obliterative coagulation is most effective with vessels less than 1 mm in diameter. *Coaptive coagulation* occurs when a vessel's lumen is occluded and the current causes a breakdown of the vascular smooth muscle followed by a fusion of the intima and fenestrated membrane. Coaptive coagulation is the most effective method for hemostasis in larger vessels. In both obliterative and coaptive coagulation, a fibrous union will eventually replace the coagulum, thereby resulting in permanent vascular occlusion.[16]

The amount of effectively coagulated tissue depends on the current power, method of application, and duration of exposure. Use of the point-source current of bipolar cautery results in significantly less tissue necrosis compared with the same current applied with a monopolar unit.[12, 22] The use of higher than normal currents results in superheating of vessels, boiling of cellular fluid, and explosion of the vessel without achieving coagulation.[16]

Clinical Use of Electrosurgery

Use of electrosurgery in human patients is based on the need for hemostasis during sharp incision and utilization of a hot scalpel.[12] The heated scalpel is useful for reducing blood loss and operative time during tumor and burn-tissue excisions. The major complications of electroincisions are delayed wound healing and increased infection rates. Fulguration remains applicable in the treatment of certain infectious and neoplastic lesions.[12, 19]

Use of electrosurgery in veterinary medicine parallels its use in people and is limited to coagulation, especially in patients with bleeding disorders. Fulguration and deroofing (removal of tissues overlying fistulous tracts) are considered useful by some surgeons in the treatment of perianal fistulas.[16, 19, 23] Success in the treatment of lesions less than 180 degrees (angle) around the anus has been described, and the major complications were recurrence of the lesion and fecal incontinence.[23]

SUTURE MATERIALS

Sutures are an integral part of surgical practice. They are often taken for granted, and their role in postoperative complications is sometimes ignored. A comprehensive discussion of the physics and biology of suture material is beyond the scope of this section, and the reader is referred to reviews of suture science.[12, 24–27] The discussion in this section will focus on the effect of suture materials on wound healing and the selection of sutures to reduce postoperative complications.

Classification of Suture Materials

Suture materials are primarily divided into two categories: absorbable and nonabsorbable sutures. *Absorbable sutures lose appreciable tensile strength within 60 days, whereas nonabsorbable sutures retain tensile strength for greater than 60 days.*[27] Sutures in each of these categories are further subdivided into natural and synthetic fibers.

Natural absorbable sutures include catgut and collagen, the latter being infrequently used. Synthetic absorbable sutures include those made of polyglycolic acid (Dexon), polyglactin 910 (Vycril), polydioxanone (PDS), and a copolymer of glycolide and trimethylene carbonate (Maxon).

Natural nonabsorbable sutures include silk and cotton. Synthetic nonabsorbable sutures include the polyamides (nylon and polymerized caprolactam), polyesters, polyolefin plastics (polypropylene and polyethylene), polybutester (Novafil), and stainless steel[24, 26, 28] (Table 15–1).

Role of Sutures in Wound Healing

During the initial wound healing stages of fibrin deposition, endothelial proliferation, and epithelial migration, wound strength is minimal. The purpose of suture material is to secure the wound edges, thereby providing a favorable healing environment without spontaneous disruption of the wound. Natural wound stability occurs 14 to 21 days following wounding, with fibroblast proliferation and collagen production. In tissues with higher collagen content, such as tendons and ligaments, weeks to months are required before moderate wound strength is obtained[24] (Figs. 15–7 and 15–8). In musculoaponeurotic (linea alba) wounds, sutures are essential for

TABLE 15–1. General Characteristics of Suture Methods

GENERIC NAME	TRADE NAME	PHYSICAL CONFIGURATION	ABSORPTION
Chromic catgut	—	Multifilament	Absorbable
Polyglycolic acid	Dexon*	Multifilament	Absorbable
Polyglactin 910	Vicryl†	Multifilament	Absorbable
Polydioxanone	PDS†	Monofilament	Absorbable
Polyglyconate	Maxon*	Monofilament	Absorbable
Silk	—	Multifilament	Nonabsorbable
Stainless steel	—	Multifilament and monofilament	Nonabsorbable
Polyester (Dacron)	Ethibond†	Multifilament	Nonabsorbable
Coated caprolactam	Braunamid‡	Multifilament	Nonabsorbable
Polyamide (nylon)	—	Multifilament and monofilament	Nonabsorbable
Polypropylene	Prolene†	Monofilament	Nonabsorbable
Polybutester	Novafil*	Monofilament	Nonabsorbable
Cotton	—	Multifilament	Nonabsorbable
Linen	—	Multifilament	Nonabsorbable

*Davis & Geck/Lederle.
†Ethicon/Pitman-Moore.
‡B. Braun Melsungen AG.
Source: Smeak DD, Wendelburg KL: Choosing suture materials for use in contaminated or infected wounds. Compend Contin Educ Pract Vet 1989; 11(4):468; reprinted with permission.

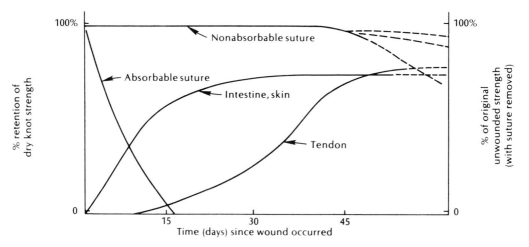

Figure 15–7. Diagram depicting loss of tensile strength for suture materials relative to gain of tensile strength during healing of wounded tissues. (From Bellinger CR: Sutures: I. The purpose of sutures and available suture materials. Compend Contin Educ Pract Vet 1982; 4(6):508, with permission.)

maintaining strength for 42 days.[29] In these tissues, sutures with retained strength characteristics, such as the synthetic nonabsorbable or newer synthetic absorbable sutures, are preferred. Experimental studies have demonstrated that in the absence of infections, suture materials have little or no overall effect on healing of skin, stomach, colon, or bladder wounds when protein and collagen synthesis and wound breaking strength are evaluated.[30–32] Factors that delay wound healing, such as infection, hypovascularity, and hypoproteinemia, will prolong the requirement for sutures.[24]

Suture Strength

Tissue strength and loading forces determine the strength of the sutures required to maintain tissue apposition and healing. Suture size, tensile strength, rate of degradation and subsequent loss of tensile strength, elastic-

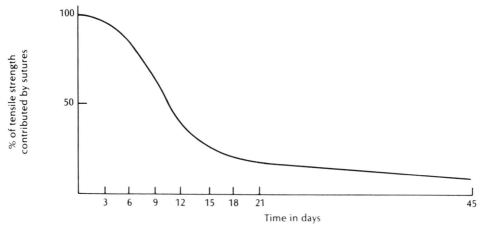

Figure 15–8. Diagram depicting the role of sutures in maintaining tensile strength of healing abdominal wounds. (From Bellinger CR: Sutures: I. The purpose of sutures and available suture materials. Compend Contin Educ Pract Vet 1982; 4(6):508, with permission.)

ity, and knot security determine the applicability of a suture material to a particular wound.[24, 28] Of the nonabsorbable sutures, stainless steel has the highest tensile strength, followed by polyester, polyethylene, caprolactam, nylon, and polypropylene.[26] Silk is the weakest suture material. Polybutester has acute breaking strength similar to nylon but is unique in its ability to elongate up to 50% of its original length at low loads. This provides dynamic properties not present in other nonabsorbable sutures.[28] Since most wound dehiscences are a result of suture materials pulling through tissue rather than suture breakage, elongation capabilities during the initial postoperative period of wound swelling may decrease the incidence of premature pull-through. This has been demonstrated experimentally, but its clinical significance is unknown.[28]

Once implanted, stainless steel retains most of its tensile strength, whereas silk loses 50% of its tensile strength by 1 year.[26, 33] Polypropylene, intermediate in tensile strength, retains its strength indefinitely once implanted.

Of the absorbable sutures, the copolymer of glycolide and trimethylene carbonate has the highest tensile strength, followed by polydioxanone. Both sutures are stronger than nylon and polypropylene.[34] Polyglactin is slightly stronger than polyglycolic acid and is followed by chromic and plain catgut.[26] Interestingly, the addition of a single throw to any of the absorbable sutures results in a loss of *in vitro* tensile strength of 35%.[34] Patterns of loss of tensile strength following implantation include polydioxanone retaining 50% of its strength at 6 weeks, glycolide and trimethylene carbonate having complete loss of tensile strength at 6 weeks,[34] and chromic catgut retaining 50% and polyglycolic acid retaining 20% of their strengths after 2 weeks.[26, 33] In clinical situations, weakness in tensile strength can be compensated somewhat by selection of larger suture size.

In comparing knot security of the nonabsorbable sutures, steel is most secure. Polypropylene, polyethylene with caprolactam, polyester, and nylon all have poor security. Silk is the worst material for knot security.

Polydioxanone appears to have better knot security than polyglycolic acid or polyglactin. Chromic catgut has the greatest knot security *in vitro,* but it swells when wet, thereby giving it very poor knot characteristics.[26]

In one study, knots of various suture materials were tested for failure after incubation with canine serum.[35] Surgeon's knots and square knots had similar properties, and catgut, polyglycolic acid, and polydioxanone granny knots were equally secure as square knots. Polydioxanone and nylon required four throws for security, whereas catgut, polypropylene, polyglycolic acid, and polyglactin required three throws. Square knots, used to start a continuous pattern, required three throws, whereas four to five throws were needed for a finishing knot.

Tissue Reaction to Sutures

Tissue response to the implantation of suture material is characterized by a foreign-body reaction. The degree of this response depends on the nature of the implant, type of tissue, amount of implant, surgical technique, and duration of implantation. Sutures are either removed, absorbed, incorporated into a fibrous capsule, or persist as part of a chronic foreign-body reaction.[24]

Among the nonabsorbable sutures, rates of reactivity from least to most are stainless steel, nylon, polypropylene and polyethylene being similar, followed by caprolactam, polyester, and silk. Silk, although classified as nonabsorbable, is eventually broken down and absorbed by phagocytosis by 2 years. Of the absorbable sutures, polydioxanone, glycolide and trimethylene carbonate, polyglactin, and polyglycolic acid all show similar tissue reactivity and are absorbed by hydrolysis. Catgut invokes a strong foreign-body reaction and is absorbed by phagocytosis.[26, 29]

In a study investigating reactions to absorbable sutures placed in the feline linea alba, catgut, polyglactin 910, and polydioxanone sutures were compared.[36] Findings were similar for all materials and involved a mild to marked purulent reaction at day 1, a fibromononuclear reaction at day 7, and fibromononuclear and granulomatous reactions at day 14.

In a study of nonabsorbable suture materials, tissues were evaluated for reactivity based on area of surrounding inflammation and differential cell count.[37] Histologic evaluation was performed at 30, 60, 90, and 120 days. Stainless steel and nylon had predominantly fibrous reactions, classified as mild and moderate. Polypropylene and coated polyamide were surrounded by moderate inflammatory responses, classified as fibromononuclear with granuloma formation around isolated material. At 120 days, silk stimulated granulomatous or pyogranulomatous tissue reactivity, with mineralization occurring around the material.

Suture Materials and Wound Infection

Suture materials, acting essentially as foreign bodies, can potentiate infection. A single silk suture increased the infectivity of *Staphylococcus pyogenes* 100,000-fold in experimentally induced infections.[38] Nylon was responsible for potentiation of experimental staphylococcal infection when used to close dead space.[39] The foreign-body response to sutures produces a protein-rich environment that potentiates bacterial growth. In addition, some suture materials permit bacterial adherence to their surfaces and allow multiplication away from host defenses. Sutures also can indirectly potentiate infection through improper surgical technique, such as increased tissue handling and trauma, excessive suture tension, and placement of an excessive amount of suture material within a wound.[40]

ACUTE INFECTION

A suture's resistance to acute infection depends on its physical form, degree of inflammatory reaction, chemical structure, capillarity, and degree of bacterial adherence. Although somewhat controversial, multifilament (braided) suture appears to have a decreased resistance to acute infection when placed into a contaminated environment compared with monofilament suture.[12, 30, 41] The causes of increased infectivity of multifilaments are the inaccessibility of bacteria within interstices of the braided suture to macrophage phagocytosis, and increased surface area of the suture compared with monofilament sutures. Natural sutures such as silk and cotton appear to have a decreased resistance to infection compared with synthetic materials.[41] In one study examining the degree of infection surrounding various contaminated suture materials in mice, stainless steel and nylon resulted in the least amount of infection. These were followed by silk, braided Dacron, polyglycolic·acid, and catgut.[42] The results were supported by a similar experiment in dogs.[43]

In general, the greater the degree of inflammation associated with implantation of a suture, the lower is the resistance to acute infection. This is modified by the chemical makeup of a suture and can be controlled surgically by the use of the least amount and smallest size of material.[40, 44] The chemical nature of a suture can affect its resistance to acute infection by substances coating the material or breakdown products of the material that are bactericidal. Lubricating coatings have been shown to have little effect on infectibility.[41] Early studies indicated that iodized catgut and benzathonium-coated sutures decreased the incidence of acute infection. Hydrolysis of polyglycolic acid releases glycolic acid and changes the pH of the surrounding tissue, which reduces bacterial infection. Nylon is also hydrolyzed and releases adipic acid and 1,6-hexanediamine, which have antibacterial activity.[40]

Braided sutures may play a role in the transport of bacteria from a contaminated to a sterile area. Surface contamination of penetrating, coated, braided polyester or polyamide sutures results in significantly greater deep or distant infections compared with noncapillary sutures.[40] Interestingly, bacterial transport within the suture material itself was of greater significance than transport on the surface, raising the question of the importance of the various surface coatings on capillary sutures.[40] As a result of these studies, recommendations were made to avoid penetration into contaminated areas, such as bowel, with capillary sutures and to avoid skin penetration with capillary sutures placed subcutaneously or intradermally.

Because suture materials are composed of glycoproteins similar to those of cell surfaces, bacteria can selectively bind to suture surfaces and have a significant effect on the incidence of acute infection. A specific example is teichoic acid, which mediates adherence of certain cocci and Enterobacteriaceae. This binding is a dynamic phenomenon that is time-dependent, reversible, and specific for the suture type and bacterial species. Uncoated polyglycolic acid, because of its hydrophilic nature, has the greatest degree of bacterial affinity. Coated polyglycolic acid, polyglactin 910, and catgut have slightly less bacterial affinity. Of the multifilament nonabsorbable sutures, siliconized polyester has greater bacterial adherence than polybutilate-coated polyester; uncoated silk has more bacterial adherence than coated silk. Monofilament nonabsorbable sutures and polydioxanone have the least bacterial adherence.[40, 45]

CHRONIC INFECTION

Suture abscess and sinus formation are surgical complications occurring late in the wound healing process. Multifilament sutures have a significantly greater propensity for delayed reactions compared with monofilament nonabsorbable sutures.[30, 40–42] This is due to fluid absorption by the multifilament materials. Monofilament sutures, such as nylon and polypropylene, have the least amount of fluid absorption, whereas multifilament sutures, such as silk and catgut, have the greatest absorption. Greater tissue reaction is associated with increased fluid absorption. Braided sutures can maintain bacterial populations for several weeks when implanted in tissue, whereas monofilament sutures have a gradual decrease in bacterial numbers after inoculation and implantation.[40]

Suture abscess formation and sinus formation are directly related to the degree of contamination present at the time of suture implantation. In a study of sinus formation following stifle joint surgery, 40 of 127 cases were associated with *Staphylococcus aureus* contamination of multifilament polyamide sutures.[46, 47] In clean procedures, there is no significant difference in the occurrence of suture abscess formation between monofilaments and multifilaments. As the degree of contamination increases, the differences in abscess and sinus formation between these two suture groups become more pronounced.[40]

Suture irritation of tissue also has been shown to affect the rates of suture abscess formation and sinus formation. Large-gauge, stiff materials placed in areas of high motion have an increased incidence of late suture complications compared with fine or soft materials placed away from motion areas.[40]

Suture Needles

The passage of a suture needle through tissue causes an inflammatory response that depends on the type of tissue, needle configuration, and needle size.[12] A taper needle passed through a parenchymatous organ, such as the liver or spleen, causes very little tissue disruption. The same needle passed through dense fascia or dermis can be excessively traumatic, thus inciting a marked inflammatory response that can delay healing and predispose to infection. A cutting needle passed through fascia or dermis causes a mild inflammatory response and is preferred for such tissues. A cutting needle passed through a parenchymatous organ, however, can create a stress line that may lead to tearing of the tissue.[25, 48]

The configuration of the cutting needle is also important. A standard cutting needle has the apex of the triangle pointing inward from the circumference of the curve. This can create a stress line outward from the placement of the suture, which can result in suture pull-out depending on the strength of the tissue. A reverse cutting needle has the apex of the triangle away from the circumference of the curve, which lessens the chances of suture pull-out but may induce tissue tearing in soft tissues such as the liver, spleen, and kidney.[25, 48]

Suture Patterns and Placement

Suture patterns and suture placement can affect wound healing by the type of tissue apposition and the degree of tension on the wound.[25] Patterns or placements that result in eversion or inversion affect healing such that cellular activity and tissue reorganization must overcome abnormal tissue alignment to regain normal strength and function. Patterns or placements that result in uneven or excessive tissue tension can result in increased inflammation or tissue necrosis at the wound edge.[12, 25] On the other hand, sutures that allow minimal or uneven tension can delay healing as a result of their inability to hold the wound in apposition against normal postoperative stresses. One study examining abdominal wound bursting strength showed running sutures to be superior to figure-of-8 or simple interrupted sutures. A figure-of-8 suture placed too tightly greatly decreased its resistance to bursting.[49]

The optimal distance between sutures needed to maximize postoperative wound strength is specific for various tissues and varies from 1 to 2 mm in the intestine to 5 to 10 mm in fascia.[25] Exceeding this distance can weaken the tissue's resistance to normal postoperative stresses and lead to wound breakdown. Sutures placed too closely can compromise blood supply and increase the foreign-body inflammatory reaction, resulting in delayed wound healing.

Optimal length of remaining suture ends above a knot was determined in one experiment to be 3 mm for silk and braided polyester with four and five knot throws, respectively.[44] Shorter suture ends resulted in increased incidence of knot loosening. Longer suture ends were assumed to be an unnecessary risk for tissue reaction.

There is considerable debate about the effect of intradermal sutures on the rate of infection and wound failure in people compared with percutaneous sutures.[12] The use of intradermal sutures in veterinary medicine is based on avoidance of self-trauma by animals during wound healing.

Suture Removal

Early suture removal is advocated to optimize wound healing. In the skin, this has traditionally been performed 7 to 10 days following placement.[12, 25] At this time, wound strength is only 10% of that of adjacent skin, so in areas of high tension, retention of sutures for up to 21 days is recommended. Any condition that may delay normal wound healing, such as hypoproteinemia or infection, will delay suture removal.[12, 25]

SURGICAL STAPLES

The first mechanical device designed for surgical wound closure was the Murphy button, developed in 1897 for intestinal anastomoses.[50] Surgical staplers date back to 1909 to a design by Humer Hutel of Budapest. This was further refined in 1921 by Aladar von Petz in Hungary. During the 1930s, numerous stapler designs were introduced, but the major advance in stapling equipment came from the Soviet Union in the 1950s.[51] In the early 1960s, Ravitch and his associates were responsible for modifying these instruments for the U.S. market with the development of instant-loading sterile cartridges.[52]

Stapling Technology

Current stapling equipment includes preloaded, sterilized, disposable staple cartridges which, with the exception of the end-to-end anastomosis device, are designed to be applied with stainless steel or alloy multiuse applicators (TA, GIA, and EEA, United States Surgical Corporation, New York, N.Y.). The gastrointestinal (GIA) and thoracoabdominal (TA) units use stainless steel staples arranged in two or three staggered rows. These staples begin with leg heights ranging from 3.0 to 4.8 mm and, after firing, compress the tissue between 1.25 and 2.0 mm, respectively (Fig. 15–9). The gastrointestinal units produce an incision between double staggered rows of similar staples (Fig. 15–10). Once fired, the staples form a B shape, which provides hemostasis without permanent damage to the microvasculature. The staggering rows also allow blood flow to tissue 2 to 3 mm beyond the staple line.[2] Cartridges are now available containing absorbable staples made of a lactide-glycolic copolymer, which can be fitted into the 55-mm TA stapler.[53] This is a two-piece interlocking staple which, when engaged, also forms a B shape.

The end-to-end anastomosis instruments (EEA) have a circumferential double row of staples and a circular knife blade. The instrument apposes two bowel ends previously closed, staples them together in an inverted

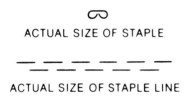

ACTUAL SIZE OF STAPLE

ACTUAL SIZE OF STAPLE LINE

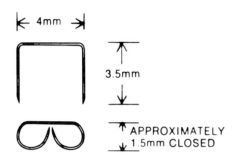

Figure 15–9. Staple pattern, dimensions, and configuration for the thoracoabdominal stapling unit (3.5-mm staples). (From Steichen FM, Ravitch MM: Stapling in Surgery. Chicago: Year Book Medical Publishers, 1984.)

4mm

3.5mm

APPROXIMATELY 1.5mm CLOSED

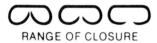

RANGE OF CLOSURE

pattern, and then cuts the overlapping tissue within the lumen. End-lumen sizes range from 11 to 21 mm. Initial staple height is 4.8 mm closed to a B-shaped staple of 2.0 mm (Fig. 15–11). These units are available in stainless steel with replaceable cartridges that are disposable. Another mechanical device for end-to-end anastomosis utilizes the telescoping action of plastic

ACTUAL SIZE OF STAPLE

ACTUAL SIZE OF STAPLE LINE.

KNIFE DIVISION

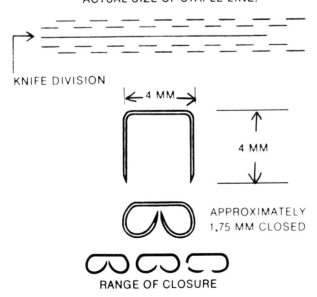

Figure 15–10. Staple pattern, dimensions, and configuration for the gastrointestinal stapling unit (4-mm staples). (From Steichen FM, Ravitch MM: Stapling in Surgery. Chicago: Year Book Medical Publishers, 1984.)

4 MM

4 MM

APPROXIMATELY 1.75 MM CLOSED

RANGE OF CLOSURE

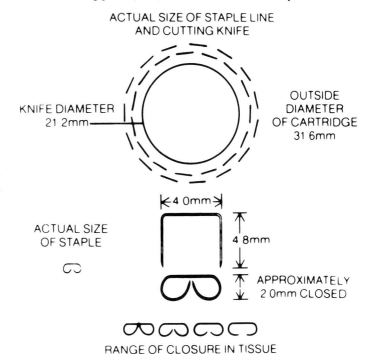

DISPOSABLE EEA 31™ Stapler and
CURVED DISPOSABLE EEA 31™ Stapler

ACTUAL SIZE OF STAPLE LINE
AND CUTTING KNIFE

KNIFE DIAMETER
21 2mm

OUTSIDE
DIAMETER
OF CARTRIDGE
31 6mm

ACTUAL SIZE
OF STAPLE

4 0mm

4 8mm

APPROXIMATELY
2 0mm CLOSED

RANGE OF CLOSURE IN TISSUE

Figure 15–11. Staple pattern, dimensions, and configuration for the end-to-end anastomosis stapling unit (31 mm). (From Steichen FM, Ravitch MM: Stapling in Surgery. Chicago: Year Book Medical Publishers, 1984.)

buttons to form a functional, sutureless anastomosis with a final lumen diameter of 12.5 mm[54] (Anastomotic Compression Button, Pfizer, Inc., Fall River, Mass.).

Multiple-use skin-stapling devices are also available.[25] Skin staples begin as an incomplete rectangle and, upon application, penetrate the skin and are formed into a complete rectangle, resulting in skin apposition. Fascial staplers, similar in design to skin staplers with the exception of a larger staple width, also have recently been introduced.

Mechanical devices for the application of stainless steel ligature clips are available in both single-load and multiple-use instruments (Surgiclips, LDS, United States Surgical Corporation, New York, N.Y.). These clips begin in a V shape, and upon application, the wings of the V are apposed on the vessel to occlude the lumen. An additional cutting instrument is available that divides between two sets of double hemostatic clips (LDS). Absorbable clips of polyglycolic acid also are available.[25, 53]

Effect of Staples on Wound Healing

In canine studies of bowel anastomoses using the functional end-to-end technique, the intestine healed in a curved fashion with a central scar in place of the previously exposed mucosa.[50, 55, 56] Minimal adhesions were present, and luminal diameter was normal. Histologic evaluations revealed inflammation at the healing wound edges that was less than reactions associated with sutured anastomoses. Granulation tissue formation also was decreased and mucosal regeneration increased with staples compared with suture techniques. No difference was found in bursting strength when comparing sutured with stapled anastomoses. The button anastomotic device mentioned previously compared favorably with the stapling device.[54]

Results in equine studies reveal distinct advantages to stapled anastomoses.[57, 58] End-to-end anastomoses performed with stapling instruments resulted in less neutrophilic infiltration, necrosis, and mucocele formation and reductions in luminar diameter, adhesion formation, and bacterial colonization compared with suturing techniques. Stapled anastomoses resulted in increased mature fibrous connective tissue and a more normal arrangement of muscle layers. Bursting strength compared favorably with that of sutured anastomoses.

When TA stapling devices were used to perform hepatic lobectomy, a decrease in microscopic hemorrhage, necrosis, and inflammation was seen at the lobectomy site compared with a suture technique.[59] Use of this device for partial lung lobectomy in the dog resulted in a lower inflammatory response, improved collagen production, and greater leakage pressures compared with suturing techniques.[60] A similar study in the horse resulted in collapse of lung tissue within 1 cm of the staple line but normal tissue beyond this extent.[61]

Studies comparing stapling of skin wounds with suture closure have shown a decrease in tensile strength for stapled wounds up to 14 to 21 days but similar strength of the wounds by 180 days.[12, 62] Early staple removal and the use of arcuate staples appear to lessen the difference between wound strength of stapled compared with sutured skin in the early postoperative period.[12] Stapled skin wounds have been shown to have a greater resistance to wound infection compared with sutured wounds.[63]

Guidelines for GIA and TA Stapling

In general, tissues that are judged by the surgeon to be questionable for anastomosis as a result of inadequate blood supply, sepsis, or underlying disease should not be stapled. There is no greater holding power or improved healing properties in stapled closures compared with sutured closures in abnormal tissues.[64] In fact, studies support the contrary in cases of staple closure involving neoplasia and bowel ischemia.[65, 66]

Another problem is attempting to staple tissues that are too thick for the instrumentation. Maximal tissue compression is obtainable with the thoracoabdominal stapler using 4.8-mm staples to compress the tissue to 2.0 mm. With edematous parenchymatous organs, 2.0 mm compression may be deleterious. Cracks in the gastric serosa or tears in the splenic or hepatic capsule indicate excessive compression. In such cases, stapling should be avoided and the organ should be oversewn.[64]

As a result of the B-shaped staple design, hemostasis is incomplete at the cut edge of stapled tissue.[64] Careful inspection should follow tissue resection and, if necessary, can be augmented with cautery or suture ligatures.

With the introduction of disposable staple cartridges, mechanical failure has been reduced to a minimum. Careful inspection, however, is warranted after stapling to evaluate tissue apposition.

An assumption is often made that stapled anastomoses resist disruption better than sutured anastomoses. In fact, owing to the smaller diameter of each staple compared with sutures, there is a greater risk of tissue laceration leading to failure if tension is applied at the anastomotic site.[64] For this reason, care must be taken to avoid any tension on stapled bowel anastomoses.

Clinical Uses and Complications of Stapling Instruments

Clinical uses of stapling instruments in human surgery include gastrointestinal procedures, lung resection, splenectomy, hepatectomy, hysterectomy, and closure of fascia and skin.[67] The use of stapling instruments in lung resection has been shown to decrease the incidence of bronchoalveolar fistula formation.[60] Complication rates are similar with gastrointestinal stapling compared with conventional methods.[52, 53, 68, 69] These complications are primarily focal abscess, stricture, or leakage at an anastomotic site. Complication rates are related to the stapling experience of the surgeon.

Clinical success in equine gastrointestinal injuries has been obtained in cecocolic anastomoses, colonic resections, jejunocecostomies, and jejuno-jejunostomies.[50, 70] Complications, such as anastomotic leakage, rupture, stenosis, or abscess formation, were similar to those with suture techniques.[50] End-to-end small intestinal anastomosis and gastrojejunostomy are not presently recommended because of the increased complication rates.[50] Successful resection of large ovarian tumors and partial lung resection have been described, although the latter was performed in normal horses. Complication rates were again similar to those with suture techniques.[61, 71]

Much of the original work with stapling instruments was performed experimentally in dogs prior to surgery in people. Clinical use of stapling devices in small animal veterinary surgery has gained popularity. Success has been achieved in partial gastrectomy for the treatment of gastric necrosis secondary to gastric dilatation and volvulus.[72] Complications directly related to the gastrectomy were not reported. Stapling technique was used in 24 open intestinal anastomoses and 2 animals had leaks and focal abscess formation.[73] Both complications were associated with an everted transverse closure. Experimentally, Billroth II gastrojejunostomies were performed, and 1 of 11 dogs had dehiscence of the staple line.[74] Clinical use of the TA staplers for lung resection was reported in 37 cases.[75] Following lobectomy, partial lobectomy, and pneumonectomy, 2 complications related directly to the stapling instrumentation were described. Breakdown of the staple line in one patient was related to cancer regrowth, and in another dog, pneumothorax occurred as a result of failure of the staples to engage properly. The authors described confidence in time with the procedure, resulting in discontinuation of a suture oversew of the staple line, a common earlier practice.

Removal of a cardiac tumor with TA stapling instruments was reported in five dogs.[76] No complications relating to the stapling procedure were documented. Use of the TA instrument also was reported in five dogs for partial hepatectomy.[77] A complication from both total and partial lobectomy was hemorrhage from the line of excision (three cases), which was easily controlled with cautery or gelatin sponge.

Skin stapling can be performed routinely to reduce operative time in high-risk patients or in prolonged procedures.[25] Long- or short-term complications have not been noted.

Summary

Advantages of stapling instruments includes speed and convenience. With proper technique, security of the stapled closure equals or exceeds that of a sutured closure. In situations where reduced surgical time is critical or accessibility for hand suturing is limited, staples are an attractive alternative to traditional suturing methods. The main disadvantages of stapling are the cost of the instrumentation and the required initial training compared with conventional suturing materials and methods.

TISSUE ADHESIVES

Cyanoacrylate

The cyanoacrylate group of tissue adhesives is used most extensively in human and veterinary surgery.[78, 79] These adhesives are considered "true" adhesives because they polymerize instantly on contact with moisture (water) to form an insoluble, flexible plastic that adheres to a wet surface. They were originally developed as rapid adhesives for domestic and industrial use. During the Vietnam war, they proved to be highly effective as instant hemostatic agents when applied as an aerosol. They were used for primary wound closure, but under contaminated field conditions, adhesives became associated with anaerobic infections. Cyanoacrylates at the "low" end of the series, such as the methyl and propyl analogues, are toxic to tissues, especially nervous tissue, and tend to cause tissue necrosis. Those at the "high" end, such as isobutyl, n-octyl, and fluoro analogues, are well tolerated by tissues and are the formulations used most commonly for medical applications.

WOUND PHYSIOLOGY

Wounds closed with cyanoacrylates have an increase in wound strength in the initial 72 hours compared with suture closure.[80] Beyond this initial period, wound strength is diminished for 6 months when cyanoacrylates are used in parenchymatous organs. In an experimental study on degradation of methylcyanoacrylate, complete breakdown by hydrolysis in tissues occurred by 120 days, along with excretion of by-products in urine and feces.[81]

In intestinal anastomoses, wounds closed by application of cyanoacrylate had less inflammatory reaction and better cellular continuity of the bowel compared with end-to-end suture closure.[82] In repair of experimental teat lacerations, cyanoacrylate closure compared favorably with suture closure except when the glue was applied deeply in a suture line.[83] In these cases, a marked foreign-body reaction was observed, and the glue acted as a barrier to the healing wound edges. From this it was concluded that successful use of the tissue adhesive depended on its ability to be extruded during the healing process.

In two studies on the effects of cyanoacrylate on bone healing, no cytotoxic response was seen, and overall healing was comparable with that of conventional stabilization methods.[84, 85] New bone formation, however, occurred around the adhesive because cyanoacrylate acted as a barrier to bone bridging. The adhesive was present and created a histologic gap 12 weeks postoperatively. This led to recommendations that cyanoacrylate be applied to multiple sites at bone-fragment edges, rather than as a continuous coating, to allow bone growth around the glue and across the fracture line.[86]

Some controversy exists regarding the susceptibility of wounds closed by cyanoacrylates to bacterial infection. In vitro application of cyanoacrylates to plates streaked with E. coli and staphylococcal organisms demonstrated a zone of inhibition proportional to the length of the alkyl side chain.[87] Skin

wounds on guinea pigs inoculated with *Staphylococcus* spp. were more susceptible to infection if closed with trifluoropropylcyanoacrylate compared·with
closure with tape.[88] Cyanoacrylate plugs contaminated with *Staphylococcus
aureus* and implanted in bone were shown to remain contaminated for 2
weeks.[89] The latter two studies prompted the recommendation for antibiotic
usage with implanted cyanoacrylates.

Clinical Uses of Cyanoacrylates

Clinical use of cyanoacrylates in human surgery was extensive during the
1960s and early 1970s.[12, 90] Repair of tracheal, lung, and esophageal wounds
did not result in clinical complications. Extensive work with intestinal surgery
resulted in clinical success depending on the technique and procedure
performed. End-to-end inverting anastomoses resulted in stricture formation
following suture and glue combinations. Similar problems of stricture formation were encountered with vascular anastomoses using cyanoacrylates.
Repair of vascular tears, however, appeared promising. Because of the high
risk to the patient with failure, clinical use of tissue glue in vascular surgery
did not become commonplace. Closure of wounds and coating of cut surfaces
of parenchymatous organs such as liver, kidney, and spleen were successful,
but scar tissue formation was increased. The use of cyanoacrylates in human
skin wounds is still controversial. In a study comparing dural closure
techniques, cyanoacrylates significantly increased wound breaking strength
when added to suture closure and showed significantly greater strength
when used alone compared with sutures.[91] Unfortunately, histologic examination revealed a marked inflammatory reaction associated with the cyanoacrylate and cortical necrosis beneath areas of its application.

In clinical veterinary medicine, cyanoacrylates have been used in teat
laceration repair,[83] replacement of osteochondral fragments,[86, 92] and augmentation of fracture repair.[93] It is also commonly used in prosthetic
implantation (total hip replacement) and in skin and subcutaneous tissue
closure.[78] In large animal surgery, it is commonly employed in hoof and
horn repair.[78] Complication rates are variable but often lower than conventional methods, with the added advantage of speed and increased wound
strength immediately after surgery.[78, 83, 86, 93]

Fibrin Glue

Interest in the use of fibrin glue as a surgical adhesive began in the early
1900s but did not progress until the 1940s with the introduction of fibrin
powder and tampons that could be applied to bleeding surfaces. Subsequent
developments included a fibrinogen–thrombin system used to anchor skin
grafts. These early products produced poor adhesion due to a lack of
concentrated fibrinogen. With the advent of clotting factor–concentrating
methods, there was a resurgence in the experimentation with fibrin glue,
and successful clinical uses such as in peripheral nerve repair were reported.
Because of concerns over viral transmission with pooled fibrinogen concen-
trates, a ban on commercial products by the FDA was instituted in 1978.
During the past decade, considerable work has been done in the development, refinement, and application testing of single-donor and autologous
fibrin sealants prepared for isolated clinical uses.[94]

The ingredients of the product are variable, but the product usually
contains two fractions (Fig. 15–12). The first is a combination of concentrated

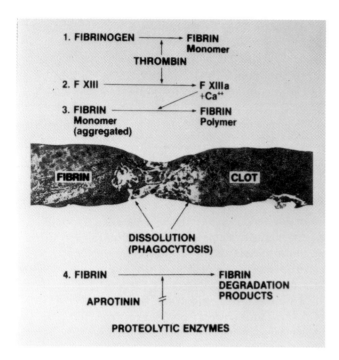

1. FIBRINOGEN ⟶ FIBRIN Monomer
   THROMBIN

2. F XIII ⟶ F XIIIa +Ca⁺⁺

3. FIBRIN Monomer (aggregated) ⟶ FIBRIN Polymer

FIBRIN   CLOT

DISSOLUTION (PHAGOCYTOSIS)

4. FIBRIN ⟶ FIBRIN DEGRADATION PRODUCTS
   APROTININ
   PROTEOLYTIC ENZYMES

Figure 15–12. Diagram depicting the physiologic basis of fibrin adhesive sealant. (From Cain JE, Dryer RF, Barton, BR: Evaluation of dural closure techniques: Suture methods, fibrin adhesive sealant, and cyanoacrylate polymer. Spine 1988; 13(7):721, with permission.)

fibrinogen, factor XIII, and various plasma proteins. The second, considered the hardener, contains thrombin and calcium chloride. When the two fractions are mixed, coagulation is initiated and a clot is formed, usually within an hour. Aprotinin may be added to slow degradation of the clot.[95]

One use of fibrin sealant is in the promotion and maintenance of coagulation to control hemorrhage from cut surfaces of parenchymatous organs.[94] In these situations, the fibrin content of the glue appears to be the essential ingredient. Another use is in the formation of an immediate seal between two surfaces by induction of the initial stages of wound healing.[94] In these applications, the fibrinogen content of the preparation appears to be the essential factor.

WOUND PHYSIOLOGY

Fibrin sealant has been shown to have a positive effect on wound healing through stimulation of fibroblast proliferation and collagen synthesis.[95] Wound strength of skin wounds repaired with fibrin sealant was shown to be greater from 0 to 4 days, equal at 4 to 20 days, and decreased beyond 20 days compared with wounds where no sealant was used.[96] Fibrin sealant has been shown to effectively inhibit wound contraction when used for attachment of skin grafts.[97]

CLINICAL USES OF FIBRIN GLUE

Successful sealant applications of fibrin glue include sealing of traumatic splenic and hepatic injuries, microvascular bleeding, and bronchial and dural fistulas.[94] Use of fibrin preparations for adhesive properties includes adherence of skin grafts over contours.[94] Additional applications such as periodontal flap construction in oral and maxillofacial surgery and the repair of peripheral nerve injuries show considerable promise.[94] In a clinical study, 8 of 10 perineal sinuses were closed successfully with the application of fibrin sealant following wound treatment.[95] Presently, studies are being conducted into the application of fibrin sealant to hepatic biopsy sites in the dog.[98] The effect of fibrin sealant on bone healing is somewhat controversial.[12] In a study evaluating the use of fibrin sealant for fixation of osteochondral fragments, resistance to fragment shearing by 14 days was comparable with that of fragments repaired with Kirschner wires.[99]

The use of fibrin glue for colonic and small bowel surgery is also controversial. Some reports indicate results comparable with those of suture techniques, whereas others cite increased complication rates.[94] In the study comparing dural closure techniques, fibrin glue was stronger than sutures and added significantly to the strength of suture closure *in vitro* when used in combination. *In vivo* tests failed to show a significant difference in strength for any of the closure techniques. Histologic changes also were similar for suture and fibrin glue closure, showing primarily a mild inflammatory reaction.[91]

At present, the use of fibrin sealant preparations in veterinary medicine is limited primarily to experimental settings because of the cost and complexity of limited-use preparations. Commercial products are currently unavailable.

Adhesive Tape

In human surgery, adhesive tape is employed frequently as a primary closure of skin wounds or as an adjunct to closure with intradermal sutures.[12] Its advantages include ease of application, superior cosmetic results, lack of a need for anesthetic, and increased early wound strength compared with suturing techniques. Another important advantage is a decreased wound infection rate by avoiding the implantation of foreign material (sutures) within the wound. The disadvantages of adhesive tape include a lack of adherence to wet surfaces, impedance in treatment of existing infections, and withholding of physiologic surface secretions. Tape is specifically applicable to linear wounds subjected to minimal static and dynamic tensions. Wounds that are under moderate tension can be apposed initially with intradermal sutures followed by tape closure of the epidermis, resulting in a more cosmetic appearance and decreasing the potential for subcutaneous infection by percutaneous sutures.[12, 100]

Clinical use of adhesive tape in veterinary medicine is limited. The primary disadvantages are rapid hair growth leading to loss of tape from the wound surface and the ease of removal by an animal.[25] In one experimental trial, adhesive tape was compared with suture closure of skin wounds in cats.[101] Cosmetic results were superior, and histologic evaluation revealed a decreased inflammatory response and increased vascularity of taped wounds compared with sutured wounds. Wound strengths were similar in taped and sutured wounds.

REFERENCES

1. Klause SE, Roberts SM: Lasers and veterinary surgery. Compend Contin Educ Pract Vet 1990; 12(11):1565–1576
2. Newman C, Jagger DH: Lasers in veterinary medicine. Proc Int Soc Optic Eng 1982; 357:38–40
3. Nasisse MP, Davidson MG: Laser therapy in veterinary ophthalmology: Perspective and potential. Semin Vet Med Surg 1988; 3(1):52–61

4. Kamat BR, Carney JM, Arndt KA, et al: Cutaneous tissue repair following CO_2 laser irradiation. J Invest Dermatol 1986; 81(2):268–271
5. Wolbarsht ML, Shi D: Mid-infrared laser surgery, in Chester AN, Mortelluci S, Scheggi AM (eds): Laser Systems in Photobiology and Photomedicine. New York: Plenum Press, 1990, pp 39–51
6. Madden JE, Edlich RF, Custer JR, et al: Studies in the management of the contaminated wound: IV. Resistance to infection of surgical wounds made by knife, electrosurgery and laser. Am J Surg 1970; 119:222–224
7. Cochrane JPS, Beacon JP, Creasey GH, Russell RGC: Wound healing after laser surgery: An experimental study. Br J Surg 1980; 67:740–743
8. Liebenberg SP, Taylor WE: The carbon-dioxide laser: Its use in pharyngeal surgery in the dog. Vet Med 1984; April:497–503
9. Lloyd KCK: Laser surgery of the upper respiratory tract, in White NA, Moore JN (eds): Current Practice of Equine Surgery. Philadelphia: JB Lippincott, 1990, pp 264–267
10. Surgical Application of Lasers. Chicago: Year Book Medical Publishers, 1984, pp 41–174
11. Bowen SG: Lasers in surgery. Practitioner 1988; 232:336–337
12. Edlich RF, Rodeheaver GT, Thacker JG: Surgical devices in wound healing management, in Cohen IK, Diegelmann RF, Lindblad WJ (eds): Wound Healing: Biological and Clinical Aspects. Philadelphia: WB Saunders, 1992, pp 581–598
13. English RV, Nasisse MP, Davidson MG: Carbon dioxide laser ablation for treatment of limbal squamous cell carcinoma in horses. J Am Vet Med Assoc 1990; 196(3):439–442
14. Anderson SM, Lippincott CL: Devocalization of dogs by carbon dioxide laser surgery. J Am Anim Hosp Assoc 1991; 27:364–366
15. Hardie EM, Stone EA, Spaulding KA, Cullen JM: Subtotal canine prostatectomy with the neodymium: yttrium–aluminum–garnet laser. Vet Surg 1990; 19(5):348–355
16. Greene JA, Knecht CD: Electrosurgery: A review. Vet Surg 1980; 9(1):27–33
17. Keenan KM, Rodeheaver GT, Kenney JG, Edlich RF: Surgical cautery revisited. Am J Surg 1984; 147:818–821
18. Link WJ, Incropera FP, Glover JL: A plasma scalpel: Comparison of tissue damage and wound healing with electrosurgical and steel scalpels. Arch Surg 1976; 111:392
19. Toombs JP, Crowe DT: Operative techniques, in Slatter DH (ed): Textbook of Small Animal Surgery. Philadelphia: WB Saunders, 1985, pp 316–320
20. Knecht CD, Clark RL, Fletcher OJ: Healing of sharp incisions and electroincisions in dogs. J Am Vet Med Assoc 1971; 159(11):1447–1452
21. Greenburg AG, Saik RP, Peskin GW: Wound dehiscence: Pathophysiology and prevention. Arch Surg 1979; 114:143–146
22. Vallfors B, Erlandson BE: Damage to nervous tissue from monopolar and bipolar electrocoagulation. J Surg Res 1980; 29:371–377
23. Goring RL, Bright RM, Stancil ML: Perianal fistulas in the dog: Retrospective evaluation of surgical treatment by deroofing and fulguration. Vet Surg 1986; 15(5):392–398
24. Bellenger CR: Sutures: I. The purpose of sutures and available suture materials. Compend Contin Educ Pract Vet 1982; 4(6):507–515
25. Bellenger CR: Sutures: II. The use of sutures and alternative methods of closure. Compend Contin Educ Pract Vet 1982; 4(7):587–600
26. Boothe HW: Suture materials and tissue adhesives, in Slatter DH (ed): Textbook of Small Animal Surgery. Philadelphia: WB Saunders, 1985, pp 334–344
27. Stashak TS, Yturraspe DJ: Considerations for selection of suture materials. Vet Surg 1978; 7(2):48–55
28. Rodeheaver GT, Nesbit WS, Edlich RF: Novafil: A dynamic suture for wound closure. Ann Surg 1986; 204(2):193–199
29. Foresman PA, Edlich RF, Rodeheaver GT: The effect of new monofilament sutures on the healing of musculoaponeurotic incisions, gastrotomies and colonic anastomoses. Arch Surg 1989; 124:708–710
30. Van Winkle W, Hastings JC, Barker E, et al: Effect of suture materials on healing of skin wounds. Surg Gynecol Obstet 1975; 140:7–12
31. Hastings JC, Van Winkle W, Barker E, et al: Effect of suture materials on healing of wounds of the stomach and colon. Surg Gynecol Obstet 1975; 140:701–707
32. Hastings JC, Van Winkle W, Barker E, et al: Effect of suture materials on healing of wounds of the bladder. Surg Gynecol Obstet 1975; 140:933–936
33. Herrmann JB: Changes in tensile strength and knot security of surgical sutures in vivo. Arch Surg 1973; 106:707–710
34. Bourne RB, Bitar H, Andreae PR, et al: In vivo comparison of four absorbable sutures: Vycril, Dexon Plus, Maxon and PDS. Can J Surg 1988; 31(1):43–45
35. Rosin E, Robinson GM: Knot security of suture materials. Vet Surg 1989; 18(4):269–273
36. Freeman LJ, Pettit GD, Robinette JA, et al: Tissue reaction to suture material in the feline linen alba: A retrospective, prospective, and histologic study. Vet Surg 1987; 16(6):440–445
37. Wood DS, Collins JE, Walshaw R: Tissue reaction to nonabsorbable suture materials in the canine linea alba: A histologic evaluation. J Am Anim Hosp Assoc 1984; 20:39–44

38. Elek SD, Conen PE: The virulence of *Staphylococcus pyogenes* for man: A study of the problems of wound infection. Br J Exp Pathol 1957; 38:573–586
39. de Holl D, Rodeheaver GT, Edgerton MT, Edlich RF: Potentiation of infection by suture closure of dead space. Am J Surg 1974; 127:716–720
40. Smeak DD, Wendelburg KL: Choosing suture materials for use in contaminated or infected wounds. Compend Contin Educ Pract Vet 1989; 11(4):467–475
41. Sharp WV, Belden TA, King PH, Teague PC: Suture resistance to infection. Surgery 1982; 91(1):61–63
42. Varma S, Ferguson HL, Breen H, Lumb WV: Comparison of seven suture materials in infected wounds: An experimental study. J Surg Res 1974; 17:165–170
43. Varma S, Lumb WV, Johnson LW, Ferguson HL: Further studies with polyglycolic acid (Dexon) and other sutures in infected experimental wounds. Am J Vet Res 1981; 42:571–574
44. James RC, MacLeod CM: Induction of staphylococcal infections in mice with small inocula introduced on sutures. Br J Exp Pathol 1961; 42:266–277
45. Chu C-C, Williams DF: Effects of physical configuration and chemical structure of suture materials on bacterial adhesion: A possible link to wound infection. Am J Surg 1984; 147:197–204
46. Dulisch ML: Suture reaction following extra-articular stifle stabilization in the dog: I. A retrospective study of 161 stifles. J Am Anim Hosp Assoc 1981; 17:569–571
47. Dulisch ML: Suture reaction following extra-capsular stifle stabilization in the dog: II. A prospective study of 66 stifles. J Am Anim Hosp Assoc 1981; 17:572–574
48. Trier WC: Considerations in the choice of surgical needles. Surg Gynecol Obstet 1979; 149:84–93
49. Poole AV, Meredith JW, Kon ND, et al: Suture technique and wound bursting strength. Am Surg 1984; 50:569–572
50. Doran RE, Allen D: The use of stapling devices in equine gastrointestinal surgery. Compend Contin Educ Pract Vet 1987; 9(8):854–860
51. Pavletic MM: Surgical stapling devices in small animal surgery. Compend Contin Educ Pract Vet 1990; 12(12):1724–1741
52. Chassin JL, Rifkind KM, Sussman B, et al: The stapled gastrointestinal tract anastomosis: Incidence of postoperative complications compared with the sutured anastomosis. Ann Surg 1978; 188(5):689–696
53. Wheeless CR: Stapling techniques in operations for malignant disease of the female genital tract. Surg Clin North Am 1984; 64(3):591–608
54. Malthaner RA, Hakki FZ, Saini N, et al: Anastomotic compression button: A new mechanical device for sutureless bowel anastomosis. Dis Colon Rectum 1990; 33:291–297
55. Steichen FM: The use of staplers in anatomical side-to-side and functional end-to-end enteroanastomoses. Surgery 1968; 64(5):948–953
56. Hess JL, McCurnin DM, Riley MG, Koehler KJ: Pilot study for comparison of chromic catgut suture and mechanically applied staples in enteroanastomoses. J Am Anim Hosp Assoc 1981; 17:409–414
57. Stoloff D, Snider TG, Crawford MP, et al: End-to-end colonic anastomosis: A comparison of techniques in normal dogs. Vet Surg 1984; 13(2):76–82
58. Stapling Techniques. General Surgery with Autosuture Instruments. Norwalk, Conn: United States Surgical Corp, 1988, pp 1–251
59. Lewis DD, Bellenger CR, Lewis DT, Latter MR: Hepatic lobectomy in the dog: A comparison of stapling and ligation techniques. Vet Surg 1990; 19(3):221–225
60. Takaio T. Use of staplers in pulmonary surgery. Surg Clin North Am 1984; 64(3):461–468
61. Boulton CH, Modransky PD, Grant BD, et al: Partial equine lung resection using a stapling instrument. Vet Surg 1986; 15(1):93–98
62. Harrison ID, Williams DF, Cuschieri A: The effect of metal clips on the tensile properties of healing skin wounds. Br J Surg 1975; 62:945–949
63. Stillman RM, Marino CA, Seligman SJ: Skin staples in potentially contaminated wounds. Arch Surg 1984; 119:821–822
64. Chassin JL, Rifkind KM, Turner JW: Errors and pitfalls in stapling gastrointestinal tract anastomoses. Surg Clin North Am 1984; 64(3):441–460
65. Sauven P, Playforth MJ, Evans M, Pollock AV: Early infective complications and late recurrent cancer in stapled colonic anastomoses. Dis Colon Rectum 1989; 32:33–35
66. Sullins KE, Stashak TS, Mero KN: Evaluation of intestinal staples for end-to-end anastomosis of the small intestine in the horse. Vet Surg 1985; 14(2):87–92
67. Ravitch MM, Steichen FM: Symposium on surgical stapling techniques, in Surgical Clinics of North America. Philadelphia: WB Saunders, 1984, pp 425–608
68. Hedberg SE, Helmy AH: Experiences with gastrointestinal stapling at the Massachusetts General Hospital. Surg Clin North Am 1984; 64(3):511–528
69. Gordon PH, Vasilevsky C: Experience with stapling in rectal surgery. Surg Clin North Am 1984; 64(3):555–566

70. Ross MW, Tate LP, Donawick WJ, Richardson DW: Cecocolic anastomosis for the surgical management of cecal impaction in horses. Vet Surg 1986; 15(1):85–92
71. Doran RE, Allen D, Gordon B: Use of stapling instruments to aid in the removal of ovarian tumors in mares. Equine Vet J 1988; 20(1):37–40
72. Clark GN, Pavletic MM: Partial gastrectomy with an automatic stapling instrument for treatment of gastric necrosis secondary to gastric dilatation–volvulus. Vet Surg 1991; 20(1):61–68
73. Ullman SL, Pavletic MM, Clark GN: Open intestinal anastomosis with surgical stapling equipment in 24 dogs and cats. Vet Surg 1991; 20(6):385–391
74. Ahmadu-Suku F, Withrow SJ, Nelson AW, et al: Billroth II gastrojejunostomy in dogs: Stapling technique and postoperative complications. Vet Surg 1988; 17(4):211–219
75. LaRue SM, Withrow SJ, Wykes PM: Lung resection using surgical staples in dogs and cats. Vet Surg 1987; 16(3):238–240
76. Wykes PM, Rouse GP, Orton EC: Removal of five canine cardiac tumors using a stapling instrument. Vet Surg 1986; 15(1):103–106
77. Lewis DD, Ellison HW, Bellah JR: Partial hepatectomy using stapling instruments. J Am Anim Hosp Assoc 1987; 23:597–602
78. Silver IA: Tissue adhesives. Vet Rec 1976; 98:405–406
79. Lehman RAW, Hayes GJ, Leonard F: Toxicity of alkyl 2-cyanoacrylates. Arch Surg 1966; 93:441–446
80. Matsumoto T, Soloway HB, Cutright DE, Hamit HF: Tissue adhesive and wound healing: Observation of wound healing (tissue adhesive vs sutures) by microscopy and microangiography. Arch Surg 1969; 98:266–271
81. Cameron JL, Woodward SC, Pulaski EJ, et al: The degradation of cyanoacrylate tissue adhesive, part I. Surgery 1965; 58:424–430
82. Linn BS, Cecil F, Conly P, et al: Intestinal anastomosis by invagination and gluing. Am J Surg 1966; 111:197–199
83. Makady FM, Whitmore HL, Nelson DR, Simon J: Effect of tissue adhesives and suture patterns on experimentally induced teat lacerations in lactating dairy cattle. J Am Vet Med Assoc 1991; 198(11):1932–1934
84. Hampel NL, Pijanowski GJ, Johnson RG: Effects of isobutyl-2-cyanoacrylate on bone healing. Am J Vet Res 1986; 47(7):1605–1610
85. Walker AM, Tomlinson JL: Use of isobutyl-cyanoacrylate adhesive in osteosynthesis: A preliminary report. Vet Surg 1984; 13(3):257–262
86. Aron DN, Gorse MJ: Clinical use of N-butyl 2-cyanoacrylate for stabilization of osteochondral fragments: Preliminary report. J Am Anim Hosp Assoc 1991; 27:203–209
87. Lehman RA, West RL, Leonard F: Toxicity of alkyl 2-cyanoacrylates: II. Bacterial growth. Arch Surg 1966; 93:447–450
88. Edlich RF, Prusak M, Madden J: Studies in the management of the contaminated wound: VIII. Assessment of tissue adhesives for repair of contaminated tissue. Am J Surg 1971; 122:394–397
89. Elson RA, Jephcott AE, McGechie DB, Verettas D: Bacterial infection in acrylic bone cement. J Bone Joint Surg 1977; 59B:452
90. Matsumoto T: Vienna international symposium: Tissue adhesives in surgery. Arch Surg 1968; 96:226–230
91. Cain JE, Dryer RF, Barton BR: Evaluation of dural closure techniques: Suture methods, fibrin adhesive sealant, and cyanoacrylate polymer. Spine 1988; 13(7):720–725
92. Gorse MJ, Aron DN, Rowland GN, et al: Evaluation of N-butyl 2-cyanoacrylate for the fixation of osteochondral fractures. Vet Comp Orthop Trauma 1991; 4:11–15
93. Kuzma AB, Hunter B: A new technique for avian fracture repair using intramedullary polymethylmethacrylate and bone plate fixation. J Am Anim Hosp Assoc 1991; 27:239–248
94. Gibble JW, Ness PM: Fibrin glue: The perfect operative sealant? Transfusion 1990; 30(8):741–747
95. Kirkegaard P, Madsen PV: Perineal sinus after removal of the rectum: Occlusion with fibrin adhesive. Am J Surg 1983; 145:791–794
96. Jorgensen PH, Jensen KH, Andreassen TT: Mechanical strength in rat skin incisional wounds treated with fibrin sealant. J Surg Res 1987; 42:237–241
97. Brown DM, Barton BR, Young VL, Pruitt BA: Decreased wound contraction with fibrin glue–treated skin grafts. Arch Surg 1992; 127:404–406
98. Wheaton LG, Meyers K: Personal communication, 1992
99. Keller J, Andreassen TT, Joyce F, et al: Fixation of osteochondral fractures: Fibrin sealant tested in dogs. Acta Orthop Scand 1985; 56:323–326
100. Conolly WB, Hunt TK, Zederfeldt B, et al: Clinical comparison of surgical wounds closed by suture and adhesive tapes. Am J Surg 1969; 117:318–321
101. Court MH, Bellenger CR: Comparison of adhesive polyurethane membrane and polypropylene sutures for closure of skin incisions in cats. Vet Surg 1989; 18(3):211–215

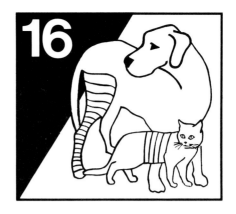

PERIOPERATIVE COMPLICATIONS OF ANESTHESIA

STEPHEN A. GREENE

Anesthetic complications during the perioperative period frequently affect patient management and outcome. A fundamental understanding of drug interactions and side effects is required to reduce or prevent patient morbidity or mortality. Prevention of intraoperative anesthetic complications is helpful in obtaining a favorable surgical outcome.

COMPLICATIONS OF ANESTHETICS

Allergic Reactions

Allergy to an anesthetic may affect the respiratory, integumentary, vascular, or gastrointestinal systems of a patient. An anaphylactic reaction requires previous exposure to an antigen (drug) and production of IgE antibodies. After the antibodies attach to mast and basophil cell membranes, the cells are sensitized to cause an anaphylactic reaction upon subsequent exposure to the same or an antigenically similar drug. Allergic reactions due to activation (classic pathway) of complement may occur during the first exposure to a drug, since no previous sensitization is required. Activation of the alternate pathway of complement can occur with a primary or secondary exposure to the drug. Thus, there are different mechanisms by which a given anesthetic drug can induce an anaphylactic reaction. Anaphylactic reactions in three dogs given thiamylal were characterized by a thick, frothy discharge from the upper airway, cyanosis, dyspnea, and tachycardia within seconds of injection.[1] Anaphylactic reactions can occur following injection of protamine (for heparin antagonism), hetastarch, dextran, and other plasma expanders. Treatment of anaphylaxis is aimed at establishing a patent airway, providing supplemental oxygen, and administering epinephrine (0.02 mg/kg) intravenously.

Anaphylactoid Reaction

An *anaphylactoid reaction* is defined as a direct effect of a drug on mast cells and basophils that stimulates release of histamine. The effects of histamine include hypotension, tachycardia, bronchial spasm, cardiac arrhythmias, and hypoxemia. While anaphylactic reactions to anesthetics are relatively rare, anaphylactoid reactions are occasionally associated with thiobarbiturates, succinylcholine, D-tubocurarine, atracurium, lidocaine, and some opioids.[2] The release of histamine is associated with administration of morphine but not fentanyl or oxymorphone. Naloxone does not inhibit morphine-induced histamine release, suggesting that the release is independent of opioid receptor binding or activation.[3]

While penicillin is a common cause of drug hypersensitivity in people, it is of practical significance only in cats, birds, and horses. During anesthesia of cats and birds, it is recommended to avoid concurrent use of penicillin.

Treatment of life-threatening anaphylactoid reactions includes airway management, delivery of oxygen, and intravenous (IV) administration of epinephrine, corticosteroids, and crystalloids. Pretreatment of susceptible animals with antihistamines (2.2 mg/kg IM) may attenuate the anaphylactoid reaction.

Radiographic contrast media injected intravenously may induce cardiovascular and respiratory reactions independent of histamine release. These agents are associated with high iodine concentrations and are hypertonic solutions which, when injected rapidly, may initially cause hypertension followed by hypotension.[4] Rapid injection of hypertonic solutions may decrease systemic vascular resistance, resulting in hypotension, particularly during anesthesia with agents that cause dose-dependent vasodilation (e.g., isoflurane or halothane).

Cell-Mediated Immune Responses

Phencyclidine is a dissociative anesthetic related to ketamine and tiletamine that binds to lymphocytes and depresses cellular immune responses.[5] However, the clinical significance of an immunosuppressant effect (if any) from ketamine or tiletamine has not been demonstrated.

Nearly all anesthetics will decrease the availability of lymphocytes.[6] Depression of T-lymphocytes has been reported during surgery and in the postoperative period.[7] In addition, decreased lymphocyte responses have been correlated with increased dose and length of anesthesia.[8] These effects may be due to the stress response associated with anesthesia and surgery. Etomidate is a nonbarbiturate, ultra-short-acting anesthetic that is associated with inhibition of corticosteroid release.[9] Etomidate-induced suppression of the corticosteroid response is generally undesirable because it inhibits the protective responses against stress associated with anesthesia and surgery.

HYPOTHERMIA

Veterinary patients are anesthetized, placed on cold surfaces, and their skin is shaved and cleansed with solutions kept at room temperature. During inhalation anesthesia, patients are ventilated with cold, dry gases. Even before the skin incision is made, these patients experience heat loss through conductive, radiant, convective, and evaporative mechanisms. Conductive heat losses are equal to the difference between skin temperature and environmental sources in direct contact with the skin. The energy required to warm irrigation fluids can dramatically decrease body temperature via this mechanism. Convective heat losses increase in proportion to the temperature difference between the body surface and the velocity of the air surrounding the patient—a phenomenon commonly referred to as the *wind-chill factor.* Convective losses are of minor significance in a properly ventilated surgical suite. Radiation of heat will increase at a rate equal to the fourth power of the temperature difference between a patient and its environment. Radiant heat loss is dramatically reduced by a single, covering layer. Evaporative heat losses occur as a result of sweating, insensible losses from the respiratory tract and skin, and evaporation of liquid antibacterial solutions applied to the skin. *Heat loss via evaporation inside large surgical incisions may equal all other sources of heat loss.*[10] Heat loss through humidification of the dry, inspired gases during inhalation anesthesia accounts for about 10% of the total heat loss during surgery in adult humans.[11] However, because the minute ventilation of very small patients is high on a per-kilogram basis, the respiratory losses represent a large percentage (up to 33%) of the total heat loss during surgery. Because of the ratio of body surface area to body weight, small patients also will have significant heat loss due to convection and radiation.

Normal thermoregulatory mechanisms in humans attempt to maintain a central body temperature within 0.4°C of normal. This threshold range may be altered by food intake, exercise, infection, thyroid disorders, thermal adaptation, and various drugs.[12] Anesthesia decreases heat production as a result of cessation of postural muscle activity and reduction of the metabolic rate. Inhaled anesthetics such as halothane and isoflurane will widen the thermoregulatory thresholds so that responses to maintain normal body temperature are initiated at a lower body temperature.[13] Vasodilator effects from tranquilizers such as acetylpromazine and inhaled anesthetics will contribute to heat loss.

Hypothermia in the perioperative period can be limited by techniques that minimize heat loss to the environment as a result of cold operating rooms, cold IV or irrigation fluids, dry and cold inspired gases, and the surgical incision. Heat loss through the breathing circuit can be decreased by using circle, rebreathing circuits when possible. Pediatric rebreathing circuits are suitable for patients weighing more than 5 kg. Addition of an active airway heater/humidifier or a passive heat/moisture exchanger to the anesthetic circuit can decrease respiratory system evaporative heat loss, especially in smaller patients.[14] Cutaneous warming will be more efficient in maintaining or restoring body temperature than airway gas warming. When using circulating warm-water blankets, attempts should be made to maximize the blanket's contact with the patient's body surface. Use of one blanket under the animal and one on top is practical. When only one circulating warm-water blanket is available, an insulating foam pad beneath the patient and the blanket on top will help to maintain normothermia. Infrared heat lamps must be used with caution because placing the lamp too close to the skin surface will create severe burns. Fluid warmers can be used for IV fluid lines, and irrigation solutions should be warmed before use. Hypothermia is most often associated with long, invasive procedures, and the surgeon must decide how aggressive to be in using some or all the warming techniques available to maintain normothermia.

HYPERTHERMIA

Hyperthermia occasionally will occur during anesthesia. It can be due to excessive warming efforts, febrile responses, hypothalamic aberrations, or malignant hyperthermia.

TABLE 16–1. Drugs in Patients Susceptible to Malignant Hyperthermia

Triggering Agents	Nontriggering Agents
Halothane	Nitrous oxide
Enflurane	Benzodiazepines
Isoflurane	Opioids
Sevoflurane	Barbiturates
Desflurane	Etomidate
Succinylcholine	Pancuronium
Amide local anesthetics	Vecuronium
Controversial Agents	Atracurium
	Epinephrine
Ketamine	Ester local anesthetics
Phenothiazines	Norepinephrine
Caffeine	Digitalis
Theophylline	Calcium
Insufficient Data	Antibiotics
	Antihistamines
Propofol	Antipyretics
	Anticholinesterases
	Oxytocin

Malignant hyperthermia (MH) is an inherited condition that involves a defect in calcium control within the sarcoplasmic reticulum of skeletal muscle.[15] Once the reaction is triggered in a susceptible individual, an uncontrollable elevation in myoplasmic calcium leads to hypermetabolism and contracture of skeletal muscle. This rapid metabolism in the muscle increases heat production and causes a rise in body temperature. Malignant hyperthermia has been reported in human beings and various breeds of dogs, cats, horses, and pigs.[15–20]

Initiating agents, or MH triggers, can be stress, excitement, high environmental temperature, or infection.[15] Volatile anesthetic agents such as halothane and isoflurane and depolarizing muscle relaxants (succinylcholine) are common triggering agents that make this disease relevant to the anesthetist[15] (Table 16–1).

The MH reaction can be variable in degree and clinical signs. The classic reaction presents initially with tachycardia and muscle rigidity. Increases in the depth and rate of respiration and depletion of the soda lime in the anesthetic circuit also can be early indicators of MH. Other clinical signs are listed in Table 16–2. Hypoxia, hyperthermia, and hyperkalemia due to muscle-cell death can lead to the cardiac arrhythmias often seen in the classic MH reaction. Laboratory evidence of severe muscle damage (increased creatine phosphokinase, aspartate transferase, and lactic dehydrogenase) and myoglobinuria may aid in the diagnosis of MH.

The halothane–caffeine contracture test has been used as a diagnostic test for MH susceptibility. For this test, muscle tissue must be obtained for *in*

TABLE 16–2. Clinical Signs of Malignant Hyperthermia

Respiratory and metabolic acidosis	Skin mottling
Hypercapnia	Muscle rigidity
Decreased mixed venous oxygen tension	Fever
Cardiac arrhythmias	Tachypnea
Hyperkalemia	Tachycardia
Hypercalcemia	Cyanosis
Unstable blood pressure	Rhabdomyolysis
Myoglobinuria	

vitro exposure to halothane, caffeine, and a combination of halothane and caffeine.

Treatment of MH relies on early recognition of the condition and prompt cooling of the patient. *Anesthesia should be terminated as soon as possible or maintained with nontriggering anesthetics* (see Table 16–1) *while the patient is aggressively cooled with a water bath and cool IV fluids.* If available, a fan should be directed toward the patient to enhance evaporative and convective heat losses. Dantrolene sodium may be effective in the treatment of MH.[21] Dantrolene decreases calcium release from the sarcoplasmic reticulum of skeletal muscle by an unknown mechanism. It must be given IV to be effective in the treatment of an acute episode. Although pharmacokinetic data for administration of dantrolene in the dog and cat are lacking, a starting dose of 1 mg/kg IV with a maximum dose of 10 mg/kg IV has been recommended.[22] In MH-suspect individuals, dantrolene can be given orally (4–5 mg/kg) as a prophylactic treatment 1 to 2 hours before anesthesia.

HYPOTENSION

The arterial pulse is a result of a wave of arterial distension that begins with the impact of each stroke volume as it is ejected into the closed arterial system. The arterial pulse pressure is the difference in pressure between systole and diastole. The two most important factors affecting the pulse pressure are (1) the left ventricular stroke volume and (2) compliance of the arterial tree. The greater the stroke volume, the greater is the volume of blood ejected into the arterial system. The effect of increased volume in the arterial system is increased blood pressure as long as arterial compliance remains constant. When changes in arterial compliance occur as a result of anesthetics, the blood pressure will be altered.

Most of the vital organs autoregulate their blood flow for a set range of blood pressure. When pressures drop below 60 mmHg, cerebral, renal, and other vascular beds cannot effectively regulate their blood flow, and organ failure may be initiated. Brief periods of hypotension (mean blood pressure less than 60 mmHg) may be tolerated by some animals better than others. Hypotension that affects oxygen delivery to nervous system tissues may be associated with neurologic deficits in the form of blindness, deafness, or altered mentation. Hypotension also may affect muscle metabolism, promoting the development of postoperative myopathy.[23] Because inhaled anesthetics are potent vasodilators, hypotension is a common complication associated with deep planes of anesthesia.

Digital palpation of an arterial pulse reflects primarily the stroke volume and may have little correlation with the actual arterial blood pressure. There are three techniques for measurement of arterial blood pressure: Doppler method, oscillometric method, and direct arterial cannulation. The Doppler method is an indirect technique based on a principle in which the frequency of an energy waveform is changed when it is reflected from a moving surface. Thus, the pitch of an amplified sound wave will be proportional to the velocity of the reflective surface. The Doppler-shifted signal is detected when the wave of blood flow causes the arterial wall to move during systole. The Doppler flow detector is moderately priced (Parks Electronics Lab, Beaverton, Oregon) and suitable for a range of veterinary patients when an appropriately sized pressure cuff is used (Fig. 16–1A). The Doppler instrument may have

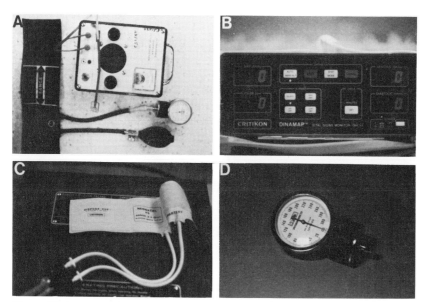

Figure 16–1. *(A)* Doppler blood pressure monitor. *(B)* Dinamap oscillometric blood pressure monitor with automated cuff inflation and deflation. *(C)* Cuff for use with the Dinamap monitor. Various cuff sizes are available for use with different limb diameters. *(D)* Aneroid manometer.

difficulty detecting signals during extreme hypotension or vasoconstriction. This technique is most accurate for measurement of the systolic arterial blood pressure. For precise measurement of blood pressure, an adjustment to the reading will be required depending on the location of the Doppler crystal above or below the level of the right atrium. For determining trends of blood pressure during a procedure, however, uncorrected values are generally adequate.

Another indirect (noninvasive) technique for measurement of blood pressure is the oscillometric method (Fig. 16–1*B*). An automated oscillometric device (Dinamap, Critikon, Tampa, Florida) has advantages over the Doppler method by maintaining accuracy yet requiring limited operator intervention. Oscillometric equipment for the measurement of blood pressure will cost more than Doppler equipment. The machine determines systolic and diastolic pressures during deflation of the pressure cuff (Fig. 16–1*C*) by detecting the oscillation of a mercury column or aneroid manometer. The mean arterial pressure is calculated from these values.

Cannulation of an artery is a direct, invasive technique for the measurement of blood pressure that is accurate and reliable. The greater metatarsal artery on the craniomedial aspect of the hock can be percutaneously catheterized using a 3- to 5-cm, 20-gauge, Teflon indwelling catheter. For surgical cases involving the hindlimb, catheterization of the lingual artery is an alternative. The catheter is connected by plastic tubing to either an electronic pressure transducer or an inexpensive aneroid manometer (Fig. 16–1*D*). The aneroid manometer will provide the mean arterial pressure value when the fluid–air interface within the pressure line is located at the level of the animal's right atrium.

In veterinary practice, hypovolemia is a common cause of hypotension. Preexisting deficits in hydration may become significant during anesthesia. Vascular fluid volume deficiencies are due to blood loss or hypoproteinemia. In addition, the potent vasodilation that occurs with high concentrations of volatile anesthetics can augment hypotension. Thus, treatment of hypotension in the anesthetized patient should be approached initially by ensuring that anesthesia is maintained at the lightest possible level. Fluid losses should be estimated, and crystalloid fluids should be administered at a rate of 10 ml/kg per hour plus two to three times the estimated volume lost as whole blood. When hypotension is severe due to hypovolemia, rapid administration of crystalloids is required (e.g., 10 to 40 ml/kg over 30 minutes).

Hypertonic solutions of saline may be administered to rapidly correct hypovolemia.[24, 25] A 7.5% saline solution should be administered at a rate of 4 ml/kg followed by infusion of lactated Ringer's solution at the maintenance rate of 10 ml/kg per hour. Electrolyte abnormalities may require alteration of this fluid therapy to allow simultaneous correction. Combinations of hypertonic saline with colloids such as dextran are beneficial in sustaining restoration of volume depletion.[26]

In cases of hypotension due to low cardiac output from poor cardiac function or myocardial depression by anesthetics, use of a catecholamine infusion may be required. Commonly used catecholamines for this purpose include ephedrine, dopamine, and dobutamine. Vigilant cardiac and blood pressure monitoring is recommended when using catecholamines during anesthesia. Tachycardia, cardiac arrhythmias, and hypertension are possible complications associated with the use of catecholamines.

HYPOXIA

Hypoxia is inadequate tissue oxygenation due to inadequate blood flow or low arterial oxygen content. *Ischemic* hypoxia is hypoxia due to inadequate blood flow. *Hypoxemic* hypoxia is hypoxia due to low oxygen content resulting from decreased hemoglobin, as in anemia, or from toxicity of methemoglobin or carboxyhemoglobin. Hypoxia may occur following complications such as pulmonary trauma, atelectasis, edema, or pneumonia. During anesthesia, hypoxia may occur as a result of drug-induced hypoventilation while breathing room air. Generally, hypoxia does not occur as a result of anesthetic-induced hypoventilation when enriched oxygen mixtures are breathed.

Obstruction of the airway may occur during anesthesia as a result of a kinked endotracheal tube or other oxygen-delivery conduit. Airway secretions may become viscous, especially following administration of anticholinergic agents, causing blockage of airways. Laryngeal spasm will completely obstruct the airway and may occur in any species, but it is most common in the cat. Laryngeal spasm in the cat most frequently occurs when anesthesia is chamber-induced using high concentrations of volatile anesthetics. The forced breathing of these inhaled anesthetics may initiate laryngospasm before the protective laryngeal reflexes are inhibited by general anesthesia. Topical application of lidocaine on the arytenoids is often effective in preventing laryngospasm in the cat. When laryngospasm occurs, use of a neuromuscular blocking agent such as atracurium (0.2 mg/kg IV) (Tracrium, Burroughs Wellcome, Research Triangle Park, North Carolina) to relax skeletal muscle is recommended. Repeated attempts to intubate a closed glottis are unlikely to succeed and may prolong the spasm or cause laryngeal edema. Laryngeal trauma that results in severe edema may necessitate tracheostomy.

During general anesthesia, hypoxia may be characterized by bradycardia, tachycardia, increased amplitude of the T wave, change in configuration of the T wave, or ST-segment depression or elevation.[27] Cyanosis may be difficult to detect until late in the course of hypoxia and may not be observed at all in patients with shock or anemia. Intraoperative hypoxia is most likely associated with the delivery of oxygen to the patient and should stimulate prompt examination of the anesthetic machine and circuit. Treatment is aimed at restoring delivery of a high inspired oxygen concentration while supporting ventilation. In patients requiring longer than 12 to 24 hours of oxygen enrichment, 40% oxygen should be delivered as a maximum to prevent oxygen toxicity.[28]

POSTOPERATIVE OLIGURIA

Dehydration, azotemia, and increased phosphate may be present in a patient with renal failure. Effects of anesthetics may be potentiated with azotemia. Lower doses are generally required for induction and maintenance of anesthesia. Anesthesia and the stress associated with surgery cause release of aldosterone, vasopressin, renin, and catecholamines. Thus, glomerular filtration rate (GFR) and renal blood flow (and therefore urine production) are generally decreased during surgery in any patient.

Intraoperative oliguria (less than 0.5 ml/kg/h) should be investigated. If the animal does not have congestive heart failure or pulmonary edema, a fluid challenge of 5 ml/kg of isotonic saline may be given. If urine production resumes, the animal was hypovolemic and fluids should be continued. If not, dopamine may be initiated as an infusion at a rate of 2 to 8 μg/kg per minute. Phenothiazine tranquilizers block dopamine receptors and alpha adrenoceptors. Thus, dopamine may be rendered ineffective in a patient given acetylpromazine.

The use of diuretics in the perioperative period is controversial. In a study of human patients, acute renal failure treated with diuretics such as mannitol and furosemide was not resolved.[29] In a dog model of uranyl nitrate–induced acute renal failure, a combination of furosemide and dopamine was effective in restoring renal blood flow and creatinine clearance, while either drug alone was not.[30] Furosemide is used to promote diuresis in patients with pulmonary edema but should not be used when the patient is known to be hypovolemic. In hypovolemia, furosemide will increase the nephrotoxicity of other agents by increasing their contact time in the renal tubules.[31] Mannitol can be given at 0.25 to 0.5 mg/kg to prevent pulmonary edema or hyponatremia if the animal does not respond to fluid administration.

PAIN

Blood levels of stress-responding hormones rise immediately after surgical incision (but not after induction of anesthesia).[32] The *stress response* to surgical trauma is a well-characterized activation of the neuroendocrine system. The severity of the stress response is quite variable and depends on the nature of the surgical trauma and associated pain.[33] In the postoperative period, it is a more complicated situation involving various physiologic responses to hypovolemia, hypothermia, etc. such that it becomes difficult to delineate precise causes of the stress response. Clinical data, however, support the concept that pain is a major component of this response.

Suppression of the stress response is achieved by inhalation or local anesthetics and opioids. Control of pain is associated with less increase in circulating catecholamine, cortisol, and glucose concentrations.[34] Pain control is indirectly associated with improved myocardial function as a result of decreased adrenergic tone causing vasodilation.[35] Lower doses of analgesics are required for prevention of pain compared with treatment once it has occurred.

Pulmonary function will normalize rapidly following adequate alleviation of pain. There is an early return to normal vital capacity and an increase in measured PaO_2 values following relief of postoperative pain.[36] Studies also have shown a slight reduction in pulmonary complications such as pneumonia and atelectasis following control of postoperative pain.[37]

Commonly used opioids in veterinary anesthesia include morphine, meperidine, butorphanol, buprenorphine, and oxymorphone (Table 16–3). Meperidine and morphine are not recommended for intravenous use because large doses may cause hypotension secondary to histamine release. The paws and pinnas of cats often become pink after morphine administration, but the side effects after intramuscular injection are minimal and duration of analgesia is longer compared with intravenous administration.

THROMBOEMBOLIC COMPLICATIONS

Major invasive surgical procedures are performed in both animal and human patients with increasing frequency. A significant complication associated with major surgical intervention in people is thromboembolic disease. It is suggested that thromboembolic disease can be attenuated by anesthetic technique in selected surgical procedures. For example, there is less intraoperative activation of fibrinolysis in patients undergoing total hip arthroplasty when they receive spinal anesthesia with tetracaine compared with patients given inhalation anesthesia.[38] Patients given epidural analgesia with bupivacaine have significantly fewer thromboembolic complications after total hip replacement compared with patients given general (intravenous) anesthesia.[39] Other investigators have shown that use of bupivacaine for epidural anesthesia during total hip replacement decreases fibrinolysis inhibition activity and decreases the capacity for activation of factor VIII compared with patients given intravenous anesthesia supplemented with nitrous oxide.[40] These results indicate a more favorable fibrinolytic status for these patients. Major lower extremity vascular surgery for patients with

TABLE 16–3. Postoperative Opioid Dosages (mg/kg, IM) and Duration of Effect

OPIOID	DOG		CAT	
	Dose	Duration	Dose	Duration
Meperidine	10	45 min	3	2 h
Morphine	0.5–1	2–4 h	0.05–0.1	3–4 h
Oxymorphone	0.2	2–4 h	0.1	2–4 h
Butorphanol	0.2–0.4	2–4 h	0.2–0.4	2–4 h
Buprenorphine	0.01–0.02	4–8 h		

atherosclerotic vascular disease given general anesthesia is associated with a hypercoagulable state postoperatively that is significantly attenuated by epidural fentanyl and bupivacaine administration.[41] The patients in this study receiving epidural anesthesia had fewer coronary artery or deep vein thromboses postoperatively than patients receiving general anesthesia.

The benefits associated with epidural anesthesia are not limited to major orthopedic or vascular surgical procedures. Women undergoing hysterectomy develop clinical signs of deep vein thrombosis with a frequency as high as 30%.[42] The factor VIII complex (F VIII:C, F VIIIR: Ag = von Willebrand factor) is increased significantly less in women undergoing hysterectomy during epidural bupivacaine anesthesia compared with those anesthetized with enflurane.[43] The authors of this study suggest that the higher factor VIII complex levels may account for the increased incidence of thromboembolic disease following hysterectomy with general anesthesia compared with epidural anesthesia.

Epidural administration of opioids for pain relief is also associated with similar benefits in terms of postoperative coagulation status and thromboembolic disease. In obese patients undergoing gastroplasty for weight reduction, those receiving epidural morphine postoperatively have fewer clinical signs of deep vein thrombosis and an earlier return to normal pulmonary function compared with patients given intramuscular morphine. It is not known if local anesthetics and opioids administered in the epidural space work via the same mechanism for neuroendocrine modulation, resulting in altered postoperative coagulation states.

In animals, little is known about the effects of specific types of surgical procedures or the influence of anesthetic technique on coagulation. In dogs, platelet aggregation was significantly decreased following administration of acetylpromazine and atropine but returned to normal during subsequent halothane anesthesia and surgery.[44] Coagulation deficiencies such as thrombocytopenia, increased prothrombin time, increased activated partial thromboplastin time, hypofibrinogenemia, increased fibrin degradation products, and decreased antithrombin III are described in association with the canine syndrome of gastric dilatation–volvulus.[45] In dogs undergoing colonic anastomosis, there was less intraoperative bleeding and more advanced healing (detected histologically) 1 and 7 days after surgery in dogs that received epidural bupivacaine and general anesthesia compared with dogs that received only general anesthesia.[46] Much work remains to be done to identify surgical procedures that pose higher risks for thromboembolic disease in animals and anesthetic techniques that will improve healing in the convalescent period.

SUMMARY

Therapeutic benefits of anesthesia include prevention and relief of pain. Anesthetics are among the most potent drugs used by veterinarians, and they require attention to factors such as variation in patient response, potential for drug interaction, and effects on organ function. In recent years, much has been learned about anesthetic drugs, methods of drug administration, and effects in our patients. While anesthetic delivery is undoubtedly safer than it was decades ago, a continuous goal is to avoid anesthetic-related morbidity and mortality. Current practices must be examined objectively and new techniques adopted that are safe and effective.

REFERENCES

1. Short CE: Allergic reactions and immune responses during anesthesia, in Short CE (ed): Principles and Practice of Veterinary Anesthesia. Baltimore: Williams & Wilkins, 1987, pp 599–606
2. Fisher MMcD: The diagnosis of acute anaphylactoid reactions to anaesthetic drugs. Anaesth Intensive Care 1981; 9:235–241
3. Stoelting RK: Pharmacology and Physiology in Anesthetic Practice. Philadelphia: JB Lippincott, 1987, p 77
4. Goldberg M: Systemic reactions to intravascular contrast media. Anesthesiology 1984; 60:46–56
5. Khansari N, Whitten HD, Fudenbeg HH: Phencyclidine-induced immunodepression. Science 1984; 225:76–78
6. Moore TC: Anesthesia-associated depression in lymphocyte traffic and its modulation. Am J Surg 1984; 147:807–812
7. Hole A, Bakke O: T-lymphocytes and the subpopulations of T-helper and T-suppressor cells measured by monoclonal antibodies (T11, T4, and T8) in relation to surgery under epidural and general anaesthesia. Acta Anaesthesiol Scand 1984; 28:296–300
8. Moore TC: Anesthesia associated depression in lymphocyte traffic: Less with regional anesthesia than with general anesthesia in sheep. Am J Surg 1984; 148:71–76
9. Kruse-Elliott KT, Swanson CR, Aucoin DP: Effects of etomidate on adrenocortical function in canine surgical patients. Am J Vet Res 1987; 48:1098–1100
10. Roe CF: Effect of bowel exposure on body temperature during surgical operations. Am J Surg 1971; 122:13–18
11. Bickler PE, Sessler DI: Efficiency of airway heat and moisture exchangers in anesthetized humans. Anesth Analg 1990; 71:415–418
12. Entrup MH, Davis FG: Perioperative complications of anesthesia. Surg Clin North Am 1991; 71:1151–1173
13. Sessler DI, Olofsson CI, Rubinstein EH, et al: The thermoregulatory threshold in humans during halothane anesthesia. Anesthesiology 1988; 68:836–842
14. Chalon J, Markham JP, Ali MM, et al: The Pall Ultipor breathing circuit filter—an efficient heat and moisture exchanger. Anesth Analg 1984; 63:566–568
15. Gronert GA: Malignant hyperthermia. Anesthesiology 1980; 53:395–423
16. Leary SL, Anderson LC, Manning PJ, et al: Recurrent malignant hyperthermia in a greyhound. J Am Vet Med Assoc 1983; 182:521–522
17. Kirmayer AH, Klide AM, Purvance JE: Malignant hyperthermia in a dog: Case report and review of the syndrome. J Am Vet Med Assoc 1984; 185:978–982
18. DeJong RH, Heavner JE, Amory DW: Malignant hyperpyrexia in the cat. Anesthesiology 1974; 41:608–609
19. Waldron-Mease E, Klein LV, Rosenberg H, Leitch M: Malignant hyperthermia in a halothane-anesthetized horse. J Am Vet Med Assoc 1981; 179:896–898
20. Hall LW, Woolf N, Bradley JWP, et al: Unusual reaction to suxamethonium chloride. Br Med J 1966; 2:1305
21. Kolb ME, Horne ML, Martz R: Dantrolene in human malignant hyperthermia. Anesthesiology 1982; 56:254–262
22. Pascoe PJ: Perioperative hyperthermia in dogs and cats. VCOT 1989; 2:67–69
23. Grandy JL, Steffey EP, Hodgson DS, Woliner MJ: Arterial hypotension and the development of postanesthetic myopathy in halothane-anesthetized horses. Am J Vet Res 1987; 48:192–197
24. Fettman MJ: Hypertonic crystalloid solutions for treating hemorrhagic shock. Compend Contin Educ Pract Vet 1985; 7:915–920
25. Muir WW, Sally J: Small-volume resuscitation with hypertonic saline solution in hypovolemic cats. Am J Vet Res 1989; 50:1883–1888
26. Allen DA, Schertel ER, Muir WW, Valentine AK: Hypertonic saline/dextran resuscitation of dogs with experimentally induced gastric dilatation–volvulus shock. Am J Vet Res 1991; 52:92–96
27. Tilley LP: Essentials of Canine and Feline Electrocardiography, 2d ed. Philadelphia: Lea & Febiger, 1985
28. Deneke SM, Fanburg BL: Normobaric oxygen toxicity of the lung. N Engl J Med 1980; 303:76–85
29. Cantarovich F, Locatelli A, Fernandez JC, et al: Furosemide in high doses in the treatment of acute renal failure. Postgrad Med J (Suppl) 1978; 47:13–19
30. Lindner A, Cutler RE, Goodman WG: Synergism of dopamine plus furosemide in preventing acute renal failure in the dog. Kidney Int 1979; 16:158–162

31. Stoelting RK: Pharmacology and Physiology in Anesthetic Practice. Philadelphia: JB Lippincott, 1987, pp 423–432
32. Engquist A, Brandt MR, Fernandes A, et al: The blocking effect of epidural analgesia on the adrenocortical and hyperglycemic responses to surgery. Acta Anaesthesiol Scand 1977; 21:330–335
33. Chernow B, Alexander R, Smallridge R, et al: Hormonal responses to graded surgical stress. Arch Intern Med 1987; 147:1273–1278
34. Benson GJ, Lin HC, Thurmon JC, et al: Assessment of analgesia by catecholamine analysis: Response to onychectomy in cats, in Short CE, van Poznak A (eds): Animal Pain. New York: Churchill Livingstone, 1992, pp 436–439
35. Klassen GA, Bramwell RS, Bromage PR, et al: Effect of acute sympathectomy by epidural anesthesia on the canine coronary circulation. Anesthesiology 1980; 52:8–15
36. Spence AA, Smith G: Postoperative analgesia and lung function: A comparison of morphine with extradural block. Br J Anaesth 1971; 43:144–148
37. Yeager MP: Outcome of pain management. Anesthesiol Clin North Am 1989; 7:241–258
38. Davis FM, McDermott E, Hickton C, et al: Influence of spinal and general anaesthesia on hemostasis during total hip arthroplasty. Br J Anaest 1987; 59:561–571
39. Modig J, Borg T, Karlstrom G, et al: Thromboembolism after total hip replacement: Role of epidural and general anesthesia. Anesth Analg 1983; 62:174–180
40. Modig J, Borg T, Bagge L, Saldeen T: Role of extradural and of general anaesthesia in fibrinolysis and coagulation after total hip replacement. Br J Anaesth 1983; 55:625–629
41. Tuman KJ, McCarthy RJ, March RJ, et al: Effects of epidural anesthesia and analgesia on coagulation and outcome after major vascular surgery. Anesth Analg 1991; 73:696–704
42. Rakoczi I, Chamone D, Collen D, Verstraete M: Prediction of postoperative leg-vein thrombosis in gynaecological patients. Lancet 1978; 1:509–510
43. Bredbacka S, Blomback M, Hagnevik K, et al: Pre- and postoperative changes in coagulation and fibrinolytic variables during abdominal hysterectomy under epidural or general anaesthesia. Acta Anaesthesiol Scand 1986; 30:204–210
44. Barr SC, Ludders JW, Looney AL, Gleed RD: Platelet function in dogs after premedication and during general anesthesia (abstract). Vet Surg 1992; 21:165
45. Millis DL, Hauptman JG: Coagulation abnormalities and gastric necrosis in canine gastric dilatation–volvulus (abstract). Vet Surg 1991; 20:342
46. Blass CE, Kirby BM, Waldron DR, et al: The effect of epidural and general anesthesia on the healing of colonic anastomoses. Vet Surg 1987; 16:75–79

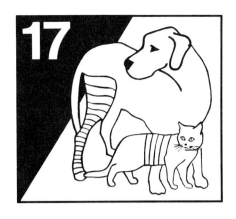

POSTOPERATIVE PHYSICAL THERAPY

CARLOS C. HODGES
ROSS H. PALMER

The primary goal of most surgical therapies is to restore function. Restoration of function following orthopedic and neurologic injury or disease depends on appropriate surgical therapy and postoperative physical therapy. In contrast to our colleagues in the fields of human medicine, we seldom have the luxury of referral for physical therapy. Therefore, maximizing our successes through physical therapy depends on knowledge of the principles involved in physical therapeutics. While the field of physical therapy is complex, the clinical application of basic principles will improve and enhance our patients' chances for recovery. The purpose of this chapter is to review basic principles and applications of physical therapy in relation to common veterinary clinical conditions.

PRINCIPLES OF PHYSICAL THERAPY

Physical therapy is the treatment of disease or injury with physical agents such as cold, heat, light, electricity, sound, and mechanical agents such as massage and exercise Physical therapy improves physical strength, range of motion, and coordination, as well as decreasing inflammation, edema, and pain. By stimulating normal physiologic responses, restoration of function can be achieved.

Local Hypothermia

Decreased tissue temperature due to local application of hypothermia causes vasoconstriction, decreased cutaneous nerve conduction velocity, and skeletal muscle relaxation.[1, 2] Vasoconstriction decreases arterial and capillary blood flow, which minimizes fluid leakage from capillary vessels. The reduction in transvascular fluid leakage effectively reduces edema formation when applied early following an acute injury.[2] Mild analgesia is induced by alteration of the nerve conduction velocity, and relief of muscle spasm is also affected.[3]

Local hypothermia has a more limited use than heat therapy but is often indicated in the early postinjury period (up to 12 to 48 hours after injury).[1] Local hypothermia is frequently accomplished in veterinary medicine by application of ice bags or cold packs. Similarly, small tanks or buckets filled with ice water (18°C, or 65°F) may be used.[4, 5] If an injured limb has open wounds or abrasions, local therapy should be performed aseptically. For this reason, cold packs applied over a sterile, water-impermeable dressing are preferable to cold water immersion. Hypothermia should be applied in short 5- to 20-minute sessions, two to four times daily.[4, 6] Hypothermia should not exceed 30 minutes per treatment because vasodilation and subsequent edema formation may follow.[1] It is often useful to apply gentle pressure wraps following local hypothermia treatment to further prevent edema.[6] Because of its vasoconstrictive action, local hypothermia should not be used on patients with peripheral vascular disease, ischemic injury, diabetes mellitus, vasculitis, or indolent wounds.[3, 5] The principles of early treatment with local hypothermia, maintenance of aseptic technique when open wounds are present, and use of numerous short sessions of treatment must be emphasized if hypothermia is to be administered effectively.

Local Hyperthermia

SUPERFICIAL HYPERTHERMIA

Heat is frequently employed in orthopedic rehabilitation. When used prior to massage and exercise, it enhances the positive effects of subsequent treatments.[3, 4, 7] Superficial heating techniques increase the temperature of the tissues to a depth of 1 to 2 cm beneath the skin surface.[2] The physiologic effects of heat are increased tissue temperature, vasodilation, and increased local circulation.[1-7] These changes cause an increase in tissue metabolic activity, which causes a further increase in tissue temperature and vasodilation, aiding in the delivery of needed tissue nutrients and in the removal of tissue waste products. Mild sedation and relief of muscular tension and pain are also achieved by heat therapy.[3, 4]

Superficial heat may be applied in 10- to 20-minute sessions, and there is little danger of overdosage if skin sensation and local circulation are normal and the patient is physically capable of moving away from the heat source.[2] A major contraindication to the use of superficial heat is the absence of skin sensation (e.g., patients with coma, spinal injury, peripheral nerve injury, general anesthesia, etc.), because the patient cannot sense or respond to excessive heat application. Because normal cutaneous and subcutaneous blood circulation is important in dissipating applied heat, decreased local blood supply (e.g., patients with epithelializing wounds, general anesthesia, etc.) is also a major contraindication for the use of superficial hyperthermia.

Superficial hyperthermia may be indicated 48 to 72 hours after an acute injury to decrease swelling, pain, and muscle spasm.[3, 4] Trauma may disrupt blood and lymphatic vessels resulting in interstitial edema. Capillary tears may be sealed within minutes, although tears in small arteries and arterioles may require 24 hours to form a secure seal. Premature application of local hyperthermia (within 48 hours of injury) can increase transvascular fluid leakage as a result of heat's vasoactive properties.[4] However, if applied at the proper time, superficial hyperthermia can increase resorption of extravasated fluid and decrease edema.

Insulated hot packs, warm moist towels, or circulating warm-water heating blankets are often used to produce superficial hyperthermia. Aseptic technique should be used when therapy is applied in the region of an open wound or abrasion. The patient should be protected from burns by insulation and feeling the skin every few minutes.[8] If the skin feels hot, more insulation must be added between the heat source and patient.[8] As a rule of thumb, if the pack is too hot to the touch, it is too hot to apply to the patient, and a few minutes should be allowed for cooling. Careful application of superficial hyperthermia will maximize its efficacy and minimize its risk.

DEEP HYPERTHERMIA

Heating of the deeper tissues through more complex therapies (e.g., short-wave diathermy, microwave, ultrasound) has a lower safety margin than the various forms of superficial heating and is used less commonly in small animal physical therapy.[2] Short-wave diathermy utilizes alternating high-frequency electric currents applied to the patient. The patient becomes part of an electrical circuit, and the electrical impedance provided by the patient's tissues transforms the energy into heat.[7] No metal can be near the field of treatment. Therefore, the treatment should not be used on patients with metal implants such as orthopedic plates, screws, pins, hemostatic clips, and pacemakers.[7] Likewise, metal treatment tables should not be used.[7] There are various techniques of short-wave diathermy application, but all techniques require training and instruction beyond the scope of this chapter.

Microwave therapy utilizes a beam of electromagnetic waves that may be reflected, scattered, refracted, or absorbed.[2, 7] The medical use of microwaves is based on selective absorption by tissues with high water content, thus allowing selective heating of certain tissues such as skeletal muscles.[7] Caution must be used when treating near the eye or edematous tissues.[7, 9] Similar to short-wave diathermy, metallic objects should not be near the treatment field.[9] Again, much research has been done with the clinical use of microwave deep heating of tissues, but proper use of the modality requires advanced training.

Ultrasound is a mechanical vibration produced at frequencies beyond the audible range of the human ear (greater than about 17,000 Hz).[7] An important characteristic of ultrasound-wave transmission is reflection, which occurs at interfaces between tissues of different acoustic impedance.[7] Burning of tissues, particularly bone, is a risk of ultrasound therapy. Powerful mechanical forces of ultrasound also can create gaseous cavitation of tissues as a result of reaction with the dissolved gases within tissues.[7] Ultrasound, like other methods of deep hyperthermia, requires proper and extensive training.

In summary, various forms of superficial heat application are available to veterinary practitioners, are relatively low-risk/high-benefit modalities, and are affordable. The more complex forms of deep hyperthermia are costly and require extensive training and expertise.

Massage

Massage increases arterial, venous, and lymphatic flow, thereby facilitating nutrient delivery and waste removal from the treated tissues.[4] Massage also can increase range of motion and locomotor comfort through stretching of adhesions and breakdown of fibrin clots between muscles and between muscles and bone.[2] Massage is often one component of combination therapy consisting of superficial hyperthermia, massage, and therapeutic exercise.

The physiologic effects of massage may be categorized as reflex or mechanical.[10] *Reflex effects* are produced in the skin by stimulation of peripheral receptors, which then transmit the impulses through the spinal cord to the brain and produce sensations of comfort and relaxation. Peripherally, these impulses cause muscular relaxation and vasoactive effects. Sedation is a major physiologic reflex effect of massage and is produced by monotonously repetitive massage without sharp variations in pressure, rate, or massage motion. Relief of mental tension is also a reflex effect of massage. *Mechanical effects* of massage include (1) assisted cardiac return of blood and lymphatic flow because massage is given with greatest force in the centripetal (toward the heart) direction and (2) measures that produce intramuscular motion. Inactive muscles of paralyzed limbs often have insufficient blood flow and exchange of nutrients, which result in severe muscle atrophy. Massage, together with active and passive exercise, minimizes atrophy induced by muscular inactivity. Massage, by itself, does not develop muscle strength and therefore is not a substitute for active exercise.

There are two major types of massage. One is called *effleurage* or stroking massage.[2, 10, 11] Effleurage is superficial and light, and is performed by running the hand lightly over the surface of the skin starting distally and proceeding toward the heart. Contact with the skin can be broken at the end of the stroke, and the therapist should maintain skin contact on the return stroke with only very light pressure. The second type of massage includes deep kneading, squeezing, and friction and is called *petrissage*.[2, 10, 11] Kneading is lifting of the soft tissues between the fingers and manipulating them in an alternating fashion such that there is motion within the muscle itself. It does not proceed in any particular direction but is used to mobilize tissue fluids and create intramuscular motion. Squeezing is performed with large muscles and consists of squeezing the muscle between two hands or between the hand and a solid object such as bone or treatment table. Friction is a circular motion performed by placing the thumb, fingertips, or heel of the hand on the skin and moving in circular loops at a moderately rapid rate with increasing pressure.

Sessions usually should be 10 to 20 minutes' duration and can be performed once every 24 to 48 hours.[11] Sessions should always begin with effleurage so that the patient can become adapted to the therapist's touch while allowing the therapist to detect areas of tenderness and spasm.[10] The massage may then progress to petrissage to facilitate breakdown of intramuscular adhesions and mobilization of interstitial fluid accumulations. The massage is concluded with effleurage to aid in blood and lymphatic flow from the treated area toward the heart and to maintain the muscular relaxation and sedative effects.

Massage has little risk and great benefit. Massage is, however, contraindicated in the presence of infection to avoid spreading the infection through tissues.[10, 11] For similar reasons, massage should be avoided in areas of malignancy.[10, 11] Massage also should be avoided in areas of acute inflammation because of pain. Caution and appropriate hygiene should be used if massage is employed on patients with contagious skin diseases and open wounds.

Exercise

PASSIVE EXERCISE

Passive exercise is accomplished by the therapist with no effort on the part of the patient and is used primarily in patients with no motor control of a limb. It also may be used in patients unwilling to use a limb because of discomfort or some disruption (patellar luxations) in normal locomotor mechanisms.[2] *Passive exercise is used to maintain normal range of motion in joints and prevent contractures.*[2, 12] *Passive exercise also improves blood and lymphatic microcirculation and stimulates sensory awareness.*[4]

The therapist moves the affected body part through unrestricted and pain-free range of motion. Excessive application of force can traumatize restricting tissues and cause further inflammation and pain. Passive physical therapy usually follows superficial hyperthermia and sometimes massage. Each joint in the limb should be treated. It usually begins away from the most seriously affected joint and progresses toward that joint, allowing the patient to become accustomed to the therapist's manipulations of the limb. Each joint can be independently treated by grasping the limb on either side of the joint and gently running the joint through extension and flexion in as complete a range of motion as the patient will allow. Each joint can be treated with 10 to 20 cycles per minute for 5 minutes, two to three times daily. If grasping the limb causes pain, wrapping the limb in a thick, soft towel may make the treatments more comfortable. After each joint has been individually treated, the entire limb is moved through a range of motion similar to ambulation.

ACTIVE EXERCISE

Active exercise is performed by the patient by voluntary movement of a body part. It is preferred over passive exercise whenever possible.[2] *Active exercise, like passive, improves tissue microcirculation, joint range of motion, and sensory awareness. Unlike passive exercise, active exercise improves muscular strength, endurance, cardiopulmonary function, and coordination.*[2]

During the recovery of a paralyzed patient, there is a gradual and progressive improvement from complete paralysis to nonambulatory paresis, weak ambulation, and finally, normal ambulation. For this reason, the exercise treatment course should logically follow the capabilities and needs of the paralyzed patient. Exercise therapy typically begins as passive exercise and then progresses to active assisted exercise and active resistive exercise.[2] *Active assisted exercise* is exercise in which the therapist assists the patient by supporting its weight to help the patient overcome the force of gravity.[2] Active assisted exercise is usually the first step in muscle reeducation. Often the patient needs a great deal of encouragement and praise during this phase of neurologic recovery. Failure during the initial steps of active assisted exercise can be devastating to the patient. Assistance by the therapist in this form of exercise may include the use of slings, harnesses, and the buoyancy provided by water tanks and pools. *Active resistive exercise* is active exercise with resistance added and can be used as a patient's strength begins to improve.[2] This form of exercise improves muscular strength, stamina, and coordination. It is accomplished by applying resistance through a desire range of motion. Human patients can be instructed to perform a particular maneuver while the therapist applies resistance to that movement. Application of resistive exercise in small animals requires considerably more creativity. One method is to apply a gentle, nonpainful, but annoying stimulus to the digits and gradually resist the animal's efforts to withdraw the limb. Obviously, this method requires a great deal of praise and positive reinforcement for the patient if continued cooperation is to be achieved. In patients with increased extensor muscle tone, the therapist can gradually apply a resistive compression to the digits in an attempt to flex the joints of the limb. Commonly, posterior paretic patients go through a stage in which they are able to stand with minimal assistance if the therapist can position them and assist with balance. At this stage, one can apply a downward force over the pelvis as a form of active resistive exercise.

Typically, paralyzed patients progress through an exercise program that begins with passive exercise and then progresses to active assisted exercise followed by active resistive exercise. Exercise sessions are performed at least twice daily. The sessions are initially very short (5 minutes) when the patient is weak but progress to sessions of 30 minutes or more. Numerous shorter sessions are preferred rather than a few lengthy sessions because patients often become resistant to therapy techniques once they are tired. Properly executed, and with encouragement, results of these treatments can be very satisfying.

Combination Therapy Programs

For each patient, multiple forms of therapy rather than a single form are often indicated. Therapy sessions can begin with superficial hyperthermia progressing to massage therapy and followed by passive or active exercise.[2-4, 7] *Whirlpools are often used to accomplish all three of these therapies* (Fig. 17–1). Whirlpools use a turbine to mix room air with bath water to attain a constant flow of agitating currents and massaging bubbles. Any temperature of water can be used, and frequently superficial hyperthermia is included in the whirlpool therapy.

When used to accomplish superficial hyperthermia, the water temperature should be 38 to 40°C (102–105°F).[13] Temperatures less than body temperature act as heat sink, whereas temperatures greater than 40°C can cause burns, excessive vasodilation, and even internal organ damage.[13]

The massage action of the circulating water and bubbles should not be relied on to accomplish massage therapy. To ensure that massage therapy is

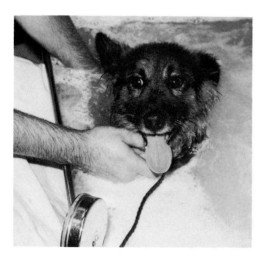

Figure 17–1. Superficial hyperthermia is included during whirlpool therapy in a dog with posterior paresis. Subsequent active/assisted physical therapy is often performed in the whirlpool session.

effective in mobilizing tissue fluids, improving tissue microcirculation, and stretching adhesions, effleurage and petrissage techniques are performed manually during whirlpool therapy sessions.

Finally, whirlpools are a very helpful form of assisted active exercise. The buoyancy helps the patient resist gravitational pull with balance. Often, the first voluntary limb movements in a patient with a spinal injury made are during whirlpool therapy. It is usually necessary to let the patient maintain balance with the whirlpool turbine turned off. Once the patient has attained balance, the jets can be turned on slowly, thus allowing the patient to balance against the water currents.

Certain precautions and principles of whirlpool therapy should be followed. Surgical patients are usually not placed in the whirlpool until their incisions have sealed (5 to 10 days after surgery). The weight-bearing surface should be nonskid so that the patient can use the tank bottom to balance. The tank should be filled with water to the level of midthorax if the therapy is designed to assist with walking. If swimming therapy is to be performed, the tank can be filled higher. A sling is often helpful in supporting patients during therapy. Each patient responds differently to water. The patient should be reassured and feel supported by the therapist when first placed in the whirlpool. The turbine must be grounded, and the electrical cord should be intact, secure, and dry. Disposable tank liners can be used to prevent contamination between patients, or the tank can be disinfected after each use. Disinfecting must include cleaning of the turbine tubes. It is recommended that bacterial cultures be obtained intermittently from parts of the whirlpool to assess cleanliness. Improperly disinfected whirlpools can be become a major source of nosocomial infections within the hospital (Chapter 11).

PHYSICAL THERAPY AT HOME

Most owners can perform basic physical therapy if they are given clear instructions and training. The owner should be taught the purpose and technique of each therapy. The owner should practice the techniques under the guidance and observation of the therapist prior to patient release from the hospital. Improperly performed, physical therapy is often ineffective and, worse yet, can be detrimental. Frequently, the owner thinks that he or she is hurting their pet although this is not occurring. For this reason, it is worthwhile to describe or demonstrate on the owner what the patient will feel. In addition, owners are encouraged to return for reevaluations 5 to 7 and 10 to 14 days after discharge. At these times, responses to therapy can be determined and programs updated. It sometimes becomes clear during reevaluations that the owner's work schedule, family commitments, and emotional attachment to the patient may render him or her incapable of performing the therapy at home.

In addition to training the owner to perform the needed therapies, it is necessary to write a thorough set of instructions, including the techniques to be used, their purpose, frequency, and duration. The owner is also instructed about pertinent precautions and signs that may indicate a problem.

Finally, and perhaps most importantly, the importance of encouragement and praise is emphasized. Often the owner quickly falls into the trap of sympathy and pity rather than a role of support, encouragement, confidence, and hope.

MEASUREMENT OF RESPONSE TO THERAPY

The key to determining the relative success or failure of any treatment program is to develop a method of measurement of response to therapy. Both *objective* and *subjective* assessments are valuable.

Objective Measurements

GONIOMETRY

Goniometry is the measurement of joint motion and is simple to perform on the limbs of most small animal patients.[14] Goniometry not only allows the therapist to detect a lack of response to treatment, but it can also permit evaluation of a mild positive response to the therapy that otherwise might go unnoticed and cause a sense of discouragement.

Measurement of angles in clinical patients can be performed by centering the protractor scale over the axis of the joint with the limbs of the goniometer centered over the longitudinal axis of the adjacent long bones (Fig. 17–2). The joint angle taken as "0 degrees" is somewhat arbitrary, and a number of systems for measurement have been described. Some regard full extension as 0 degrees, whereas others consider it 180 degrees. A common veterinary reference defines 0 degrees as the joint angle with the patient in normal standing position. Extension and flexion range of motion deviate from this zero point.[15] Using this system, the normal range of motion in the joints of the limbs of dogs and cats is known (Fig. 17–3).

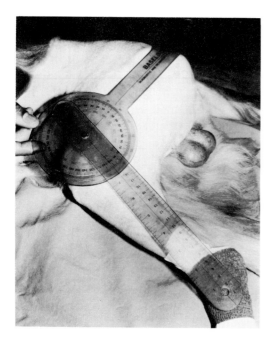

Figure 17–2. Proper use of a goniometer. The protractor scale is centered over the axis of the joint, and the limb of the goniometer is centered over the longitudinal axis of adjacent bones.

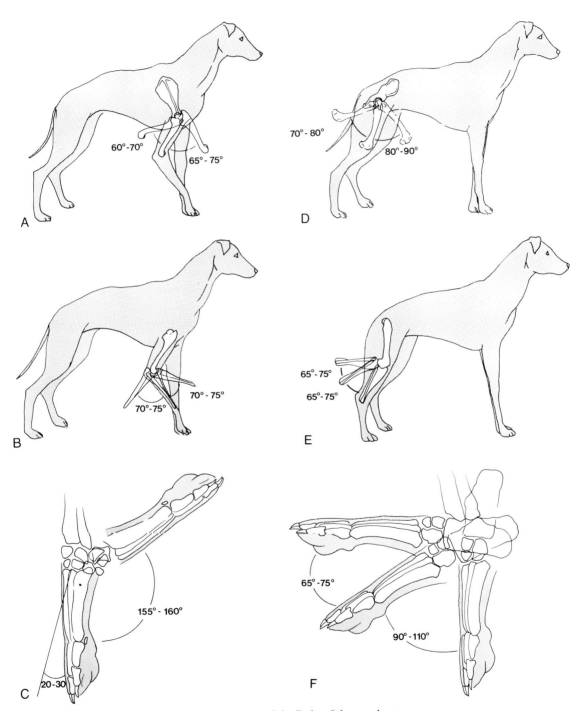

Figure 17–3. Normal ranges of motion in the joints of the limbs of dogs and cats.

MEASUREMENT OF MUSCLE MASS

A number of methods to measure body muscle mass and mass of a particular muscle group have been developed. A simple and reasonably reliable method is girth measurement of a given muscle mass. In measuring girth of a muscle mass, it is important to use specific landmarks to maintain consistent evaluations. For example, the girth of the thigh musculature decreases from the hip region down to the stifle joint; therefore, specific landmarks should be used to ensure repeatability of measurement. A metric tape measure can be used to record girth in centimeters. Girth measurement is not specific for any given muscle, so concurrent atrophy of one muscle group and hypertrophy of another may show no change in overall girth. A greater limitation of girth measurement is that it tells nothing of muscular performance, the ultimate assessment of therapy.

MEASUREMENT OF MUSCLE STRENGTH

Patient cooperation provides physicians with a tremendous advantage in measurement of muscle strength. It is difficult to instruct clinical small animal patients to cooperate, although research animals have been conditioned to perform a variety of tasks.

A method that can be used to assess relative changes in strength of withdrawal muscles begins by positioning the patient in lateral recumbency. A spring weight scale is attached to the end of the foot with adhesive tape. A gentle but noxious stimulus is applied to the toes so the patient withdraws the limb while the scale (attached to the toes) is held rigidly by hand or is attached to the wall. Using this method, the withdrawal force of the animal can be determined. In order for this method to be accurate, the only motion during withdrawal should be in the limb (i.e., the patient may not slide along the floor), the scale must be firmly held, and the scale must be securely attached to the toes. Another source of potential error is the inconsistency in the withdrawal response to a noxious stimulus. This method is simple, quick, and useful in monitoring trends of a given patient. It is of little value for comparing patients.

A similar method can be used to assess the strength of extensor muscles. The patient's limb is placed on a compression weight scale. Gentle pressure is applied to the shoulder or pelvis. This downward pressure is gradually increased until the patient begins to buckle or collapse on the limb. The force at the time of collapse is recorded. This technique also can be used with the patient in lateral recumbency if the patient will resist flexion of the limb.

MEASUREMENT OF SPEED, ENDURANCE, AND AGILITY IN THE ATHLETE

The considerations for the athletic animal are very similar to those for human patients. There is a given level of performance that is expected of the patient upon recovery. Any reduction in performance from that level is *disability*. For the racing dog, objective time trials are used to assess the success of treatment or stage of recovery. Similarly, various field trials are used to assess the recovery from disability in hunting dogs. Recognition of the difference between the performance animal and the companion animal is necessary to determine from the owner the desired level of performance before therapy is initiated. The owner must be given an accurate prognosis for *attaining the desired level of performance*.

GAIT-ANALYSIS SYSTEMS

Sophisticated gait-analysis systems, which correlate video recordings of gait with force-plate measurements, have been used to objectively evaluate normal gaits, response to surgical procedures, and diagnosis of lameness.[16, 17] Similar computerized systems have been used to classify body motions into defined finite movements and are tremendously valuable in training human athletes. Although these systems will likely become more and more valuable in applied clinical research, their use in the daily assessment of small animal patients is not yet a reality.

Subjective Measurements

Subjective measurements are often criticized because of intraobserver and interobserver variations. That is, from observation to observation, the same observer may falsely note improvement in patient status as a result of wishful thinking, mood changes, and time of day when, in reality, there is no improvement. Likewise, one observer may note one level of function one day, and on the return hospital visit, a second observer may report another level of function, but the two observations have no comparative basis. While often criticized, subjective observations can be valuable and practical because evaluation by the owner ultimately determines the level of client satisfaction.

Certain principles of subjective observation can minimize potential errors. Observations should be made by the same observer(s) when possible. Multiple observers at each assessment decrease the impact of intraobserver bias. Observations made too frequently often "hide" the progression or regression of function. For this reason, the owner is often too close to see changes in the level of performance. The owner should, therefore, be asked to compare the level of performance in terms of 2-week reference frames rather than day-to-day evaluations. Preferably, recheck examinations can be scheduled so the veterinarian can make and record subjective observations. When possible, observers should compare the injured body part with a normal body part. For example, if an animal has muscular atrophy and weakness due to a unilateral sciatic nerve injury, the contralateral "normal" limb can be used for comparisons of muscle size, strength, range of motion, etc. Grading scales can be developed to assess performance. Such scales have been developed for assessment of spinal injury/recovery, muscle strength, and lameness (Tables 17–1 through 17–3).

TABLE 17–1. Spinal Injury/Recovery Scale

GRADE	NEUROLOGIC EXAMINATION FINDINGS
0	Normal; no spinal pain
1	Spinal pain; no neurologic deficits
2	Mild paresis; patient is ambulatory without assistance
3	Profound paresis; patient cannot ambulate without assistance
4	Paralysis; deep pain perception intact
5	Paralysis; absence of deep pain perception
6	Progressive paralysis; ascending/descending myelomalacia

TABLE 17–2. Muscle-Strength Scale

GRADE	EXAMINATION FINDINGS
0	Zero strength; complete paralysis.
1	Trace strength; muscle contraction can be seen or palpated, but strength is insufficient to produce motion even with gravity.
2	Poor strength; the muscle can move the joint through a full range of motion only if a part is positioned so that force of gravity is assisting motion.
3	Fair strength; the muscle can move the joint through a full range of motion against gravity.
4	Good strength; the muscle can move the joint through a full range of motion against gravity and moderate resistance applied by the examiner.
5	Normal strength; the muscle can move the joint through a full range of motion against gravity and full resistance applied by the examiner.

CLINICAL APPLICATIONS OF PHYSICAL THERAPY

Orthopedic Injuries

DISTAL DIAPHYSEAL FEMORAL FRACTURES

Quadriceps contracture (quadriceps "tie-down") is a devastating complication of surgical and nonsurgical treatment of the distal aspect of the femur fractures in skeletally immature patients.[3, 18, 19] Quadriceps contracture is characterized by hyperextension of the affected stifle joint with reduced flexion of both the hock and stifle joints (Fig. 17–4). Many treatments for this contracture have been described, but clinical improvement is inconsistent and costly. Prevention of quadriceps contracture is preferable to treatment.

Proper and timely physical therapy should be recommended for any patient at risk of developing quadriceps contracture. Factors that place an animal at risk are age less than 1 year, fractures involving the distal third of the femur, fracture comminution, and associated soft-tissue damage.[19] In these patients, local hypothermia is used immediately following injury and fracture fixation to decrease inflammation, edema formation, and pain. Two to 3 days after surgical repair, superficial hyperthermia with gentle application of warm, moist towels is used to ease muscle spasm and pain, and to improve tissue microcirculation. Massage therapy and passive exercise are started, very gently at first, as soon as the patient will comfortably allow it (3 to 5 days after surgery). Once the incision is sealed, whirlpool therapy can be used. The pet owner should be thoroughly instructed about the need for physical therapy, and its importance must be emphasized. Two recheck examinations are performed in the first 10 days after surgery. Failure to recognize developing quadriceps contracture in the first 3 weeks after surgery makes treatment with physical therapy very difficult.[3, 19]

Alternatively, a 90–90 flexion sling, which maintains the stifle joints and

TABLE 17–3. Lameness Scale

GRADE	EXAMINATION FINDINGS
0	Normal gait
1	Normal standing and walking; lameness while running
2	Normal standing; slight lameness while walking; obvious lameness while running
3	Incomplete weight-bearing while standing; lameness while walking and running
4	Poor functional limb use; limb carried most of the time

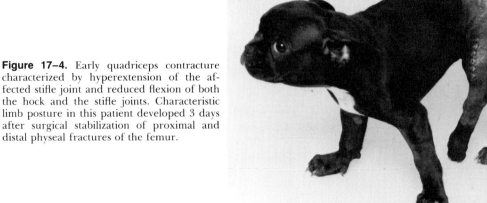

Figure 17–4. Early quadriceps contracture characterized by hyperextension of the affected stifle joint and reduced flexion of both the hock and the stifle joints. Characteristic limb posture in this patient developed 3 days after surgical stabilization of proximal and distal physeal fractures of the femur.

tarsus in 90 degrees of flexion, can be applied immediately after surgery and maintained for 7 to 10 days[19] (Fig. 17–5). Typically, patients will begin to extend their stifle joints from the flexed position within several days after sling removal.[19]

DISTAL DIAPHYSEAL HUMERAL FRACTURES

Reduced elbow extension is a common complication following surgical reduction and stabilization of intraarticular fractures of the elbow joint. Typically, these patients will carry the injured limb with the elbow slightly flexed (Fig. 17–6). The patients often flex and extend the shoulder to swing the limb but seldom completely extend the elbow. Rigid internal fixation and accurate anatomic reduction improve the prognosis for functional recovery because they permit early institution of physical therapy. Timely use of hypothermia, hyperthermia, massage, and exercise to decrease inflammation,

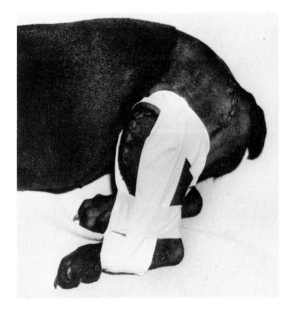

Figure 17–5. A 90–90 flexion sling used to maintain the stifle and tarsus in 90 degrees of flexion after surgery.

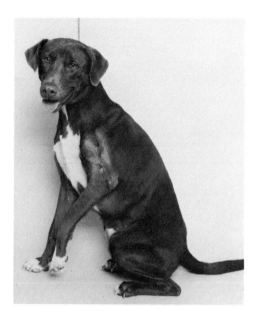

Figure 17–6. An animal with an intraarticular elbow fracture characterized by reduced elbow extension and muscle atrophy.

muscle spasm, and pain while improving tissue circulation and range of motion can dramatically improve return of function. Active exercise with these patients can sometimes be encouraged by slowly walking on inclines or stairs. Judicious use of analgesic and anti-inflammatory medications is also beneficial. Occasionally, once fracture healing has begun to occur (2 to 4 weeks after surgery depending on the age of the animal), a small syringe cap or marble is taped under the toes of the normal limb to encourage use of the injured limb. Such sessions are limited to 5 to 10 minutes, and the patient is not left unattended. In addition, wheelbarrowing can be performed by supporting the animal and lifting up the hindlimbs, thereby encouraging and forcing the animal to use the forelimbs.

Occasionally, an animal presented for suture removal and reevaluation (7 to 10 days postoperatively) has loss of elbow joint extension. With these animals, a spica splint is applied for 2 to 3 weeks. The primary objectives of the spica splint are to maintain joint extension and not lose flexion. Short-term use of a spica splint has yielded favorable results if the splint is used on an individual case basis with specific objectives in mind. If loss of extension can be prevented through active exercise and physical therapy, a splint is not necessary.

Neurologic Diseases

Veterinarians are frequently presented with neurologically disabled patients as a result of intervertebral disk disease, caudal cervical spondylomyelopathy, diskospondylitis, spinal fractures, ischemic myelopathy, and degenerative myelopathy. The physical therapy plan must be designed in accordance with the disease or injury responsible for the disability. As an example, active exercise cannot be encouraged in the nonoperated patient with intervertebral disk disease within 3 to 4 weeks after onset of neurologic deficits. Surgical decompression of the spinal cord, however, often permits earlier and more aggressive physical therapy. Likewise, surgical stabilization of spinal fractures often permits earlier and more aggressive physical therapy than nonsurgical management.

AMBULATORY POSTERIOR PARESIS/TETRAPARESIS

While these patients are able to ambulate, the goals of therapy are to improve their strength, coordination, and sensory awareness to restore more normal locomotor function. Active exercise therapy, both assisted and resistive, is valuable in treating these patients. The therapist (owner, veterinarian, or technician) *must* develop and establish a friendship with the patient to keep the animal actively involved in the therapy.

The weight-bearing surface of the treatment area must not be slippery or abrasive. Clean, soft, short grass is ideal. Treatment sessions begin by encouraging the patient to attain and maintain a standing posture, and assistance is given only when needed. When the patient begins to fatigue, it should be encouraged to stand just a little longer. After appropriate rest, the patient is encouraged to walk while the therapist provides only enough balance and resistance to gravity to keep the patient moving. Active resistive exercise is then used to develop both balance and strength. If the animal is capable of standing unassisted, the therapist can gently push laterally against the animal's hip or shoulder to disrupt its balance. The push should be gentle enough that the animal is not knocked over but firm enough to force the patient to shift its weight. When the patient has obtained its balance again, lateral pressure is released again, forcing the patient to regain balance. This therapy is repeated several times from each side of the patient. With the patient in a standing position, a gentle downward force can be placed over the shoulder and pelvis, thereby forcing the patient to resist by pushing up. When the therapist feels the patient begin to fatigue, the downward pressure is slowly released. The therapist must be very perceptive of the patient during the therapy sessions, making sure to push the patient to its performance limit without exceeding it. The value of praise and encouragement for the patient's efforts cannot be overemphasized.

NONAMBULATORY POSTERIOR PARESIS/PLEGIA

Physical therapy is aimed at maintaining range of motion in the joints, increasing strength, reeducating muscles, developing coordination, and preventing the formation of dependent edema and decubital ulcers. Assisting these patients, particularly large dogs, can be extremely challenging. Many owners are not capable of performing the therapy, and extended hospitalization may be necessary.

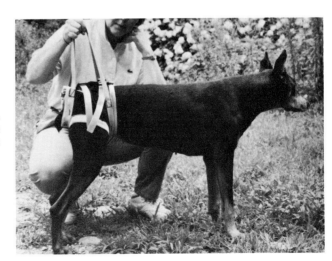

Figure 17–7. A walkabout sling used in an animal with posterior paresis. The adjustable sling is constructed with nylon straps and a neoprene harness.

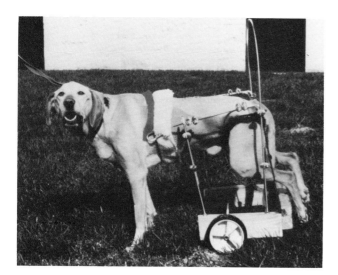

Figure 17–8. A cart used to support a dog with posterior paralysis. The cart is constructed with flexible aluminum rods, abdominal slings, and small wheels.

Whirlpools are used frequently for the combination of hyperthermia, massage, and buoyancy provided by the water. The buoyancy helps resist the gravitational force on the patient and encourages voluntary movement. Frequently, the first voluntary limb movement in neurologically disabled patients is detected during whirlpool therapy. Small dogs may be encouraged to walk or swim. Although there is often not enough room for mobility, large dogs can be encouraged to stand and maintain their balance against changing water currents. Massage and passive exercise also can be instituted during the whirlpool treatment. Addition of an antiseptic solution to the water helps control bacterial contamination from urine and feces.

A variety of slings have been used to assist patients with ambulation (Walkabout Harness, Aptos, Calif.) (Fig. 17–7). The response of patients to these slings is variable, although most animals find them comfortable and helpful in learning to walk. Occasionally, patients are more active without a sling. A variety of carts are also available (K9 Carts, Berwyn, Pa.; Kitty Kart, Madison, Wisc.) (Fig. 17–8). The carts increase patient mobility and help prevent decubital ulcers and abrasions. *We discourage the use of carts for small dogs and cats during the first 3 to 4 months after disability because patients depend on the cart and are less enthusiastic about their physical therapy.* If disability extends beyond 3 to 4 months, however, carts can be of tremendous help. Carts may be useful sooner in therapy of larger patients to assist mobility. Manufacturers have designed carts specifically for both dogs and cats. Mobile slings are often used with nonambulatory tetraparetic/plegic patients and serve a similar purpose as carts. These mobile slings are particularly helpful in supporting large-breed dogs, which are very difficult to assist. Placing the patient in the sling several times a day also helps prevent decubital ulcer formation. Once the patient is supported in a sling, the therapist can provide encouragement while assisting the patient with rising, standing, or walking.

Nonambulatory patients, particularly large dogs, often become discouraged and reluctant to try standing or walking. Although difficult, the therapist must persistently maintain enthusiasm and encouragement because there is little hope if both the patient and the therapist become discouraged.

REFERENCES

1. Gucker T: The use of heat and cold in orthopedics, in Light SH (ed): Therapeutic Heat and Cold. Baltimore, Md: Waverly Press, 1965, pp 398–407
2. Marone PJ: Orthopaedic rehabilitation, in Gartland JJ (ed): Fundamentals of Orthopaedics, 4th ed. Philadelphia: WB Saunders, 1987, pp 409–424
3. Anderson GI: Fracture disease and related contractures. Vet Clin North Am 1991; 21:845–858
4. Tangner PH: Physical therapy in small animal patients: Basic principles and application. Compend Contin Educ Vet Pract 1984; 6:933–936
5. Downer AH: Extremity immersion bath technique, in Downer AH (ed): Physical Therapy for Animals: Selected Techniques. Springfield, Ill: Charles C Thomas, 1978, pp 84–86
6. Downer AH, Spear VL: Physical therapy in the management of long bone fractures in small animals. Vet Clin North Amer 1975; 5:157–164
7. Lehmann JF, Delateur BJ: Diathermy and superficial heat, laser and cold therapy, in Kottke FJ, Lehmann JF (eds): Krusen's Handbook of Physical Medicine and Rehabilitation, 4th ed. Philadelphia: WB Saunders, 1990, pp 283–367
8. Downer AH: Hot packs, in Downer AH (ed): Physical Therapy for Animals: Selected Techniques. Springfield, Ill: Charles C Thomas, 1978, pp 36–44
9. Downer AH: Microwave, in Downer AH (ed): Physical Therapy for Animals: Selected Techniques. Springfield, Ill: Charles C Thomas, 1978, pp 57–62
10. Knapp ME: Massage, in Kottke FJ, Lehmann JF (eds): Krusen's Handbook of Physical Medicine and Rehabilitation, 4th ed. Philadelphia: WB Saunders, 1990, pp 433–435
11. Downer AH: Massage, in Downer AH (ed): Physical Therapy for Animals: Selected Techniques. Springfield, Ill: Charles C Thomas, 1978, pp 163–168
12. Kottke FJ: Therapeutic exercise to maintain mobility, in Kottke FJ, Lehmann JF (eds): Krusen's Handbook of Physical Medicine and Rehabilitation, 4th ed. Philadelphia: WB Saunders, 1990, pp 436–451
13. Downer AH: Whirlpools, in Downer AH (ed): Physical Therapy for Animals: Selected Techniques. Springfield, Ill: Charles C Thomas, 1978, pp 29–35
14. Cole TM, Tobis JS: Management of musculoskeletal function, in Kottke FJ, Lehmann JF (eds): Krusen's Handbook of Physical Medicine and Rehabilitation, 4th ed. Philadelphia: WB Saunders, 1990, pp 20–71
15. Newton CD: Joint range of motion: Average of ten mixed-breed dogs and ten domestic short-haired cats, in Newton CD, Nunamaker DM (eds): Textbook of Small Animal Orthopedics. Philadelphia: JB Lippincott, 1985, p 1106
16. Budsberg SC: Force plate analysis in normal walking dogs. Vet Surg 1987; 16:85–91
17. Anderson GI, Hearne T, Taves C: Force plate gait analysis in normal and dysplastic dogs before and after total hip replacement: An experimental study (abstract) Vet Surg 1988; 17:27
18. Bardet JF, Hohn RD: Quadriceps contracture in dogs. J Am Vet Med Assoc 1983; 183:680–685
19. Aron DN, Crowe DT: The 90–90 flexion splint for prevention of stifle joint stiffness with femoral fracture repairs. J Am Anim Hosp Assoc 1987; 23:447–454

INDEX

Note: Page numbers in *italics* refer to illustrations; page numbers followed by t refer to tables.